# CALCULATE
## with CONFIDENCE

### Eighth Edition

Deborah C. Morris, RN, BSN, MA, LNC

Professor Emeritus
Department of Nursing and Allied Health Sciences
Bronx Community College of the City University of New York (CUNY)
Bronx, New York

ELSEVIER

Elsevier
3251 Riverport Lane
St. Louis, Missouri 63043

CALCULATE WITH CONFIDENCE, EDITION 8                    ISBN: 978-0-323-69695-1

---

**Notice**

---

Previous editions copyrighted 2018, 2014, 2010, 2006, 2002, 1998, and 1994.

**Library of Congress Control Number: 2021939337**

*Senior Content Strategist:* Yvonne Alexopoulos
*Senior Content Development Manager:* Lisa Newton
*Senior Content Development Specialist:* Danielle Frazier
*Publishing Services Manager:* Julie Eddy
*Book Production Specialist:* Clay S. Broeker
*Design Direction:* Julia Dummitt

Printed in the United States of America

Last digit is the print number:  9  8  7  6  5  4  3  2  1

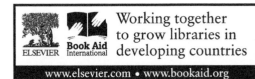

*To my children, Cameron, Kimberly, Kanin, and Cory,
thanks for your love and support. You light up my life.
To my mother, your love, support, guidance, and
nurturing helped me to become the person I am today.
To my husband, Reggie, thank you for all the hard
work you did in helping me with the current and
previous editions of this text. Your support and
encouragement kept me on track and focused.*

*To the two special additions and loves of my life,
my two grandsons, Ryan and Eison, you touch my life
more than you know.*

*Thank you to friends, nursing colleagues, and students
past and present. To future and current practitioners of
nursing, I hope this book will be valuable in teaching
the principles of dosage calculation and reinforcing the
importance of safety in administration of medications
to all clients regardless of the setting.*

# Reviewers

**Bridgette Cotton, DNP, MSN, RN**
Assistant Professor
Goldfarb School of Nursing
Barnes-Jewish College
St. Louis, Missouri

**Paula Denise Silver, PharmD, MEd, BS**
Medical Instructor
School of Health Science
ECPI University
Newport News, Virginia

**Bobbi Steelman, CPhT, MAEd**
Pharmacy Technician Educator
American National University
Bowling Green, Kentucky

# Preface to the Instructor

Safety is a priority in the delivery of health care. To advance client safety and its importance in health care delivery worldwide, several organizations are involved in reinforcing the promotion of client safety in health care, which includes emphasis on improving safety in medication administration. These organizations include the Institute of Medicine (IOM), the Institute for Safe Medication Practices (ISMP), and The Joint Commission (TJC).

The Quality and Safety Education for Nurses (QSEN) looks at six competencies, two of which are relevant to medication administration: safety and informatics. *Safety* refers to reducing the risk of harm to clients, and *informatics* refers to technology used to mitigate errors. Safety and informatics will be referred to in this text where applicable. The text uses the term *client* to denote one who is the recipient of health care and can also be referred to as *patient, resident,* and *health care consumer.*

The eighth edition of *Calculate with Confidence* not only teaches the aspects of dosage calculation, it also emphasizes the importance of safety in medication administration. *Calculate with Confidence* is written to meet the needs of nursing students as well as nurses returning to the workforce after being away from the clinical setting. It is also suitable for courses within nursing curricula whose content reflects the calculation of dosages and solutions. The text can generally be used as a reference by any health care professional whose responsibilities include safe administration of medications and solutions to clients in diverse clinical settings.

*Calculate with Confidence,* eighth edition, has incorporated feedback from users of previous editions, including students, instructors, and reviewers. This edition has maintained a style similar to previous editions. The text presents three methods of dosage calculation—dimensional analysis, formula method, and ratio and proportion. Each method is illustrated, empowering students to choose the method that suits their learning style and works for them. It also enables the instructor to teach a preferred method or multiple methods to students.

The new edition responds to changes in the health care field and includes the introduction of new medications, discussion of new methods for medication administration, and an emphasis on clinical reasoning in prevention of medication errors. Principles of QSEN have been incorporated where applicable. An ample number of practice problems that include the shading of syringes where indicated continues to be featured to allow for visualization of dosages, reinforcement of clinical thinking skills, and prevention of medication errors. Safety alerts are also incorporated throughout the chapters to further reinforce the importance of error prevention in medication administration. Despite technological advances in equipment, health care professionals must continue to use clinical reasoning skills and have a consistent focus on safety to minimize the risk of harm to clients. Answers to practice problems include rationales to enhance understanding of principles and answers related to dosages. Answers have been placed at the end of chapters to allow for immediate feedback.

In response to the increased need for competency in basic math as an essential prerequisite for dosage calculation, practice problems in the basic math section are provided to allow the student to identify his or her strengths and weaknesses in basic math areas that provide the foundation for math skills applied in dosage calculation.

The once controversial use of calculators is now a more accepted practice, and they are used on many nursing examinations, including the NCLEX; however, their use is individualized. Many health care agencies have policies that require the use of calculators to verify calculations (e.g., critical care calculations) to avoid medication errors. A basic handheld calculator that has functions of addition, subtraction, multiplication, division, and a square root key is usually sufficient for medical dosage calculation, and students should know how to use such a calculator.

## ORGANIZATION OF CONTENT

The eighth edition continues to be organized in a progression from simple topics to more complex ones, making content relevant to the needs of the student and using realistic practice problems to enhance learning and make material clinically applicable.

The 24 chapters are arranged into 5 units.

**Unit One** includes Chapters 1 through 4. This unit provides a review of basic arithmetic skills, including fractions, decimals, ratio and proportion, and percentages. A Pre-Test and Post-Test are included. This unit allows the student to determine his or her weaknesses and strengths in arithmetic and provides a review of basic math, which includes fractions, decimals, percents, and ratio and proportion. Ample practice problems as well as word problems are included in the basic math sections.

**Unit Two** includes Chapters 5 through 8. Chapters 5 through 7 introduce the student to the three systems of measurement: metric, household, and apothecary. The metric system is emphasized, and some aspects of household measures are discussed because of their implications for care at home. The apothecary system is discussed in terms of its non-use, and the error-prone abbreviations from this system to avoid in this system have been placed in Appendix A. Chapter 8 provides conversions relating to temperature, length, weight, and military time. Calculation of intake and output (I&O) is included (both basic and complex). A brief discussion of completion times for IV therapy is also presented.

**Unit Three** includes Chapters 9 through 15. This unit provides essential information that is needed as a foundation for dosage calculation and safe medication administration. Chapter 9 includes an expanded discussion of medication errors; routes of medication administration; equipment used in medication administration; the six basic rights of medication administration, as well as additional rights to be considered when administering medications; and the nursing role in preventing medication errors. Chapter 10 presents the abbreviations used in medication administration and interpretation of medication orders. Chapter 11 introduces students to medication administration records and has been updated to include the various medication distribution systems. Chapter 12 provides the student with the skills necessary to read medication labels to calculate dosages. Medication labels include medications in current use as well as some of the newer medication labels on the market. The important skill of reading labels is developed by providing practice with identification of information on labels. Resources that include TJC's official "Do Not Use" list and ISMP's list of Error-Prone Abbreviations, Symbols, and Dose Designations are emphasized and have been included in the appendices, along with other resources. Emphasis is placed on the nurse's responsibility to stay abreast of standards regarding medication orders to ensure client safety and prevent errors in medication administration. Chapters 13 through 15 introduce the various methods used for dosage calculation (ratio and proportion, formula method, and dimensional analysis). Practice problems are provided for each method, giving the student the opportunity to practice the various methods and choose the one preferred.

**Unit Four** includes Chapters 16 through 19. In Chapter 16, the student learns the principles and calculations related to oral medications (solid and liquids). In Chapter 17, the student learns about the various types of syringes and the skills needed for calculating injectable medications. Chapter 18 introduces concepts of solutions. Calculations associated with reconstituted solutions for injectable and oral medications are discussed. Calculations associated with preparation of noninjectable solutions, including nutritional feedings, determining the strength of solutions, and calculation of solutions, are also included. Chapter 19 introduces the student to insulin types, including U-500 insulin and the U-500 insulin syringe. The chapter has been expanded to include discussion of insulin pens, the use of the sliding scale, and glucose monitoring systems. The methods of dosage calculation are illustrated in the chapters (ratio and proportion, formula method, and dimensional analysis), and practice problems are provided in each chapter.

**Unit Five** includes Chapters 20 through 24. Chapters 20 and 21 provide a discussion of equipment used in the administration of intravenous (IV) fluids and IV solutions, as well as associated calculations related to IV therapy. Content includes a focus on safety with IV administration, recalculating IV flow rate with an alternative method of determining the percentage of variation, and determining infusion and completion time for IV therapy. IV labels have been added throughout the chapter, with a discussion of additives to IV solutions. Chapter 22 presents a discussion of heparin and new heparin labels. Heparin weight-based protocol has been expanded to include adjusting IV heparin based on activated partial thromboplastin time (aPTT). Chapter 23 provides the student with the skills necessary to calculate critical care IV medications. Titration of IV flow rates for titrated medications is explained, as well as how to develop a titration table. Additional practice problems have also been added to the chapter. Chapter 24 provides the student with the skills and principles for calculation of pediatric and adult dosages and verification of safe dosages based on weight. Determining the body surface area (BSA) using a nomogram and formula is discussed, and calculation and verification of safe dosages based on BSA is also included. Calculation of daily fluid maintenance, also referred to as daily fluid requirement (DFR), for children has also been included, as have practice problems.

Safety Alerts, Tips for Clinical Practice, Practice Problems, Clinical Reasoning scenarios, and Points to Remember are included throughout the text. A Comprehensive Post-Test is included at the end of the text and includes practice problems covering content from all 24 chapters. A Drug Label Index is also included.

## NEW FEATURES TO THE EIGHTH EDITION

- A change in format in some chapters for ease of reading.
- Updates in the chapter on Medication Administration that include the "culture of safety" and the Risk Evaluation and Mitigation Strategy (REMS).
- Discussion of Clinical Decision-Making Support Systems (CDSS) and Computerized Provider Order Entry (CPOE).
- Updated labels that include current medications on the market are provided throughout the text, along with discussion of the Black Box Warning.
- An update of the Insulin chapter with current insulin labels provided by Eli Lilly and Company and an updated discussion of insulin syringes, which includes the U-500 insulin syringe.
- Current heparin labels in the Heparin Calculations chapter and throughout the text.
- Labels presented in easily readable format.
- Addition of case studies in select chapters to help prepare students for the Next-Generation NCLEX (NGN).
- Updates to Medication Distribution Systems.
- Calculation and verification of safe dosages using BSA.
- Updates in the chapters on IV therapy that include calculations and equipment used to administer IV fluids.

## ANCILLARIES

*Evolve Resources* for *Calculate with Confidence,* eighth edition, are available to enhance student instruction. These online resources can be found at http://evolve.elsevier.com/GrayMorris/.

These resources correspond with the chapters of the main book and includes the following:
- Updated Student Review Questions and Test Bank Questions to coincide with the chapters, as well as sample NCLEX Review Questions.
- Elsevier's Interactive Drug Calculation Application, version 1: This interactive drug calculation application provides hands-on, interactive practice for the user to master drug calculations. Users can select the mode (Study, Exam, or Comprehensive Exam) and then the category for study and exam modes. There are eight categories that cover the main drug calculation topics. Users are also able to select the number of problems they want to complete and their preferred drug calculation method. A calculator is available for easy access within any mode, and the application also provides history of the work done by the user. There are 750 practice problems in this application.

It is my hope that this book will be a valuable asset to current and future practitioners. May it help you calculate dosages accurately and with confidence, using calculation and critical thinking skills to ensure that medications are administered safely to all clients regardless of the setting. This is both a priority and a primary responsibility of the nurse.

*Deborah C. Morris*

# Acknowledgments

I would like to extend sincere gratitude and appreciation to those individuals from both the past and present who have inspired and encouraged me throughout the writing of the editions of this text. Who knew that this text would now be in its eighth edition? First and foremost, thank you to my family for all of your support during the writing of every edition. A special thanks to my daughter-in-law, who we call Marcy (Marcella Willis-Gray, MD), for taking the time out of your busy schedule to answer questions relating to medication orders and guiding me to the source to obtain an electronic medication administration record (eMAR) for use in this edition.

I am particularly thankful for the encouragement and support of present and former colleagues at Bronx Community College of the City University of New York (CUNY). Thanks to Professor Lois Augustus, former chairperson of the Department of Nursing and Allied Health Sciences, for your friendship and encouragement. Thank you to Mr. Clarence Hodge (Lecturer) who currently teaches Pharmacology Computations; your feedback has been invaluable. Thank you to Professor Helen Papas-Kavalis, a friend and colleague, for sharing your pediatric expertise when needed. A special note of thanks and sincere appreciation to Professor Ellen Hoist, a colleague and a friend, who provided me with support, mentoring, and encouragement from the beginning with the first edition of this text, when I expressed doubt of editions beyond the first. You could see the potential even when I expressed doubt.

Thanks to former Chairpersons of the Department of Mathematics and Computer Sciences at Bronx Community College, Professor Germana Glier, and the late Dr. Gerald S. Lieblich, whose mathematical expertise was invaluable. A special thanks to the late Dr. Andrew McInerney, a colleague and friend (who also was a former Chairperson) for all of your suggestions and validation of answers in the mathematical portion of this text. Your help was invaluable, and you will always be missed.

Thanks to past and present students at Bronx Community College in the Department of Nursing and Allied Health Sciences who provided the inspiration for me to write this text. You helped me to have an appreciation for the problems students encounter with basic math and the calculation of medication dosages.

I am especially grateful to the staff at Elsevier for their support and help in planning, writing, and producing the eighth edition of this text. A special thanks to Danielle M. Frazier and Yvonne Alexopoulos; thank you for your patience and understanding during a difficult time when I needed it most while doing the revisions. Thanks also to Tracey Schriefer and Clay S. Broeker for their work in producing the text.

To all of my friends, and especially to Anna Nunnally, my friend who always says I am her sis, thanks for your encouragement and admiration and for always saying "you can do it." To my friend the late Frank A. Rucker, your encouragement, inspiring words, and admiration for me as an author will always remain with me.

I wish to acknowledge and thank Eli Lilly and Company for providing current images of medication labels for reproduction in this text. I also want to thank the companies that provided images of medication equipment and documents for use in this edition. Thanks to Omnicell for the image of their Automated Dispensing Cabinet (ADC) and Becton Dickinson and Company (BD) for the image of the Flow Controller. Thank you to Epic for providing the image of an eMAR and to ISMP and TJC for granting permission for documents used in the text.

Thank you all!

*Deborah C. Morris*

# Contents

# UNIT ONE

# Math Review

An essential role of the nurse is providing safe medication administration to all clients. To accurately perform dosage calculations, the nurse must have knowledge of basic math, regardless of the problem-solving method used in calculation. Knowledge of basic math is a necessary component of dosage calculation that nurses need to know to prevent medication errors and ensure the safe administration of medications to all clients, regardless of the setting. Serious harm to clients can result from a mathematical error during calculation and administration of a medication dosage. The nurse must practice and be proficient in the basic math used in dosage calculations. Knowledge of basic math is a prerequisite for the prevention of medication errors and ensures the safe administration of medications.

Although calculators are accessible for basic math operations, the nurse needs to be able to perform the processes involved in basic math. Even when a calculator is used, checking the accuracy of an answer often requires nurses to employ the skill of estimating an answer quickly in their heads. Calculators may indeed be recommended for complex calculations to ensure accuracy and save time; the types of calculations requiring their use are presented later in this text. However, because the basic math required for less complex calculations is often simple and can be done without the use of a calculator, it is a realistic expectation that each practitioner should be competent in the performance of basic math operations without its use. Performing basic math operations enables the nurse to think logically and critically about the dosage ordered and the dosage calculated.

# PRE-TEST

This test is designed to evaluate your ability in the basic math areas reviewed in Unit One. The test consists of 72 questions. If you are able to complete the pre-test with 100% accuracy, you may want to bypass Unit One. Any problems answered incorrectly should be used as a basis for what you might need to review. The purposes of this test and the review that follows are to build your confidence in basic math skills and to help you avoid careless mistakes when you begin to perform dosage calculations.

Identify the fraction(s) equal to 1.

1. $\dfrac{26}{25}, \dfrac{3}{4}, \dfrac{8}{8}$ _____

Identify the fraction as a proper fraction, an improper fraction, or a mixed number.

2. $\dfrac{13}{7}$ _____  5. $3\dfrac{5}{8}$ _____

3. $\dfrac{7}{12}$ _____  6. $\dfrac{14}{14}$ _____

4. $8\dfrac{2}{7}$ _____  7. $\dfrac{5}{21}$ _____

Change the following fractions to whole or mixed numbers and reduce if necessary.

8. $\dfrac{28}{14}$ _____  10. $\dfrac{48}{10}$ _____

9. $\dfrac{20}{8}$ _____

Reduce the following fractions to lowest terms.

11. $\dfrac{14}{21}$ _____  14. $\dfrac{24}{30}$ _____

12. $\dfrac{25}{100}$ _____  15. $\dfrac{24}{36}$ _____

13. $\dfrac{2}{150}$ _____

Perform the indicated operations; reduce to lowest terms where necessary.

16. $\dfrac{2}{3} \div \dfrac{3}{9} =$ _____  23. $2\dfrac{1}{6} - 1\dfrac{1}{4} =$ _____

17. $4 \div \dfrac{3}{4} =$ _____  24. $9 - \dfrac{3}{5} =$ _____

18. $\dfrac{2}{5} + \dfrac{1}{9} =$ _____  25. $4\dfrac{1}{4} - 1\dfrac{3}{4} =$ _____

19. $7\dfrac{1}{7} - 2\dfrac{5}{6} =$ _____  26. $7\dfrac{1}{5} - 1\dfrac{3}{4} =$ _____

20. $4\dfrac{2}{3} \times 4 =$ _____  27. $7 - \dfrac{9}{16} =$ _____

21. $3\dfrac{5}{6} + 5\dfrac{2}{3} =$ _____  28. $3\dfrac{3}{10} - 1\dfrac{7}{10} =$ _____

22. $5\dfrac{6}{7} + 3\dfrac{5}{7} =$ _____

Change the following fractions to decimals; express your answer to the nearest tenth.

29. $\dfrac{6}{7}$ _____

31. $\dfrac{2}{3}$ _____

30. $\dfrac{6}{20}$ _____

32. $\dfrac{7}{8}$ _____

Indicate the largest fraction in each group.

33. $\dfrac{3}{4}, \dfrac{4}{5}, \dfrac{7}{8}$ _____

34. $\dfrac{7}{12}, \dfrac{11}{12}, \dfrac{4}{12}$ _____

Perform the indicated operations with decimals. Provide the exact answer; do not round off.

35. $20.1 + 67.35 =$ _____

37. $4.6 \times 8.72 =$ _____

36. $0.008 + 5 =$ _____

38. $56.47 - 8.7 =$ _____

Divide the following decimals; express your answer to the nearest tenth.

39. $7.5 \div 0.004 =$ _____

41. $84.7 \div 2.3 =$ _____

40. $45 \div 1.9 =$ _____

Indicate the largest decimal in each group.

42. $0.674, 0.659$ _____

44. $0.25, 0.6, 0.175$ _____

43. $0.375, 0.37, 0.38$ _____

Solve for $x$, the unknown value.

45. $8 : 2 = 48 : x$ _____

47. $\dfrac{1}{10} : x = \dfrac{1}{2} : 15$ _____

46. $x : 300 = 1 : 150$ _____

48. $0.1 : 1 = 0.2 : x$ _____

Round off to the nearest tenth.

49. $0.43$ _____

51. $1.47$ _____

50. $0.66$ _____

Round off to the nearest hundredth.

52. $0.735$ _____

54. $1.227$ _____

53. $0.834$ _____

Complete the table below, expressing the measures in their equivalents where indicated. Reduce to lowest terms where necessary.

| | Percent | Decimal | Ratio | Fraction |
|---|---|---|---|---|
| 55. | 6% | _____ | _____ | _____ |
| 56. | _____ | _____ | 7 : 20 | _____ |
| 57. | _____ | _____ | _____ | $5\frac{1}{4}$ |
| 58. | _____ | 0.015 | _____ | _____ |

Find the following percentages. Express your answer to the hundredths place as indicated.

59. 5% of 95 _____

60. $\frac{1}{4}$% of 2,000 _____

61. 2 is what % of 600 _____

62. 20 is what % of 100 _____

63. 30 is what % of 164 _____

64. A client is instructed to take $1\frac{1}{2}$ teaspoons of a cough syrup three (3) times a day. How many teaspoons of cough syrup will the client take each day? _____

65. A tablet contains 0.75 milligrams (mg) of a medication. A client receives three (3) tablets a day for five (5) days. How many mg of the medication will the client receive in five (5) days? _____

66. A client took 0.44 micrograms (mcg) of a medication every morning and 1.4 mcg each evening for five (5) days. What is the total amount of medication taken? _____

67. Write a ratio that represents that every tablet in a bottle contains 0.5 milligrams (mg) of a medication. _____

68. Write a ratio that represents 60 milligrams (mg) of a medication in 1 milliliter (mL) of a liquid. _____

69. A client takes 10 milliliters (mL) of a medication three (3) times a day. How long will 120 mL of medication last? _____

70. A client weighed 275 pounds (lb) before dieting. After dieting, the client weighed 250 lb. What is the percentage of change in the client's weight? _____

71. A client was prescribed 10 milligrams (mg) of a medication for a week. After a week, the health care provider reduced the medication to seven (7) mg. What was the percentage of decrease in medication? _____

72. A client received 22.5 milligrams (mg) of a medication in tablet form. Each tablet contained 4.5 mg of medication. How many tablets were given to the client? _____

**Answers on p. 5**

## ⭐ ANSWERS

1. 8/8

2. improper fraction

3. proper fraction

4. mixed number

5. mixed number

6. improper fraction

7. proper fraction

8. 2

9. $\frac{20}{8} = 2\frac{4}{8} = 2\frac{1}{2}$

10. $\frac{48}{10} = 4\frac{8}{10} = 4\frac{4}{5}$

11. $\frac{2}{3}$

12. $\frac{1}{4}$

13. $\frac{1}{75}$

14. $\frac{4}{5}$

15. $\frac{2}{3}$

16. 2

17. $5\frac{1}{3}$

18. $\frac{23}{45}$

19. $4\frac{13}{42}$

20. $18\frac{2}{3}$

21. $9\frac{3}{6} = 9\frac{1}{2}$

22. $8\frac{11}{7} = 9\frac{4}{7}$

23. $\frac{11}{12}$

24. $8\frac{2}{5}$

25. $2\frac{2}{4} = 2\frac{1}{2}$

26. $5\frac{9}{20}$

27. $6\frac{7}{16}$

28. $1\frac{6}{10} = 1\frac{3}{5}$

29. 0.9

30. 0.3

31. 0.7

32. 0.9

33. $\frac{7}{8}$

34. $\frac{11}{12}$

35. 87.45

36. 5.008

37. 40.112

38. 47.77

39. 1,875

40. 23.7

41. 36.8

42. 0.674

43. 0.38

44. 0.6

45. $x = 12$

46. $x = 2$

47. $x = 3$

48. $x = 2$

49. 0.4

50. 0.7

51. 1.5

52. 0.74

53. 0.83

54. 1.23

| | Percent | Decimal | Ratio | Fraction |
|---|---|---|---|---|
| 55. | 6% | 0.06 | 3 : 50 | $\frac{3}{50}$ |
| 56. | 35% | 0.35 | 7 : 20 | $\frac{7}{20}$ |
| 57. | 525% | 5.25 | 21 : 4 | $5\frac{1}{4}$ |
| 58. | 1.5% | 0.015 | 3 : 200 | $\frac{3}{200}$ |

59. 4.75

60. 5

61. 0.33%

62. 20%

63. 18.29%

64. $4\frac{1}{2}$ teaspoons

65. 11.25 milligrams (mg)

66. 9.2 micrograms (mcg)

67. 0.5 mg : 1 tablet or 0.5 mg/1 tablet

68. 60 mg : 1 mL or 60 mg/1 mL

69. 4 days

70. 9%

71. 30%

72. 5 tablets

# CHAPTER 1
# Fractions

## Objectives

*After reviewing this chapter, you should be able to:*
1. Compare the size of fractions
2. Add fractions
3. Subtract fractions
4. Divide fractions
5. Multiply fractions
6. Reduce fractions to lowest terms

Health care professionals need to have an understanding of fractions. Fractions may be seen in medical orders, client records, prescriptions, documentation relating to care given to clients, and literature related to health care. Nurses often encounter fractions when converting metric to household measures in dosage calculation.

Fractions may be used occasionally in the writing of a medication order or used by the pharmaceutical manufacturer on a medication label (which usually includes the metric equivalent). In 2010 the Institute for Safe Medication Practices (ISMP) president Michael R. Cohen edited the abridged edition of the book *Medication Errors,* which contained this statement: "Occasionally using fractions instead of metric designation could help prevent errors." In 2020, 10 years later, this statement still is very true. For example, the dosage embossed on 2.5-mg Coumadin tablets is "2½ mg" and on 7.5 mg is "7½ mg" (see Figures 1.1 and 1.2). The use of "2½ mg" and "7½ mg" prevents confusion with "25" mg and "75" mg, respectively, eliminating the possibility of a patient receiving a massive overdose of this anticoagulation medication.

As you will see later in the text, some methods of solving dosage calculations rely on expressing relationships in a fraction format. Therefore proficiency with fractions can be beneficial in a variety of situations.

A fraction represents a part of a whole (Figure 1.3). It is written as two quantities: an upper number referred, to as the **numerator** (parts of the whole), and a **denominator,** the bottom part of the fraction that represents the whole. The numerator and denominator are separated by a horizontal line. The horizontal line above the denominator is a division sign; therefore a fraction may also be read as the numerator divided by the denominator.

$$\frac{\text{Numerator}}{\text{Denominator}} \leftarrow \text{horizontal bar (division sign)}$$

Examples: Suppose you have to administer a medication that is scored (marked) for division into four parts to a client, and you must administer one part of the tablet. The denominator represents the whole tablet, and the numerator represents the amount you administer. The fraction, or part, of the tablet you administer is written as:

$$\frac{\text{Numerator}}{\text{Denominator}} = \frac{1 \text{ part}}{4 \text{ parts}} = \frac{1}{4}$$

This number is read as one-fourth. The denominator is 4 because 4 parts make up the whole. If you administer one part, you administer $\frac{1}{4}$ of the tablet.

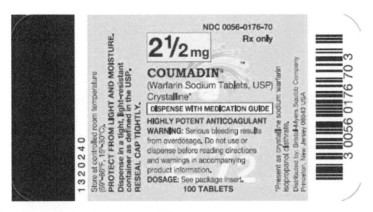

**Figure 1.1** Coumadin 2.5 mg (expressed as 2½ mg).

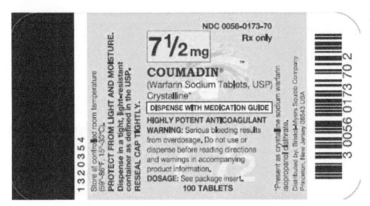

**Figure 1.2** Coumadin 7.5 mg (expressed as 7½ mg).

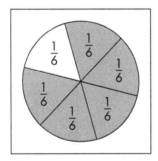

**Figure 1.3** The shaded part of the circle, which is 5 parts, reflects the numerator, and the total number of parts (6) is the denominator. Therefore $\frac{5}{6}$ means 5 of 6 equal parts.

Occasionally fractions may be used to show the relationship between part of a group and the whole group. For example, you are working on a surgical unit, and in a group of 18 clients who had surgery, 7 developed infections. The number of clients in the full group, 18, is the whole, or the denominator. You write the fraction of clients who developed infections as:

$$\frac{\text{Part (numerator)}}{\text{Whole (denominator)}} = \frac{\text{Clients who developed infections}}{\text{Whole group}} = \frac{7}{18}$$

## Types of Fractions

There are various types of fractions:

**Proper Fraction:** Numerator is less than the denominator, and the fraction has a value of less than 1.

Examples:   $\frac{1}{8}, \frac{5}{6}, \frac{7}{8}, \frac{1}{150}$

**Improper Fraction:** Numerator is larger than, or equal to, the denominator, and the fraction has a value of 1 or greater than 1.

Examples:     $\dfrac{3}{2}, \dfrac{7}{5}, \dfrac{300}{150}, \dfrac{4}{4}$

**Mixed Number:** Whole number and a proper fraction in which the total value of the mixed number is greater than 1.

Examples:     $3\dfrac{1}{3}, 5\dfrac{1}{8}, 9\dfrac{1}{6}, 25\dfrac{7}{8}$

**Complex Fraction:** Numerator, denominator, or both are fractions. The value may be less than, greater than, or equal to 1.

Examples:     $\dfrac{3\frac{1}{2}}{2}, \dfrac{\frac{1}{3}}{\frac{1}{2}}, \dfrac{2}{1\frac{1}{4}}, \dfrac{2}{\frac{1}{150}}$

**Whole Numbers:** Have an unexpressed denominator of one (1).

Examples:     $1 = \dfrac{1}{1}, 3 = \dfrac{3}{1}, 6 = \dfrac{6}{1}, 100 = \dfrac{100}{1}$

## Converting Fractions

An improper fraction can be changed to a mixed number or whole number by dividing the numerator by the denominator. If there is a remainder, that number is placed over the denominator, and the answer is reduced to lowest terms.

Examples:     $\dfrac{6}{5} = 6 \div 5 = 1\dfrac{1}{5}, \dfrac{100}{25} = 100 \div 25 = 4, \dfrac{10}{8} = 10 \div 8 = 1\dfrac{2}{8} = 1\dfrac{1}{4}$

A mixed number can be changed to an improper fraction by multiplying the whole number by the denominator, adding it to the numerator, and placing the sum over the denominator.

Example:     $5\dfrac{1}{8} = \dfrac{(5 \times 8) + 1}{8} = \dfrac{41}{8}$

## Comparing Fractions

Comparing the size of fractions is important in the administration of medications. It helps the new practitioner learn the value of medication dosages early on. Fractions can be compared if the numerators are the same by comparing the denominators or if the denominators are the same by comparing the numerators. These rules are presented in Box 1.1.

---

**BOX 1.1   Rules for Comparing Size of Fractions**

Here are some basic rules to keep in mind when comparing fractions.

1. If the numerators are the same, the fraction with the smaller denominator has the greater value.

Example 1:     $\dfrac{1}{2}$ is larger than $\dfrac{1}{3}$

Example 2:     $\dfrac{1}{150}$ is larger than $\dfrac{1}{300}$

2. If the denominators are the same, the fraction with the larger numerator has the greater value.

Example 1:     $\dfrac{3}{4}$ is larger than $\dfrac{1}{4}$

Example 2:     $\dfrac{3}{100}$ is larger than $\dfrac{1}{100}$

Two or more fractions with different denominators can be compared by changing both fractions to fractions with the same denominator (see Box 1.1). This is done by finding the lowest common denominator (LCD), or the lowest number evenly divisible by the denominators of the fractions being compared.

**Example:** Which is larger, $\frac{3}{4}$ or $\frac{4}{5}$?

**Solution:** The lowest common denominator is 20, because it is the smallest number that can be divided by both denominators evenly. Change each fraction to the same terms by dividing the lowest common denominator by the denominator and multiplying that answer by the numerator. The answer obtained from this is the new numerator. The numerators are then placed over the lowest common denominator.

**For the fraction $\frac{3}{4}$:** $20 \div 4 = 5$; $5 \times 3 = 15$; therefore $\frac{3}{4}$ becomes $\frac{15}{20}$.

**For the fraction $\frac{4}{5}$:** $20 \div 5 = 4$; $4 \times 4 = 16$; therefore $\frac{4}{5}$ becomes $\frac{16}{20}$.

Therefore $\frac{4}{5}\left(\frac{16}{20}\right)$ is larger than $\frac{3}{4}\left(\frac{15}{20}\right)$.

Box 1.2 presents fundamental rules of fractions.

### BOX 1.2 Fundamental Rules of Fractions

In working with fractions, there are some fundamental rules that we need to remember.
1. When the numerator and denominator of a fraction are both multiplied or divided by the same number, the value of the fraction remains unchanged.

**Examples:** $\frac{1}{2} = \frac{1 \times (2)}{2 \times (2)} = \frac{2}{4} = \frac{2 \times (25)}{4 \times (25)} = \frac{50}{100}$, etc.

$\frac{50}{100} = \frac{50 \div (10)}{100 \div (10)} = \frac{5}{10} = \frac{5 \div (5)}{10 \div (5)} = \frac{1}{2}$, etc.

As shown in the examples, common fractions can be written in various forms, provided that the numerator, divided by the denominator, always yields the same number (quotient). The particular form of a fraction that has the smallest possible whole number for its numerator and denominator is called the *fraction in its lowest terms*. In the example, therefore $^{50}/_{100}$, $^{5}/_{10}$, or $^{2}/_{4}$ is $^{1}/_{2}$ in its lowest terms.
2. To change a fraction to its lowest terms, divide its numerator and its denominator by the largest whole number that will divide both evenly.

**Example:** Reduce $\frac{128}{288}$ to lowest terms.

$$\frac{128}{288} = \frac{128 \div 32}{288 \div 32} = \frac{4}{9}$$

**Note:** When you do not see the largest number that can be divided evenly at once, the fraction may have to be reduced by using repeated steps.

**Example:** $\frac{128}{288} = \frac{128 \div 4}{288 \div 4} = \frac{32}{72} = \frac{32 \div 8}{72 \div 8} = \frac{4}{9}$

**Note:** If both the numerator and denominator cannot be divided evenly by a whole number, the fraction is already in lowest terms. Fractions should always be expressed in their lowest terms.
3. LCD (lowest common denominator) is the smallest whole number that can be divided evenly by all of the denominators within the problem.

**Examples:** $\frac{1}{3}$ and $\frac{5}{12}$: 12 is evenly divisible by 3; therefore 12 is the LCD.

$\frac{3}{7}$, $\frac{2}{14}$, and $\frac{2}{28}$: 28 is evenly divisible by 7 and 14; therefore 28 is the LCD.

## ▦ PRACTICE **PROBLEMS**

Circle the fraction with the least value in each of the following sets.

1. $\dfrac{6}{30}$   $\dfrac{4}{5}$
    6. $\dfrac{4}{8}$   $\dfrac{1}{8}$   $\dfrac{3}{8}$

2. $\dfrac{5}{4}$   $\dfrac{6}{8}$
    7. $\dfrac{1}{40}$   $\dfrac{1}{10}$   $\dfrac{1}{5}$

3. $\dfrac{1}{75}$   $\dfrac{1}{100}$   $\dfrac{1}{150}$
    8. $\dfrac{1}{300}$   $\dfrac{1}{200}$   $\dfrac{1}{175}$

4. $\dfrac{6}{18}$   $\dfrac{7}{18}$   $\dfrac{8}{18}$
    9. $\dfrac{4}{24}$   $\dfrac{5}{24}$   $\dfrac{10}{24}$

5. $\dfrac{4}{5}$   $\dfrac{17}{85}$   $\dfrac{3}{5}$
    10. $\dfrac{4}{3}$   $\dfrac{1}{2}$   $\dfrac{1}{6}$

Circle the fraction with the greater value in each of the following sets.

11. $\dfrac{6}{8}$   $\dfrac{5}{9}$
    16. $\dfrac{2}{5}$   $\dfrac{6}{5}$   $\dfrac{3}{5}$

12. $\dfrac{7}{6}$   $\dfrac{2}{3}$
    17. $\dfrac{1}{8}$   $\dfrac{4}{6}$   $\dfrac{1}{4}$

13. $\dfrac{1}{72}$   $\dfrac{6}{12}$   $\dfrac{1}{24}$
    18. $\dfrac{7}{9}$   $\dfrac{5}{9}$   $\dfrac{8}{9}$

14. $\dfrac{1}{10}$   $\dfrac{1}{6}$   $\dfrac{1}{8}$
    19. $\dfrac{1}{10}$   $\dfrac{1}{50}$   $\dfrac{1}{150}$

15. $\dfrac{1}{75}$   $\dfrac{1}{125}$   $\dfrac{1}{225}$
    20. $\dfrac{2}{15}$   $\dfrac{1}{15}$   $\dfrac{6}{15}$

**Answers on p. 21**

## Reducing Fractions

Fractions should always be reduced to their lowest terms.

> **RULE**
> To reduce a fraction to its lowest terms, the numerator and denominator are each divided by the largest number by which they are both evenly divisible.

**Example 1:**  Reduce the fraction $\dfrac{6}{20}$.

**Solution:**   Both numerator and denominator are evenly divisible by 2.

$$\frac{6}{20} \div \frac{2}{2} = \frac{3}{10}$$

$$\frac{6}{20} = \frac{3}{10}$$

**Example 2:** Reduce the fraction $\dfrac{75}{100}$.

**Solution:** Both numerator and denominator are evenly divisible by 25.

$$\frac{75}{100} \div \frac{25}{25} = \frac{3}{4}$$

$$\frac{75}{100} = \frac{3}{4}$$

## PRACTICE **PROBLEMS**

Reduce the following fractions to their lowest terms.

21. $\dfrac{10}{15} =$ _____

22. $\dfrac{7}{49} =$ _____

23. $\dfrac{64}{128} =$ _____

24. $\dfrac{100}{150} =$ _____

25. $\dfrac{20}{28} =$ _____

26. $\dfrac{14}{98} =$ _____

27. $\dfrac{10}{18} =$ _____

28. $\dfrac{24}{36} =$ _____

29. $\dfrac{10}{50} =$ _____

30. $\dfrac{9}{27} =$ _____

31. $\dfrac{9}{9} =$ _____

32. $\dfrac{15}{45} =$ _____

33. $\dfrac{124}{155} =$ _____

34. $\dfrac{12}{18} =$ _____

35. $\dfrac{36}{64} =$ _____

**Answers on p. 21**

## Adding Fractions

> **RULE**
>
> To add fractions with the same denominator, add the numerators, place the sum over the denominator, and reduce to lowest terms.

**Example 1:**

$$\frac{1}{6} + \frac{4}{6} = \frac{5}{6}$$

**Example 2:**

$$\frac{1}{6} + \frac{3}{6} + \frac{4}{6} = \frac{8}{6}$$

$$\frac{8}{6} = \frac{4}{3} = 1\frac{1}{3}$$

> **NOTE**
>
> In addition to reducing to lowest terms in Example 2, the improper fraction was changed to a mixed number.

> **RULE**
>
> To add fractions with different denominators, change fractions to their equivalent fraction with the lowest common denominator, add the numerators, write the sum over the common denominator, and reduce if necessary.

Example 1: $\frac{1}{4} + \frac{1}{3}$

Solution: The lowest common denominator is 12. Change to equivalent fractions.

$$\frac{1}{4} = \frac{3}{12}$$

$$+\frac{1}{3} = \frac{4}{12}$$

$$\frac{7}{12}$$

Example 2: $\frac{1}{2} + 1\frac{1}{3} + \frac{2}{4}$

Solution: Change the mixed number $1\frac{1}{3}$ to $\frac{4}{3}$. Find the lowest common denominator, change fractions to equivalent fractions, add, and reduce if necessary. The lowest common denominator is 12.

$$\frac{1}{2} = \frac{6}{12}$$

$$\frac{4}{3} = \frac{16}{12}$$

$$+\frac{2}{4} = \frac{6}{12}$$

$$\frac{28}{12} = 2\frac{4}{12} = 2\frac{1}{3}$$

## Subtracting Fractions

> **RULE**
> To subtract fractions with the same denominator, subtract the numerators, and place this amount over the denominator. Reduce to lowest terms if necessary.

Example 1: $\frac{5}{4} - \frac{3}{4} = \frac{2}{4} = \frac{1}{2}$

Example 2: $2\frac{1}{6} - \frac{5}{6}$

Solution: Change the mixed number $2\frac{1}{6}$ to $\frac{13}{6}$

$$\frac{13}{6} - \frac{5}{6} = \frac{8}{6} = \frac{4}{3} = 1\frac{1}{3}$$

> **RULE**
> To subtract fractions with different denominators, find the lowest common denominator, change to equivalent fractions, subtract the numerators, and place the sum over the common denominator. Reduce to lowest terms if necessary.

Example 3:                                          $\dfrac{15}{6} - \dfrac{3}{5}$

Solution:     The lowest common denominator is 30. Change to equivalent fractions, and
              subtract.

$$\dfrac{15}{6} = \dfrac{75}{30}$$

$$-\dfrac{3}{5} = \dfrac{18}{30}$$

$$\dfrac{57}{30} = 1\dfrac{27}{30} = 1\dfrac{9}{10}$$

Example 4:  $2\dfrac{1}{5} - \dfrac{4}{3}$

Solution:     Change the mixed number $2\dfrac{1}{5}$ to $\dfrac{11}{5}$. Find the lowest common denomina-

              tor, change to equivalent fractions, subtract, and reduce if necessary.
              The lowest common denominator is 15.

$$\dfrac{11}{5} = \dfrac{33}{15}$$

$$-\dfrac{4}{3} = \dfrac{20}{15}$$

$$\dfrac{13}{15}$$

## Subtracting a Fraction From a Whole Number

> **RULE**
>
> To subtract a fraction from a whole number, follow these steps:
> 1. Borrow 1 from the whole number and change it to a fraction, creating a mixed number.
> 2. Change the fraction so that it has the same denominator as the fraction to be subtracted.
> 3. Subtract the fraction from the mixed number.
> 4. Reduce if necessary.

Example 1:  Subtract $\dfrac{7}{12}$ from 6.

$$6 = 5 + \dfrac{1}{1} = 5\dfrac{12}{12}$$

$$-\dfrac{7}{12} = \dfrac{7}{12}$$

$$5\dfrac{5}{12}$$

## Subtracting Fractions Using Borrowing

> **RULE**
>
> To subtract fractions using borrowing, use the following steps:
> 1. Change both fractions to the same denominator if necessary.
> 2. Borrow 1 from the whole number and change it to the same denominator as the fraction in the mixed number. Add the two fractions together.
> 3. Subtract the fractions and the whole numbers.
> 4. Reduce if necessary.

Example 2: $5\dfrac{1}{4} - 3\dfrac{3}{4}$

In the above example, because $\dfrac{3}{4}$ is larger than $\dfrac{1}{4}$, subtraction of the fractions is not possible. Both fractions have the same denominator; no changes need to be made. Therefore borrow 1 from the whole number part (5), and add the 1 to the fractional part $\left(\dfrac{1}{4}\right)$.

This results in

$$5\dfrac{1}{4} = 4 + \dfrac{1}{1} + \dfrac{1}{4} = 4 + \dfrac{4}{4} + \dfrac{1}{4} = 4\dfrac{5}{4}$$

$$5\dfrac{1}{4} = 4\dfrac{5}{4}$$
$$-3\dfrac{3}{4} = 3\dfrac{3}{4}$$
$$\rule{3cm}{0.4pt}$$
$$1\dfrac{5-3}{4} = 1\dfrac{2}{4} = 1\dfrac{1}{2}$$

Example 3: Subtract $4\dfrac{3}{4}$ from $9\dfrac{2}{3}$.

Both fractions need to be changed to the same denominator of 12:

$$9\dfrac{2}{3} = 9\dfrac{8}{12} \text{ and } 4\dfrac{3}{4} = 4\dfrac{9}{12}$$

Subtraction of the fractions is not possible because $\dfrac{9}{12}$ is larger than $\dfrac{8}{12}$.

Therefore borrow 1 from 9.

$$9\dfrac{8}{12} = 8 + \dfrac{1}{1} + \dfrac{8}{12} = 8 + \dfrac{12}{12} + \dfrac{8}{12} = 8\dfrac{20}{12}$$

Now subtract:

$$9\dfrac{2}{3} = 9\dfrac{8}{12} = 8\dfrac{20}{12}$$
$$-4\dfrac{3}{4} = 4\dfrac{9}{12} = 4\dfrac{9}{12}$$
$$\rule{3cm}{0.4pt}$$
$$4\dfrac{11}{12}$$

## Multiplying Fractions

**RULE**

1. Cancel terms if possible.
2. Multiply the numerators, multiply the denominators.
3. Reduce the result (product) to the lowest terms, if necessary.

Notice in this example that the numerator and denominator of any of the fractions involved in multiplication may be cancelled when they can be divided by the same number (cross-cancellation).

Example 1:
$$\frac{3}{\overset{\cancel{4}}{2}} \times \frac{\overset{1}{\cancel{2}}}{5} = \frac{3}{10}$$

Example 2:
$$\frac{2}{4} \times \frac{3}{4}$$

Solution: Reduce $\frac{2}{4}$ to $\frac{1}{2}$ and then multiply.

$$\frac{1}{2} \times \frac{3}{4} = \frac{3}{8}$$

Example 3:
$$6 \times \frac{5}{6}$$

$$\frac{\overset{1}{\cancel{6}}}{1} \times \frac{5}{\underset{1}{\cancel{6}}} = 5$$

*or*

$$\frac{6 \times 5}{6} = \frac{30}{6} = 5$$

Example 4:
$$3\frac{1}{3} \times 2\frac{1}{2}$$

Solution: Change mixed numbers to improper fractions. Proceed with multiplication.

$$3\frac{1}{3} = \frac{10}{3}; 2\frac{1}{2} = \frac{5}{2}$$

$$\frac{10}{3} \times \frac{5}{2} = \frac{50}{6} = 8\frac{2}{6} = 8\frac{1}{3}$$

*or*

$$\frac{\overset{5}{\cancel{10}}}{3} \times \frac{5}{\underset{1}{\cancel{2}}} = \frac{25}{3} = 8\frac{1}{3}$$

## Dividing Fractions

**RULE**

1. To divide fractions, invert (turn upside down) the second fraction (divisor); change ÷ to ×.
2. Cancel terms, if possible.
3. Multiply fractions.
4. Reduce where necessary.

Example 1:
$$\frac{3}{4} \div \frac{2}{3}$$

Solution:
$$\frac{3}{4} \times \frac{3}{2} = \frac{9}{8} = 1\frac{1}{8}$$

Example 2:
$$1\frac{3}{5} \div 2\frac{1}{10}$$

Solution:     Change mixed numbers to improper fractions. Proceed with steps of division.

$$1\frac{3}{5} = \frac{8}{5}; 2\frac{1}{10} = \frac{21}{10}$$

$$\frac{8}{\overset{1}{\cancel{5}}} \times \frac{\overset{2}{\cancel{10}}}{21} = \frac{16}{21}$$

Example 3:
$$5 \div \frac{1}{2}$$

Solution:
$$5 \times \frac{2}{1} = \frac{10}{1} = 10$$

*or*

$$\frac{5}{1} \times \frac{2}{1} = \frac{10}{1} = 10$$

With dosage calculations that involve division, the fractions may be written as follows: $\frac{1/4}{1/2}$. In this case, $\frac{1}{4}$ is the numerator and $\frac{1}{2}$ is the denominator. Therefore the problem is set up as: $\frac{1}{4} \div \frac{1}{2}$, which becomes $\frac{1}{\underset{2}{\cancel{4}}} \times \frac{\overset{1}{\cancel{2}}}{1} = \frac{1}{2}$.

---

## 🖩 PRACTICE **PROBLEMS**

Change the following improper fractions to mixed numbers, and reduce to lowest terms.

36. $\dfrac{18}{5} =$ _____     39. $\dfrac{35}{12} =$ _____

37. $\dfrac{60}{14} =$ _____     40. $\dfrac{112}{100} =$ _____

38. $\dfrac{13}{8} =$ _____

Change the following mixed numbers to improper fractions.

41. $1\dfrac{4}{25} =$ _____     44. $3\dfrac{3}{8} =$ _____

42. $4\dfrac{2}{8} =$ _____     45. $15\dfrac{4}{5} =$ _____

43. $4\dfrac{1}{2} =$ _____

Add the following fractions and mixed numbers, and reduce fractions to lowest terms.

46. $\dfrac{2}{3} + \dfrac{5}{6} =$ _____     49. $7\dfrac{2}{5} + \dfrac{2}{3} =$ _____

47. $2\dfrac{1}{8} + \dfrac{2}{3} =$ _____     50. $12\dfrac{1}{2} + 10\dfrac{1}{3} =$ _____

48. $2\dfrac{3}{10} + 4\dfrac{1}{5} + \dfrac{2}{3} =$ _____

Subtract and reduce fractions to lowest terms.

51. $\dfrac{4}{3} - \dfrac{3}{7} =$ _____

52. $3\dfrac{3}{8} - 1\dfrac{3}{5} =$ _____

53. $\dfrac{15}{16} - \dfrac{1}{4} =$ _____

54. $2\dfrac{5}{6} - 2\dfrac{3}{4} =$ _____

55. $\dfrac{1}{8} - \dfrac{1}{12} =$ _____

56. $14 - \dfrac{5}{9} =$ _____

57. $3\dfrac{3}{10} - 1\dfrac{7}{10} =$ _____

Multiply the following fractions and mixed numbers, and reduce to lowest terms.

58. $\dfrac{2}{3} \times \dfrac{4}{5} =$ _____

59. $\dfrac{6}{25} \times \dfrac{3}{5} =$ _____

60. $\dfrac{1}{50} \times 3 =$ _____

61. $2\dfrac{5}{8} \times 2\dfrac{3}{4} =$ _____

62. $\dfrac{5}{12} \times \dfrac{4}{9} =$ _____

Divide the following fractions and mixed numbers, and reduce to lowest terms.

63. $2\dfrac{6}{8} \div 1\dfrac{2}{3} =$ _____

64. $\dfrac{1}{60} \div \dfrac{1}{2} =$ _____

65. $6 \div \dfrac{2}{5} =$ _____

66. $\dfrac{7}{8} \div \dfrac{7}{8} =$ _____

67. $3\dfrac{1}{3} \div 1\dfrac{7}{12} =$ _____

**Answers on p. 21**

## ◉ CHAPTER **REVIEW**

Change the following improper fractions to mixed numbers, and reduce to lowest terms.

1. $\dfrac{10}{8} =$ _____

2. $\dfrac{30}{4} =$ _____

3. $\dfrac{67}{10} =$ _____

4. $\dfrac{11}{4} =$ _____

5. $\dfrac{64}{15} =$ _____

6. $\dfrac{100}{13} =$ _____

Change the following mixed numbers to improper fractions.

7. $7\dfrac{3}{8} =$ _____

8. $8\dfrac{4}{10} =$ _____

9. $3\dfrac{1}{5} =$ _____

10. $12\dfrac{3}{4} =$ _____

11. $6\dfrac{5}{7} =$ _____

Add the following fractions and mixed numbers. Reduce to lowest terms.

12. $\frac{2}{5} + \frac{1}{3} + \frac{7}{10} =$ _____

13. $\frac{1}{4} + \frac{1}{6} + \frac{1}{8} =$ _____

14. $6\frac{1}{4} + \frac{2}{9} + \frac{1}{36} =$ _____

15. $10\frac{1}{6} + 12\frac{4}{6} =$ _____

16. $1\frac{4}{5} + 7\frac{9}{10} + 3\frac{1}{2} =$ _____

Subtract the following fractions and mixed numbers. Reduce to lowest terms.

17. $2\frac{1}{4} - 1\frac{1}{2} =$ _____

18. $\frac{4}{5} - \frac{1}{6} =$ _____

19. $\frac{4}{5} - \frac{1}{4} =$ _____

20. $4\frac{1}{6} - 1\frac{1}{3} =$ _____

21. $\frac{8}{5} - \frac{1}{3} =$ _____

22. $\frac{5}{6} - \frac{7}{12} =$ _____

23. $48\frac{6}{11} - 24 =$ _____

24. $39\frac{11}{18} - 8\frac{3}{6} =$ _____

Multiply the following fractions and mixed numbers. Reduce to lowest terms.

25. $\frac{1}{3} \times \frac{4}{12} =$ _____

26. $2\frac{7}{8} \times 3\frac{1}{4} =$ _____

27. $36 \times \frac{3}{4} =$ _____

28. $\frac{5}{4} \times \frac{2}{4} =$ _____

29. $\frac{10}{25} \times \frac{5}{3} =$ _____

30. $\frac{1}{2} \times \frac{3}{4} \times \frac{3}{5} =$ _____

31. $\frac{3}{5} \times 3\frac{1}{8} =$ _____

32. $2\frac{2}{5} \times 4\frac{1}{6} =$ _____

33. $2 \times 4\frac{3}{8} =$ _____

34. $\frac{2}{5} \times \frac{5}{4} =$ _____

Divide the following fractions and mixed numbers. Reduce to lowest terms.

35. $2\frac{1}{3} \div 4\frac{1}{6} =$ _____

36. $25 \div 12\frac{1}{2} =$ _____

37. $\frac{7}{8} \div 2\frac{1}{4} =$ _____

38. $\frac{4}{6} \div \frac{1}{2} =$ _____

39. $\frac{3}{10} \div \frac{5}{25} =$ _____

40. $3 \div \frac{2}{5} =$ _____

41. $\frac{15}{30} \div 10 =$ _____

42. $\frac{3}{4} \div \frac{3}{8} =$ _____

43. $12 \div \frac{2}{3} =$ _____

44. $\frac{7}{8} \div 14 =$ _____

45. $\frac{15}{8} \div 5 =$ _____

Arrange the following fractions in order from largest to the smallest.

46. $\frac{3}{16}, \frac{1}{16}, \frac{5}{16}, \frac{14}{16}, \frac{7}{16}$

47. $\frac{5}{12}, \frac{5}{32}, \frac{5}{8}, \frac{5}{6}, \frac{5}{64}$

Apply the principles of borrowing, and subtract the following:

48. $2 - \dfrac{10}{21} =$ _____

49. $9\dfrac{1}{4} - \dfrac{3}{4} =$ _____

50. $5\dfrac{1}{2} - 3\dfrac{3}{4} =$ _____

51. A client is instructed to drink 20 ounces of water within 1 hour. The client has only been able to drink 12 ounces. What portion of the water remains? (Express your answer as a fraction reduced to lowest terms.) _____

52. A child's oral Motrin Suspension contains 100 milligrams per teaspoonful. 20 milligrams represents what part of a dosage? _____

53. A client is receiving 240 milliliters of Ensure by mouth as a supplement. The client consumes 200 milliliters. What portion of the Ensure remains? (Express your answer as a fraction reduced to lowest terms.) _____

54. A client takes $1\frac{1}{2}$ tablets of medication four times per day for 4 days. How many tablets will the client have taken at the end of the 4 days? _____

55. A juice glass holds 120 milliliters. If a client drinks $2\frac{1}{3}$ glasses, how many milliliters did the client consume? _____

56. On admission a client weighed $150\frac{3}{4}$ lb. On discharge the client weighed $148\frac{1}{2}$ lb. How much weight did the client lose? _____

57. How many hours are there in $3\frac{1}{2}$ days? _____

58. A client consumed the following: $2\frac{1}{4}$ ounces of tea, $\frac{1}{3}$ ounce of juice, $1\frac{1}{2}$ ounces of Jell-O. What is the total number of ounces consumed by the client?

    _____

59. One tablet contains 200 milligrams of pain medication.

    How many milligrams are in $3\frac{1}{2}$ tablets? _____

60. A bottle of medicine contains 30 doses. How many doses are in $2\frac{1}{2}$ bottles? _____

61. The nurse gave a client $\frac{3}{4}$ tablespoons (tbs) of medication with breakfast, $\frac{1}{2}$ tbs at lunch, $\frac{1}{2}$ tbs at dinner, and $1\frac{1}{4}$ tbs at bedtime. How much medication did the nurse administer? _____

62. A client weighed $160\frac{1}{2}$ pounds (lb) at the previous visit to the doctor. At this visit, the client weighs $2\frac{3}{4}$ lb more. How many lb does the client weigh? _____

63. At the beginning of a shift there are $5\frac{1}{4}$ bottles of hand sanitizer available. At the end of the shift, $3\frac{1}{2}$ bottles are left. How much was used? _____

64. A client was given a 16-ounce container of water to drink throughout the day. If the client drank $\frac{7}{8}$ of the container, how many ounces did the client drink? _____

65. How many $1\frac{1}{2}$-ounce doses of medication are there in a 24-ounce bottle?
   _____

66. A bottle contains 36 tablets. If a client took $\frac{1}{3}$ of the tablets, how many tablets are left? _____

67. A client drank $4\frac{3}{4}$ ounces of juice, $5\frac{1}{2}$ ounces of coffee, and $4\frac{1}{4}$ ounces of water. How much fluid did the client drink? _____

68. One tablet contains 400 milligrams of medication. A client was given $1\frac{1}{2}$ tablets for 5 days. How many milligrams of medication did the client receive in 5 days? _____

69. An order is written for a client to receive $1\frac{1}{2}$ ounces of a powdered medication dissolved in water. The client drank $\frac{3}{4}$ ounces of the medication. How much more medication must be given to the client? _____

70. An infant grew $\frac{3}{4}$ inch in the first month, $\frac{1}{2}$ inch in the second month, $\frac{7}{8}$ inch in the third month, and $1\frac{1}{8}$ inches in the fourth month. How many inches has the infant grown? _____

71. For 4 days a client received $2\frac{1}{2}$ ounces of medication 4 times per day. How many ounces did the client receive over 4 days? _____

72. A bottle contains 24 ounces of a liquid pain medication. If a typical dose is $\frac{3}{4}$ ounce, how many doses are there in the bottle? _____

73. A nurse worked $9\frac{3}{4}$ hours on Monday, $11\frac{1}{2}$ hours on Tuesday, and $10\frac{3}{4}$ hours on Wednesday. How many hours did she work for the 3 days? _____

74. A nurse needs $\frac{1}{2}$ hour to complete an intake interview form on each new client. How many intake interview forms can the nurse complete in $2\frac{1}{2}$ hours?
   _____

75. A client drinks $\frac{3}{4}$ of a glass of juice that contains 180 milliliters. How many milliliters of juice did the client drink? _____

76. A client is instructed to drink the equivalent of 8 glasses of water daily. How many times will the client need to drink $\frac{1}{2}$ glass of water? _____

77. One tablet contains 150 milligrams of medication. How many milligrams are in $3\frac{1}{2}$ tablets? _____

78. A client at home was instructed to take $\frac{3}{4}$ ounce of medication with meals. The nurse learns that the client took $\frac{2}{3}$ ounce. Did the client take too little, too much, or just the right amount? _____

79. A client has taken $\frac{3}{4}$ of a bottle of tablets that contained 100 tablets. How many tablets has the client taken? _____

80. A client drank $3\frac{1}{2}$ cups of water from a cup that held 210 milliliters. How many milliliters did the client drink? _____

**Answers on p. 22**

## ⭐ ANSWERS

### Chapter 1
**Answers to Practice Problems**

1. LCD = 30; therefore $\frac{6}{30}$ has the lesser value.

2. LCD = 8; therefore $\frac{6}{8}$ has the lesser value.

3. $\frac{1}{150}$ has the lesser value; the denominator (150) is larger.

4. $\frac{6}{18}$ has the lesser value; the numerator (6) is smaller.

5. $\frac{17}{85}$ has the lesser value; reduced to $\frac{1}{5}$; the numerator (1) is smaller.

6. $\frac{1}{8}$ has the lesser value; the numerator (1) is smaller.

7. $\frac{1}{40}$ has the lesser value; the denominator (40) is larger.

8. $\frac{1}{300}$ has the lesser value; the denominator (300) is larger.

9. $\frac{4}{24}$ has the lesser value; the numerator (4) is smaller.

10. LCD = 6; therefore $\frac{1}{6}$ has the lesser value.

11. LCD = 72; therefore $\frac{6}{8}$ has the higher value.

12. LCD = 6; therefore $\frac{7}{6}$ has the higher value.

13. LCD = 72; therefore $\frac{6}{12}$ has the higher value.

14. $\frac{1}{6}$ has the higher value; the denominator (6) is smaller.

15. $\frac{1}{75}$ has the higher value; the denominator (75) is smaller.

16. $\frac{6}{5}$ has the higher value; the numerator (6) is larger.

17. LCD = 24; therefore $\frac{4}{6}$ has the higher value.

18. $\frac{8}{9}$ has the higher value; the numerator (8) is larger.

19. $\frac{1}{10}$ has the higher value; the denominator (10) is smaller.

20. $\frac{6}{15}$ has the higher value; the numerator (6) is larger.

21. $\frac{10 \div 5}{15 \div 5} = \frac{2}{3}$

22. $\frac{7 \div 7}{49 \div 7} = \frac{1}{7}$

23. $\frac{64 \div 32}{128 \div 32} = \frac{2}{4} = \frac{1}{2}$

24. $\frac{100 \div 50}{150 \div 50} = \frac{2}{3}$

25. $\frac{20 \div 4}{28 \div 4} = \frac{5}{7}$

26. $\frac{14 \div 14}{98 \div 14} = \frac{1}{7}$

27. $\frac{10 \div 2}{18 \div 2} = \frac{5}{9}$

28. $\frac{24 \div 12}{36 \div 12} = \frac{2}{3}$

29. $\frac{10 \div 10}{50 \div 10} = \frac{1}{5}$

30. $\frac{9 \div 9}{27 \div 9} = \frac{1}{3}$

31. $\frac{9 \div 9}{9 \div 9} = \frac{1}{1} = 1$

32. $\frac{15 \div 15}{45 \div 15} = \frac{1}{3}$

33. $\frac{124 \div 31}{155 \div 31} = \frac{4}{5}$

34. $\frac{12 \div 6}{18 \div 6} = \frac{2}{3}$

35. $\frac{36 \div 4}{64 \div 4} = \frac{9}{16}$

36. $3\frac{3}{5}$

37. $4\frac{2}{7}$

38. $1\frac{5}{8}$

39. $2\frac{11}{12}$

40. $1\frac{3}{25}$

41. $\frac{29}{25}$

42. $\frac{34}{8}$

43. $\frac{9}{2}$

44. $\frac{27}{8}$

45. $\frac{79}{5}$

46. $1\frac{1}{2}$

47. $2\frac{19}{24}$

48. $7\frac{1}{6}$

49. $8\frac{1}{15}$

50. $22\frac{5}{6}$

51. $\frac{19}{21}$

52. $1\frac{31}{40}$

53. $\frac{11}{16}$

54. $\frac{1}{12}$

55. $\frac{1}{24}$

56. $13\frac{4}{9}$

57. $1\frac{3}{5}$

58. $\frac{8}{15}$

59. $\frac{18}{125}$

60. $\frac{3}{50}$

61. $7\frac{7}{32}$

62. $\frac{5}{27}$

63. $1\frac{13}{20}$

64. $\frac{1}{30}$

65. 15

66. 1

67. $2\frac{2}{19}$

## Answers to Chapter Review

1. $1\frac{2}{8} = 1\frac{1}{4}$

2. $7\frac{2}{4} = 7\frac{1}{2}$

3. $6\frac{7}{10}$

4. $2\frac{3}{4}$

5. $4\frac{4}{15}$

6. $7\frac{9}{13}$

7. $\frac{59}{8}$

8. $\frac{84}{10}$

9. $\frac{16}{5}$

10. $\frac{51}{4}$

11. $\frac{47}{7}$

12. LCD = 30; $1\frac{13}{30}$

13. LCD = 24; $\frac{13}{24}$

14. LCD = 36; $\frac{234}{36} = 6\frac{18}{36} = 6\frac{1}{2}$

15. $22\frac{5}{6}$

16. LCD = 10; $13\frac{2}{10} = 13\frac{1}{5}$

17. LCD = 4; $\frac{3}{4}$

18. LCD = 30; $\frac{19}{30}$

19. LCD = 20; $\frac{11}{20}$

20. LCD = 6; $\frac{17}{6} = 2\frac{5}{6}$

21. LCD = 15; $\frac{19}{15} = 1\frac{4}{15}$

22. LCD = 12; $\frac{3}{12} = \frac{1}{4}$

23. $24\frac{6}{11}$

24. LCD = 18; $31\frac{1}{9}$

25. $\frac{4}{36} = \frac{1}{9}$

26. $9\frac{11}{32}$

27. 27

28. $\frac{10}{16} = \frac{5}{8}$

29. $\frac{50}{75} = \frac{2}{3}$

30. $\frac{9}{40}$

31. $1\frac{7}{8}$

32. 10

33. $8\frac{3}{4}$

34. $\frac{1}{2}$

35. $\frac{42}{75} = \frac{14}{25}$

36. 2

37. $\frac{7}{18}$

38. $1\frac{1}{3}$

39. $1\frac{25}{50} = 1\frac{1}{2}$

40. $7\frac{1}{2}$

41. $\frac{15}{300} = \frac{1}{20}$

42. 2

43. 18

44. $\frac{1}{16}$

45. $\frac{3}{8}$

46. $\frac{14}{16}, \frac{7}{16}, \frac{5}{16}, \frac{3}{16}, \frac{1}{16}$

47. $\frac{5}{6}, \frac{5}{8}, \frac{5}{12}, \frac{5}{32}, \frac{5}{64}$

48. $1\frac{11}{21}$

49. $8\frac{2}{4} = 8\frac{1}{2}$

50. $1\frac{3}{4}$

51. $\frac{2}{5}$ of water remains

52. $\frac{1}{5}$ the dosage

53. $\frac{1}{6}$ of Ensure remains

54. 24 tablets

55. 280 milliliters

56. $2\frac{1}{4}$ lb

57. 84 hours

58. $4\frac{1}{12}$ ounces

59. 700 milligrams

60. 75 doses

61. 3 tbs

62. $163\frac{1}{4}$ lb

63. $1\frac{3}{4}$ bottles

64. 14 ounces

65. 16 ($1\frac{1}{2}$ ounce doses in the bottle)

66. 24 tablets

67. $14\frac{1}{2}$ ounces

68. 3,000 milligrams

69. $\frac{3}{4}$ ounce

70. $3\frac{1}{4}$ inches

71. 40 ounces

72. 32 ($\frac{3}{4}$ ounce doses in the bottle)

73. 32 hours

74. 5 interview forms

75. 135 milliliters

76. 16 times

77. 525 milligrams

78. Too little

79. 75 tablets

80. 735 milliliters

# CHAPTER 2
## Decimals

## Objectives

*After reviewing this chapter, you should be able to:*
1. Read decimals
2. Write decimals
3. Compare the size of decimals
4. Convert fractions to decimals
5. Convert decimals to fractions
6. Add decimals
7. Subtract decimals
8. Multiply decimals
9. Divide decimals
10. Round decimals to the nearest tenth
11. Round decimals to the nearest hundredth

Medication dosages and other measurements in the health care system use metric measures, which are based on the decimal system. An understanding of decimals is crucial to the calculation of dosages. In the administration of medications, nurses calculate dosages that contain decimals in addition to encountering labels that may have dosage strengths expressed as decimals. Some examples include Coreg, terbutaline, Flomax, and clonidine. See example labels in Figures 2.1 and 2.2 with dosage strengths expressed in decimal format.

Decimal points in dosages have been cited as a major source of medication errors. A misunderstanding of the value of a dosage expressed as a decimal or the omission of a decimal point can result in a serious medication error. Decimals should be written with great care to prevent misinterpretation of a value. A clear understanding of the importance of decimal points and their value will assist the nurse in the prevention of medication errors.

A decimal is a fraction that has a denominator that is a multiple of 10. A decimal fraction is written as a decimal by the use of a decimal point (.). The decimal point is used to indicate place value. Some examples are as follows:

| Fraction | Decimal Number |
|---|---|
| $\dfrac{3}{10}$ | 0.3 |
| $\dfrac{18}{100}$ | 0.18 |
| $\dfrac{175}{1,000}$ | 0.175 |

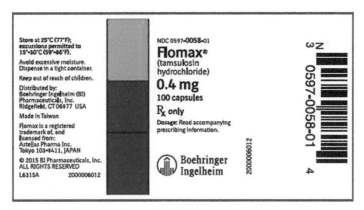

**Figure 2.1** Flomax, each capsule is 0.4 mg.

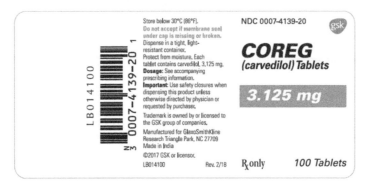

**Figure 2.2** Coreg, each tablet is 3.125 mg.

The decimal point represents the center that separates whole and fractional amounts. The position of the numbers in relation to the decimal point indicates the place of value of numbers.

- The whole number is placed to the **left** of the decimal point. These numbers have a value of one (1) or greater.
- Decimal fractions are written to the **right** of the decimal point and represent a value that is less than one (1) or part of one. The words for all decimal fractions end in -*th(s)*.

The easiest way to understand decimals is to memorize the place values (Box 2.1).

---

**BOX 2.1  Decimal Place Values**

The decimal value is determined by its position to the right of the decimal point.

| Hundred-thousands (100,000) | Ten-thousands (10,000) | Thousands (1,000) | Hundreds (100) | Tens (10) | Ones (Units) (1) | Decimal point | Tenths (0.1) | Hundredths (0.01) | Thousandths (0.001) | Ten-thousandths (0.0001) | Hundred-thousandths (0.00001) |
|---|---|---|---|---|---|---|---|---|---|---|---|
| 6 | 5 | 4 | 3 | 2 | 1 | . | 1 | 2 | 3 | 4 | 5 |

**Whole Numbers to the Left**                    **Decimal Numbers to the Right**

**Example 1:** 0.3 = three tenths

**Example 2:** 0.03 = three hundredths

**Example 3:** 0.003 = three thousandths

---

**SAFETY ALERT!**

When there is no whole number before a decimal point, place a zero (0) to the left of the decimal point to emphasize that the number is a decimal fraction and has a value less than 1. This will emphasize its value and prevent errors in interpretation and avoid errors in dosage calculation. This zero does not change the value of the number. This has been emphasized by the Institute for Safe Medication Practices (ISMP) and is a requirement of the accrediting body for health care organizations, The Joint Commission (TJC), when writing decimal fractions in medical notation and is part of TJC's official "Do Not Use" list.

---

The source of many medication errors is misplacement of a decimal point or incorrect interpretation of a decimal value.

## Reading and Writing Decimals

**RULE**

To read the decimal numbers, read:
1. The whole number
2. The decimal point as "and"
3. The decimal fraction by naming the value of the last decimal place
Notice that the words for all decimal fractions end in -th(s).

**Example 1:** The decimal number 1.125 is read as "one and one hundred twenty-five thousandths."

**Example 2:** The number 12.5 is read as "twelve and five tenths."

**Example 3:** The number 10.03 is read as "ten and three hundredths."

**RULE**

When reading decimal numbers in which a zero is placed before the decimal, such as in a decimal fraction (whose value is less than 1), read the number alone, without stating the zero.

**Example 1:** The number 0.4 is read as "four tenths."

**Example 2:** The number 0.175 is read as "one hundred seventy-five thousandths."

**TIPS FOR CLINICAL PRACTICE**

An exception to this is in an emergency situation when a nurse must take a verbal order over the phone from a prescriber. When repeating back an order for a medication involving a decimal, the zero should be read aloud to prevent a medication error.

**Example:** "Zero point 4" would be the verbal interpretation of Example 1 and "zero point 175" of Example 2. In addition to repeating the order back, the receiver of the order should write down the complete order or enter it into a computer, then read it back, and receive confirmation of the order from the individual giving the order.

**RULE**

To write a decimal number, write the following:
1. The whole number (If there is no whole number, write zero [0] to the left of the decimal.)
2. The decimal point to indicate the place value of the rightmost number
3. The decimal portion of the number to the right of the decimal

**Example 1:** Written, seven and five tenths = 7.5

**Example 2:** Written, one hundred twenty-five thousandths = 0.125

**Example 3:** Written, five tenths = 0.5

**RULE**

When writing decimals, placing a zero after the last digit of a decimal fraction does not change its value and is not necessary.

**Example:**    0.37 = 0.370

**SAFETY ALERT!**

When writing decimals, trailing zeros should not be placed at the end of the number to avoid misinterpretation of a value. This is also a recommendation of the Institute for Safe Medication Practices (ISMP) and is a part of The Joint Commission's (TJC) official "Do Not Use" List. TJC forbids the use of trailing zeros for medication orders or other medication-related documentation. Omitting trailing zeros decreases the potential for giving a client 10 times the ordered dose or more. Exception: A trailing zero may be used only when required to demonstrate the level of precision of the value being reported, such as for laboratory results, imaging studies that report the size of lesions, or catheter/tube sizes.

Because the last zero does not change the value of the decimal, it is not necessary. For example, the required notation is 0.37, not 0.370, and 30, not 30.0, which could be interpreted as 370 and 300, respectively, if the decimal point is not clear or is missed.

**RULE**

Zeros added before or after the decimal point of a decimal number may change its value.

**Example 1:** 0.375 ≠ (is not equal to) 0.0375

**Example 2:** 2.025 ≠ 20.025

However, .7 = 0.7 and 15 = 15.0, but you should write 0.7 (with a leading zero) and 15 (without a trailing zero).

---

## ▦ PRACTICE **PROBLEMS**

Write each of the following numbers in word form.

1. 8.35 _____

2. 11.001 _____

3. 4.57 _____

4. 5.0007 _____

5. 10.5 _____

6. 0.163 _____

Write each of the following in decimal form.

7. four tenths _____

8. eighty-four and seven
   hundredths _____

9. seven hundredths _____

10. two and twenty-three
    hundredths _____

11. five hundredths _____

12. nine thousandths _____

**Answers on p. 39**

## Comparing the Value of Decimals

It is essential to be able to compare decimal amounts and know which has the greater or lesser value in the calculation of dosages. This helps prevent errors in dosage and gives the nurse an understanding of the size of a dosage (i.e., 0.5 mg, 0.05 mg).

> **SAFETY ALERT!**
> Understanding the value of decimals helps ensure accuracy and prevents misinterpretation of values. There is an appreciable difference between 0.5 milligram (mg) and 0.05 milligram. In fact, 0.5 mg is 10 times larger than 0.05 mg. In dosage calculations, a misinterpretation of the value of decimals can result in serious consequences.

> **RULE**
> When decimal numbers contain whole numbers, the whole numbers are compared to determine which is greater.

**Example 1:** 4.8 is greater than 2.9

**Example 2:** 11.5 is greater than 7.5

**Example 3:** 7.37 is greater than 6.94

> **RULE**
> If the whole numbers being compared are the **same** (e.g., 5.6 and 5.2) or if there is **no whole number** (e.g., 0.45 and 0.37), then the number in the **tenths** place determines which decimal is greater.

**Example 1:** 0.45 is greater than 0.37

**Example 2:** 1.75 is greater than 1.25

> **RULE**
> If the whole numbers are the same or zero and the numbers in the **tenths place** are the **same**, then the decimal with the higher number in the **hundredths place** has the greater value, and so forth.

**Example 1:** 0.67 is greater than 0.66

**Example 2:** 0.17 is greater than 0.14

## ⊞ PRACTICE **PROBLEMS**

Circle the decimal with the largest value in the following:

13. 0.5         0.15        0.05            16. 0.175        0.1         0.05

14. 2.66        2.36        2.87            17. 7.02         7.15        7.35

15. 0.125       0.375       0.25            18. 0.067        0.087       0.077

**Answers on p. 39**

## Adding and Subtracting Decimals

> **RULE**
> To add or subtract decimals, place the numbers in columns so that the decimal points are lined up directly under one another and add or subtract from right to left. Zeros may be added at the end of the decimal fraction, making all decimals of equal length, but unnecessary zeros should be eliminated in the final answer.

> **SAFETY ALERT!**
> Eliminate unnecessary zeros in the final answer to avoid confusion and prevent errors in misinterpretation of values.

**Example 1:**  Add 16.4 + 21.8 + 13.2

$$
\begin{array}{r}
16.4 \\
21.8 \\
+\,13.2 \\
\hline
51.4
\end{array} = 51.4
$$

**Example 2:**  Add 2.25 + 1.75

$$
\begin{array}{r}
2.25 \\
+\,1.75 \\
\hline
4.00
\end{array} = 4
$$

**Example 3:**  Subtract 2.6 from 18.6

$$
\begin{array}{r}
18.6 \\
-\,2.6 \\
\hline
16.0
\end{array} = 16
$$

**Example 4:**  Add 11.2 + 16

$$
\begin{array}{r}
11.2 \\
+\,16.0 \\
\hline
27.2
\end{array} = 27.2
$$

**Example 5:**  Subtract 3.78 from 12.84

$$
\begin{array}{r}
12.84 \\
-\,3.78 \\
\hline
9.06
\end{array} = 9.06
$$

**Example 6:**  Subtract 0.007 from 0.05

$$
\begin{array}{r}
0.050 \\
-\,0.007 \\
\hline
0.043
\end{array} = 0.043
$$

**Example 7:**  Add 6.54 + 2.26

$$
\begin{array}{r}
6.54 \\
+\,2.26 \\
\hline
8.80
\end{array} = 8.8
$$

**Example 8:**  Add 0.7 + 0.75 + 0.23 + 2.324

$$
\begin{array}{r}
0.700 \\
0.750 \\
0.230 \\
+\,2.324 \\
\hline
4.004
\end{array} = 4.004
$$

**Example 9:**  Subtract 0.2 from 0.375

$$
\begin{array}{r}
0.375 \\
-\,0.200 \\
\hline
0.175
\end{array} = 0.175
$$

## PRACTICE **PROBLEMS**

Add the following decimals.

19.  4.7 + 5.3 + 8.4 = _____

20.  38.52 + 0.029 + 1.9 = _____

21.  0.7 + 3.25 = _____

22.  2.2 + 1.67 = _____

Subtract the following decimals.

23.  3.67 − 0.75 = _____

24.  64.3 − 21.2 = _____

25.  0.08 − 0.045 = _____

26.  6.75 − 0.87 = _____

**Answers on p. 39**

## Multiplying Decimals

> **RULE**
>
> To multiply decimals, multiply as with whole numbers. In the answer (product), count off from right to left as many decimal places as there are in the numbers being multiplied. Zeros may also be added to the left if necessary.

**Example 1:**            1.2 × 3.2

$$
\begin{array}{r}
1.2 \quad \text{(1 decimal place)}\\
\times\,3.2 \quad \text{(1 decimal place)}\\
\hline
24\phantom{.}\\
36\phantom{..}\\
\hline
384.
\end{array}
$$

**Answer:**    3.84

In Example 1, 1.2 has one number after the decimal, and 3.2 also has one. Therefore you will need to place the decimal point two places to the left in the answer (product).

> **RULE**
> When there are insufficient numbers in the answer for correct placement of the decimal point, add as many zeros as needed to the left of the answer.

**Example 2:**                           $1.35 \times 0.65$

$$
\begin{array}{r}
1.35 \quad \text{(2 decimal places)} \\
\times 0.65 \quad \text{(2 decimal places)} \\
\hline
675 \\
810 \\
\hline
8775. \\
\end{array}
$$

**Answer:**    0.8775

In Example 2, 1.35 has two numbers after the decimal, and 0.65 also has two. Therefore you will need to place the decimal point four places to the left in the answer (product), and add a zero in front of the decimal point.

**Example 3:**                           $0.11 \times 0.33$

$$
\begin{array}{r}
0.11 \quad \text{(2 decimal places)} \\
\times 0.33 \quad \text{(2 decimal places)} \\
\hline
33 \\
33 \\
\hline
0363. \\
\end{array}
$$

**Answer:**    0.0363

In Example 3, four decimal places are needed (two numbers after each decimal in 0.11 and 0.33), but there are only three numbers in the product. A zero must be placed to the left of these numbers for correct placement of the decimal point. Place a zero before the decimal point.

**Example 4:**                           $1.6 \times 0.05$

$$
\begin{array}{r}
1.6 \quad \text{(1 decimal place)} \\
\times 0.05 \quad \text{(2 decimal places)} \\
\hline
080. \\
\end{array}
$$

**Answer:**    $0.080 = 0.08$

In Example 4, three decimal places are needed (1.6 has one number after the decimal and 0.05 has two), so a zero has to be placed between the decimal point and 8 to allow for enough places. The unnecessary zero is eliminated in the final answer, and a zero is placed before the decimal point.

## Multiplication by Decimal Movement

> **RULE**
> This method may be preferred when doing metric conversions because it is based on the decimal system. Multiplying by 10, 100, 1,000, and so forth can be done by moving the decimal point to the right the same number of places as there are zeros in the number by which you are multiplying.

When multiplying by 10, move the decimal one place to the right; by 100, two places to the right; by 1,000, three places to the right; and so forth.

**Example 1:** $1.6 \times 10 = 16$ (The multiplier 10 has 1 zero; decimal point moved 1 place to the right.)

**Example 2:** $5.2 \times 100 = 520$ (The multiplier 100 has 2 zeros; decimal point moved 2 places to the right.)

**Example 3:** $0.463 \times 1,000 = 463$ (The multiplier 1,000 has 3 zeros; decimal point moved 3 places to the right.)

**Example 4:** $6.64 \times 10 = 66.4$ (The multiplier 10 has 1 zero; decimal point moved one place to the right.)

> **! SAFETY ALERT!**
> When multiplying decimals, be sure the decimal is placed in the correct position in the answer (product). Misplacement of decimal points can lead to a critical medication error.

## ⊞ PRACTICE **PROBLEMS**

Multiply the following decimals.

27. $3.15 \times 0.015 =$ _____

28. $3.65 \times 0.25 =$ _____

29. $9.65 \times 1,000 =$ _____

30. $8.9 \times 0.2 =$ _____

31. $14.001 \times 7.2 =$ _____

**Answers on p. 39**

## Dividing Decimals

Division of decimals is done in the same manner as division of whole numbers except for placement of the decimal point. Incorrect placement of the decimal point changes the numerical value and can cause errors in calculation. Errors made in the division of decimals are commonly caused by improper placement of the decimal point, incorrect placement of numbers in the quotient (answer), and omission of necessary zeros in the quotient.

The parts of a division problem are as follows:

$$\text{Divisor)}\overline{\text{Dividend}}^{\text{Quotient}}$$

The number being divided is called the **dividend,** the number being divided into the dividend is the **divisor,** and the answer is the **quotient.**

Symbols used to indicate division are as follows:

1. $\overline{)}$

    **Example:**      $9\overline{)27}$      Read as 27 divided by 9.

2. $\div$

    **Example:**      $27 \div 9$      Read as 27 divided by 9.

3. The horizontal bar with the dividend on the top and the divisor on the bottom

    **Example:**      $\dfrac{27}{9}$      Read as 27 divided by 9.

4. The slanted bar with the dividend to the left and the divisor to the right

Example:                               $^{27}/_9$                    Read as 27 divided by 9.

## Dividing a Decimal by a Whole Number

> **RULE**
>
> To divide a decimal by a whole number, place the decimal point in the quotient directly above the decimal point in the dividend. Proceed to divide as with whole numbers.

**Example:**    Divide 17.5 by 5

$$
\begin{array}{r}
3.5 \\
5\overline{)17.5} \\
-15 \\
\hline
25 \\
-25 \\
\hline
0
\end{array}
$$

**Answer:**    3.5

## Dividing a Decimal or a Whole Number by a Decimal

> **RULE**
>
> To divide by a decimal, the decimal point in the divisor is moved to the right until the number is a whole number. The decimal point in the dividend is moved the same number of places to the right, and zeros are added as necessary. Proceed to divide as with whole numbers.

**Example:**    Divide 6.96 by 0.3

**Step 1:**                      $6.96 \div 0.3 = 0.3\overline{)6.96}$

$3\overline{)69.6}$   (after moving decimals in the divisor the same number of places as the dividend)

**Step 2:**

$$
\begin{array}{r}
23.2 \\
3\overline{)69.6} \\
-6 \\
\hline
9 \\
-9 \\
\hline
6 \\
-6 \\
\hline
0
\end{array}
$$

**Answer:**    23.2

## Division by Decimal Movement

> **RULE**
>
> To divide a decimal by 10, 100, or 1,000, move the decimal point to the **left** the same number of places as there are zeros in the divisor.

**Example 1:**  $0.46 \div 10 = 0.046$ (The divisor 10 has 1 zero; the decimal point is moved 1 place to the left.)

**Example 2:**  $0.07 \div 100 = 0.0007$ (The divisor 100 has 2 zeros; the decimal point is moved 2 places to the left.)

**Example 3:** 0.75 ÷ 1,000 = 0.00075 (The divisor 1,000 has 3 zeros; the decimal point is moved 3 places to the left.)

## Rounding Off Decimals

The determination of how many places to carry your division when calculating dosages is based on the equipment being used. Some syringes are marked in **tenths** and some in **hundredths.** As you become familiar with the equipment used in dosage calculation, you will learn how far to carry your division and when to round off. To ensure accuracy, most calculation problems require that you carry your division at least **two decimal places (hundredths place)** and **round off to the nearest tenth.**

> **NOTE**
> In some instances, such as critical care or pediatrics, it may be necessary to compute decimal calculations to thousandths (three decimal places) and round to hundredths (two decimal places). These areas may require this level of accuracy.

> **RULE**
> To express an answer to the nearest tenth, carry the division to the hundredths place (two places after the decimal). If the number in the hundredths place **is 5 or greater,** add 1 to the tenths place. If the number **is less than 5,** drop the number to the right of the desired decimal place.

**Example 1:** Express 4.15 to the nearest tenth.

**Answer:** 4.2 (The number in the hundredths place is 5, so the number in the tenths place is **increased by one.** 4.1 becomes 4.2.)

**Example 2:** Express 1.24 to the nearest tenth.

**Answer:** 1.2 (The number in the hundredths place is less than 5, so the number in the **tenths place does not change.** The 4 is dropped.)

**Example 3:** Express 0.98 to the nearest tenth.

**Answer:** 1.0 = 1 (The number in the hundredths place is 8, so the number in the tenths place is **increased by one.** 0.9 becomes 1. The zero at the end of this decimal is dropped, because it is unnecessary and can cause potential confusion.)

> **RULE**
> To express an answer to the nearest hundredth, carry the division to the thousandths place (three places after the decimal). If the number in the thousandths place is **5 or greater,** add one to the hundredths place. If the number **is less than 5,** drop the number to the right of the desired decimal place.

**Example 1:** Express 0.176 to the nearest hundredth.

**Answer:** 0.18 (The number in the thousandths place is 6, so the number in the hundredths place is **increased by one.** 0.17 becomes 0.18.)

**Example 2:** Express 0.554 to the nearest hundredth.

**Answer:** 0.55 (The number in the thousandths place is less than 5, so the number in **the hundredths place does not change.**) The 4 is dropped.

**Example 3:** Express 0.40 to the nearest hundredth.

**Answer:** 0.4 (There is a 0 in the hundredths place. When this is rounded to the hundredths, the final zero should be dropped. It is not necessary to clarify the number and can cause potential confusion.)

## 🖩 PRACTICE **PROBLEMS**

Divide the following decimals. Carry division to the hundredths place where necessary. Do not round off.

32. $2 \div 0.5 =$ _____

33. $1.4 \div 1.2 =$ _____

34. $63.8 \div 0.9 =$ _____

35. $39.6 \div 1.3 =$ _____

36. $1.9 \div 3.2 =$ _____

Express the following decimals to the nearest tenth.

37. 3.57 _____

38. 0.95 _____

39. 1.98 _____

Express the following decimals to the nearest hundredth.

40. 3.550 _____

41. 0.607 _____

42. 0.738 _____

Divide the following decimals.

43. $0.005 \div 10 =$ _____

44. $0.004 \div 100 =$ _____

Multiply the following decimals.

45. $58.4 \times 10 =$ _____

46. $0.5 \times 1,000 =$ _____

**Answers on p. 39**

## Changing Fractions to Decimals

> **RULE**
> To change a fraction to a decimal, divide the numerator by the denominator and add zeros as needed. If the numerator doesn't divide evenly into the denominator, carry division three places.

Example 1:
$$\frac{2}{5} = 5\overline{)2} = 5\overline{)2.0}^{\,0.4}$$

Example 2:
$$\frac{3}{8} = 8\overline{)3} = 8\overline{)3.000}^{\,0.375}$$

Changing fractions to decimals can also be a method of comparing fraction size. The fractions being compared are changed to decimals, and the rules relating to comparing decimals are then applied. (See Comparing the Value of Decimals, p. 27.)

**Example:**     Which fraction is larger, $\frac{1}{3}$ or $\frac{1}{6}$?

**Solution:**     $\frac{1}{3} = 0.333 \ldots$ as a decimal

$\frac{1}{6} = 0.166 \ldots$ as a decimal

**Answer:**     $\frac{1}{3}$ is therefore the larger fraction.

## Changing Decimals to Fractions

**RULE**

To convert a decimal to a fraction, write the decimal number as a whole number in the numerator of the fraction, and express the denominator of the fraction as a power of 10. Place the number 1 in the denominator of the fraction, and add as many zeros as there are places to the right of the decimal point. Reduce to lowest terms if necessary. (See Reading and Writing Decimals, p. 25.)

**Example 1:**  0.4 is read "four tenths" and written $\frac{4}{10}$, which $= \frac{2}{5}$ when reduced.

**Example 2:**  0.65 is read "sixty-five hundredths" and written $\frac{65}{100}$, which $= \frac{13}{20}$ when reduced.

**Example 3:**  0.007 is read "seven thousandths" and written $\frac{7}{1,000}$.

Notice that the number of places to the right of the decimal point is the same as the number of zeros in the denominator of the fraction.

---

## ▦ PRACTICE **PROBLEMS**

Change the following fractions to decimals, and carry the division three places as indicated. Do not round off.

47. $\frac{3}{4}$ _____     49. $\frac{1}{2}$ _____

48. $\frac{5}{9}$ _____

Change the following decimals to fractions, and reduce to lowest terms.

50. 0.75 _____     52. 0.04 _____

51. 0.0005 _____     **Answers on p. 39**

---

> ⚙ **POINTS TO REMEMBER**
> - Read decimals carefully.
> - When the decimal fraction is **not** preceded by a whole number (e.g., .12), **always place a "0"** to the left of the decimal (0.12) to avoid interpretation errors and to avoid overlooking the decimal point.
> - Never follow a whole number with a decimal point and zero. This could result in a medication error because of misinterpretation (e.g., 3, not 3.0).
> - Add zeros to the right as needed for making decimals of equal spacing for addition and subtraction. These zeros do not change the value. Eliminate unnecessary zeros at the end in the final answer.
> - Adding zeros at the end of a decimal (except when called for to create decimals of equal length for addition or subtraction) can result in error (e.g., 1.5, not 1.50).
> - Adding zeros after the decimal point can change the value (e.g., 1.5 is not equal to 1.05, nor is it the same number).
> - To convert a fraction to a decimal, divide the numerator by the denominator.
> - To convert a decimal to a fraction, write the decimal number as a whole number in the numerator and the denominator as a power of 10. Reduce to lowest terms (e.g., $0.05 = \frac{5}{100} = \frac{1}{20}$).
> - Double-check work to avoid errors.

---

## ◎ CHAPTER **REVIEW**

Identify the decimal with the largest value in the following sets.

1. 0.4, 0.44, 0.444 _____

2. 0.8, 0.7, 0.12 _____

3. 1.32, 1.12, 1.5 _____

4. 0.1, 0.05, 0.2 _____

5. 0.725, 0.357, 0.125 _____

Arrange the following decimals from smallest to largest.

6. 0.5, 0.05, 0.005 _____

7. 0.123, 0.1023, 1.23 _____

8. 0.64, 4.6, 0.46 _____

9. 5.15, 5.05, 5.55 _____

10. 0.73, 0.307, 0.703 _____

Perform the indicated operations. Give exact answers.

11. 3.005 + 4.308 + 2.47 = _____

12. 20.3 + 8.57 + 0.03 = _____

13. 5.886 − 3.143 = _____

14. 8.17 − 3.05 = _____

15. 3.8 − 1.3 = _____

Solve the following. Carry division to the hundredths place where necessary.

16. 5.7 ÷ 0.9 = _____

17. 3.75 ÷ 2.5 = _____

18. 1.125 ÷ 0.75 = _____

19. 0.15 × 100 = _____

20. 15 × 2.08 = _____

21. 472.4 × 0.002 = _____

Express the following decimals to the nearest tenth.

22. 1.75 _____

23. 0.13 _____

Express the following decimals to the nearest hundredth.

24. 1.427 _____    25. 0.147 _____

Change the following fractions to decimals. Carry division three decimal places as necessary.

26. $\dfrac{8}{64}$ _____    28. $6\dfrac{1}{2}$ _____

27. $\dfrac{3}{50}$ _____

Change the following decimals to fractions, and reduce to lowest terms.

29. 1.01 _____    30. 0.065 _____

Add the following decimals.

31. You are to give a client one tablet labeled 0.15 milligram (mg) and one labeled 0.025 mg. What is the total dosage of these two tablets?    _____

32. If you administer two tablets labeled 0.04 milligram (mg), what total dosage will you administer?    _____

33. You have two tablets, one labeled 0.025 milligram (mg) and the other 0.1 mg. What is the total dosage of these two tablets?    _____

34. You have just administered 3 tablets with dose strength of 1.5 milligrams (mg) each. What was the total dosage?    _____

35. If you administer two tablets labeled 0.6 milligram (mg), what total dosage will you administer?    _____

Multiply the following numbers by moving the decimal.

36. $0.08 \times 10 =$ _____    37. $0.002 \times 100 =$ _____

Divide the following numbers, and round to the nearest hundredth.

38. $0.13 \div 0.25 =$ _____    40. $6.45 \div 10 =$ _____

39. $4 \div 4.1 =$ _____

Round the following decimals to the nearest thousandth.

41. 4.2475 _____    43. 7.8393 _____

42. 0.5673 _____    44. 2.3249 _____

45. A client's water intake is 1.05 liters (L), 0.65 L, 2.05 L, and 0.8 L. What is the total intake in liters? _____

46. A client's creatinine level on admission was 2.5 milligrams per deciliter (mg/dL). By discharge the creatinine level dropped 0.9 mg. What is the client's current creatinine level? _____

47. A baby weighed 4.85 kilograms (kg) at birth and now weighs 7.9 kg. How many kilograms did the baby gain? _____

48. A client received a series of injections of medication in milliliters (mL): 1.5 mL, 2.3 mL, and 2.1 mL. What was the total amount of medication (in mL) the client received? _____

49. A client's sodium intake at one meal was the following: 0.002 gram (g), 0.35 g. How many grams of sodium did the client consume? _____

50. True or False? 2.4 grams (g) = 2.04 g _____

51. 0.7 milligram (mg) of a medication has been ordered. The recommended maximum dosage of the medication is 0.35 mg, and the minimum recommended dosage is 0.175 mg. Is the dosage ordered within the allowable limits? _____

52. A client weighed 85.4 kilograms (kg) in January. In February, the client gained 1.8 kg. In March, the client gained 2.3 kg. How much did the client weigh at the end of March? _____

53. If a dosage of medication is 2.5 milliliters (mL), how much medication is needed for 25 dosages? _____

54. A client received 17.5 milligrams (mg) of a medication in tablet form. Each tablet contained 3.5 mg of medication. How many tablets were given to the client? _____

55. A client received a total of 4.5 grams (g) of a medication. If the client received the total over a 3-day period and was given 3 doses per day, what was the strength of each dose? _____

56. A client is brought to the emergency room with a body temperature of 95.3°F. If the normal body temperature is 98.6°F, how far below normal was the client's temperature? _____

57. A vial holds a total of 7.5 milliliters (mL) of medication. If two injections are withdrawn from the vial (1.6 mL and 0.8 mL), how much medication is left in the vial? _____

58. One dose of flu vaccine is 0.5 milliliter (mL). How much vaccine is needed to vaccinate 30 walk-ins at a clinic? _____

59. A client's hemoglobin was 13.8 grams (g) before surgery. During surgery, the hemoglobin dropped 4.5 g. What was the hemoglobin value after it dropped? _____

60. For a certain medication, the safe dosage should be greater than or equal to 0.7 gram (g) but less than or equal to 2 g. Which of the following dosages fall within the range? (More than one answer is correct.)

    0.8 g, 0.25 g, 2.5 g, 1.25 g

61. In a 24-hour period, a premature infant drank 5.5 milliliters (mL), 15 mL, 5.25 mL, 15 mL, 6 mL, and 12.5 mL. How many mL did the infant drink in 24 hours? _____

62. A baby weighed 3.7 kilograms (kg) at birth. The baby now weighs 5.65 kg. How many kg did the baby gain? _____

63. A client receives a dosage of 5.5 milliliters (mL) of medication 4 times a day. How much medication would the client receive in 7 days? _____

64. A client received 17.5 milligrams (mg) of medication in tablet form. Each tablet contains 2.5 mg of medication. How many tablets were given to the client? _____

65. The doctor prescribed 1.5 tablets of a medication to be administered to a client 4 times a day for 7 days. How many tablets were prescribed? _____

**Answers below**

---

## ⭐ ANSWERS

### Chapter 2
### Answers to Practice Problems

1. eight and thirty-five hundredths
2. eleven and one thousandth
3. four and fifty-seven hundredths
4. five and seven ten thousandths
5. ten and five tenths
6. one hundred sixty-three thousandths

| | | | | | |
|---|---|---|---|---|---|
| 7. 0.4 | 15. 0.375 | 23. 2.92 | 31. 100.8072 | 39. 2 | 47. 0.75 |
| 8. 84.07 | 16. 0.175 | 24. 43.1 | 32. 4 | 40. 3.55 | 48. 0.555 |
| 9. 0.07 | 17. 7.35 | 25. 0.035 | 33. 1.16 | 41. 0.61 | 49. 0.5 |
| 10. 2.23 | 18. 0.087 | 26. 5.88 | 34. 70.88 | 42. 0.74 | 50. $\frac{3}{4}$ |
| 11. 0.05 | 19. 18.4 | 27. 0.04725 | 35. 30.46 | 43. 0.0005 | |
| 12. 0.009 | 20. 40.449 | 28. 0.9125 | 36. 0.59 | 44. 0.00004 | 51. $\frac{1}{2,000}$ |
| 13. 0.5 | 21. 3.95 | 29. 9,650 | 37. 3.6 | 45. 584 | |
| 14. 2.87 | 22. 3.87 | 30. 1.78 | 38. 1 | 46. 500 | 52. $\frac{1}{25}$ |

### Answers to Chapter Review

| | | | |
|---|---|---|---|
| 1. 0.444 | 19. 15 | 35. 1.2 mg | 51. No, 0.7 mg is outside the allowable limits of the safe dosage range of 0.175 mg to 0.35 mg. It is twice the allowable maximum dosage. |
| 2. 0.8 | 20. 31.2 | 36. 0.8 | |
| 3. 1.5 | 21. 0.94 | 37. 0.2 | |
| 4. 0.2 | 22. 1.8 | 38. 0.52 | |
| 5. 0.725 | 23. 0.1 | 39. 0.98 | 52. 89.5 kg |
| 6. 0.005, 0.05, 0.5 | 24. 1.43 | 40. 0.65 | 53. 62.5 mL |
| 7. 0.1023, 0.123, 1.23 | 25. 0.15 | 41. 4.248 | 54. 5 tablets |
| 8. 0.46, 0.64, 4.6 | 26. 0.125 | 42. 0.567 | 55. 0.5 g per dose |
| 9. 5.05, 5.15, 5.55 | 27. 0.06 | 43. 7.839 | 56. 3.3°F |
| 10. 0.307, 0.703, 0.73 | 28. 6.5 | 44. 2.325 | 57. 5.1 mL |
| 11. 9.783 | 29. $1\frac{1}{100}$ | 45. 4.55 L | 58. 15 mL |
| 12. 28.9 | | 46. 1.6 mg/dL | 59. 9.3 g |
| 13. 2.743 | 30. $\frac{13}{200}$ | 47. 3.05 kg | 60. 0.8 g, 1.25 g |
| 14. 5.12 | | 48. 5.9 mL | 61. 59.25 mL |
| 15. 2.5 | 31. 0.175 mg | 49. 0.352 g | 62. 1.95 kg |
| 16. 6.33 | 32. 0.08 mg | 50. False | 63. 154 mL |
| 17. 1.5 | 33. 0.125 mg | | 64. 7 tablets |
| 18. 1.5 | 34. 4.5 mg | | 65. 42 tablets |

# CHAPTER 3
# Ratio and Proportion

## Objectives

*After reviewing this chapter, you should be able to:*

1. Define ratio and proportion
2. Define means and extremes
3. Set up a ratio and proportion in linear and fraction format
4. Calculate problems for a missing term (*x*) using ratio and proportion

Ratio and proportion is one logical method for calculating medications. It can be used to calculate all types of medication problems. Nurses use ratios to calculate and to check medication dosages. Some medications express the strength of the solution by using a ratio. Example: An epinephrine label may state 1 : 1,000. Ratios are used in hospitals to determine the client-to-nurse ratio. Example: If there are 28 clients and 4 nurses on a unit, the ratio of clients to nurses is 28 : 4 or "28 to 4" or 7 : 1. As with fractions, ratios should be stated in lowest terms. Like a fraction, which indicates the division of two numbers, a ratio indicates the division of two quantities. The use of ratio and proportion is a logical approach to calculating medication dosages and other clinical calculations.

## Ratios

A ratio is used to indicate a relationship between two numbers.

### Linear Format

Numbers that are related can be written in a **linear format.** A ratio set up in a linear format uses a colon (:) to show the relationship between the two numbers. These numbers are separated by a colon (:).

Example: 3 : 4 The linear format is read as "three is to four."
The colon indicates division; therefore a ratio is a fraction.

### Fraction Format

A ratio can also be written in a **fraction format** to indicate a relationship between numbers. When writing a ratio in the fraction format, a line (-) is used to show the relationship between the numbers. The numbers or terms of the ratio are the numerator and the denominator.

> **RULE**
>
> The numerator is always the quantity written to the left of the colon (the first quantity), and the denominator is always to the right of the colon (second quantity). Like fractions, ratios should be stated in lowest terms.

Example 1:  3 : 4 (3 is the numerator, 4 is the denominator, and the ratio can be written in the fraction format as $\frac{3}{4}$). The fraction format is read as "three divided by four."

**Example 2:** In a nursing class, if there are 25 male students and 75 female students, what is the ratio of male students to female students? 25 male students to 75 female students = 25 male students per 75 female students = $\dfrac{25}{75} = \dfrac{1}{3}$. This is the same as a ratio of 25:75 or 1:3.

## Ratio Measures in Solutions

Some medications express the strength of the solution by using a ratio. Ratio measures are commonly seen in solutions. Ratios represent parts of medication per parts of solution, for example, 1:10,000 (this means 1 part medication to 10,000 parts solution).

**Example 1:** A 1:5 solution contains 1 part medication in 5 parts solution.

**Example 2:** A solution that is 1 part medication in 2 parts solution would be written as 1:2.

**Ratio strengths are always expressed in lowest terms.**

> ### TIPS FOR CLINICAL PRACTICE
> The more solution a medication is dissolved in, the less potent the strength becomes. For example, a ratio strength of 1:1,000 (1 part medication to 1,000 parts solution) is more potent than a ratio strength of 1:10,000 (1 part medication to 10,000 parts solution). A misunderstanding of these numbers and what they represent can have serious consequences.

## Proportions

A proportion is an equation of two ratios of equal value. The terms of the first ratio have a relationship to the terms of the second ratio. As shown with ratios, a proportion can be written in different formats (linear or fraction).

**Example 1:** 3 : 4 :: 6 : 8 (A double [:] colon is used to show the relationship between the two ratios and is read as "as.") Read as "three is to four as six is to eight."

**Example 2:** 3:4 = 6:8 (An equal [=] sign can be used in the place of a double colon.) Read as "three is to four equals six is to eight."

**Example 3:** $\dfrac{3}{4} = \dfrac{6}{8}$ (Written as a fraction, the equal [=] sign is used to show the relationship between the two ratios.) Read as "three-fourths equals six-eighths."

When a proportion is written in linear format, it proves that the ratios are equal and that the proportion is true and can be done mathematically.

**Example:**

$$5:25 = 10:50$$

*or*

$$5:25::10:50$$

The terms in a linear proportion are called the *means* and *extremes*. Confusion of these terms can result in an incorrect answer. To avoid confusion of terms in proportions, remember **m** for the middle terms **(means)** and **e** for the end terms **(extremes)** of the proportion. Let's refer to our example to identify these terms.

The extremes are the outer or end numbers (previous example: 5, 50), and the means are the inner or middle numbers (previous example: 25, 10).

**Example:**

$$\underset{\underset{\text{extremes}}{\rule{0pt}{0pt}}}{\overset{\overset{\text{means}}{\rule{0pt}{0pt}}}{5:25 = 10:50}}$$

> **RULE**
>
> In a proportion, the product of the means (the two inner, or middle, numbers) equals the product of the extremes (the two outer, or end, numbers). To find the product of the means and extremes, you multiply.

In other words, the answers obtained when you multiply the means and extremes are equal.

> **NOTE**
>
> The product of the means, 250, equals the product of the extremes, 250, proving the ratios are equal and the proportion is true.

**Example:**                            $5:25 = 10:50$

$$25 \times 10 = 50 \times 5$$

means      extremes
$$250 = 250$$

Because ratios are the same as fractions, the same proportion can be expressed as a fraction like this:

$$\frac{5}{25} = \frac{10}{50}$$

The fractions are equivalent, or equal.

The numerator of the first fraction and the denominator of the second fraction are the extremes. The denominator of the first fraction and the numerator of the second fraction are the means.

**Example:**            $\dfrac{5 \text{ (extreme)}}{25 \text{ (mean)}} = \dfrac{10 \text{ (mean)}}{50 \text{ (extreme)}}$

Cross-multiply to find the equal products of the means and extremes.

$$\frac{5}{25} = \frac{10}{50}$$

$$5 \times 50 = 10 \times 25$$

$$250 = 250$$

## Solving for x in Ratio and Proportion

Because the product of the means always equals the product of the extremes, if three numbers of the two ratios are known, the fourth number can be found. The unknown quantity may be any of the four terms. In a proportion problem, the unknown quantity is represented by $x$. After multiplying the means and extremes, the unknown $x$ is usually placed on the left side of the equation. Begin with the product containing the $x$, which will result in the $x$ being isolated on the **left** and the answer on the **right.**

**Example:**    $12:9 = 8:x$

**Steps:**    $12x = 72$

$\dfrac{12x}{12} = \dfrac{72}{12}$

$x = \dfrac{72}{12}$

$x = 6$

1. Multiply the extremes and then the means. (This results in $x$ being placed on the left side of the equation.)

2. Divide both sides of the equation by the number preceding the $x$, in this instance 12, without changing the relationship. The number used for division should always be the number preceding the unknown ($x$), so that when this step is completed, the unknown ($x$) will stand alone on the left side of the equation.

**Proof:**     Place the answer obtained for $x$ in the equation, and multiply to be certain that the product of the means equals the product of the extremes.

$$12 : 9 = 8 : 6$$

$$9 \times 8 = 12 \times 6$$

$$72 = 72$$

Solving for $x$ with a proportion in a fraction format can be done by cross-multiplication to determine the value of $x$.

**Example:**     $\dfrac{4}{3} = \dfrac{12}{x}$

**Steps:**     $4x = 36$          1. Cross-multiply to obtain the product of the means and extremes.

$\dfrac{4x}{4} = \dfrac{36}{4}$          2. Divide both sides by the number preceding $x$ (in this example, 4) to obtain the value for $x$.

$x = \dfrac{36}{4}$

$x = 9$

**Proof:**     Place the value obtained for $x$ in the equation; the cross-products should be equal.

$$\frac{4}{3} = \frac{12}{9}$$

$$4 \times 9 = 12 \times 3$$

$$36 = 36$$

Solving for $x$ in proportions that involve decimals in the equation can be done by the same process.

**Example:**     $25 : 5 = 1.5 : x$

**Steps:**     $25x = 5 \times 1.5$          1. Multiply the extremes and then the means. (The $x$ will be placed on the left side of the equation.)

$\dfrac{25x}{25} = \dfrac{7.5}{25}$          2. Divide both sides by the number preceding $x$ (in this example, 25) to obtain the value for $x$.

$x = \dfrac{7.5}{25}$

$x = 0.3$

**Proof:**          $25 : 5 = 1.5 : 0.3$

$$25 \times 0.3 = 5 \times 1.5$$

$$7.5 = 7.5$$

Solving for $x$ in proportions that involve fractions in the equation can be done by the same process.

**Example:** $\frac{1}{2} : x = \frac{1}{5} : 1$

**Steps:** $\frac{1}{5} \times x = \frac{1}{2} \times 1$     1. Multiply the means and then the extremes. (The $x$ will be placed on the left side of the equation.)

$\frac{1}{5}x = \frac{1}{2}$

$\dfrac{\frac{1}{5}x}{\frac{1}{5}} = \dfrac{\frac{1}{2}}{\frac{1}{5}}$

$x = \frac{1}{2} \div \frac{1}{5}$

2. Divide *both* sides by the number preceding $x$ (in this example, $\frac{1}{5}$). Division of the two fractions becomes multiplication, and the second fraction is inverted. Multiply numerators and denominators.

$x = \frac{1}{2} \times \frac{5}{1}$

$x = \frac{5}{2} = 2.5 \text{ or } 2\frac{1}{2}$     3. Reduce the final fraction to solve for $x$.

**Proof:**

$$\frac{1}{2} : 2\frac{1}{2} = \frac{1}{5} : 1$$

$$1 \times \frac{1}{2} = 2\frac{1}{2} \times \frac{1}{5} = \frac{5}{2} \times \frac{1}{5}$$

$$\frac{1}{2} = \frac{5}{10} = \frac{1}{2}$$

$$\frac{1}{2} = \frac{1}{2}$$

> **RULE**
>
> If the answer is expressed in fraction format for $x$, it must be reduced to **lowest terms**. Division should be carried **two decimal places** when an answer does not work out evenly and may have to be **rounded to the nearest tenth** to prove the answer correct.

## Applying Ratio and Proportion to Dosage Calculation

Now that we have reviewed the basic definitions and concepts relating to ratio and proportion, let's look at how this might be applied in dosage calculation.

In dosage calculation, ratio and proportion may be used to represent **the weight of a medication that is in tablet or capsule form.**

**Example 1:**     1 tab : 0.125 mg *or* $\dfrac{1 \text{ tab}}{0.125 \text{ mg}}$

This may also be expressed by stating the weight of the medication first:

$$0.125 \text{ mg} : 1 \text{ tab } \textit{ or } \dfrac{0.125 \text{ mg}}{1 \text{ tab}}$$

This means that 1 tablet contains 0.125 mg or is equal to 0.125 mg of medication.

**Example 2:** If a capsule contains a dosage of 500 mg, this could be represented by a ratio as follows:

$$1 \text{ cap} : 500 \text{ mg } \textit{ or } \dfrac{1 \text{ cap}}{500 \text{ mg}}$$

This may also be expressed stating the weight of the medication first:

$$500 \text{ mg} : 1 \text{ cap } \textit{ or } \dfrac{500 \text{ mg}}{1 \text{ cap}}$$

Another use of ratio and proportion in dosage calculation is to express liquid medications used for oral administration and for injection. When stating a dosage of a liquid medication, a ratio expresses the **weight (strength) of a medication in a certain volume of solution.**

**Example 1:** A solution that contains 250 mg of medication in each **1 mL** could be written as:

$$250 \text{ mg} : \textbf{1 mL} \ or \ \frac{250 \text{ mg}}{\textbf{1 mL}}$$

**1 mL** contains 250 mg of medication.

**Example 2:** A solution that contains 80 mg of medication in each **2 mL** would be written as:

$$80 \text{ mg} : \textbf{2 mL} \ or \ \frac{80 \text{ mg}}{\textbf{2 mL}}$$

**2 mL** contains 80 mg of medication.

---

> **⚠ SAFETY ALERT!**
>
> When using ratio and proportion in dosage calculation, do not forget the units of measurement. Including units in the dosage strength will help you avoid some common errors. For example, if you have two solutions of a medication, one of the solutions contains 1 gram (g) of the medication in 25 milliliters (mL); the other contains 1 milligram (mg) of the medication in 25 milliliters (mL). Notice that although both of these solution strengths have a ratio of 1:25, they are obviously different from each other. To clearly distinguish between them and avoid error, the unit of measurement should be included. The first solution should be written as 1 g:25 mL. The second solution is written as 1 mg:25 mL.

Proving mathematically that ratios are equal and the proportion is true is important with medications. This can be illustrated by using the previous medication strength examples.

**Example 1:** 1 cap:500 mg = 2 cap:1,000 mg

If 1 cap contains 500 mg, 2 cap will contain 1,000 mg.

$$\overset{\text{extremes}}{1 \text{ cap} : 500 \text{ mg} = 2 \text{ cap} : 1,000 \text{ mg}}_{\text{means}}$$

$$500 \times 2 = 1,000 \times 1$$
$$1,000 = 1,000$$

**Example 2:** 2 mL:80 mg = 1 mL:40 mg

$$80 \times 1 = 2 \times 40$$
$$80 = 80$$

*Note:* When ratio and proportion are used to calculate a medication dosage or to make a conversion of units, three of the four numbers will be known, and a proportion is set up to solve for the fourth number (the unknown). This will be demonstrated in later chapters on conversions and dosage calculations.

---

> **⚙ POINTS TO REMEMBER**
>
> - Proportions represent two ratios that are equal and have a relationship to each other.
> - When three values are known, the fourth can be easily calculated.
> - When solving for the unknown ($x$), regardless of which term of the equation is the unknown, the unknown value ($x$) is usually placed on the left side. Begin with the product containing $x$, so $x$ can be isolated on the left side and the answer on the right side.
> - Ratios and proportions can be stated in linear or fraction format.
> - Ratio can be used to state the amount of medication contained in a volume of solution, tablet, or capsule. When using ratio and proportion in dosage calculation, include the units of measurement in the dosage strength.
> - Proportions in linear format are solved by multiplying the means and extremes.
> - Ratios are always stated in their lowest terms.
> - Double-check work.

## ▦ PRACTICE **PROBLEMS**

Express the following solution strengths as ratios.

1. 1 part medication to 100 parts solution _____

2. 1 part medication to 3 parts solution _____

Identify the strongest solution in each of the following:

3. 1:2, 1:20, 1:200 _____

4. 1:1,000, 1:5,000, 1:10,000 _____

5. Assume that the ratio of clients to nurses is 15 to 2. Express the ratio in fraction and linear format. _____

Express the following dosages as ratios in linear format. Include the unit of measurement and the numerical value.

6. An injectable liquid that contains 100 mg in each 0.5 mL _____

7. A tablet that contains 0.25 mg of medication _____

8. An oral liquid that contains 1 g in each 10 mL _____

9. A capsule that contains 500 mg of medication _____

Determine the value for $x$ in the following problems. Express your answer to the nearest tenth as indicated.

10. $12.5:5 = 24:x$ _____     13. $1/300:3 = 1/120:x$ _____

11. $1.5:1 = 4.5:x$ _____     14. $x:12 = 9:6$ _____

12. $750/3 = 600/x$ _____

**Answers on p. 49**

## ◉ CHAPTER **REVIEW**

Express the following fractions as linear ratios. Reduce to lowest terms.

1. $\dfrac{2}{3}$ _____          4. $\dfrac{1}{5}$ _____

2. $\dfrac{1}{9}$ _____          5. $\dfrac{5}{10}$ _____

3. $\dfrac{6}{8}$ _____          6. $\dfrac{2}{10}$ _____

Express the following ratios as fractions. Reduce to lowest terms.

7. $3:7$ _____          10. $8:6$ _____

8. $4:6$ _____          11. $3:4$ _____

9. $1:7$ _____

Solve for $x$ in the following proportions. Carry division two decimal places as necessary.

12. $20:40 = x:10$ _____

13. $\dfrac{1}{4}:\dfrac{1}{2} = 1:x$ _____

14. $0.12:0.8 = 0.6:x$ _____

15. $\dfrac{1}{250}:2 = \dfrac{1}{150}:x$ _____

16. $x:9 = 5:10$ _____

17. $\dfrac{1}{4}:1.6 = \dfrac{1}{8}:x$ _____

18. $\dfrac{1}{2}:2 = \dfrac{1}{3}:x$ _____

19. $125:0.4 = 50:x$ _____

20. $x:1 = 0.5:5$ _____

21. $\dfrac{2.2}{x} = \dfrac{8.8}{5}$ _____

22. $0.5:0.15 = 0.3:x$ _____

23. $\dfrac{16}{40} = \dfrac{22}{x}$ _____

24. $20:40 = x:15$ _____

25. $\dfrac{x}{26} = \dfrac{10.1}{13}$ _____

26. $12:1 = x:5.5$ _____

27. $\dfrac{60}{1} = \dfrac{x}{2\frac{1}{4}}$ _____

Set up the following problems as a proportion and solve. Include labels in the setup and in the answer.

28. If 150 milligrams (mg) of medication are in 2 capsules (caps), how many mg of medication are in 10 caps? _____

29. If 60 milligrams (mg) of a medication are in 500 milliliters (mL), how many mL of solution contain 36 mg of medication? _____

30. If 1 kilogram (kg) equals 2.2 lb, how many kg are in 61.6 lb? _____

31. If one glass of milk contains 280 milligrams (mg) of calcium, how many mg of calcium are in $2\frac{1}{2}$ glasses of milk? _____

32. The prescriber orders 0.25 milligram (mg) of a medication. The medication is available in 0.125-mg tablets. How many tablets will you give? _____

Express the following dosages as ratios. Be sure to include the units of measure and numerical value. Do not reduce the ratio.

33. A capsule that contains 250 mg of medication _____

34. An oral solution that contains 125 mg in each 5 mL _____

35. An injectable solution that contains 40 mg in each mL _____

36. An injectable solution that contains 1,000 mcg in each 2 mL _____

37. An injectable solution that contains 1 g in each 3.6 mL _____

38. A tablet that contains 0.4 mg of medication _____

39. A capsule that contains 1 g of medication _____

40. An oral liquid that contains 0.5 mg in each milliliter _____

Express the following strengths as ratios.

41. 1 part medication to 2,000 parts solution _____

42. 1 part medication to 400 parts solution _____

43. 1 part medication to 50 parts solution _____

Identify the weakest solution in each of the following:

44. 1:50, 1:500, 1:5,000 _____

45. 1:3, 1:6, 1:60 _____

Set up the following word problems as proportions and solve. Include labels in the setup and in the answer.

46. The prescriber orders 15 milligrams (mg) of a medication for every 10 lb of a client's weight. How many mg of medication will be given for a person who weighs 120 lb? _____

47. There are 40 milligrams (mg) of medication in every 5 milliliters (mL) of liquid. How much liquid is required to administer 120 mg of medication? _____

48. The ratio of male to female clients in a nursing facility is 3 to 5. If there are 40 women in the facility, how many men are there? _____

49. If 3 ounces (oz) of medicine must be mixed with 7 oz of water, how many ounces of water are needed for 12 oz of medicine? _____

50. A client's weight is reported as 65 kilograms (kg). How many pounds (lb) does the client weigh? (1 kg = 2.2 lb) _____

51. If 100 grams (g) of ice cream contain 20 g of fat, how many g of fat are in 275 g of ice cream? _____

52. A survey indicates that 8 out of 10 people suffer from colds each year. If there are 48,000 people in the area, how many people will suffer from colds? _____

53. A nurse counts a client's pulse at 19 beats in 15 seconds. If the nurse counts the client's pulse for 1 minute, how many beats would there be in 1 minute? (1 minute = 60 seconds) _____

54. If 30 milligrams (mg) of medication are in 2 tablets (tabs), how many mg of medication are in 10 tabs? _____

55. A client receives 275 milligrams (mg) of medication given evenly over $5\frac{1}{2}$ hours. How many mg of the medication does the client receive per hour? _____

56. A client is receiving an intravenous medication at a rate of 6.25 milligrams (mg) per minute. After 50 minutes, how many mg of medications has the client received? _____

57. A label on a dinner roll wrapper reads, "2.5 grams (g) of fiber per $\frac{3}{4}$ ounce (oz) serving." If a client eats $1\frac{1}{2}$ ounces of dinner rolls, how many g of fiber will the client consume? _____

58. If 100 milliliters (mL) of solution contain 20 milligrams (mg) of medication, how many mg of the medication will be in 650 mL of the solution? _____

59. The label on a bag of popcorn reads, "140 calories per serving; one serving is 4 cups." If you consume $1\frac{1}{2}$ cups, how many calories did you consume? _____

60. If 40 vitamin tablets (tabs) contain 5,000 milligrams (mg), how many tabs are needed for a dosage of 375 mg? _____

**Answers below and on p. 50**

---

## ⭐ ANSWERS

### Chapter 3
### Answers to Practice Problems

1. $1:100$
2. $1:3$
3. $1:2$
4. $1:1,000$
5. $\frac{15}{2}$, $15:2$

6. 100 mg:0.5 mL, 0.5 mL:100 mg
7. 0.25 mg:1 tab, 1 tab:0.25 mg
8. 1 g:10 mL, 10 mL:1 g
9. 500 mg:1 cap, 1 cap:500 mg
10. $x = 9.6$

11. $x = 3$
12. $x = 2.4$
13. $x = 7.5$
14. $x = 18$

### Answers to Chapter Review

1. $2:3$
2. $1:9$
3. $3:4$
4. $1:5$
5. $1:2$
6. $1:5$
7. $\frac{3}{7}$
8. $\frac{2}{3}$
9. $\frac{1}{7}$
10. $1\frac{1}{3}$
11. $\frac{3}{4}$

12. $x = 5$
13. $x = 2$
14. $x = 4$
15. $x = 3.33$
16. $x = 4.5$
17. $x = 0.8$
18. $x = 1.33$ *or* $\frac{4}{3}$
19. $x = 0.16$

20. $x = 0.1$
21. $x = 1.25$
22. $x = 0.09$
23. $x = 55$
24. $x = 7.5$
25. $x = 20.2$
26. $x = 66$
27. $x = 135$

28. 150 mg:2 caps $= x$ mg:10 caps *or*

$$\frac{150 \text{ mg}}{2 \text{ caps}} = \frac{x \text{ mg}}{10 \text{ caps}}$$

$x = 750$ mg

29. 60 mg:500 mL $= 36$ mg:$x$ mL *or*

$$\frac{60 \text{ mg}}{500 \text{ mL}} = \frac{36 \text{ mg}}{x \text{ mL}}$$

$x = 300$ mL

30. 1 kg:2.2 lb $= x$ kg:61.6 lb *or*

$$\frac{1 \text{ kg}}{2.2 \text{ lb}} = \frac{x \text{ kg}}{61.6 \text{ lb}}$$

$x = 28$ kg

31. 1 glass:280 mg $= 2\frac{1}{2}$ glasses:$x$ mg *or*

$$\frac{1 \text{ glass}}{280 \text{ mg}} = \frac{2\frac{1}{2} \text{ glasses}}{x \text{ mg}}$$

$x = 700$ mg

32. 0.125 mg:1 tab $= 0.25$ mg:$x$ tab *or*

$$\frac{0.125 \text{ mg}}{1 \text{ tab}} = \frac{0.25 \text{ mg}}{x \text{ tab}}$$

$x = 2$ tabs

33. 250 mg:1 cap *or* 1 cap:250 mg
34. 125 mg:5 mL *or* 5 mL:125 mg
35. 40 mg:1 mL *or* 1 mL:40 mg
36. 1,000 mcg:2 mL *or* 2 mL:1,000 mcg
37. 1 g:3.6 mL *or* 3.6 mL:1 g
38. 0.4 mg:1 tab *or* 1 tab:0.4 mg
39. 1 g:1 cap *or* 1 cap:1 g
40. 0.5 mg:1 mL *or* 1 mL:0.5 mg
41. $1:2,000$
42. $1:400$
43. $1:50$

44. $1:5,000$

45. $1:60$

46. $15 \text{ mg}:10 \text{ lb} = x \text{ mg}:120 \text{ lb}$ *or*

$$\frac{15 \text{ mg}}{10 \text{ lb}} = \frac{x \text{ mg}}{120 \text{ lb}}$$

$x = 180 \text{ mg}$

47. $40 \text{ mg} : 5 \text{ mL} = 120 \text{ mg} : x \text{ mL}$ *or*

$$\frac{40 \text{ mg}}{5 \text{ mL}} = \frac{120 \text{ mg}}{x \text{ mL}}$$

$x = 15 \text{ mL}$

48. $3 \text{ males}:5 \text{ females} = x \text{ males}:40 \text{ females}$ *or*

$$\frac{3 \text{ males}}{5 \text{ females}} = \frac{x \text{ males}}{40 \text{ females}}$$

$x = 24 \text{ males}$

49. $3 \text{ oz medicine}:7 \text{ oz water} = 12 \text{ oz medicine}:x \text{ oz water}$
*or*

$$\frac{3 \text{ oz medicine}}{7 \text{ oz water}} = \frac{12 \text{ oz medicine}}{x \text{ oz water}}$$

$x = 28 \text{ oz}$

50. $1 \text{ kg} : 2.2 \text{ lb} = 65 \text{ kg} : x \text{ lb}$
*or*

$$\frac{1 \text{ kg}}{2.2 \text{ lb}} = \frac{65 \text{ kg}}{x \text{ lb}}$$

$x = 143 \text{ lb}$

51. $100 \text{ g ice cream}:20 \text{ g fat} = 275 \text{ g ice cream}:x \text{ g fat}$
*or*

$$\frac{100 \text{ g ice cream}}{20 \text{ g fat}} = \frac{275 \text{ g ice cream}}{x \text{ g fat}}$$

$x = 55 \text{ g}$

52. $8 \text{ cold sufferers}:10 \text{ people} = x \text{ cold sufferers}:48,000 \text{ people}$
*or*

$$\frac{8 \text{ cold suffers}}{10 \text{ people}} = \frac{x \text{ cold sufferers}}{48,000 \text{ people}}$$

$x = 38,400 \text{ people}$

53. $19 \text{ beats}:15 \text{ seconds} = x \text{ beats}:60 \text{ seconds}$ *or*

$$\frac{19 \text{ beats}}{15 \text{ seconds}} = \frac{x \text{ beats}}{60 \text{ seconds}}$$

$x = 76 \text{ beats}$

54. $30 \text{ mg} : 2 \text{ tabs} = x \text{ mg} : 10 \text{ tabs}$ *or*

$$\frac{30 \text{ mg}}{2 \text{ tabs}} = \frac{x \text{ mg}}{10 \text{ tabs}}$$

$x = 150 \text{ mg}$

55. $275 \text{ mg}:5\frac{1}{2} \text{ hours} = x \text{ mg}:1 \text{ hour}$ *or*

$$\frac{275 \text{ mg}}{5\frac{1}{2} \text{ hours}} = \frac{x \text{ mg}}{1 \text{ hour}}$$

$x = 50 \text{ mg}$

56. $6.25 \text{ mg}:1 \text{ minute} = x \text{ mg}:50 \text{ minutes}$ *or*

$$\frac{6.25 \text{ mg}}{1 \text{ minute}} = \frac{x \text{ mg}}{50 \text{ minutes}}$$

$x = 312.5 \text{ mg}$

57. $2.5 \text{ g}:\frac{3}{4} \text{ oz} = x \text{ g}:1\frac{1}{2} \text{ oz}$ *or*

$$\frac{2.5 \text{ g}}{\frac{3}{4} \text{ oz}} = \frac{x \text{ g}}{1\frac{1}{2} \text{ oz}}$$

$x = 5 \text{ g}$

58. $20 \text{ mg}:100 \text{ mL} = x \text{ mg}:650 \text{ mL}$ *or*

$$\frac{20 \text{ mg}}{100 \text{ mL}} = \frac{x \text{ g}}{650 \text{ mL}}$$

$x = 130 \text{ mg}$

59. $140 \text{ calories}:4 \text{ cups} = x \text{ calories}:1\frac{1}{2} \text{ cups}$ *or*

$$\frac{140 \text{ calories}}{4 \text{ cups}} = \frac{x \text{ calories}}{1\frac{1}{2} \text{ cups}}$$

$x = 52.5 \text{ calories or } 52\frac{1}{2} \text{ calories}$

60. $5,000 \text{ mg}:40 \text{ tabs} = 375 \text{ mg}:x \text{ tabs}$ *or*

$$\frac{5,000 \text{ mg}}{40 \text{ tabs}} = \frac{375 \text{ mg}}{x \text{ tabs}}$$

$x = 3 \text{ tabs}$

# CHAPTER **4**
# **Percentages**

## Objectives

*After reviewing this chapter, you should be able to:*

1. Define percent
2. Convert percents to fractions
3. Convert percents to decimals
4. Convert percents to ratios
5. Convert decimals to percents
6. Convert fractions to percents
7. Convert fractions to ratios
8. Determine the percent of numbers

Percents, as decimals and fractions, are a way to express the relationship of parts to a whole. Percent (%) means parts per hundred. A percentage is the same as a fraction in which the denominator is 100, and the numerator indicates the part of 100 that is being considered.

The symbol used to indicate a percent (%) is placed after the number, as in 40%. The example 40% (40 percent) means 40 out of 100. Percents can be more than 100% (such as 200%) or less than 1% (0.1%). A percent may also contain a decimal (0.6%), a fraction ($\frac{1}{2}$%), or a mixed number (14$\frac{1}{2}$%).

**Example:** $4\% = 4 \text{ percent} = \dfrac{4}{100} \text{ (4 per 100)} = 0.04$

Health care professionals see percentages written with medications (e.g., magnesium sulfate 50%, lidocaine 2%). Solutions for the eye and topical (for external use) ointments, lotions, and creams use percentages to express dosage strength. For example, hydrocortisone cream is available in 1% and 2.5%. Timolol ophthalmic solutions are available in 0.25% and 0.5%.

In addition, nurses and other health professionals frequently administer solutions with the concentration expressed as a percent, such as intravenous (IV) solutions (e.g., 5% dextrose in water). IV means directly into a person's vein.

Percents may also be used by nurses when it is required to calculate percentages of partial quantities (e.g., to determine the percentage of a diet of fluids that a client consumed).

In current practice, percentage solutions are prepared by the pharmacy, and people can purchase solutions or components of the solutions over the counter. Some institutions require nurses to prepare solutions in house (in the hospital) as well as in home care for clients being cared for at home. Understanding percentages provides the foundation for preparing and calculating dosages for medications that are ordered in percentages.

Percentages are also used in the assessment of burns. The size of a burn (percentage of injured skin) is determined by using the rule of nines in an adult. The basis of the rule is that the body is divided into anatomical sections, each of which represents 9% or a multiple of 9% of the total body surface area (BSA). The total BSA is represented by 100%. Another method used is the age-specific burn diagram or chart. Burn size is expressed as a percentage of the total BSA. In children, age-related charts are used because their body proportions differ from those of an adult.

Let's get an understanding of the relationship of ratios, percents, fractions, and decimals by showing how to convert from one to another.

## Converting Percentages to Fractions, Decimals, and Ratios

**RULE**

To convert a percent to a fraction:
1. Drop the percent sign.
2. Write the number as the numerator (top number in a fraction).
3. Write 100 as the denominator (bottom number in a fraction).
4. Reduce the fraction to lowest terms.

**Example 1:**  $8\% = \dfrac{8}{100}$, reduced is $\dfrac{2}{25}$

**Example 2:**  $\dfrac{1}{4}\% = \dfrac{1}{4} \div 100 = \dfrac{1}{4} \times \dfrac{1}{100} = \dfrac{1}{400}$

**RULE**

To convert a percent to a decimal:
1. Drop the percent sign.
2. Divide the number by 100; this is the same as moving the decimal point two places to the left (add zeros as needed).

**Example 1:** $25\% = \dfrac{25}{100} = 25 \div 100 = .25 = 0.25$

**Example 2:** $1.4\% = \dfrac{1.4}{100} = 1.4 \div 100 = .014 = 0.014$

**Example 3:** $75\% = \dfrac{75}{100} = \dfrac{3}{4}$  (lowest terms). Divide the numerator of the fraction (3) by the denominator (4).

$$4\overline{)3.00}^{\,0.75} = 0.75$$

Example 3 is an alternative method. Drop the percent sign. Write the remaining number as the numerator. Write "100" as the denominator. Reduce the result to lowest terms. Divide the numerator by the denominator to obtain a decimal.

**RULE**

To convert a percent to a ratio:
1. Drop the percent sign.
2. Write the number as a fraction (place it in the numerator).
3. Write 100 as the denominator.
4. Reduce the fraction to lowest terms.
5. Place the numerator as the first term of the ratio and the denominator as the second term.
6. Separate the two terms with a colon (:).

Example 1: $$10\% = \frac{10}{100} = \frac{1}{10} = 1:10$$

Example 2: $$80\% = \frac{80}{100} = \frac{4}{5} = 4:5$$

**RULE**

To convert a fraction to a percent:
1. Multiply the fraction by 100.
2. Reduce if necessary.
3. Add the percent sign (%).
    OR
1. Convert the fraction to a decimal.
2. Multiply decimal by 100, which is the same as moving the decimal point two places to the right.
3. Add the percent sign (%).

**Example 1:** $\frac{3}{4}$ changed to a percent is    *or*    $\frac{3}{4}$ changed to a decimal is

$$\frac{3}{4} \times \frac{100}{1} = \frac{300}{4} = \frac{75}{1} = 75$$

$$4\overline{)3.00}\phantom{}^{0.75}$$

$$0.75 \times 100 = 0.\underset{\smile}{75} = 75\%$$

Add percent sign: 75%          Add percent sign: 75%

**Example 2:** $5\frac{1}{2}$ changed to a percent is

Change to an improper fraction: $\frac{11}{2}$   *or*   Change to an improper fraction: $\frac{11}{2}$

$$2\overline{)11.0}\phantom{}^{5.5}$$

$$\frac{11}{2} \times \frac{100}{1} = \frac{1,100}{2} = \frac{550}{1} = 550$$       $$5.5 \times 100 = 5.\underset{\smile}{50} = 550$$

Add percent sign: 550%          Add percent sign: 550%

**RULE**

To convert a decimal to a percent:
1. Multiply the decimal number by 100, which is the same as moving the decimal point two places to the right. Add zeros if necessary.
2. Add the percent sign (%).

**Example 1:** Change 0.45 to %.

Move the decimal point two places to the right.

Add the percent sign:

$$0.\underset{\smile}{45}. = 45\%$$

**Example 2:** Convert 2.35 to %.

Move the decimal point two places to the right.

Add the percent sign:

$$2.\underset{\smile}{35} = 235\%$$

Another method that can be used to convert a decimal to a percent can be done as follows:

> **RULE**
> To convert a decimal to a percent:
> 1. Change the decimal to a fraction, then follow the steps to convert a fraction to a percent.
> 2. If the percent does not end as a whole number, express the percent with the remainder as a fraction, to the nearest whole percent, or to the nearest tenth of a percent.

Example:     $0.625 = \dfrac{625}{1,000} = \dfrac{5}{8} = 62\dfrac{1}{2}\%,\ 63\%,\ \text{or}\ 62.5\%$

$$\dfrac{625}{1,000} = \dfrac{5}{8};\ \dfrac{5}{8} \times \dfrac{100}{1} = \dfrac{500}{8} = 62.5\%$$

> **RULE**
> To convert a ratio to a percent:
> 1. Convert the ratio to a fraction, and proceed with the steps for changing a fraction to a percent.
>    *or*
> 1. Convert the ratio to a fraction.
> 2. Convert the fraction to a decimal.
> 3. Convert the decimal to a percent.

Example:     $1:4 = \dfrac{1}{4},\ \dfrac{1}{4} \times \dfrac{100}{1} = 25$   *or*          $1:4 = \dfrac{1}{4}$

$$4\overline{)1.00}^{\ 0.25}$$

$0.25 \times 100 = 0.\underset{\smile}{25}. = 25\%$

Add percent sign: 25%          Add percent sign: 25%

---

## ⊞ PRACTICE **PROBLEMS**

Change the following percents to fractions, and reduce to lowest terms.

1. 1% _____          4. 150% _____

2. 2% _____          5. 3% _____

3. 50% _____

Change the following percents to decimals. Round to two decimal places, as indicated.

6. 10% _____          9. 14.2% _____

7. 35% _____          10. $\dfrac{6}{7}\%$ _____

8. 50% _____

Change each of the following percents to a ratio. Express in lowest terms.

11. 25% _____          14. 4.5% _____

12. 11% _____          15. $\dfrac{2}{5}\%$ _____

13. 75% _____

Change the following fractions to percents.

16. $\dfrac{2}{5}$ _____

17. $\dfrac{11}{4}$ _____

18. $\dfrac{1}{2}$ _____

19. $\dfrac{1}{4}$ _____

20. $\dfrac{7}{10}$ _____

Convert the following decimals to percents.

21. 1.32 _____

22. 0.02 _____

23. 0.8 _____

24. 2.3 _____

25. 0.013 _____

Change the following ratios to percents.

26. 1:25 _____

27. 3:4 _____

28. 1:10 _____

29. 1:100 _____

30. 1:2 _____

**Answers on p. 64**

## Percentage Measures

As previously stated, **intravenous (IV) solutions are ordered in percentage strengths, and nurses need to be familiar with their meaning (e.g., 1,000 milliliters [mL] 5% dextrose in water). Percentage solution means the number of grams (g) of solute per 100 mL of diluent.**

**Example 1:**  1,000 mL IV of 5% dextrose and water contains 50 g (grams) of dextrose

$$\% = \text{g per 100 mL; therefore } 5\% = 5 \text{ g per 100 mL}$$

$$5 \text{ g} : 100 \text{ mL} = x \text{ g} : 1,000 \text{ mL}$$

$$x = 50 \text{ g dextrose}$$

**Example 2:**  250 mL IV of 10% dextrose contains 25 g (grams) of dextrose

$$\% = \text{g per 100 mL; therefore } 10\% = 10 \text{ g per 100 mL}$$

$$10 \text{ g} : 100 \text{ mL} = x \text{ g} : 250 \text{ mL}$$

$$x = 25 \text{ g dextrose}$$

## ▦ PRACTICE **PROBLEMS**

Determine the number of grams of medication and dextrose as indicated in the following solutions.

31. How many grams of medication will 500 mL of a 10% solution contain?

_____

32. How many grams of dextrose will 1,000 mL of a 10% solution contain?

_____

33. How many grams of dextrose will 250 mL of a 5% solution contain?

_____

34. How many grams of medication will 100 mL of a 50% solution contain?

_____

35. How many grams of dextrose will 150 mL of a 5% solution contain?

_____

**Answers on p. 64**

## Comparing Percents and Ratios

Nurses as well as other health care professionals administer solutions that may be expressed as percents or ratios. Intravenous solutions come in varying percentages. Example: 0.45%, 5%. It is important to be clear on the numbers and quantities they represent. An IV solution that is 5% is more potent or concentrated than a 0.45% solution. Converting percentages and ratios to equivalent decimals can clarify values so that professionals can compare concentrations.

Like IV fluids, ointments, creams, and lotions can be available in different percentage strengths, and nurses need to be clear on the quantities they represent as well. A 0.025% ointment is more potent or concentrated than one that is 0.02%.

**Example 1:**  $0.45\% = \dfrac{0.45}{100} = 0.45 \div 100 = .00.45 = = 0.0045$

**Example 2:**  $5\% = \dfrac{5}{100} = 5 \div 100 = .05. = 0.05$ (greater value, stronger concentration than 0.0045)

**Compare solution concentrations expressed as a ratio, such as 1:1,000 and 1:10,000.**

**Example 1:**  $1:1,000 = \dfrac{1}{1,000} = 0.001$ (1:1,000 is a stronger concentration than 1:10,000)

**Example 2:**  $1:10,000 = \dfrac{1}{10,000} = 0.0001$

**(!) SAFETY ALERT!**
The higher the percentage strength, the stronger the solution or ointment. A misunderstanding of these numbers (%) can have serious consequences.

**Example:**     10% IV solution is more potent than 5%. A solution of 5% is more potent than 0.9%. **Always check the percentage of IV solution prescribed.**

## ⊞ PRACTICE **PROBLEMS**

Identify the strongest solution, ointment, or cream in each of the following:

36. Ophthalmic solution 0.1%, 0.5%, 1% _____

37. Ointment 0.025%, 0.3%, 0.5% _____

38. Cream 0.02%, 0.025%, 0.25% _____

39. Solution 1:30, 1:300, 1:3 _____

40. Solution 0.33%, 0.9%, 0.45% _____

**Answers on p. 64**

## Determining the Percent of a Quantity

Nurses may find it necessary to determine a given percentage or part of a quantity.

>  **RULE**
> To determine a given percent of a number:
> 1. First convert the percent to a decimal or fraction.
> 2. Multiply the decimal or fraction by the number.

**Example 1:** A client reports drinking 25% of an 8-ounce cup of tea. Determine what amount 25% of 8 ounces is.

**Solution:**  Change the percentage to a decimal:

$$25\% = \frac{25}{100} = .25 = 0.25$$

Multiply the decimal by the number:

$$0.25 \times 8 \text{ ounces} = 2 \text{ ounces}$$

Therefore 25% of 8 ounces = 2 ounces

The percent of a quantity may also be determined using a ratio and proportion written in linear or fraction format. For example, using the above problem:

$$25 : 100 = x : 8 \quad or \quad \frac{25}{100} = \frac{x}{8}$$

Either one of these formats would net the same answer.

**Example 2:**                    40% of 90

**Solution:**                    $40\% = \dfrac{40}{100} = .40 = 0.4$

$$0.4 \times 90 = 36$$

Therefore 40% of 90 = 36
*or*
40 : 100 = x : 90 *or* 40/100 = x/90

## Determining What Percent One Number Is of Another

>  **RULE**
> To determine what percent one number is of another, it is necessary to make a fraction with the numbers.
> 1. The **denominator** (bottom number) of the fraction is the number following the word "of" in the problem.
> 2. The other number is the **numerator** (top number) of the fraction.
> 3. Convert the fraction to a decimal, and then convert to a percentage.

**Example 1:** 12 is what percentage of 60? *or* What percentage of 60 is 12?

**Solution:**    Make a fraction using the two numbers:

$$\frac{12}{60}$$

Convert the fraction to a decimal:

$$60\overline{)12.0}^{\,0.2}$$

Convert the decimal to a percentage:

$$0.2 \times 100 = 0.20. = 20\%$$

Therefore 12 = 20% of 60 *or* 20% of 60 = 12

**Example 2:** 1.2 is what percentage of 4.8? *or* What percentage of 4.8 is 1.2?

**Solution:** Make a fraction using the two numbers:

$$\frac{1.2}{4.8}$$

Convert the fraction to a decimal:

$$4.8\overline{)1.200}^{\,0.25}$$

Convert the decimal to a percentage:

$$0.25 \times 100 = 0.25. = 25\%$$

Therefore 1.2 = 25% of 4.8 *or* 25% of 4.8 = 1.2

**Example 3:** $3\frac{1}{2}$ is what percentage of 8.5? *or* What percentage of 8.5 is $3\frac{1}{2}$?

**Solution:** Make a fraction using the two numbers:

$$\frac{3\frac{1}{2}}{8.5} = \frac{3.5}{8.5}$$

Convert the fraction to a decimal:

$$
\begin{array}{r}
0.4117 \\
8.5\overline{)3.50000} \\
-340 \\
\hline
100 \\
-85 \\
\hline
150 \\
-85 \\
\hline
650 \\
-595 \\
\hline
55
\end{array}
$$

Convert the decimal to a percentage:

$$0.412 \times 100 = 0.412 = 41.2\%$$

Therefore $3\frac{1}{2}$ = 41.2% of 8.5 *or* 41.2% of 8.5 = $3\frac{1}{2}$

## ⊞ PRACTICE **PROBLEMS**

41. A client drinks 30% of a bowl of broth that holds 200 milliliters (mL). How many mL did the client drink? _____

42. A client drinks 80% of a 5-ounce (oz) cup of ginger ale. How many oz did the client drink? _____

Perform the indicated operations. Round decimals to the hundredths place.

43. 60% of 30 _____        49. 0.7% of 60 _____

44. 20% of 75 _____        50. 75% of 165 _____

45. 2 is what percentage of 200? _____        51. 25 is what percentage of 40? _____

46. 50 is what percentage of 500? _____        52. 1.3 is what percentage of 5.2? _____

47. 40 is what percentage of 1,000? _____        53. $\frac{1}{4}$% of 68 _____

48. 3% of 842 _____        54. What percentage of 8.4 is $3\frac{1}{2}$? _____

**Answers on p. 64**

## Calculating the Percent of Change

It may be useful to determine a percent of change (increase or decrease). For example, you might want to know if an increase or decrease in a client's weight is a significant increase or decrease.

> **RULE**
>
> To determine the percent of change:
> 1. Make a fraction of change $= \dfrac{\text{change}}{\text{old}}$
> 2. Multiply the fraction by 100 to change the fraction to a percent OR change the fraction to a decimal and multiply decimal by 100, which is the same as moving the decimal point two places to the right.
> 3. Add the percent sign.

Example 1:  A client's weight before surgery was 176 lb. Following 2 weeks of bed rest, the client's weight was 184.8 lb. What was the percent of increase in the client's weight?

Solution:  The increase $= 184.8$ lb $- 176$ lb $= 8.8$ lb

Fraction of change $= \dfrac{8.8}{176}$

$\dfrac{8.8}{176} \times 100 = \dfrac{880}{176} = 5\%$

*or*

Change fraction to a decimal, multiply by 100.

Fraction of change $= \dfrac{8.8}{176}$

$\dfrac{8.80}{176} = 0.05 \qquad 0.05 \times 100 = 0.05. = 5\%$

The percent of increase in the client's weight was 5%.

**Example 2:** A client was drinking 40 ounces of water per day, but this was reduced by 10 ounces per day. What is the percent of change?

**Solution:** The decrease = 40 ounces − 30 ounces = 10 ounces

Fraction of change $= \dfrac{10}{40} = 25\%$

$\dfrac{10}{40} \times 100 = \dfrac{1,000}{40} = 25\%$

*or*

Change fraction to a decimal, multiply by 100.

Fraction of change $= \dfrac{10}{40}$

$40\overline{)10.00}\phantom{xx}$ 0.25 $= 0.25 \times 100 = 0.25. = 25\%$
$\phantom{xx}-80$
$\phantom{xxxx}200$

##  PRACTICE **PROBLEMS**

55. A client's weight before dieting was 300 lb. After one month of dieting, the client's weight was 240 lb. What was the percent of decrease in the client's weight? _____

56. A client was taking 400 milligrams (mg) of a pain medication. The doctor increased the dosage to 600 mg. What is the percent of increase in the dosage? _____

57. Physical therapy increases a client's pulse rate. The client's rate before the physical therapy was 60 beats per minute. At the completion of physical therapy, the rate is 75 beats per minute. What is the percent of increase in the pulse rate? _____

58. The number of nurses on the night shift has increased from 4 to 6. What is the percent of increase? _____

59. The population at a small assisted-living facility dropped from 150 to 135 residents. What was the percent of decrease in population? _____

60. In February, 2,500 cases of flu were reported. In June of the following year, 900 cases of flu were reported. What is the percent decrease in reported cases of flu? _____

**Answers on p. 64**

Answers on p. 64

---

**POINTS TO REMEMBER**

- Fractions, decimals, ratios, and percents are related equivalents.
- Express ratios in lowest terms.
- **To convert a percent to a fraction,** drop the % sign and place the remaining number as the numerator, write 100 as the denominator, and reduce the fraction to lowest terms.
- **To convert a percent to a decimal,** drop the % sign and divide by 100.
- **To convert a percent to a ratio,** first convert the percent to a fraction in lowest terms. Then, place the numerator as the first term of the ratio and the denominator as the second term. Separate the two terms with a colon (:).
- **To convert a fraction to a percent,** multiply the fraction by 100, reduce if necessary, and add the % sign **OR** convert the fraction to a decimal, multiply the decimal by 100, and add the % sign.

- **To convert a decimal to a percent,** multiply the decimal by 100 and add the % sign **OR** change the decimal to a fraction, then follow the steps to convert a fraction to a percent. If the percent does not terminate as a whole number, express the percent with the remainder as a fraction to the nearest whole percent, or to the nearest tenth of a percent.
- **To convert a ratio to a percent,** convert the ratio to a fraction and proceed with the steps for changing a fraction to a percent **OR** convert the ratio to a fraction, convert the resulting fraction to a decimal and then to a percent.
- Percentage solutions means the number of grams of solute per 100 milliliters of diluent.
- The higher the percentage strength, the stronger the solution, ointment, or cream.
- To determine the given percent or part of a quantity, convert the percent to a decimal or fraction. Multiply the decimal or fraction by the number. This can also be done using any of the formats for ratio and proportion.
- **To calculate the percent of change,** make a fraction of the change $= \dfrac{\text{change}}{\text{old}}$ and multiply the fraction by 100 to change the fraction to a percent **OR** change the fraction to a decimal, multiply by 100, and add the % sign.

## ○ CHAPTER **REVIEW**

Complete the table below. Express each of the following measures in their equivalents where indicated. Reduce fractions and ratios to lowest terms; round decimals to hundreths.

| | Percent | Ratio | Fraction | Decimal |
|---|---|---|---|---|
| 1. | 52% | _____ | _____ | _____ |
| 2. | 71% | _____ | _____ | _____ |
| 3. | _____ | _____ | $\dfrac{7}{100}$ | _____ |
| 4. | _____ | 1:50 | _____ | _____ |
| 5. | _____ | _____ | _____ | 0.06 |
| 6. | _____ | _____ | $\dfrac{7}{10}$ | _____ |
| 7. | _____ | _____ | $\dfrac{61}{100}$ | _____ |
| 8. | _____ | 7:1,000 | _____ | _____ |
| 9. | 5% | _____ | _____ | _____ |
| 10. | 2.5% | _____ | _____ | _____ |

Perform the indicated operations.

11. A client reports drinking 40% of a 12-ounce can of ginger ale. How many ounces did the client drink? _____

12. 40% of 140 _____    13. 100 is what percentage of 750? _____

14. $\frac{1}{2}$ is what percentage of 60? _____    15. 15% of 250 _____

16. What percentage of 6.4 is 1.6? _____

17. Which of the following solutions is strongest: 0.0125%, 0.25%, 0.1%? _____

Change each of the following percentages to a ratio, and reduce to lowest terms.

18. 16% _____    19. 45% _____

20. A client is on a 1,000 milliliters (mL) fluid restriction per 24 hours. At breakfast and lunch, the client consumed 40% of the fluid allowance. How many mL did the client

consume? _____

21. A client drank 75% of a 12-ounce can of ginger ale. How many ounces did the client

drink? _____

22. A client consumes 55% of a bowl of chicken broth at lunch. The bowl holds

180 milliliters (mL). How many mL did the client consume? _____

23. In a class of 30 students, 6 students did not pass an exam. What percentage of the

students did not pass the exam? _____

24. At the first prenatal visit, a client weighed 140 pounds. At the second visit, the client

had a 5% weight increase. How many pounds did the client gain? _____

25. An infant consumed 55% of an 8-ounce bottle of formula. How many ounces of

formula did the infant consume? _____

26. In a portion of turkey that is 100 grams (g), there are 23 g of protein and 4 g of fat.

What percentage of the portion is protein? _____

What percentage of the portion is fat? _____

27. A nursing review test has 130 questions, and you answer 120 correctly. What is

your score, as a percentage? _____

28. A client's intake for the day was 2,000 calories, and 600 of the calories came from fat.

What percentage of the client's intake came from fat? _____

29. A client began receiving 325 milligrams (mg) of a medication. The prescriber increased the dosage of medication by 10%. What will the new dosage be?

_____ mg

30. The recommended daily allowance (RDA) of a vitamin is 14 milligrams (mg). If a multivitamin provides 55% of the RDA, how many mg of the vitamin would the client receive from the multivitamin? _____

31. A client's pulse rate decreases from 80 beats per minute to 72 beats per minute. What is the percent of decrease? _____

32. A client's medication is increased from 400 milligrams (mg) to 500 mg. What is the percent of increase in the dosage? _____

33. A client's weight increased from 120 lb to 132 lb. What was the percent of increase in body weight? _____

34. A client's intake decreased from 2,500 milliliters (mL) per day to 2,000 mL per day. What was the percent of decrease? _____

35. The number of capsules a client received each day has decreased from 3 capsules each day to 2 capsules per day. What is the percent of decrease? _____

36. If a client ate 400 calories at breakfast, what percentage of a 2,000-calorie diet was consumed? _____

37. A newborn weighed 3,751 grams (g) at birth and 3,352 g prior to discharge. What is the percentage of weight loss? _____

38. In August of one year, 15 cases of heat stroke were treated in the emergency room. In August of the next year, 12 cases of heat stroke were treated. What is the percent of decrease in cases of heat stroke? _____

39. A client is on a 2,000-calorie-per-day diet. If lunch accounts for 45% of a client's daily calories, how many calories can the client have for lunch? _____

Convert the following percents to decimals.

40. 4.4% _____    41. 103% _____

Convert the following decimals to percents.

42. 0.32 _____    43. 0.06 _____

Identify the strongest in each of the following.

44. 1 : 10, 1 : 100, 1 : 200 _____    45. 1 : 25, $\frac{1}{5}$, 0.02% _____

**Answers on p. 64**

# ⭐ ANSWERS

## Chapter 4
### Answers to Practice Problems

1. $\frac{1}{100}$

2. $\frac{1}{50}$

3. $\frac{1}{2}$

4. $1\frac{1}{2}$

5. $\frac{3}{100}$

6. 0.1

7. 0.35

8. 0.5

9. 0.14

10. 0.0086

11. 1:4

12. 11:100

13. 3:4

14. 4.5:100

15. 0.4:100

16. 40%

17. 275%

18. 50%

19. 25%

20. 70%

21. 132%

22. 2%

23. 80%

24. 230%

25. 1.3%

26. 4%

27. 75%

28. 10%

29. 1%

30. 50%

31. 50 g

32. 100 g

33. 12.5 g

34. 50 g

35. 7.5 g

36. 1%

37. 0.5%

38. 0.25%

39. 1:3

40. 0.9%

41. 60 mL

42. 4 oz

43. 18

44. 15

45. 1%

46. 10%

47. 4%

48. 25.26

49. 0.42

50. 123.75

51. 62.5%

52. 25%

53. 0.17

54. 41.67%

55. 20%

56. 50%

57. 25%

58. 50%

59. 10%

60. 64%

### Answers to Chapter Review

| | Percent | Ratio | Fraction | Decimal |
|---|---|---|---|---|
| 1. | 52% | 13:25 | $\frac{13}{25}$ | 0.52 |
| 2. | 71% | 71:100 | $\frac{71}{100}$ | 0.71 |
| 3. | 7% | 7:100 | $\frac{7}{100}$ | 0.07 |
| 4. | 2% | 1:50 | $\frac{1}{50}$ | 0.02 |
| 5. | 6% | 3:50 | $\frac{3}{50}$ | 0.06 |
| 6. | 70% | 7:10 | $\frac{7}{10}$ | 0.7 |
| 7. | 61% | 61:100 | $\frac{61}{100}$ | 0.61 |
| 8. | 0.7% | 7:1,000 | $\frac{7}{1,000}$ | 0.007 |
| 9. | 5% | 1:20 | $\frac{1}{20}$ | 0.05 |
| 10. | 2.5% | 1:40 | $\frac{1}{40}$ | 0.03 |

11. 4.8 oz

12. 56

13. 13.3%

14. 0.83%

15. 37.5

16. 25%

17. 0.25%

18. 4:25

19. 9:20

20. 400 mL

21. 9 oz

22. 99 mL

23. 20%

24. 7 lb

25. 4.4 oz

26. 23% protein, 4% fat

27. 92.3%

28. 30%

29. 357.5 mg

30. 7.7 mg

31. 10%

32. 25%

33. 10%

34. 20%

35. 33.3% or $33\frac{1}{3}$%

36. 20%

37. 10.6%

38. 20%

39. 900 calories

40. 0.044

41. 1.03

42. 32%

43. 6%

44. 1:10

45. $\frac{1}{5}$

# POST-TEST

After completing Unit One of this text, you should be able to complete this test. The test consists of a total of 75 questions. If you miss any questions in any section, review the chapter relating to that content.

1. There are 6 nurses and 48 clients at a nursing facility. What is the ratio of nurses to clients expressed as a fraction?

2. Write the following information as a proportion: 30 milligrams (mg) is to 1 dosage as 120 mg is to 4 dosages.

3. Identify the numerator and denominator in the following fraction:

   $$\frac{0.26}{1.2}$$

   Numerator: _____

   Denominator: _____

4. A client drank 6 ounces (oz) of an 8-oz glass of juice. What percentage did the client drink?

5. 800 milligrams (mg) of a medication were prescribed for a client. A week later, the medication was reduced to 600 mg. What was the percent of decrease in the medication?

6. The tablets your client is to receive are labeled 0.1 milligram (mg), and you are to administer $4\frac{1}{2}$ tablets. What is the total dosage?

7. Convert the fraction $3\frac{3}{5}$ to a percent.

8. Convert the ratio 2 : 3 to a fraction and a percent. State the percent to the nearest whole percent. Fraction: _____ Percent: _____

9. A solution of 100 milliliters (mL) contains 10 grams (g) of dextrose. How many g of dextrose are in 1,000 mL of this solution?

10. A client drank $8\frac{1}{2}$ ounces (oz) of juice, and $6\frac{3}{4}$ oz of coffee for breakfast. How many oz did the client drink?

Reduce the following fractions to lowest terms.

11. $\frac{8}{6}$ _____

14. $\frac{10}{15}$ _____

12. $\frac{22}{33}$ _____

15. $\frac{16}{10}$ _____

13. $\frac{27}{63}$ _____

Perform the indicated operations with fractions; reduce to lowest terms where indicated.

16. $\frac{5}{6} \div \frac{7}{10} =$ _____

19. $5\frac{1}{5} - 3\frac{4}{7} =$ _____

17. $5\frac{1}{2} \div 4\frac{1}{2} =$ _____

20. $\frac{5}{4} + \frac{2}{9} =$ _____

18. $6\frac{1}{3} \times 4 =$ _____

21. $\frac{4}{9} + \frac{7}{9} =$ _____

22. $1\dfrac{1}{3} + \dfrac{5}{7} =$ _____

24. $7\dfrac{1}{4} - 2\dfrac{1}{3} =$ _____

23. $7\dfrac{1}{2} \times \dfrac{3}{4} =$ _____

25. $2 - \dfrac{10}{21} =$ _____

Change the following fractions to decimals; express each answer to the nearest tenth.

26. $\dfrac{8}{7}$ _____

28. $\dfrac{1}{15}$ _____

27. $\dfrac{1}{8}$ _____

29. $\dfrac{12}{13}$ _____

Indicate the largest fraction in each group.

30. $\dfrac{1}{2}, \dfrac{2}{3}, \dfrac{5}{9}$ _____

31. $\dfrac{3}{4}, \dfrac{7}{10}, \dfrac{5}{8}$ _____

Perform the indicated operations with decimals. Provide exact answers.

32. $16.7 + 21 =$ _____

34. $10.57 \times 10 =$ _____

33. $0.007 + 17.4 =$ _____

35. $36.8 - 3.86 =$ _____

Divide the following decimals; express each answer to the nearest tenth.

36. $67.8 \div 0.8 =$ _____

38. $5.01 \div 10 =$ _____

37. $9 \div 0.4 =$ _____

Indicate the largest decimal in each group.

39. $0.85, 0.085$ _____

41. $0.478, 0.445, 0.493$ _____

40. $3.002, 0.39, 0.399$ _____

Solve for $x$, the unknown value.

42. $10 : 20 = x : 8$ _____

44. $0.3 : x = 1.8 : 0.6$ _____

43. $500 : x = 200 : 1$ _____

45. $\dfrac{1}{4} : x = \dfrac{1}{8} : 2$ _____

Round off to the nearest tenth.

46. $0.57$ _____

48. $1.42$ _____

47. $0.99$ _____

Round off to the nearest hundredth.

49. $0.677$ _____

51. $1.222$ _____

50. $0.832$ _____

Complete the table below. Express each of the measures in their equivalents where indicated. Reduce fractions and ratios to lowest terms; round decimals to hundredths.

| | Percent | Decimal | Ratio | Fraction |
|---|---|---|---|---|
| 52. | _____ | _____ | 1:10 | _____ |
| 53. | 60% | _____ | _____ | _____ |
| 54. | $66\frac{2}{3}\%$ | _____ | _____ | _____ |
| 55. | 25% | _____ | _____ | _____ |

Find the percentage.

56. 9% of 200 _____    59. 5 is what percent of 2,000? _____

57. 2.5% of 750 _____    60. 25 is what percent of 65? _____

58. 30 is what percent of 45? _____

Express the following solution strengths as ratios.

61. 1 part medication to 80 parts solution _____

62. 1 part medication to 300 parts solution _____

63. 1 part medication to 20 parts solution _____

Identify the strongest solution in each of the following:

64. 1:80, 1:800, 1:8,000 _____    65. 1:1,000, 1:2,000, 1:5,000 _____

66. A client who weighed 81.5 kilograms (kg) lost 3.75 kg. How much does the client weigh now? _____

67. A client's weight increased from 175 pounds (lb) to 210 lb. What was the percent of increase in the client's weight? _____

68. A client is receiving 0.6 milligram (mg) of a medication four (4) times a day. How many mg would the client receive after $2\frac{1}{2}$ days? _____

69. If 6 oz of medication must be mixed with 15 oz of water, how many oz of water is needed for four (4) oz of medication? _____

70. A client is taking two (2) tablets twice a day for 14 days. The tablet contains 2.2 mg. How much medication did the client receive? _____

71. A client should have received 3.25 grams (g) of medication. In error the nurse administered 32.5 g. How much more medication did the client receive? _____

72. Write a ratio that represents 20 milligrams (mg) of a medication in 100 milliliters (mL) of liquid. _____

73. A client's weight decreased from 150 pounds (lb) to 132 lb. What is the percent of decrease in the client's weight? _____

74. A client receives a total of 13.5 milligrams (mg) from nine (9) tablets. What is the dosage strength of each tablet? _____

75. Write a ratio that represents every capsule in a bottle contains 0.75 milligram (mg).
_____

**Answers on p. 68**

## ⭐ ANSWERS

1. $\dfrac{1}{8}$

2. $\dfrac{30 \text{ mg}}{1 \text{ dosage}} = \dfrac{120 \text{ mg}}{4 \text{ dosages}}$

   *or* 30 mg : 1 dosage = 120 mg : 4 dosages

3. 0.26, 1.2

4. 75%

5. 25%

6. 0.45 mg

7. 360%

8. Fraction: $\dfrac{2}{3}$; Percent: 67%

9. 100 g

10. $15\dfrac{1}{4}$ oz

11. $1\dfrac{1}{3}$

12. $\dfrac{2}{3}$

13. $\dfrac{3}{7}$

14. $\dfrac{2}{3}$

15. $1\dfrac{3}{5}$

16. $1\dfrac{4}{21}$

17. $1\dfrac{2}{9}$

18. $25\dfrac{1}{3}$

19. $1\dfrac{22}{35}$

20. $1\dfrac{17}{36}$

21. $\dfrac{11}{9} = 1\dfrac{2}{9}$

22. $2\dfrac{1}{21}$

23. $5\dfrac{5}{8}$

24. $4\dfrac{11}{12}$

25. $1\dfrac{11}{21}$

26. 1.1

27. 0.1

28. 0.1

29. 0.9

30. $\dfrac{2}{3}$

31. $\dfrac{3}{4}$

32. 37.7

33. 17.407

34. 105.7

35. 32.94

36. 84.8

37. 22.5

38. 0.5

39. 0.85

40. 3.002

41. 0.493

42. $x = 4$

43. $x = 2.5$ *or* $2\dfrac{1}{2}$

44. $x = 0.1$ *or* $\dfrac{1}{10}$

45. $x = 4$

46. 0.6

47. 1

48. 1.4

49. 0.68

50. 0.83

51. 1.22

| | Percent | Decimal | Ratio | Fraction |
|---|---|---|---|---|
| 52. | 10% | 0.1 | 1:10 | $\dfrac{1}{10}$ |
| 53. | 60% | 0.6 | 3:5 | $\dfrac{3}{5}$ |
| 54. | $66\dfrac{2}{3}$% | 0.67 | 67:100 | $\dfrac{67}{100}$ |
| 55. | 25% | 0.25 | 1:4 | $\dfrac{1}{4}$ |

56. 18

57. 18.75

58. $66\dfrac{2}{3}$% *or* 66.7% *or* 67%

59. 0.25%

60. 38.46% *or* 38.5% *or* 38%

61. 1:80

62. 1:300

63. 1:20

64. 1:80

65. 1:1,000

66. 77.75 kilograms (kg)

67. 20%

68. 6 milligrams (mg)

69. 10 oz

70. 123.2 milligrams (mg)

71. 29.25 grams (g)

72. 20 mg:100 mL *or* 1 mg:5 mL *or* 20 mg/100 mL; 1 mg/5 mL

73. 12%

74. 1.5 milligrams (mg)

75. 0.75 mg:1 capsule *or* 0.75 mg/1 capsule

# UNIT TWO

# Systems of Measurement

For the nurse to be competent in the administration of medications, the nurse must be knowledgeable in the most frequently used and preferred measurement system to order, measure, and administer medications. The metric system is the preferred system of measurement used in health care. Because the metric system is the preferred system for health care, knowledge of the metric system is imperative. Let's begin with the discussion of the metric system.

# CHAPTER 5
## Metric System

## Objectives

*After reviewing this chapter, you should be able to:*

1. Express metric measures correctly using rules of the metric system
2. State common equivalents in the metric system
3. Convert measures within the metric system

To administer medications safely to clients, it is important to have a thorough knowledge of the system of measurements used in medication administration. Understanding common equivalents and the systems of measurement used in medication administration will help in the prevention of **medication errors** related to incorrect dosages.

Historically, there were three different systems of measure used in medication administration: the apothecary, household, and metric systems. As stated, the metric system is the preferred system of measurement for medications and measurements used in the health care setting. For example, newborn weights are recorded in grams (g) and kilograms (kg); centimeters (cm) are used in obstetrics to express fundal height (upper portion of the uterus) and to measure incisions. As a nurse, more than 90% of the medication calculations you will encounter in the clinical setting will involve the metric system.

The metric system is an international decimal system of weights and measures that was introduced in France in the late seventeenth and eighteenth centuries. It is also referred to as the *International System of Units*. The International System of Units, universally abbreviated SI (from the French Le Systéme International d Unités), is the modern metric system of measurement. The abbreviations of this system of metric notations are the most widely accepted. The benefit of the metric system lies in its simplicity and accuracy because it is based on the decimal system. The nurse will find that medication calculation and administration skills involve familiarity and accuracy with the metric system to administer medications safely.

Prescribers should use the metric system for prescribing medications to prevent medication errors. The Joint Commission (TJC), U.S. Food and Drug Administration (FDA), and Institute for Safe Medication Practices (ISMP) concur that the metric system should be used to prevent medication errors. This includes writing prescriptions in the metric system, and all FDA-approved prescription medication labels provide metric dosage.

## Particulars of the Metric System

1. The metric system is based on the decimal system, in which divisions and multiples of 10 are used. Therefore a lot of math can be done by decimal point movement.
2. Three basic units of measure are used in the metric system, as shown in Table 5.1.

| TABLE 5.1 Basic Units of Metric Measurement | | |
|---|---|---|
| Table of Measure | Basic Unit | Abbreviation |
| Weight (solid) | gram | g |
| Volume (liquid) | liter | L |
| Length | meter | m |

Dosages are calculated by using metric measurements that relate to weight and volume. Meter (m), which is the base unit used for linear (length) measurement, is the least used measurement for dosage calculations but is important in the health care setting. Linear measurements are commonly used to measure the height of an individual, for serial abdominal girth (the circumference of the abdomen, usually measured at the umbilicus), the circumference of an infant's head, length of an amount of medicated ointment or paste, and for pressure ulcer measurements. These are examples of important measures that can be seen in the health care setting. Most length measurements seen in the health care setting are millimeters (mm) and centimeters (cm).

3. Common prefixes in this system denote the numerical value of the unit being discussed. Memorization of these prefixes is necessary for quick and accurate calculations. The prefixes in bold in Table 5.2 are the ones used most often in health care for dosage calculations. However, some of the prefixes may be used to express other values, such as laboratory values. *Kilo* is a common prefix used to identify a measure larger than the basic unit. The other common prefixes used in medication administration are smaller units: *centi, milli,* and *micro.*

Let's look at the following example to see how the prefixes may be used.

**Example:** 67 milligrams

Prefix—*milli*—means measure in thousandths of a unit.
*Gram* is a unit of weight.
Therefore 67 milligrams = 67 thousandths of a gram.

4. Regardless of the size of the unit, the name of the basic unit is incorporated into the measure (see Table 5.1). This allows easy recognition of the unit of measure.

**Example 1:** milli**liter**—The word *liter* indicates you are measuring volume (*milli* indicates 1/1,000 of that volume).

**Example 2:** kilo**gram**—The word *gram* indicates you are measuring weight (*kilo* indicates 1,000 of that weight; 1 kilogram = 1,000 grams).

**Example 3:** kilo**liter**—The word *liter* indicates you are measuring volume (*kilo* indicates 1,000 of that volume; 1 kiloliter = 1,000 liters).

**Example 4:** deci**liter**—The word *liter* indicates that you are measuring volume (*deci* indicates 0.1 of that volume [liter], or 100 milliliters). "Female's normal hemoglobin is 12 to 16 g/dL," means there are 12 to 16 grams of hemoglobin contained in 100 milliliters of blood.

**Example 5:** cubic milli**meter** ($mm^3$)—cubic millimeter is a unit of volume of three-dimensional space (length × width × height). In a normal individual the white blood cell count ranges between 5,000 and 10,000 cells per cubic millimeter of blood. Therefore 1 $mm^3$ of blood contains between 5,000 and 10,000 white blood cells (5,000/$mm^3$ and 10,000/$mm^3$).

| TABLE 5.2 | Common Prefixes Used in Health Care | |
|---|---|---|
| **Prefix** | **Numerical Value** | **Meaning** |
| **Kilo*** | 1,000 | one thousand times |
| Hecto | 100 | one hundred times |
| Deka | 10 | ten times |
| Deci | 0.1 | one tenth |
| **Centi*** | 0.01 | one hundredth part of |
| **Milli*** | 0.001 | one thousandth part of |
| **Micro*** | 0.000001 | one millionth part of |

*Prefixes used most often in medication administration.

> **SAFETY ALERT!**
>
> Do not confuse units of measure in the metric system for weight, volume, and length that have similar names. Milligram is a unit of weight; milliliter is a unit of volume; and millimeter is a unit of length.

> **POINTS TO REMEMBER**
>
> It is important to memorize the prefixes and the amounts they represent. A mnemonic to help remember the important metric prefixes' order from largest measurement to smallest is: **K**itty **H**awk **D**oesn't **D**rink **C**anned **M**ilk **M**uch.
>
> kilo, hecto, deka, deci, centi, milli, micro

5. The abbreviation for a unit of measure in the metric system is often the first letter of the word. Lowercase letters are used more often than capital letters.

**Example 1:** g = gram

**Example 2:** m = meter

The exception to this rule is liter, for which a capital letter is used.

**Example 3:** liter = L

6. When prefixes are used in combination with the basic unit, the first letter of the prefix and the first letter of the unit of measure are written together in lowercase letters.

**Example 1:** Milligram—abbreviated as *mg*. The *m* is taken from the prefix *milli* and the *g* from *gram*, the unit of weight.

**Example 2:** Microgram—abbreviated as **mcg.** Microgram is also abbreviated using the Greek symbol ($\mu$g). Use of this symbol for micrograms ($\mu$g) should not be used for communicating medical information, including medication orders. It can be misinterpreted as mg (milligrams), resulting in a thousandfold overdose.

> **SAFETY ALERT!**
>
> The abbreviation μg for microgram is listed on the Institute for Safe Medication Practice (ISMP) list of Error-Prone Abbreviations, Symbols, and Dose Designations (2015). Confusion of the symbol used for microgram with the abbreviation for milligram could cause a critical error in dosage calculation. These units differ from each other in value by 1,000.

**Example 3:** Milliliter—abbreviated as **mL.** Note that when *L (liter)* is used in combination with a prefix, it **remains capitalized.** Milliliter (mL) is a small volume, it is one-thousandth of a liter, and is commonly used in dosage calculation.

> **⚠ SAFETY ALERT!**
>
> You may see gram abbreviated as *Gm* or *gm*, liter as lowercase *l*, and milliliter as *ml*. These abbreviations are outdated and can lead to misinterpretation. Use only the standardized SI abbreviations. Use *g* for gram, *L* for liter, and *mL* for milliliter. Cubic centimeter, abbreviated *cc*, was used interchangeably for mL. Using *cc* for *mL* should not be done and has been misinterpreted for zeros (OO) or units (U). In addition, cc is not a measure of volume; it is the amount of space occupied by a milliliter (mL). The use of the abbreviation *U* is prohibited and must be spelled out (unit). It has been mistaken for zero (0) and the number 4 (four). When in doubt about an abbreviation being used, never assume; ask the prescriber for clarification.

> **⚠ SAFETY ALERT!**
>
> It is critical to differentiate between the SI abbreviations for milligram (mg) and milliliter (mL). At a quick glance these abbreviations appear similar; however, confusing these two units can result in lethal consequences for a client.

Box 5.1 lists the common metric abbreviations.

---

**BOX 5.1  Common Metric Abbreviations**

gram = g
microgram = mcg
milligram = mg
kilogram = kg
liter = L
*deciliter = dL
milliliter = mL

*Seen in the expression of laboratory values (e.g., hemoglobin, creatinine levels).

---

## Rules of the Metric System

Certain rules specific to the metric system are important to remember (Box 5.2). **These rules are critical to the prevention of errors and ensure accurate interpretation of metric notations when used in medication orders. (Never assume.)** Ask for clarification if you are not sure of the abbreviation or notation to prevent an error.

> **⚠ SAFETY ALERT!**
>
> As part of the National Patient Safety Goals, TJC set up specific guidelines for the use of leading and trailing zeros. This is also a recommendation of ISMP. A zero should always be placed in front of the decimal when the quantity is less than a whole number **(leading zero)**. When the quantity expressed is preceded by a whole number, zeros are not placed after the number **(trailing zeros)**. This rule is critical to preventing misinterpretation and medication errors. Always double-check the placement of decimals and zeros.

**Example 1:** .52 mL is written as 0.52 mL to **reinforce the decimal** and avoid being misread as 52 mL. Lack of a leading zero before the decimal point could result in the decimal point being missed and cause a critical error in dosage interpretation.

**Example 2:** 2.5 mL is written as 2.5 mL, not 2.50 mL. **Addition of unnecessary zeros can lead to errors in reading;** 2.50 mL may be misread as 250 mL instead of 2.5 mL. Unnecessary zeros can also result in the decimal point being missed and cause a critical error in dosage interpretation.

**BOX 5.2 Metric System Rules**

1. Use Arabic numbers to express quantities in this system.

   **Example:** 1, 1,000, 0.5

2. Express parts of a unit or fractions of a unit as decimals.

   **Example:** 0.4 g, 0.5 L $\left(\text{not } \frac{2}{5} \text{ g}, \frac{1}{2} \text{ L}\right)$

3. Always write the quantity, whether in whole numbers or in decimals, before the abbreviation or symbol for a unit of measure.

   **Example:** 1,000 mg, 0.75 mL (not mg 1,000, mL 0.75)

4. Use a full space between the numeral and abbreviation.

   **Example:** 2 mL, 1 L (not 2mL, 1L)

5. Always place a leading zero to the left of the decimal point if there is no whole number. Eliminate trailing zeros to the right of the decimal point.

   **Example:** 0.4 mL, 2 mg (not .4 mL, 2.0 mg)

6. Do not use the abbreviation $\mu$g for microgram; it might be mistaken for mg. Remember mg is 1,000 times larger.

7. Do not use the abbreviation *cc* for mL. This abbreviation can be misinterpreted as zeros. mL is the acceptable unit for volume.

   **Example:** 2 mL (not 2 cc)

8. Avoid periods after the abbreviation for a unit of measure to avoid the possibility of it being misread for the number 1 in a poorly handwritten order.

   **Example:** mg (not mg.)

9. Place commas in values at 1,000 or above. ISMP recommends this to improve readability.

   **Example:** 100,000 units (not 100000 units)

10. Do not add "s" on a unit of measure to make it plural; this could lead to misinterpretation.

    **Example:** mg (not mgs)

---

## PRACTICE **PROBLEMS**

Applying the guidelines relating to the use of leading and trailing zeros, express the following values correctly.

1. .750 g _____

2. 1.70 mL _____

3. .68 L _____

4. 7.0 kg _____

5. .002 mg _____

**Answers on p. 80**

## Units of Measure

Understanding common equivalents in the metric system can assist the nurse in preventing medication errors related to incorrect dosage.

### Weight

The gram is the basic unit of weight. Medications may be ordered in grams or fractions of a gram, such as milligram or microgram.

   1. The milligram is 1,000 times smaller than a gram:

$$1 \text{ g} = 1,000 \text{ mg}$$

2. The microgram is 1,000 times smaller than a milligram and 1 million times smaller than a gram. The word *micro* also means tiny or small. Micrograms are tiny parts of a gram (i.e., 1,000 mcg = 1 mg). A milligram is 1,000 times larger than a microgram. It takes 1 million mcg to make 1 g.

3. The kilogram is very large and is not used for measuring medications. A kilogram is 1,000 times larger than a gram (i.e., 1 kg = 1,000 g). This measure is often used to denote weights of clients, on which medication dosages are based. This is the only unit you will see used to identify a unit larger than the basic unit.

## Volume

1. The **liter** is the basic unit.

$$1 \text{ L} = 1,000 \text{ mL}$$

2. The **milliliter** is 1,000 times smaller than a liter. It is abbreviated as *mL*.

$$1 \text{ mL} = 0.001 \text{ L}$$

3. As previously stated, **cubic centimeter** (cc) should not be used because of misinterpretation. The cubic centimeter is the amount of space that 1 mL of liquid occupies. Remember, mL is the correct term for volume. The use of cc for mL is currently prohibited by many health care organizations. TJC has also suggested that institutions prohibit the use of the abbreviation cc and add it to their "Do Not Use" List. ISMP also includes cc as an abbreviation that should not be used. Figure 5.1 shows metric measures that may be seen on a medication cup. ***Note:*** *mL* markings on the medicine cup indicate a capacity of 30 mL.

Although pint and quart are not metric measures, they have metric equivalents. For example, a quart is approximately the size of a liter: 1 quart ≈ 1,000 mL and 1 pint ≈ 500 mL. Although pint and quart are not measures used in medication administration, you may need them to calculate a solution, especially in home care. For pharmacological purposes, the equivalents stated for pint and quart are used.

Box 5.3 presents the metric units of measure used most often for dosage calculations and measurement of health status. This text will use the standardized abbreviations for metric units throughout.

| BOX 5.3 Metric Equivalents to Memorize | |
|---|---|
| **Weight** | **Volume** |
| 1 kilogram (kg) = 1,000 grams (g) | 1 liter (L) = 1,000 milliliters (mL) |
| 1 gram (g) = 1,000 milligrams (mg) | 1 milliliter (mL) = 0.001 liter (L) |
| 1 milligram (mg) = 1,000 micrograms (mcg) | |
| | **Length** |
| | 1 meter (m) = 100 centimeters (cm) = 1,000 mm |
| | 1 millimeter (mm) = 0.001 meter (m) = 0.1 cm |

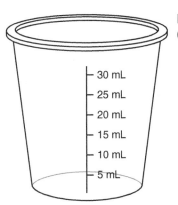

**Figure 5.1** Medicine cup showing volume measure in milliliters (mL).

- 30 mL
- 25 mL
- 20 mL
- 15 mL
- 10 mL
- 5 mL

## Conversions Between Metric Units

Because the metric system is based on the decimal system, conversions between one metric system unit and another can be done by moving the decimal point. The number of places to move the decimal point depends on the equivalent. In the metric system the most common terms used are the kilogram, gram, milligram, microgram, liter, milliliter, and centimeter. To **convert** or make a **conversion** means to change from one unit to another. This converting can be simply changing a measure to its equivalent in the same system. Changing from grams to milligrams illustrates a metric measure changed to another metric measure. Each metric unit in common use for *medication administration* differs from the next by a factor of 1,000. Metric conversions can therefore be made by dividing or multiplying by **1,000.** A way to remember how far to move the decimal point is this: There are three (3) zeros in 1,000, and the decimal point is moved three places, the same as the number of zeros in the conversion (1,000). Knowledge of the size of a unit is important when converting by moving the decimal because this determines whether division or multiplication is necessary to make the conversion.

To make conversions within the metric system, remember the common conversion factors (1 kg = 1,000 g, 1 g = 1,000 mg, 1 mg = 1,000 mcg, and 1 L = 1,000 mL) and the following rules:

> **RULE**
> To convert a **smaller** unit of measure to a **larger** one, **divide** by moving the decimal point **three places to the left.**

**Example 1:**  100 mL = ___ L          (conversion factor: 1,000 mL = 1 L)
              (smaller)    (larger)

100 mL = .100 = 0.1 L   **(Placing zero in front of the decimal is important.)**

**Example 2:**  50 mg = ___ g           (conversion factor: 1,000 mg = 1 g)
              (smaller)   (larger)

50 mg = .050 = 0.05 g  **(Placing zero in front of the decimal is important.)**

> **RULE**
> To convert a **larger** unit of measure to a **smaller** one, **multiply** by moving the decimal **three places to the right.**

**Example 1:**  0.75 g = ___ mg          (conversion factor: 1 g = 1,000 mg)
              (larger)    (smaller)

0.75 g = 0.750 = 750 mg

**Example 2:**  0.04 kg = ___ g          (conversion factor: 1 kg = 1,000 g)
              (larger)    (smaller)

0.04 kg = 0.040 = 40 g

> **SAFETY ALERT!**
> When converting quantities within the metric system from one unit of measure to another, pay close attention to the decimal point. Moving the decimal point incorrectly (in the wrong direction) can result in a dangerous error.

## PRACTICE **PROBLEMS**

Convert the following metric measures by moving the decimal.

6. 300 mg = _____ g      16. 529 mg = _____ g

7. 6 mg = _____ mcg      17. 645 mcg = _____ mg

8. 0.7 L = _____ mL      18. 347 L = _____ mL

9. 180 mcg = _____ mg    19. 238 g = _____ mcg

10. 0.02 mg = _____ mcg  20. 3,500 mL = _____ L

11. 4.5 L = _____ mL     21. 0.04 kg = _____ g

12. 4.2 g = _____ mg     22. 658 kg = _____ g

13. 0.9 g = _____ mg     23. 51 mL = _____ L

14. 3,250 mL = _____ L   24. 1.6 mg = _____ mcg

15. 42 g = _____ kg      25. 28 mL = _____ L

**Answers on p. 80**

### POINTS TO REMEMBER

- The liter and the gram are the basic units used for medication administration.
- Conversion factors must be memorized to do conversions. The common conversion factors in the metric system are 1 kg = 1,000 g, 1 g = 1,000 mg, 1 mg = 1,000 mcg, and 1 L = 1,000 mL.
- mL is the correct term to use in relation to volume, not cc:
- Express answers using the following rules of the metric system:
  1. Fractional metric units are expressed as a decimal.
  2. Place a **leading zero** in front of the decimal point when the quantity is less than a whole number to prevent potential dosage error.
  3. Omit **trailing zeros** to avoid misreading of a value and potential error in dosage.
  4. The abbreviation for a measure is placed after the quantity.
  5. Place a full space between the numeral and abbreviation.
  6. Use standard SI abbreviations.
- Converting common metric units used in medication administration from one unit of measure to another is done by multiplying or dividing by 1,000. The decimal point is moved the same number of zeros in the conversion (1,000), always 3 places.
- Answers should be stated with the unit of measure as the label.
- Place commas in amounts of 1,000 or above.
- Never guess at the meaning of a metric notation; ask for clarification.

## CHAPTER **REVIEW**

1. List the three units of measurement used in the metric system.

   a. _____       c. _____

   b. _____

2. Which is larger, kilogram or milligram? _____

3. 1 mL = _____ L

4. What units of measure are used in the metric system for:

   a. liquid capacity? _____     b. weight? _____

5. 1,000 mg = _____ g       7. 1,000 mcg = _____ mg

6. 1 L = _____ mL        8. 1 kg = _____ g

Using the rules of the metric system, state the acceptable abbreviations for the following units of measure.

9. liter _____     12. gram _____

10. microgram _____     13. kilogram _____

11. milliliter _____

Provide the meaning for the following prefixes.

14. kilo _____     15. milli _____

Using abbreviations and the rules of the metric system, express the following quantities correctly.

16. Six tenths of a gram _____     21. Five thousandths of a gram _____

17. Fifty kilograms _____     22. Six hundredths of a gram _____

18. Four tenths of a milligram _____     23. Two and six tenths milliliters _____

19. Four hundredths of a liter _____     24. One hundred milliliters _____

20. Four and two tenths micrograms ____     25. Three hundredths of a milliliter _____

Convert the following metric measures by moving the decimal.

26. 950 mcg = _____ mg     35. 0.015 g = _____ mg

27. 58.5 L = _____ mL     36. 250 mcg = _____ mg

28. 130 mL = _____ L     37. 8 kg = _____ g

29. 276 g = _____ mg     38. 2 kL = _____ L

30. 550 mL = _____ L     39. 5 L = _____ mL

31. 56.5 L = _____ mL     40. 0.75 L = _____ mL

32. 205 g = _____ kg     41. 0.33 g = _____ mg

33. 0.025 kg = _____ g     42. 750 mg = _____ g

34. 0.056 L = _____ mL     43. 6.28 kg = _____ g

44. 36.5 mg = _____ g          55. 4.5 g = _____ mg

45. 2.2 mg = _____ g           56. 8.6 mg = _____ mcg

46. 400 g = _____ kg           57. 250,000 mcg = _____ mg

47. 0.024 L = _____ mL         58. 40 mg = _____ g

48. 100 mg = _____ g           59. 0.65 kg = _____ g

49. 150 g = _____ mg           60. 37.5 mcg = _____ mg

50. 85 mcg = _____ mg          61. 0.026 mg = _____ mcg

51. 1.25 L = _____ mL          62. 36,000 mg = _____ g

52. 0.05 mg = _____ mcg        63. 0.125 g = _____ mg

53. 120 mg = _____ g           64. 5,524 g = _____ kg

54. 475 mL = _____ L           65. 8,500 mcg = _____ mg

Which of the following is stated correctly using metric abbreviations and rules?

66. .5 g, 0.5 gm, .5 gm, 0.5 g _____

67. 4 KG, 4.0 Kg, Kg 04, 4 kg _____

68. 1500.0 mg, 1,500 MG, 1,500 mg, 1500 mg

69. 1.5 mm, 1.50 mm, $1\frac{1}{2}$ mm, 1.5 Mm

70. cm 2, 2.0 cm, 2 cm, 0.2 cm

71. 80.0 mcg, 080 mcg, 80 mcg, mcg 80

72. mL .7, .7 mL, mL 0.7, 0.7 mL

73. Lasix 20.0 mg, Lasix 20 mg, Lasix 20 MG, Lasix mg 20 _____

74. Gentamicin $1\frac{1}{2}$ mL, gentamicin 1.5 ml, gentamicin 1.5 mL,

    gentamicin $1\frac{1}{2}$ ml _____

75. Ampicillin 500 mg, ampicillin 500.0 mg, ampicillin 500 MG,

    ampicillin mg 500 _____

**Answers on p. 80**

evolve

**80**    UNIT TWO **Systems of Measurement**

## ★ ANSWERS

### Chapter 5

**Answers to Practice Problems**

1.  0.75 g
2.  1.7 mL
3.  0.68 L
4.  7 kg
5.  0.002 mg
6.  0.3 g
7.  6,000 mcg
8.  700 mL
9.  0.18 mg
10. 20 mcg
11. 4,500 mL
12. 4,200 mg
13. 900 mg
14. 3.25 L
15. 0.042 kg
16. 0.529 g
17. 0.645 mg
18. 347,000 mL
19. 238,000,000 mcg
20. 3.5 L
21. 40 g
22. 658,000 g
23. 0.051 L
24. 1,600 mcg
25. 0.028 L

### Answers to Chapter Review

1.  gram (g), liter (L), meter (m)
2.  kilogram (kg)
3.  0.001 L
4.  a. L (liter), mL (milliliter)
    b. g (gram), mg (milligram), mcg (microgram), kg (kilogram)
5.  1 g
6.  1,000 mL
7.  1 mg
8.  1,000 g
9.  L
10. mcg
11. mL
12. g
13. kg
14. one thousand times
15. the thousandth part of
16. 0.6 g
17. 50 kg
18. 0.4 mg
19. 0.04 L
20. 4.2 mcg
21. 0.005 g
22. 0.06 g
23. 2.6 mL
24. 100 mL
25. 0.03 mL
26. 0.95 mg
27. 58,500 mL
28. 0.13 L
29. 276,000 mg
30. 0.55 L
31. 56,500 mL
32. 0.205 kg
33. 25 g
34. 56 mL
35. 15 mg
36. 0.25 mg
37. 8,000 g
38. 2,000 L
39. 5,000 mL
40. 750 mL
41. 330 mg
42. 0.75 g
43. 6,280 g
44. 0.0365 g
45. 0.0022 g
46. 0.4 kg
47. 24 mL
48. 0.1 g
49. 150,000 mg
50. 0.085 mg
51. 1,250 mL
52. 50 mcg
53. 0.12 g
54. 0.475 L
55. 4,500 mg
56. 8,600 mcg
57. 250 mg
58. 0.04 g
59. 650 g
60. 0.0375 mg
61. 26 mcg
62. 36 g
63. 125 mg
64. 5.524 kg
65. 8.5 mg
66. 0.5 g
67. 4 kg
68. 1,500 mg
69. 1.5 mm
70. 2 cm
71. 80 mcg
72. 0.7 mL
73. Lasix 20 mg
74. Gentamicin 1.5 mL
75. Ampicillin 500 mg

# CHAPTER 6
# Apothecary and Household Systems and Additional Measures Used in Medication Administration

## Objectives

*After reviewing this chapter, you should be able to:*

1. Identify reasons for non-use of apothecary measures and symbols
2. State the common household equivalents
3. State specific rules that relate to the household system
4. Identify measures in the household system
5. Define other measures used in medication administration:
   - milliequivalent (mEq)
   - international units
   - unit

## Apothecary System

The apothecary system of measurement is an English system and considered to be one of the oldest systems of measure. It is also referred to as the *fractional system* because parts of units are expressed by using fractions, with the exception of the fraction one-half, which is expressed as *ss* or $\overline{ss}$. The unusual notations, which can be confusing, inclusion of fractions, Roman numerals, and medication errors resulting from its use have caused concern about the use of the apothecary system.

Although the metric system is the preferred system, you may still see remnants of the apothecary system on medication cups (dram). Ounce, which is apothecary, is still used today as part of the household system; however, the apothecary symbol for ounce ($\overline{3}$) should not be used. Some medication labels may still include both apothecary and metric measures. However, many of the newer labels include metric measures only. Many of the newer syringes in use today no longer include a minim scale.

The Institute for Safe Medication Practices (ISMP) has recommended that all medications be prescribed and calculated with metric measures. The United States Pharmacopeia (USP) does not recognize the apothecary system as an official system for measurement of medication dosages. Because of the difficulty encountered with using the apothecary system, the medication errors resulting from its use, and the recommendations of TJC, ISMP, and the Food and Drug Administration (FDA or USFDA), the apothecary system measures and rules will not be focused on. The FDA is often referred to as the "consumer watchdog." The FDA is responsible for protecting and promoting public health through regulation and supervision of products that include food and prescriptions and over-the-counter medications. See Appendix A for discussion of apothecary units, their metric equivalents, and the symbols and abbreviations in the apothecary system that have been identified as error prone and should not be used.

## Household System

Household measures are used most often in the home care setting and less frequently in the clinical setting. The household system is derived from the apothecary system, the least accurate system of measure, and includes approximate equivalents. Conversions between household and metric are based on approximate equivalents, as can be seen with pints and quarts. For example, there are 32 ounces in a quart, which is generally accepted to be 1 liter (1,000 mL). The measures encountered most often include measures such as ounce, tablespoon, and teaspoon, which still appear on most medication cups. With medication errors being one of the most common causes of client harm, and reporting of errors caused by confusion between variable measuring systems, there has been a push by various national organizations to use metric measurements and eliminate these measures to reduce the possibility of errors. It is possible that these measures may be eliminated in the near future.

Dating back to 2009, the ISMP issued a call for practitioners to move to sole use of the metric system for measuring over-the-counter (OTC) and prescription oral doses. In 2011 the ISMP issued its "Statement on the Use of Metric Measurements to Prevent Errors with Oral Liquids." This statement recommended the exclusive use of metric units when prescribing, dispensing, and administering medications, not teaspoon or non-metric measurements (ISMP, 2011). National Alert Network (NAN), which publishes alerts from the National Medication Errors Reporting Program, operated by ISMP, in "Move Toward Full Use of Metric Dosing: Eliminate Dosage Cups That Measure Liquids in Fluid Drams. Use Cups That Measure mL" (June 30, 2015), indicated the recommendation to prevent mix-ups between variable measurement systems. Multiple national organizations have called for the adoption of the metric system (milliliter) as the standard for prescribing and measuring doses of liquid medications. In addition to ISMP and FDA, these organizations include American Academy of Pediatrics (AAP), Centers for Disease Control and Prevention (CDC), and American Pharmacists Association (APhA).

Despite recommendations and some progress toward measuring and prescribing liquids in mL, in 2020 there are still dosing devices used that have household measures, and clients often use utensils in the home to take prescribed medications. Capacities of utensils such as a teaspoon, a tablespoon, and a cup vary from one house to another. When calculating doses or interpreting the health care provider's instructions for the client at home, the nurse must remember that household measures are used. Consequently, the nurse must be able to calculate equivalents for adaptation in the home, even though medication administration spoons, droppers, and medication measuring cups (Figure 6.1) are available.

### Particulars of the Household System

1. There are no standard rules for expressing household measures, which accounts for variations in their use.
2. Standard cookbook abbreviations are used in this system.
3. Arabic numbers and fractions are used to express quantities.
4. The smallest unit of measure in the household system is the drop (gtt).
5. The unit ounce used to measure liquid is sometimes referred to as fluid ounce.

See Box 6.1 for household measures and metric equivalents to memorize.

Metric/household

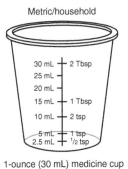

1-ounce (30 mL) medicine cup

**Figure 6.1**   Medicine cup showing metric/household measurements.

## BOX 6.1　Household/Metric Equivalents

| Unit | Abbreviation | Equivalent | Metric Equivalent |
|---|---|---|---|
| teaspoon | t (tsp) | ---------- | 5 mL |
| tablespoon | T (tbs) | 1 T = 3 t | 15 mL |
| ounce (fluid) | oz | 1 oz = 2 T | 30 mL |
| cup (standard measuring) | C | 1 cup = 8 oz | 240 mL |
| pint | pt | 1 pt = 2 cups (16 oz) | 500 mL* |
| quart | qt | 1 qt = 4 cups = 2 pt = 32 oz | 1,000 mL* |
| pound (weight) | lb | 1 lb = 16 oz | 2.2 lb = 1 kg (1,000 g) |

*Note:* The unit "ounce," which is used to measure liquid volume, is sometimes referred to as "fluid ounce."
*Approximate equivalent in the metric system.

### SAFETY ALERT!

Although household utensils may be most familiar to clients, they may invite inaccuracies with medication dosages. Using ordinary household utensils may constitute a safety risk because ordinary household utensils do not come in standard sizes.

- To ensure accurate dosages at home, utensils used should be marked or calibrated. Determine what kind of measuring devices the client is using at home and teach their proper use. Advise clients and their families to use the measuring device provided with the medication or purchase calibrated devices from the pharmacy as opposed to using their kitchen teaspoon, for example.
- Review the household equivalents and abbreviations. Do not confuse the abbreviations for teaspoon (t) and tablespoon (T). 1 teaspoon = 5 mL, and 1 tablespoon = 15 mL; confusing the abbreviations and their equivalents could result in a threefold error.
- Drops should never be used as a measure for medications, because the size of drops varies according to the diameter of the utensil and therefore can be inaccurate. When drops are ordered, the dropper often comes with the medication and should be used only for that medication.
- Anything less than a teaspoon should be measured in a syringe-type device that has no needle, not in a measuring cup.

## Other Medication Measurements Used in Dosage Calculation

Other measurements that may be used to indicate the strength or potency of certain medications include unit, international unit, milliunit, and milliequivalent (mEq). The quantity or amount is expressed using Arabic numbers, with the unit of measure following.

**Units** express the amount of medication present in 1 milliliter (mL) of solution and are specific to the medication for which they are used. Units measure a medication in terms of its action. Medications such as heparin, insulin, and penicillin are measured in the United States Pharmacopeia unit (USP unit). USP unit has been standardized between manufacturers and has been determined by the United States Pharmacopeia (USP). USP is a government agency that sets standards for medications.

**International unit** represents a unit of potency used to measure things such as vitamins and chemicals. These International units represent the amount of medication needed to produce a certain effect and are standardized by international agreement.

**Milliunit** is 1/1,000 of a unit. 1 unit is equal to 1,000 milliunits. Nurses may need to convert units to milliunits. For example, oxytocin (Pitocin) is available in units (10 USP units per 1 mL). Very small doses of oxytocin may be ordered in milliunits. When oxytocin is used to augment labor, the intravenous infusion rate can be 0.5 to 2 milliunits per minute (0.0005 = 0.002 USP units).

**Milliequivalents (mEq)** are used to measure electrolytes (e.g., potassium) and the ionic activity of a medication. The milliequivalent is one thousandth (1/1,000) of the equivalent weight of an ion. The chemist or pharmacist defines milliequivalents as an expression of the number of grams of medication contained in 1 mL of normal solution. Other electrolytes measured in mEq include calcium, magnesium, and sodium.

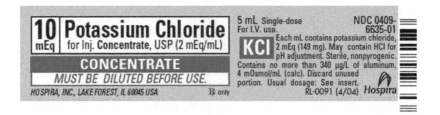

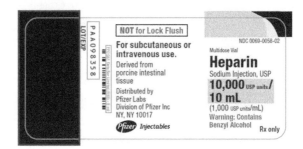

**Figure 6.2** Medication labels showing milliequivalents and units.

The nurse does not have to memorize conversions for the international unit, USP unit, or milliequivalent, because medications that are ordered in these measurements are also prepared and administered in the same system. For example, medications that are ordered in units (such as insulin) will be available in units. Potassium is ordered in milliequivalents and available in milliequivalents. Figure 6.2 shows sample labels of medications in milliequivalents and units.

> ⚠ **SAFETY ALERT!**
> The abbreviations U and IU are prohibited and must be written out (units and international units). The abbreviation U and IU are included on TJC's official "Do Not Use" List (2019) and ISMP's list of Error-Prone Abbreviations, Symbols, and Dose Designations.

> ⚙ **POINTS TO REMEMBER**
> - Teaspoon and tablespoon are common measures used in the household system.
> - For safety, encourage clients to use the measuring device that comes with the medication or a measuring device purchased from the pharmacy.
> - There are no rules for stating household measures.
> - The household system uses fractions and Arabic numerals.
> - Conversions between metric and household measures are approximate equivalents.
> - Dosages less than a teaspoon should be measured with a syringe-type device that does not have a needle attached.
> - When possible, convert household measures to metric measures.
> - When in doubt about an unfamiliar unit or one that is not used often, consult a reference or an equivalency table.
> - No conversion is necessary for unit, international unit, and milliequivalent. Medications prescribed in these measures are available in the same system.
> - 1 unit = 1,000 milliunits. Nurses may have to convert units to milliunits.

---

## 🖩 PRACTICE **PROBLEMS**

Write the abbreviations for the following measures.

1. ounce _____

2. tablespoon _____

3. pint _____

4. teaspoon _____

5. pound _____

6. quart _____

Use Box 6.1 to determine the following equivalents.

7. $\frac{1}{2}$ oz = _____ mL    12. 8 oz = _____ cup

8. 2 tsp = _____ mL    13. 1 oz = _____ T

9. 45 mL = _____ tbs    14. 3 tbs = _____ mL

10. $\frac{1}{2}$ pt = _____ oz    15. 3 pt = _____ mL

11. 90 mL = _____ oz

Write the following amounts correctly using numerals and abbreviations where indicated.

16. 10 ounces _____

17. fifteen units _____

18. sixty-five pounds _____

19. twenty milliequivalents _____

20. two and one-half teaspoons _____

21. three quarts _____

22. fourteen and one-quarter ounces _____

23. ten tablespoons _____

24. What household measure might be used to give $\frac{1}{2}$ ounce of cough syrup?

_____

25. The nurse encouraged a client with diarrhea to drink 40 ounces of water per day.

How many cups does this represent? _____

26. Medications such as penicillin and insulin are commonly measured in _____.

27. The unit used to measure the concentration of serum electrolytes such as potassium and sodium is _____ and is abbreviated _____.

**Answers on p. 86**

---

## ⊙ CHAPTER **REVIEW**

Express the following using numerals and abbreviations where indicated.

1. one-third ounce _____    5. three and one-half quarts _____

2. three million units _____    6. forty-five milliequivalents _____

3. five and one-quarter teaspoons _____    7. five ounces _____

4. ten thousand units _____

Complete the following.

8. Pound is a unit of _____.

9. The abbreviation for drop is _____.

10. T is the abbreviation for _____.

11. The abbreviation t is used for _____.

12. 1 t = _____ mL

13. 1 oz = _____ mL

14. 1 cup = _____ oz

15. 1 tbs = _____ mL

16. 1 pt = _____ oz

17. 1 qt = _____ oz

Express the following notations in words.

18. $8\frac{1}{4}$ oz _____

19. 30 mEq _____

20. 2 pt _____

21. $15\frac{1}{2}$ lb _____

22. 8 tbs _____

23. True or False? The household system of measurement is commonly used for client dosages at home. _____

24. True or False? Units can be abbreviated as U. _____

25. True or False? Household measures are approximate equivalents. _____

**Answers on p. 87**

---

ⓔvolve

For additional information, refer to the Conversions and Equivalents section of the Elsevier's Interactive Drug Calculation Application, Version 1, on Evolve.

---

## ⭐ ANSWERS

### Chapter 6

### Answers to Practice Problems

| | | | | |
|---|---|---|---|---|
| 1. oz | 8. 10 mL | 14. 45 mL | 20. 2½ t, 2½ tsp (varies) | 24. 1 T, 1 tbs (varies) |
| 2. T, tbs | 9. 3 tbs | 15. 1,500 mL | 21. 3 qt, qt 3 | 25. 5 cups |
| 3. pt | 10. 8 oz | 16. 10 oz, oz 10 | 22. 14¼ oz, oz 14¼ | 26. units |
| 4. t, tsp | 11. 3 oz | 17. 15 units | 23. 10 T, 10 tbs (varies) | 27. milliequivalent; mEq |
| 5. lb | 12. 1 cup | 18. 65 lb | | |
| 6. qt | 13. 2 T | 19. 20 mEq | | |
| 7. 15 mL | | | | |

## Answers to Chapter Review

1. $\frac{1}{3}$ oz, oz $\frac{1}{3}$

2. 3,000,000 units

3. $5\frac{1}{4}$ t, $5\frac{1}{4}$ tsp (varies)

4. 10,000 units

5. $3\frac{1}{2}$ qt, qt $3\frac{1}{2}$

6. 45 mEq

7. 5 oz, oz 5

8. weight

9. gtt

10. tablespoon

11. teaspoon

12. 5 mL

13. 30 mL

14. 8 oz

15. 15 mL

16. 16 oz

17. 32 oz

18. eight and one-quarter ounces

19. thirty milliequivalents

20. two pints

21. fifteen and one-half pounds

22. eight tablespoons

23. True

24. False

25. True

# CHAPTER 7
## Converting Within and Between Systems

## Objectives

*After reviewing this chapter, you should be able to:*
1. State the equivalent metric and household approximate equivalents
2. Convert a unit of measure to its equivalent within the same system
3. Convert a unit of measure from one system of measurement to its equivalent in another system of measurement

## Equivalents Among Metric and Household Systems

As noted in earlier chapters dealing with the systems of measure, some measures in one system have equivalents in another; however, equivalents are not exact measures, and there are discrepancies. Several tables have been developed illustrating conversions/equivalents. Sometimes drug companies use different equivalents for a measure.

In the health care system, it is imperative that nurses be proficient in converting among the different systems of measure. Nurses are becoming increasingly responsible for administration of medications to clients and teaching clients and family outside of the conventional hospital setting (e.g., home care). Nurses have become more involved in discharge planning and are responsible for ensuring that the client can safely self-administer medications in the correct dosage. Table 7.1 lists some of the equivalents. You may need to convert between systems. Memorize these common equivalents!

## Converting

The term *convert* means to change from one form to another. Converting can mean changing a measure to its equivalent in the same system or changing a measurement from one system to another system, which is called *converting between systems*. The measurement obtained when converting between systems is **approximate, not exact.** Thus, certain equivalents have been established to ensure continuity.

One of the most important skills needed for calculating dosages is the nurse's ability to make conversions when necessary to administer the ordered amount of medication. The

---

| TABLE 7.1 | Approximate Equivalents to Remember |
|---|---|

1 t = 5 mL
1 T = 3 t = 15 mL
1 oz = 30 mL (2 T)
1 pt = 16 oz (500 mL)
1 qt = 32 oz (2 pt), (1,000 mL)
1 cup (measuring) = 8 oz
16 oz = 1 lb
2.2 lb = 1 kg (1,000 g)
1 in = 2.5 cm

*Note:* Equivalents in the table are those used most often. The preferred and accurate unit for liquid measurements is milliliter (mL).

nurse therefore must understand the system of measurement and be able to convert within the same system and from one system to another with accuracy.

Before beginning the actual process of converting, the nurse should learn the approximate equivalents in the equivalents to remember in Table 7.1 and apply the following important points to make converting simple.

### POINTS TO REMEMBER

1. Memorization of the equivalents/conversions is essential.
2. Think of memorized equivalents/conversions as essential conversion factors, or as a ratio.

   **Example:**   1,000 mg = 1 g is called a conversion factor.
   1,000 mg : 1 g is a ratio.

3. Follow basic math principles, regardless of the conversion method used.
4. Answers should be expressed by applying specific rules that relate to the system to which you are converting.

   **Example:**   The metric system uses decimals; the household system uses fractions.

5. THINK CRITICALLY—select the appropriate equivalent to make conversions (see Table 7.1).

## Methods of Converting
### Moving the Decimal Point

Moving the decimal point is discussed in Chapter 5. Because the metric system is based on the decimal system, conversions within the metric system can be done easily by moving the decimal point. This method cannot be applied in the household system because decimal points are not often used in the system (with the exception of pounds). **Remember the two rules for moving decimal points:**

### RULE

To convert a smaller unit of measure to a larger one in the metric system, divide or move the decimal point three places to the left.

Example:                              350 mg = _____ g
                                  (smaller)   (larger)

Solution:    After determining that mg is the smaller unit and that you are converting to a larger unit (g), recall the conversion factor that allows you to change milligrams to grams (1 g = 1,000 mg). Therefore 350 is divided by 1,000 by moving the decimal point three places to the left, indicating 350 mg = 0.35 g.

$$350mg = .350 = 0.35 \text{ g}$$

*Note:* The final answer is expressed in decimal form. Remember to always place a leading zero (0) in front of the decimal point to indicate a value that is less than 1.

### RULE

To convert a larger unit of measure to a smaller one in the metric system, multiply or move the decimal point three places to the right.

Example:                              0.85 L = _____ mL
                                  (larger)   (smaller)

Solution:      After determining that L is the larger unit and you are converting to a smaller unit (mL), recall the conversion factor that allows you to change liters to milliliters (1 L = 1,000 mL). Therefore 0.85 is multiplied by 1,000 by moving the decimal point three places to the right, indicating 0.85 L = 850 mL.

$$0.850 \text{ L} = 0.850. = 850 \text{ mL}$$

Note the addition of a zero here to allow movement of the decimal point the correct number of places.

---

## ⊞ PRACTICE **PROBLEMS**

For additional practice in converting by decimal movement, convert the following metric measures to the equivalent units indicated.

1. 600 mL = _____ L

2. 0.016 g = _____ mg

3. 15 kg = _____ g

4. 3 mcg = _____ mg

5. 25 mg = _____ g

6. 0.16 kg = _____ g

7. 1.9 L = _____ mL

8. 0.5 g = _____ kg

9. 0.006 mg = _____ mcg

10. 650 mL = _____ L

**Answers on p. 106**

### Using Ratio and Proportion

Using ratio and proportion is one of the easiest ways to make conversions, whether within the same system or between systems. The basics on how to state ratios and proportions and how to solve them when looking for one unknown are presented in Chapter 3. To make conversions using ratio and proportion, a proportion that expresses a numerical relationship between the two systems must be set up. A proportion may be written in linear format or as a fraction when making conversions. Regardless of the format used, there are some basic rules to follow when using this method.

**RULE**

**Rules for Ratio and Proportion**
1. State the known equivalent first (memorized equivalent).
2. Add the incomplete ratio on the other side of the equal sign, making sure the units of measurement are written in the same sequence.

**Example:**                    mg : g = mg : g

3. Label all terms in the proportion, including x. (These labels are not carried when multiplying or dividing.)
4. Solve the problem by using the principles for solving ratios and proportions. (The product of the means equals the product of the extremes.)
5. The final answer for x should be labeled with the appropriate unit of measure or desired unit.

When the method of ratio and proportion are used to make conversions, as with any method used, the known equivalents must be memorized. Stating the proportion in the fraction format may be a way of avoiding confusion with the terms (means and extremes). However, regardless of the format used, the terms must correspond to each other in value and have a relationship. Division should always be carried at least two decimal places to ensure accuracy.

Example:                                 8 mg = _____ g

Solution:    State the known equivalent first, then add the incomplete ratio, making sure
             the units are in the same sequence. Label all the terms in the proportion,
             including $x$.

$$1{,}000 \text{ mg} : 1 \text{ g} \quad = \quad 8 \text{ mg} : x \text{ g}$$

$$\text{(known equivalent)} \quad = \quad \text{(unknown)}$$

Read as "1,000 mg is to 1 g as 8 mg is to $x$ g."

Once the proportion is stated, solve it by multiplying the means (inner terms) and then the
extremes (outer terms). Place the "$x$" product on the left side of the equation.

Result:

$$\overbrace{1{,}000 \text{ mg} : 1 \text{ g} = 8 \text{ mg} : x \text{ g}}^{\text{means}}$$
$$\underbrace{\phantom{1{,}000 \text{ mg} : 1 \text{ g} = 8 \text{ mg} : x \text{ g}}}_{\text{extremes}}$$

$$1{,}000 \times x = 1 \times 8$$

$$\frac{1{,}000\, x}{1{,}000} = \frac{8}{1{,}000}$$

$$x = \frac{8}{1{,}000}$$

$$x = 0.008 \text{ g}$$

Because the measure you are converting to is metric, the fraction is changed to a decimal
by dividing 8 by 1,000 to obtain an answer of 0.008 g. However, because the measures are
metric in this example, perhaps moving the decimal point would be the preferred method
as opposed to actual division.

An alternate way of stating the problem illustrated in the previous example would be
stating it as a fraction and cross-multiplying to solve for $x$.

$$\frac{1{,}000 \text{ mg}}{1 \text{ g}} \times \frac{8 \text{ mg}}{x \text{ g}}$$

$$1{,}000\, x = 8$$

$$\frac{1{,}000\, x}{1{,}000} = \frac{8}{1{,}000}$$

$$x = 0.008 \text{ g}$$

Another way of writing a ratio and proportion to eliminate errors is to set up the conversion problem in a fraction format.

Place the conversion factor first (numerator), and place the problem underneath matching up the units (the denominator); then cross-multiply to solve for $x$.

Example:                              8 mg = ____ g

$$\frac{1{,}000 \text{ mg}}{8 \text{ mg}} \times \frac{1 \text{ g}}{x \text{ g}}$$

$$1{,}000\, x = 8$$

$$\frac{1{,}000\, x}{1{,}000} = \frac{8}{1{,}000}$$

$$x = 0.008 \text{ g}$$

The remainder of this chapter will show examples of the methods used in converting
within the same system and between systems.

## Converting Within the Same System

Converting within the same system is often seen with metric measures; however, it can be done using the household system of measurement, such as one household measure being converted to an equivalent within the household system. Any one of the methods discussed can be used, but movement of decimal points is limited to the metric system as shown in previous examples. Ratio and proportion can be used for all systems set up in a fraction or linear format as illustrated.

**Dimensional Analysis.**  Dimensional analysis is a conversion method that has been used in chemistry and other sciences and will be discussed in more detail in Chapter 15. Dimensional analysis involves manipulation of units to get the desired unit. This method can be used for conversion in all systems. As with other methods discussed, you must know the conversion factor (equivalent).

### Steps for Converting Using Dimensional Analysis:
1. Identify the desired unit you are converting to.
2. Write the conversion factor (equivalent) in fraction format so that the desired unit is in the numerator of the fraction. This is written first in the equation, followed by a multiplication sign ($\times$). (Notice the unit in the numerator is the same as the unit you desire.)
3. Write the unit in the successive numerator to match the unit of measure in the previous denominator.
4. Cancel the alternate denominator/numerator units to leave the unit desired (being calculated).
5. Perform the mathematical process indicated.

**Example:**   (metric)   (metric)

$$0.12 \text{ kg} \quad \text{to} \quad \text{g}$$

**Solution:**  You want to cancel the kilograms and obtain the equivalent amount in grams. Begin by identifying the unknown, in this case, g. Because 1 kg = 1,000 g, the fraction that will allow you to cancel kg is $\dfrac{1,000 \text{ g}}{1 \text{ kg}}$.

$$x \text{ g} = \frac{1,000 \text{ g}}{1 \text{ kg}} \times \frac{0.12 \text{ kg}}{1}$$

**Note:** The unit you want to cancel is always written in the denominator of the fraction. Then proceed by placing as the next numerator the same label as the first denominator, in this case, kg.

**Note:** Placing a 1 under a number does not change its value.

$$\text{Cancel the units } x \text{ g} = \frac{1,000 \text{ g}}{1 \text{ k\!g}} \times \frac{0.12 \text{ k\!g}}{1}$$

$$1,000 \times 0.12 = 120$$

$$x = 120 \text{ g}$$

**Answer:**   0.12 kg is equivalent to 120 g.

---

### 🖩 PRACTICE **PROBLEMS**

Convert the following measures to the equivalent units indicated.

11. 1,700 mL = _____ L       13. 1.4 L = _____ mL

12. 4 kg = _____ g       14. 1 mL = _____ L

15. 4.5 mg = _____ mcg      21. 1,600 mL = _____ L

16. 0.004 L = _____ mL      22. 0.015 L = _____ mL

17. 6.5 L = _____ mL      23. 0.18 g = _____ mg

18. 60 g = _____ kg      24. 25 mcg = _____ mg

19. 600 mg = _____ g      25. 5.2 g = _____ kg

20. 0.736 mg = _____ mcg      **Answers on p. 106**

## Converting Between Systems

The methods presented previously can be used to change a measure in one system to its equivalent in another, or the conversion factor method can be used. This method requires that you consider the size of units. To convert from a larger unit to a smaller unit of measure, you multiply by the conversion factor as shown in Example 1. To convert from a smaller to a larger unit of measure, you must divide by the conversion factor.

**Example 1:**                (household)  (metric)

$$4 \text{ oz} = \text{\_\_\_\_\_ mL}$$

(large)       (small)

---

### ✓ Solution Using Conversion Factor Method

Equivalent: 1 oz = 30 mL

Conversion factor is 30.

An ounce is larger than a milliliter.

Multiply 4 by 30 to obtain 120.

**Answer:**      120 mL

*Alternative:* Express the conversion in proportion format and solve for *x*. (One way to remember this method is to remember that it is the known or have : want to know or have.)

---

### ✓ Solution Using Ratio and Proportion

$$1 \text{ oz} : 30 \text{ mL} = 4 \text{ oz} : x \text{ mL}$$

$$x = 30 \times 4 = 120$$

$$x = 120 \text{ mL}$$

*or*

$$\frac{1 \text{ oz}}{30 \text{ mL}} = \frac{4 \text{ oz}}{x \text{ mL}}$$

$$x = 4 \times 30 = 120$$

$$x = 120 \text{ mL}$$

*or*

$$\frac{1 \text{ oz}}{4 \text{ oz}} = \frac{30 \text{ mL}}{x \text{ mL}}$$

## ✓ Solution Using Dimensional Analysis

Here you want to cancel oz to find the equivalent amount in mL. Because 1 oz = 30 mL, the fraction you desire so that you can cancel oz is:

$$\frac{30 \text{ mL}}{1 \text{ oz}}$$

Therefore:

$$x \text{ mL} = \frac{30 \text{ mL}}{1 \cancel{\text{oz}}} \times 4 \cancel{\text{oz}}$$

$$x = 30 \times 4 = 120$$

$$x = 120 \text{ mL}$$

120 mL is equivalent to 4 oz

Example 2:                    (household)   (metric)

110 lb = _____ kg

## ✓ Solution Using Conversion Factor Method

Equivalent: 1 kg = 2.2 lb

Conversion factor is 2.2.

A pound is smaller than a kilogram; 110 is divided by 2.2.

Answer:     50 kg

## ✓ Solution Using Ratio and Proportion

$$1 \text{ kg} : 2.2 \text{ lb} = x \text{ kg} : 110 \text{ lb}$$

$$\frac{2.2x}{2.2} = \frac{110}{2.2}$$

$$x = 50 \text{ kg}$$

or

$$\frac{1 \text{ kg}}{2.2 \text{ lb}} = \frac{x \text{ kg}}{110 \text{ lb}}$$

or

$$\frac{1 \text{ kg}}{x \text{ kg}} = \frac{2.2 \text{ lb}}{110 \text{ lb}}$$

## ✓ Solution Using Dimensional Analysis

Here you want to cancel lb to find the equivalent amount in kg. Because 1 kg = 2.2 lb, the fraction you desire so that you can cancel lb is:

$$\frac{1 \text{ kg}}{2.2 \text{ lb}}$$

Therefore:

$$x \, kg = \frac{1 \, kg}{2.2 \, \cancel{lb}} \times \frac{110 \, \cancel{lb}}{1}$$

$$x = \frac{110}{2.2}$$

$$x = 50 \, kg$$

Example 3:                    (metric)   (household)

$$55 \, cm = \underline{\hspace{2cm}} \, in$$

---

### ✓ Solution Using Conversion Factor Method

Equivalent: 1 in = 2.5 cm

Conversion factor is 2.5

A cm is smaller than an inch (in); 55 is divided by 2.5.

Answer:      22 in

---

### ✓ Solution Using Ratio and Proportion

$$2.5 \, cm : 1 \, in = 55 \, cm : x \, in$$

$$\frac{2.5x}{2.5} = \frac{55}{2.5}$$

$$x = 22 \, in$$

*or*

$$\frac{2.5 \, cm}{1 \, in} = \frac{55 \, cm}{x \, in}$$

*or*

$$\frac{2.5 \, cm}{55 \, cm} = \frac{1 \, in}{x \, in}$$

---

### ✓ Solution Using Dimensional Analysis

Here you want to cancel cm to find the equivalent amount in inches (in). Because 2.5 cm = 1 in, the fraction you desire so that you can cancel cm is:

$$\frac{1 \, in}{2.5 \, cm}$$

Therefore:

$$x \, in = \frac{1 \, in}{2.5 \, \cancel{cm}} \times \frac{55 \, \cancel{cm}}{1}$$

$$x = \frac{55}{2.5}$$

$$x = 22 \, in$$

Answer:      22 in is equivalent to 55 cm

## Calculating Intake and Output

The nurse often converts between systems to calculate a client's **intake and output**. Intake and output is abbreviated **I&O**. *Intake* refers to the monitoring of fluids a client takes orally (p.o.), by feeding tube, or parenterally. Oral intake includes fluids and solids that become liquid at body and room temperature, such as gelatin and Popsicles. Intake also includes water, broth, tea, juice, and coffee. Water taken with medications is also considered intake. Solids such as bread, cereal, or meats are not considered in fluid intake. Intravenous (IV) fluids and continuous and intermittent intravenous piggyback (IVPB) and blood components are considered intake. One of the main purposes of IVPB is to infuse medications on an intermittent basis (e.g., antibiotics q6h). It can also be used to infuse additional fluids. The medication is diluted in a specific volume of IV fluid. The nurse documents the volume of fluid administered in the IVPB as parenteral fluid on the I&O, and the medication administered on the medication record. Liquid output refers to fluids that exit the body, such as diarrhea, vomitus (emesis), gastric suction, urine, and drainage from postsurgical wounds or other tubes. A client's intake and output are usually recorded on a special form called an *intake and output flow sheet* (or I&O flow sheet or record) (Figure 7.1), which varies from institution to institution. In some institutions where the charting is computerized, the I&O may be recorded in the computer. A variety of clients require I&O monitoring, such as those whose fluids are restricted and those who are receiving diuretic or intravenous (IV) therapy.

Intake and output may still be recorded at some institutions using cubic centimeters or milliliters. The preferred term for volume is milliliters. Milliliters will be used throughout this text. When measuring output, the nurse uses a graduated receptacle calibrated in metric measures (mL), and conversions are not necessary. Oral intake usually must be converted from household measures to metric measures before it can be recorded. Each time a client takes oral liquids, even those administered with medications, the amount and time are recorded on the appropriate form. The total intake and output are recorded at the end of each shift and also totaled for a 24-hour period.

| Juice glass | – 180 mL | Jell-O cup | – 150 mL |
|---|---|---|---|
| Water glass | – 210 mL | Ice cream | – 120 mL |
| Coffee cup | – 240 mL | Creamer | – 30 mL |
| Soup bowl | – 180 mL | | |
| Small water cup | – 120 mL | | |

Addressograph with Client Information

Date ___*October 30, 2020*___

| INTAKE | | | | | | OUTPUT | | | | |
|---|---|---|---|---|---|---|---|---|---|---|
| ORAL | | | IV | | | | | | OTHER | |
| TIME | TYPE | AMT | TIME | TYPE | AMOUNT ABSORBED | TIME | URINE | STOOL | | |
| 8A | Juice | 60 mL | | | | | | | | |
| | Coffee | 120 mL | | | | | | | | |
| | Milk | 250 mL | | | | | | | | |
| | | | | | | | | | | |
| | | | | | | | | | | |
| | | | | | | | | | | |
| | | | | | | | | | | |
| | | | | | | | | | | |

**Figure 7.1** Sample I&O flow sheet.

Conversion of a client's intake is usually required when recording measurements such as a bowl or coffee cup. Each agency usually has an I&O sheet with a ledger that indicates the standard measurement for the utensils used in its facility. For example, it may indicate that a standard cup is 6 oz or a coffee cup is 180 mL. A client's oral intake is calculated in the same manner as other conversion problems. After each item is converted, the items are added together for the total intake. Intake and output are based on the conversion factor 1 oz = 30 mL.

**Example 1:** Calculate the client's intake for breakfast in milliliters. Assume that the glass holds 6 oz and the cup holds 8 oz. The client had the following for breakfast at 8 AM:

| Items | Conversion Factors |
|---|---|
| ⅓ glass of apple juice | 1 oz = 30 mL |
| 2 sausages* | 1 pint = 500 mL |
| 1 boiled egg* | 1 cup = 8 oz |
| ½ cup of coffee | 1 glass = 6 oz |
| ½ pint of milk | |

*The 2 sausages and 1 boiled egg are not part of fluid intake.

## Solution:

1. ⅓ glass of apple juice

$$1 \text{ glass} = 6 \text{ oz}; \frac{1}{3} \text{ of } 6 \text{ oz} = 2 \text{ oz}$$

Therefore 1 oz = 30 mL, 2 oz × 30 mL = 60 mL

### ✓ Solution Using Ratio and Proportion

1 oz : 30 mL = 2 oz : $x$ mL, $x$ = 60 mL (ratio and proportion)

### ✓ Solution Using Dimensional Analysis

$$x \text{ mL} = \frac{30 \text{ mL}}{1 \text{ oz}} \times \frac{2 \text{ oz}}{1}$$

2. ½ cup of coffee

$$1 \text{ cup} = 8 \text{ oz}; \frac{1}{2} \text{ of } 8 \text{ oz} = 4 \text{ oz}$$

Therefore 4 oz × 30 = 120 mL

### ✓ Solution Using Ratio and Proportion

1 oz : 30 mL = 4 oz : $x$ mL, $x$ = 120 mL

### ✓ Solution Using Dimensional Analysis

$$x \text{ mL} = \frac{30 \text{ mL}}{1 \text{ oz}} \times \frac{4 \text{ oz}}{1}$$

3. ½ pint of milk

$$1 \text{ pint} = 500 \text{ mL}; \frac{1}{2} \text{ of } 500 \text{ mL} = 250 \text{ mL}$$

4. Total mL = 60 mL + 120 mL + 250 mL = 430 mL

Another solution would be to total the number of ounces (6 oz in this example). Convert ounces to milliliters, and add the half pint of milk (expressed in milliliters).

---

### ✓ Solution Using Ratio and Proportion

$$1 \text{ oz} : 30 \text{ mL} = 6 \text{ oz} : x \text{ mL}$$

$$x = 180 \text{ mL}$$

$$180 \text{ mL} + 250 \text{ mL} = 430 \text{ mL}$$

---

### ✓ Solution Using Dimensional Analysis

$$x \text{ mL} = \frac{30 \text{ mL}}{1 \cancel{\text{ oz}}} \times \frac{6 \cancel{\text{ oz}}}{1}$$

The conversions are recorded on an I&O flow sheet (or record) next to the time ingested. The I&O sheet in Figure 7.1 is filled out with the data for this sample problem.

8:00 AM      juice, 60 mL      coffee, 60 mL      milk, 250 mL

Let's look at a more complex I&O calculation. This can be done applying the same principles and methods shown in the previous example:

**Example:**   A client receives 75 mL/hr of IV fluid from 7 AM to 3 PM. The client also consumes the following:

**Breakfast:**   3 oz juice
$1\frac{1}{2}$ cups coffee (cup = 8 oz)
**Lunch:**   $\frac{3}{4}$ bowl of broth (bowl = 6 oz)
4 oz gelatin dessert

At 3 PM the client's foley catheter is emptied of 800 mL of urine and a surgical drain emptied of 75 mL.

(a)  How many milliliters will you record for the intake? _____

(b)  How many milliliters will you record for the output? _____

### Solution:

1. 75 mL/hr of IV fluid from 7 AM to 3 PM

   7 AM to 3 PM = 8 hr      75 mL × 8 = 600 mL/8 hr

2. **Oral intake:**

   - 3 oz juice, 1 oz = 30 mL, 3 × 30 mL = 90 mL
   - $1\frac{1}{2}$ cups coffee, 1 cup = 8 oz; $1\frac{1}{2}$ × 8 oz = 12 oz;
     therefore 1 oz = 30 mL = 12 × 30 = 360 mL
   - $\frac{3}{4}$ bowl of broth, 1 bowl = 6 oz; $\frac{3}{4}$ of 6 oz = $4\frac{1}{2}$ oz;
     1 oz = 30 mL, $4\frac{1}{2}$ × 30 = 135 mL
   - 4 oz gelatin, 1 oz = 30 mL, 4 × 30 = 120 mL

3. Add the milliliters to get the total intake

   600 mL IV fluid + 705 mL oral intake (90 mL + 360 mL + 135 mL + 120 mL)

   Total intake is:      600 mL (IV)
                    + 705 mL (oral)
                       1,305 mL

*Note:* This could have also been done using any of the methods shown in the previous example. Here you could have also gotten the total ounces, which is $23\frac{1}{2}$ in this example (then converted ounces to milliliters and added the IV solution in milliliters to get the total).

4. The output is in milliliters; no conversion is needed.
   **Add the mL:** 800 mL (urine) + 75 mL (surgical drain) = 875 mL
   Total intake recorded = 1,305 mL
   Total output recorded = 875 mL

In addition to oral intake, if a client is receiving IV therapy, the amount of IV fluid given is also recorded on the I&O flow sheet (or record). When an IV bottle or bag is hung or added, the nurse indicates the time and the type and amount of fluid in the appropriate column on the sheet (or record). When the IV fluid has infused or the IV is changed, the nurse records the actual amount of fluid **infused,** or **absorbed.**

In a situation in which a bag or bottle of IV fluid is not completed by the end of the shift, the nurse beginning the next shift is informed of how much fluid is left in the bag. At some institutions, the amount is also indicated on the I&O flow sheet (or record) with the abbreviation LIB (left in bag or bottle). As already stated, IV fluids given intermittently such as IVPB are also recorded as parenteral intake and recorded every shift on the I&O indicating the amount of fluid that that has been administered in the IVPB.

**Example:** The nurse hangs a 1,000 mL bag of DsW at 7 AM. The client also receives 1 g of an antibiotic in 100 mL of 0.9% normal saline (NS) at 9 AM. The nurse records the 100 mL as being absorbed. At 3 PM, 150 mL is left in the IV bag. The nurse records 850 mL was absorbed from the IV and indicates 150 mL is LIB. Refer to the sample I&O form in Figure 7.2, which shows how this example is charted.

| Juice glass – 180 mL | Small water cup – 120 mL |
|---|---|
| Water glass – 210 mL | Jell-O cup – 150 mL |
| Coffee cup – 240 mL | Ice cream – 120 mL |
| Soup bowl – 180 mL | Creamer – 30 mL |

Client information

**Date:** September 21, 2020

| INTAKE | | | | | | OUTPUT | | | |
|---|---|---|---|---|---|---|---|---|---|
| Time | Type | Amt | Time | IV/ blood type | Amount absorbed | Time | Urine | Stool | Other |
|  |  |  | 7A | D5W 1,000 mL | 850 mL |  |  |  |  |
|  |  |  | 9A | IVPB | 100 mL |  |  |  |  |
|  |  |  |  |  |  |  |  |  |  |
|  |  |  |  |  |  |  |  |  |  |
|  |  |  |  |  |  |  |  |  |  |
|  |  |  |  |  |  |  |  |  |  |
|  |  |  |  |  |  |  |  |  |  |
|  |  |  |  |  |  |  |  |  |  |
| 8 hr total |  |  |  |  | 950 mL |  |  |  |  |
|  |  |  | 3P | D5W 150 mL LIB |  |  |  |  |  |

**Figure 7.2** Charting IV fluids on an I&O flow sheet. *IVPB,* Intravenous piggyback; *LIB,* left in bag.

I&O flow sheets usually have a place for recording p.o. intake and IV intake and a column or columns for output. Figure 7.3 shows a sample 24-hour I&O flow sheet illustrating the charting of intake.

As discussed, output is also recorded on the I&O form. The most commonly measured output is urine. After a client's output is recorded, sometimes the nurse needs to compute an average. The most important average nurses compute in most health care settings is the hourly urine output. The **hourly** urine output for an adult to maintain proper renal function is 30 mL/hr to 50 mL/hr. Usually, the hourly amount is more significant than each voiding. To find the hourly average of urinary output, take the total and divide by the number of hours.

Example: $\dfrac{400 \text{ mL of urine}}{8 \text{ hr}} = 50 \text{ mL of urine/hr}$

The charting of I&O varies at each institution. Always check the policies to ensure compliance with a particular institution.

| Juice glass – 180 mL | Small water cup – 120 mL |
|---|---|
| Water glass – 210 mL | Jell-O cup – 150 mL |
| Coffee cup – 240 mL | Ice cream – 120 mL |
| Soup bowl – 180 mL | Creamer – 30 mL |

**Client information**

**Date:** September 21, 2020

| INTAKE | | | | | OUTPUT | | | | |
|---|---|---|---|---|---|---|---|---|---|
| Time | Type | Amt | Time | IV/ blood type | Amount absorbed | Time | Urine | Stool | Other |
| 8A | juice | 240 mL | 7A | D5W 1,000 mL | 850 mL | 8A | 400 mL | | |
| | milk | 120 mL | 12n | IVPB | 50 mL | 10A | 450 mL | | |
| | coffee | 200 mL | | | | 1³⁰/P | 450 mL | | |
| 9³⁰/A | water | 60 mL | | | | | | | |
| 12P | broth | 180 mL | | | | | | | |
| | juice | 120 mL | | | | | | | |
| 1P | water | 120 mL | | | | | | | |
| | | | | | | | | | |
| 8 hr total | | 1,040 mL | | | 900 mL | | 1,300 mL | | |
| 5P | tea | 100 mL | 3P | D5W 150 mL  LIB | 150 mL | 4p | 425 mL | | |
| | broth | 360 mL | 5P | D5W 1,000 mL | 750 mL | 7p | 400 mL | | |
| | ice-cream | 120 mL | 6P | IVPB | 50 mL | 9³⁰/P | 350 mL | | |
| 9 P | water | 240 mL | | | | | | | |
| | | | | | | | | | |
| | | | | | | | | | |
| 8 hr total | | 820 mL | | | 950 mL | | 1,175 mL | | |
| 1A | water | 120 mL | 11P | D5W 250 mL  LIB | 250 mL | | | | |
| 5A | tea | 200 mL | | | | 2A | 350 mL | | |
| | | | 12A | IVPB | 50 mL | 5A | 150 mL | | |
| | | | 3A | D5W 1,000 mL | 500 mL | | | | |
| | | | 6A | IVPB | 50 mL | | | | |
| | | | | | | | | | |
| | | | | | | | | | |
| 8 hr total | | 320 mL | | | 850 mL | | 500 mL | | |
| 24 hr total | | 2,180 mL | | | 2,700 mL | | 3,275 mL | | |

Total intake 24 hr: (4,880 mL)    (2,180 mL + 2,700 mL)

Total output 24 hr: (3,275 mL)    (1,300 mL + 1,175 mL + 800 mL)

**Figure 7.3** I&O flow sheet (completed 24 hours). *IVPB,* Intravenous piggyback; *LIB,* left in bag.

## ▦ PRACTICE **PROBLEMS**

Convert the following to the equivalent measures and express answer to two decimal places as indicated.

26. 60 lb = _____ kg        34. 178.2 lb = _____ kg

27. 187.5 cm = _____ in        35. 20 mL = _____ tsp

28. 66 lb = _____ kg        36. 3 oz = _____ T

29. $3\frac{1}{2}$ pt = _____ oz        37. 4 qt = _____ mL

30. 7 oz = _____ mL        38. 72 kg = _____ lb

31. 250 mL = _____ qt        39. 3 in = _____ cm

32. 45 mL = _____ tbs        40. 2.4 L = _____ mL

33. 10 cm = _____ in

Compute how much IV fluid you would document on an I&O form as being absorbed from a 1,000-mL bag if the following amounts remain.

41. 300 mL _____        43. 100 mL _____

42. 450 mL _____

Compute the average hourly urinary output in the following situations (round to nearest whole number).

44. 650 mL in 8 hr _____        46. 1,000 mL in 24 hr _____

45. 250 mL in 8 hr _____        47. 1,240 mL in 24 hr _____

48. A client's output for the 3 to 11 PM shift was as follows:

   325 mL of urine at 4:00 PM
    75 mL of vomitus at 7:00 PM
   225 mL of urine at 8:00 PM
   200 mL of nasogastric (NG) drainage at 11:00 PM
    50 mL of wound drainage at 11:00 PM
   What is the total output in milliliters? _____

49. What is the client's output in liters in question 48? _____

50. If 375 mL of a 500-mL bag of IV solution were absorbed on the 3 to 11 PM shift, the nurse records that 375 mL was absorbed. How many milliliters are recorded as left in bag (LIB)? _____

51. A client had the following during an 8-hour shift:

   • 125 mL/hr of IV fluid from 7 AM to 1 PM
   • 250 mL of packed red blood cells from 1 PM to 3 PM

   **Breakfast:**    $2\frac{1}{2}$ cup of coffee (cup = 6 oz)
                     $\frac{1}{2}$ glass of juice (glass = 4 oz)
   **Lunch:**       $1\frac{1}{2}$ bowls of broth (bowl = 6 oz)
                     3 oz milk

The client voided four times during the shift:

350 mL, 275 mL, 450 mL, and 300 mL of urine

Calculate the I&O for the 8-hour shift in milliliters

a. Intake mL _____

b. Output mL _____

**Answers on p. 106**

---

**POINTS TO REMEMBER**

- Regardless of the method used for converting, **memorizing equivalents** is a necessity.
- Answers stated in fraction format should be **reduced** as necessary.
- When more than one equivalent is learned for a unit of measure, use the **most common equivalent** for the measure or use the number that divides equally without a remainder.
- Division should be carried to the hundredths place or two decimal places to ensure accuracy, and it is not rounded.
- Decimal point movement as a method for converting is limited to the metric system; ratio and proportion, dimensional analysis, and conversion factor method can be used for all systems of measure.
- Oral intake is converted before placing data on an I&O flow sheet (or record). The amount is usually recorded in cubic centimeters at some institutions; however, milliliter is the correct unit for volume. Conversion factor for I&O is 1 oz = 30 mL.
- Always check the policy of the institution regarding I&O and the charting of it.
- The most common units of measure used to calculate dosages are metric units of measurement.

---

## ◉ CHAPTER **REVIEW**

Convert the following to the equivalent measures indicated.

1. 0.007 g = _____ mg    12. 1.6 L = _____ mL

2. 1 mg = _____ g    13. 47 kg = _____ lb

3. 6,000 g = _____ kg    14. 3 mL = _____ L

4. 5 mL = _____ L    15. 75 lb = _____ kg

5. 0.45 L = _____ mL    16. 36 mg = _____ g

6. 45 mL = _____ oz    17. $4\frac{1}{2}$ pt = _____ mL

7. 1.8 mg = _____ mcg    18. 0.25 mg = _____ mcg

8. 23 g = _____ kg    19. 82 kg = _____ g

9. 6.5 mcg = _____ mg    20. 6,172 g = _____ kg

10. $3\frac{1}{2}$ oz = _____ mL    21. 200 mL = _____ tsp

11. 1,200 mL = _____ oz    22. 102 lb = _____ kg

23. 204 g = _____ kg        32. 67.5 mL = _____ t

24. 1.5 L = _____ mL        33. 66.25 cm = _____ in

25. 200 mcg = _____ mg        34. 16 t = _____ mL

26. 48.6 L = _____ mL        35. 20 oz = _____ mL

27. 0.7 L = _____ mL        36. 16 mcg = _____ mg

28. $9\frac{1}{2}$ oz = _____ T        37. 75 tsp = _____ mL

29. 4 tsp = _____ mL        38. 10 mL = _____ oz

30. 1.8 mg = _____ g        39. 4 kg = _____ lb

31. 2 tbs = _____ mL        40. 3.25 mg = _____ mcg

Calculate the fluid intake in milliliters. Use the following equivalents for the problems below: 1 cup = 8 oz, 1 glass = 4 oz.

41. Client had the following at lunch:
    4 oz fruit cocktail
    1 tuna fish sandwich
    $\frac{1}{2}$ cup of tea
    $\frac{1}{4}$ pt of milk

    Total mL = _____

42. Calculate the following individual items and give the total number of milliliters:
    3 Popsicles (3 oz each)
    $\frac{1}{2}$ qt iced tea
    $1\frac{1}{2}$ glasses water
    12 oz soft drink

    Total mL = _____

43. Client had the following:
    8 oz milk
    6 oz orange juice
    4 oz water with medication

    Total mL = _____

44. Client had the following:
    10 oz of coffee
    8 oz water
    6 oz vegetable broth

    Total mL = _____

45. Client had the following:
    $\frac{3}{4}$ glass of milk
    4 oz water
    2 oz beef broth

    Total mL = _____

46. A client had the following at lunch:
    $\frac{1}{4}$ glass of apple juice
    8 oz chicken broth
    6 oz gelatin dessert
    $1\frac{3}{4}$ cups of coffee

    Total mL = _____

Convert the following amounts of fluid to milliliters.

47. $9\frac{1}{2}$ oz = _____ mL        48. $\frac{3}{4}$ C (8 oz cup) = _____ mL

Compute how much IV fluid you would document on an I&O form as being absorbed from a 1,000-mL bag if the following amounts are left in the bag.

49. 275 mL _____        51. 75 mL _____

50. 550 mL _____

Compute the average hourly urinary output in each of the following situations (round to nearest whole number).

52. 500 mL in 8 hr _____    54. 700 mL in 8 hr _____

53. 640 mL in 24 hr _____

Compute how much IV fluid you would document on an I&O form as being absorbed from a 500-mL bag if the following amounts are left in the bag.

55. 125 mL _____

56. 225 mL _____

57. A client received 1,750 mL of IV fluid. How many liters of IV fluid did the client receive? _____

58. A client has an order for 125 mcg of digoxin. How many milligrams will you administer to the client? _____

59. The prescriber directs a client to take 15 oz of the laxative agent GoLYTELY. The cup holds 6 oz. How many cups will the client have to drink? _____

60. A client has an order for 1,500 mL of water by mouth every 24 hours. How many ounces is this? _____

61. A client had an output of 1.1 L. How many milliliters is this? _____

62. The prescriber orders 2 ounces of a liquid medication for a client. How many tablespoons should the client take? _____ tbs

63. A client is given a prescription for 7.5 mL of a cough suppressant every four hours. The client will be using a measuring device that is calibrated in teaspoons. How much medication should the client take for each dose? _____ tsp

64. A client weighed 95 kg on the initial visit to the clinic. When the client reported for the subsequent visit the client reported losing 11 lb. What is the client's current weight in kg? _____ kg

65. A client is instructed to drink 2,500 mL of water per day. How many quarts of water should the client be instructed to drink? _____ qt

66. An infant's head circumference is 45 cm. The parents ask for the equivalent in inches. You tell the parents their infant's head circumference is _____ in.

67. A client drank 24 ounces of water. How many cups did the client drink? _____ cups

68. A client needs to drink $1\frac{1}{2}$ ounces of an elixir per day. How many tablespoons would this be equivalent to? _____ tbs

69. A client consumed $2\frac{1}{2}$ pints of water in a day. How many cups of water is this equivalent to? _____ cups

70. An infant drinks 4 ounces of a ready-to-feed formula every 3 hours during the day and night. The formula comes in a quart container. How many quarts of formula should the mother buy for a 7-day supply? _____ qt

71. Calculate the total fluid intake in mL for 24 hours.

    **Breakfast:**  5 oz milk
    2 oz orange juice
    4 oz water with medication
    **Lunch:**      12 oz ginger ale
    **Snack:**      10 oz hot tea
    2 oz gelatin dessert
    **Dinner:**     4 oz water
    6 oz apple juice
    3 oz chicken broth
    **Snack:**      3 oz Jell-O
    8 oz iced tea
    6 oz water with medication

    Total = _____ mL

72. Calculate the client intake for 12 hours (7 AM to 7 PM).
    The client receives intravenous fluids at 100 mL/hr from 7 AM to 3 PM, 300 mL of packed red blood cells from 3 PM to 5 PM, and 50 mL/hr of IV fluid from 5 PM to 7 PM.

    **Breakfast:**  4 oz orange juice
    8 oz hot tea
    **Lunch:**      8 oz milk
    **Dinner:**     4 oz hot tea

73. How many milliliters will you record on the I&O for the intake? _____
    A client's intake and output was the following for 8 hours:

    *Intake:*
    1.2 L of IV fluid

    **Breakfast:**  1½ cups of tea (cup = 6 oz)
    **Lunch:**      1 can ginger ale (can = 12 oz)
    **Dinner:**     1 bowl chicken broth (bowl = 6 oz)

    *Output:*
    Foley catheter: 1,200 mL of urine
    Surgical drain: 100 mL
    Calculate the I&O in milliliters.

    a. Total intake _____

    b. Total output _____

**Answers on p. 106**

# ⭐ ANSWERS

## Chapter 7
### Answers to Practice Problems

1. 0.6 L
2. 16 mg
3. 15,000 g
4. 0.003 mg
5. 0.025 g
6. 160 g
7. 1,900 mL
8. 0.0005 kg
9. 6 mcg
10. 0.65 L
11. 1.7 L

12. 4,000 g
13. 1,400 mL
14. 0.001 L
15. 4,500 mcg
16. 4 mL
17. 6,500 mL
18. 0.06 kg
19. 0.6 g
20. 736 mcg
21. 1.6 L
22. 15 mL

23. 180 mg
24. 0.025 mg
25. 0.0052 kg
26. 27.27 kg
27. 75 in, in 75
28. 30 kg
29. 56 oz, oz 56
30. 210 mL
31. 1/4 qt, qt 1/4
32. 3 tbs, tbs 3
33. 4 in, in 4

34. 81 kg
35. 4 tsp, tsp 4
36. 6 T, T 6
37. 4,000 mL
38. 158.4 lb *or*
   $158\frac{2}{5}$ lb, lb 158.4
   *or* lb $158\frac{2}{5}$
39. 7.5 cm
40. 2,400 mL
41. 700 mL

42. 550 mL
43. 900 mL
44. 81 mL/hr
45. 31 mL/hr
46. 42 mL/hr
47. 52 mL/hr
48. 875 mL
49. 0.875 L
50. 125 mL
51. a. 1,870 mL
    b. 1,375 mL

### Answers to Chapter Review

1. 7 mg
2. 0.001 g
3. 6 kg
4. 0.005 L
5. 450 mL
6. oz $1\frac{1}{2}$, $1\frac{1}{2}$ oz
7. 1,800 mcg
8. 0.023 kg
9. 0.0065 mg
10. 105 mL
11. 40 oz, oz 40
12. 1,600 mL
13. 103.4 lb, $103\frac{2}{5}$ lb
14. 0.003 L
15. 34.09 kg

16. 0.036 g
17. 2,250 mL
18. 250 mcg
19. 82,000 g
20. 6.172 kg
21. 40 tsp, tsp 40
22. 46.36 kg
23. 0.204 kg
24. 1,500 mL
25. 0.2 mg
26. 48,600 mL
27. 700 mL
28. T 19, 19 T
29. 20 mL
30. 0.0018 g
31. 30 mL
32. $13\frac{1}{2}$ t, t $13\frac{1}{2}$

33. $26\frac{1}{2}$ in, in $26\frac{1}{2}$
34. 80 mL
35. 600 mL
36. 0.016 mg
37. 375 mL
38. $\frac{1}{3}$ oz, oz $\frac{1}{3}$
39. 8.8 lb, $8\frac{4}{5}$ lb
40. 3,250 mcg
41. 245 mL
42. 1,310 mL
43. 540 mL
44. 720 mL
45. 270 mL
46. 870 mL
47. 285 mL

48. 180 mL
49. 725 mL
50. 450 mL
51. 925 mL
52. 63 mL/hr
53. 27 mL/hr
54. 88 mL/hr
55. 375 mL
56. 275 mL
57. 1.75 L
58. 0.125 mg
59. $2\frac{1}{2}$ cups
60. 50 oz, oz 50
61. 1,100 mL
62. T 4, 4 T

63. t $1\frac{1}{2}$, tsp $1\frac{1}{2}$, $1\frac{1}{2}$ t, $1\frac{1}{2}$ tsp
64. 90 kg
65. qt $2\frac{1}{2}$, $2\frac{1}{2}$ qt
66. 18 in, in 18
67. 3 cups
68. tbs 3, T 3, 3 tbs, 3 T
69. 5 cups
70. qt 7, 7 qt
71. 1,950 mL
72. 1,920 mL
73. a. 2,010 mL
    b. 1,300 mL

ⓔvolve

For additional information, refer to the Conversions and Equivalents section of the Elsevier's Interactive Drug Calculation Application, Version 1, on Evolve.

# Additional Conversions Useful in the Health Care Setting

## Objectives

*After reviewing this chapter, you should be able to:*

1. Convert between Celsius and Fahrenheit temperature
2. Convert between units of length: inches, centimeters, and millimeters
3. Convert between units of weight: pounds and kilograms, pounds and ounces to kilograms
4. Convert between traditional and international time

## Converting Between Celsius and Fahrenheit

Most health care facilities use electronic digital temperature thermometers, which instantly convert between the two scales (*Celsius* and *Fahrenheit*), rather than mercury thermometers. The mercury in glass thermometers, which was once the standard device, has been eliminated from health care facilities because of the environmental hazards of mercury. However, such devices do not eliminate the need for the nurse to understand the important difference between Celsius and Fahrenheit. In addition, it may be necessary for the nurse to explain to clients or families how to convert from one to another. Another factor is the recognition that all persons involved in client care do not have a "universal" measurement for temperature; therefore Fahrenheit or Celsius may be used.

Let's look first at some general information that will help you understand the formulas used.

### Differentiating Between Celsius and Fahrenheit

To differentiate which scale is being used (Fahrenheit or Celsius), the temperature reading is followed by an *F* or *C*. *F* indicates Fahrenheit, and *C* indicates Celsius. (*Note:* Celsius was formerly known as *centigrade*.)

Examples:    98°F
                36°C

The freezing point of water on the Fahrenheit scale is **32°F,** and the boiling point is **212°F.** The freezing point of water on the Celsius scale is **0°C,** and the boiling point is **100°C.**

The difference between the freezing and boiling points on the Fahrenheit scale is **180°,** whereas the difference between these points on the Celsius scale is **100°.**

The differences between Fahrenheit and Celsius in relation to the freezing and boiling points led to the development of appropriate conversion formulas. Figure 8.1 shows two thermometers reflecting the relationship of pertinent values between the two scales. The glass thermometers shown in Figure 8.1 are for illustration purposes only. As previously stated, electronic digital thermometers are commonly used in health care settings.

The **32° difference** between the freezing point on the scales is used for converting temperature from one scale to the other. As previously stated, there is a **180°** difference between the boiling and freezing points on the Fahrenheit thermometer and **100°** between the boiling

**Figure 8.1** Celsius and Fahrenheit temperature scales. (From Clayton BD, Willihnganz M: *Basic pharmacology for nurses*, ed. 17, St. Louis, 2017, Mosby.)

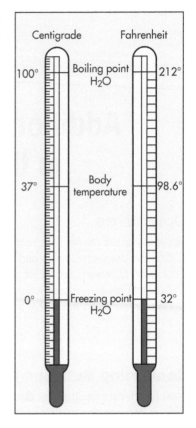

and freezing points on the Celsius scale. These differences can be set as a ratio, 180 : 100. Therefore consider the following:

$$180 : 100 = \frac{180}{100} = \frac{9}{5}$$

The fraction $\frac{9}{5}$ expressed as a decimal is 1.8; therefore you will see this constant used in temperature conversions.

## Formulas for Converting Between Fahrenheit and Celsius Scales

**RULE**

To convert from Celsius to Fahrenheit, multiply by 1.8 and add 32.

$$°F = 1.8(°C) + 32$$

*or*

$$°F = \frac{9}{5}(°C) + 32$$

**Example:**  Convert 37.5°C to °F.

$$°F = 1.8(37.5) + 32$$
$$°F = 67.5 + 32$$
$$°F = 99.5°$$

*or*

$$°F = \frac{9}{5}(37.5) + 32$$
$$°F = 67.5 + 32$$
$$°F = 99.5°$$

**RULE**

To convert from Fahrenheit to Celsius, subtract 32 and divide by 1.8.

$$°C = \frac{°F - 32}{1.8} \qquad or \qquad °C = (°F - 32) \div \frac{9}{5}$$

**Example:** Convert 68°F to °C.

$$°C = \frac{68 - 32}{1.8} \qquad\qquad °C = (68 - 32) \div \frac{9}{5}$$

$$°C = \frac{36}{1.8} \qquad or \qquad °C = 36 \div \frac{9}{5}$$

$$°C = 20° \qquad\qquad °C = (36) \times \frac{5}{9}$$

$$°C = 20°$$

**Note:** Thermometers are calibrated in tenths when converting between Fahrenheit and Celsius; if necessary, carry the math process to the hundreds and round to tenths.

## ▦ PRACTICE **PROBLEMS**

Convert the following temperatures as indicated (round your answer to tenths).

1. 4°C = _____ °F     4. 101.3°F = _____ °C

2. 101°F = _____ °C     5. 37.5°C = _____ °F

3. 38.1°C = _____ °F

Change the given temperatures in the following statements to their corresponding equivalents in °C or °F (round your answer to tenths).

6. Store medication at room temperature: 20° to 25°C. _____ °F

7. Notify health care provider for temperature greater than 101°F. _____ °C

8. Store vaccine serum at 7°F. _____ °C

9. Normal adult body temperature is 37°C. _____ °F

10. Do not store IV solutions at less than 46°F. _____ °C

**Answers on p. 120**

In addition to temperature conversions, other measures that may be encountered in the health care setting relate to linear measurement. As with temperature conversion, even though there are devices that instantly convert these measures, nurses need to understand the process. For the purpose of this chapter, we will focus on millimeters (mm) and centimeters (cm).

### Metric Measures Relating to Length

In health care settings, metric measures relating to length include the following:
- Diameter of the pupil of the eye may be described in millimeters (mm); the normal diameter of pupils is 3 to 7 mm. Charts may show pupillary size in millimeters.
- Accommodation of pupils is tested by asking a client to gaze at a distant object (e.g., a far wall) and then at a test object (e.g., a finger or pencil) held by the examiner approximately 10 centimeters (cm) (4 in) from the bridge of the client's nose.
- A baby's head and chest circumference are expressed in centimeters.
- Gauze for dressings is available in different size squares measured in centimeters. Example: 10 × 10 cm (4 × 4 in); 5 × 5 cm (2 × 2 in)
- Length of an incision may be expressed in measures such as centimeters.

Refer to the conversions in Box 8.1.

| BOX 8.1 Conversions Relating to Length |
| --- |
| 1 cm = 10 mm<br>1 in = 2.54 cm* |

*The approximate conversion of 1 in = 2.5 cm is used for conversions.

Now let's try some conversions using these equivalents.

**Example 1:** A client's incision measures 25 mm. How many centimeters is this?

**Conversion factor:** 1 cm = 10 mm

**Solution:** Think: mm is smaller and cm is larger. Divide by 10, or move the decimal point one place to the left.

$$25 \div 10 = 2.5 \text{ cm } or \text{ } 25_{,} = 2.5 \text{ cm}$$

**Answer:** 2.5 cm

**Example 2:** Convert 30 cm to inches (in).

**Conversion factor:** 1 in = 2.5 cm

**Solution:** Think: smaller to larger (divide).

$$30 \div 2.5 = 12 \text{ in}$$

**Answer:** 12 in

**Example 3:** An infant's head circumference is 35.5 cm. How many millimeters is this?

**Conversion factor:** 1 cm = 10 mm

**Solution:** Think: larger to smaller (multiply). Multiply by 10, or move the decimal point one place to the right.

$$35.5 \times 10 = 355 \text{ mm } or \text{ } 35.5 = 355 \text{ mm}$$

**Answer:** 355 mm

*Any methods presented in previous chapters may be used for converting. Decimal movement, however, is limited to conversions of one metric measure to another.

## PRACTICE **PROBLEMS**

Convert the following to the equivalent indicated.

11. A gauze pad for a dressing is

10 cm _____ in

12. A client's incision measures

45 mm _____ cm

13. An infant's head circumference is

    37.5 cm _____ mm

14. A newborn is $20\frac{1}{2}$ in long

    _____ cm

15. 14.8 in = _____ cm

16. 6.5 cm = _____ in

17. 100 in = _____ cm

18. An infant's chest circumference is

    32 cm _____ in

19. An infant's head circumference is

    38 cm _____ in

20. A newborn is 20 in long

    _____ cm

    **Answers on p. 120**

## Conversions Relating to Weight

Determination of body weight is important for calculating dosages in adults, children, and, because of the immaturity of their systems, even more so in infants and neonates. This chapter focuses on converting weights for adults and children. Medications such as heparin are more therapeutic when based on weight in kilograms. The most frequently used calculation method for pediatric medication administration is milligrams per kilogram. Some medications are calculated in micrograms per kilogram.

Because medication dosages in drug references are usually based on kilograms, it is essential to be able to convert from pounds to kilograms. However, the nurse also needs to know how to do the opposite (convert from kilograms to pounds). In addition, because a child's weight may be in pounds and ounces, conversion of these units to kilograms is also important. Knowledge of weight conversions is an important part of general nursing knowledge.

### Converting Pounds to Kilograms

> **RULE**
>
> Equivalent: 2.2 lb = 1 kg
> To convert lb to kg, divide by 2.2 (think smaller to larger).
> The answer is rounded to the nearest tenth.

**Example 1:** A child weighs 65 lb. Convert to kilograms.

$$65 \div 2.2 = 29.54 = 29.5 \text{ kg}$$

**Example 2:** An adult weighs 135 lb. Convert to kilograms.

$$135 \div 2.2 = 61.36 = 61.4 \text{ kg}$$

### Converting Weight in Pounds and Ounces to Kilograms

**Step 1:** Convert the ounces to the nearest tenth of a pound, and **add** this to the total pounds.

Equivalent: 16 oz = 1 lb

**Step 2:** Convert the total pounds to kilograms, and round to the nearest tenth.

Equivalent: 2.2 lb = 1 kg

**Example 1:** A child's weight is 10 lb, 2 oz.

Think: smaller to larger.

$2 \text{ oz} \div 16 = 0.12 = 0.1 \text{ lb}$

$10 \text{ lb} + 0.1 \text{ lb} = 10.1 \text{ lb}$

Think: smaller to larger.

$10.1 \div 2.2 = 4.59 = 4.6 \text{ kg}$

**Example 2:** A child's weight is 7 lb, 4 oz.

$4 \text{ oz} \div 16 = 0.25 = 0.3 \text{ lb}$

$7 \text{ lb} + 0.3 \text{ lb} = 7.3 \text{ lb}$

$7.3 \div 2.2 = 3.31 = 3.3 \text{ kg}$

---

##  PRACTICE **PROBLEMS**

Convert the following weights to kilograms (round to the nearest tenth).

21. 6 lb, 5 oz = _____ kg        23. 10 lb, 4 oz = _____ kg

22. 12 lb, 2 oz = _____ kg       24. 7 lb, 12 oz = _____ kg

Convert the following weights in pounds to kilograms (round to the nearest tenth where indicated).

25. 20 lb = _____ kg        28. 121 lb = _____ kg

26. 64 lb = _____ kg        29. 85 lb = _____ kg

27. 22 lb = _____ kg        **Answers on p. 120**

### Converting Kilograms to Pounds

> **RULE**
> Equivalent: 2.2 lb = 1 kg
> To convert kilograms to pounds, multiply by 2.2. (Think: larger to smaller.)
> Answer is expressed to the nearest tenth.

**Example 1:** A child weighs 24.7 kg. Convert to pounds.

$$(24.7) \times 2.2 = 54.34 = 54.3 \text{ lb}$$

**Example 2:** An adult weighs 72.2 kg. Convert to pounds.

$$(72.2) \times 2.2 = 158.84 = 158.8 \text{ lb}$$

Any of the methods presented in Chapter 7 can be used for converting pounds to kilograms and kilograms to pounds, except decimal movement. Remember, pounds can be expressed using a decimal.

## ▦ PRACTICE **PROBLEMS**

Convert the following weights in kilograms to pounds (round to the nearest tenth where indicated).

30. 20 kg = _____ lb     33. 10.4 kg = _____ lb

31. 46 kg = _____ lb     34. 34.9 kg = _____ lb

32. 98.2 kg = _____ lb     35. 5.8 kg = _____ lb

**Answers on p. 120**

## Military Time

Another conversion that is necessary for the nurse to know because it is being used more frequently is the conversion of traditional time using the 24-hour clock. The 24-hour clock is commonly referred to as *military time, international time,* or *24-hour time.* Although some watches and clocks are manufactured with traditional time and military time visible on the face to eliminate confusion, it is important to understand how to read and write military time for avoiding errors.

### Traditional Time 12-Hour Clock

- Provides a source for error in medication administration.
- Uses 12 numbers (1–12) to represent morning and evening hours (Figure 8.2).
- Each time occurs twice a day. For example, the hour 7:00 is recorded as both 7:00 AM and 7:00 PM. The abbreviation "AM" means ante meridian or before noon; "PM" means post meridian or after noon. The times 7 AM and 7 PM may look very similar if the A and P are not clear or not written, which could result in errors and the client receiving the medication at the wrong time.
- The use of the colon (:) to separate hours from minutes. Hours are represented by Arabic numbers to the left of the colon, and minutes are to the right of the colon. For example, 11:30 (11 = hours, 30 = minutes).
- Day starts at 12:00 AM, and ends at 11:59 PM.

### Military Time 24-Hour Clock

- Military time is a 24-hour clock. Uses 0 to 24 to represent the hours of the day (Figure 8.3).
- Main advantage of using military time is that it prevents errors in documentation and medication errors because numbers are not repeated. Each time occurs once per day. Example 7:00 AM is written as 0700, whereas 7:00 PM is written as 1900.
- Use of a four-digit number without the colon and AM and PM. The first two digits represent the hours; the last two digits, the minutes. For example, 1130 (11 = hours, 30 = minutes).
- The day begins after 0000 (midnight); the first minute of the day is 0001, and the day ends at 2400 (midnight). The minutes between 2400 (midnight) and 0100 (1:00 AM) are written as 0001, 0002…0058, 0059.
- Both 0000 and 2400 represent midnight. The time 0000 is commonly used by the military and read as "zero hundred"; 2400 is read as "twenty-four hundred."
- Although still referred to as military time, a more accurate term is "international time."

Many health care facilities are using military time in documentation such as nursing notes and medication administration records and to document treatments. Use of military time prevents misinterpretation about when a therapeutic measure is due, such as medications, and is less problematic.

### Rules for Conversion to Military Time (International Time)

**RULE**

To convert AM time: omit the colon and AM and ensure that a 4-digit number is written, adding a zero in the beginning as needed.

**Example:**    8:45 AM = 0845

**RULE**

To convert PM time: omit the colon and PM; add 1200 to time.

**Example:**    7:50 PM = 750 + 1200 = 1950

### Rules for Converting to Traditional Time

**RULE**

To convert AM time: insert the colon, add AM, and delete any zero in front of number.

**Example:**    0845 = 8:45 AM

**RULE**

To convert PM time: subtract 1200, insert the colon, and add PM.

**Example:**    1950 = 1950 − 1200 = 7:50 PM

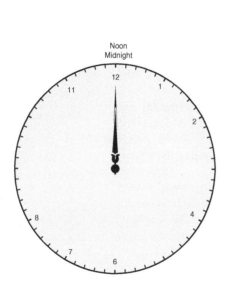

**Figure 8.2** Traditional 12-hour clock.

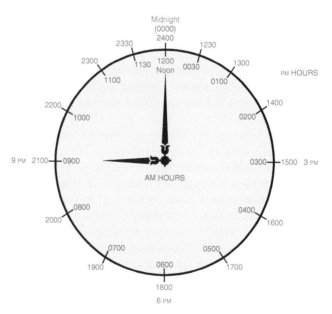

**Figure 8.3** 24-hour clock.

## ▦ PRACTICE **PROBLEMS**

Convert the following traditional times to military (international) time.

36. 7:30 AM = _____

37. 10:30 AM = _____

38. 8:10 PM = _____

39. 5:45 PM = _____

40. 12:16 AM = _____

41. 6:20 AM = _____

42. 1:30 PM = _____

43. 11:45 AM = _____

44. 11:58 PM = _____

45. 2:10 AM = _____

Convert the following military (international) times to traditional (AM/PM) time.

46. 0207 = _____

47. 1743 = _____

48. 0004 = _____

49. 0240 = _____

50. 1259 = _____

51. 0525 = _____

52. 1620 = _____

53. 1050 = _____

54. 1830 = _____

55. 1200 = _____

**Answers on p. 120**

## Calculating Completion Times

As you will see in Chapter 21, the nurse can determine the time an intravenous (IV) bag will be completed or empty using military time (international time) or traditional time depending on institutional policy. Now that we have discussed the conversion of time, let's briefly look at how to determine completion times in military and traditional time. This will be discussed in more detail in Chapter 21.

**Determining Completion Time in Military (International Time).** Calculation of completion time is easier when military time is used to set up and work the problem.

- Identify the start time of the IV using military time.
- Add the infusion time in hours and minutes to the start time.
- If the added infusion time exceeds 2400, subtract 2400 from the total. As the saying goes, there are only 24 hours in a day, and the day ends at 2400. Subtracting 2400 will give you the correct completion time, which would be the next day.
- When calculating the completion time, if the minutes are equal to or greater than 60 minutes, subtract 60 from the number of minutes and then add the equivalent 1 hour (60 minutes = 1 hour) to the hours.

**Example 1:** An IV is started at 0800 to be completed in 6 hours. Determine the completion time.

- Add the infusion time to the 0800-start time.

$$\begin{array}{r} 0800 \\ + 0600 \\ \hline \end{array}$$

**Completion time:** 1400 or 2:00 PM.

**Example 2:** An IV is started at 0650 to be completed in 4 hours and 30 minutes. Determine the completion time.

- Add the infusion time to the 0650-start time.

$$
\begin{array}{r}
0650 \\
+\ 0430 \\
\hline
1080 \text{ (the minutes are greater than 60; 80 minutes)}
\end{array}
$$

$$
\begin{array}{r}
1080 \\
-\ 0060 \text{ minutes (1 hour)} \\
\hline
1020 \\
+\ 0100 \text{ (add the 1 hour obtained when you} \\
\text{subtracted the 60 minutes)}
\end{array}
$$

**Completion time:** 1120 or 11:20 AM

**Example 3:** An IV is started at 2100 to be completed in 10 hours. Determine the completion time.

- Add the infusion time to the 2100-start time.

$$
\begin{array}{r}
2100 \\
+\ 1000 \\
\hline
3100 \text{ (the time here is greater than 2400)}
\end{array}
$$

$$
\begin{array}{r}
3100 \\
-\ 2400 \\
\hline
\end{array}
$$

**Completion time:** 0700 or 7:00 AM (the next day)

### Traditional Time Calculations

**Example 1:** An IV medication is to infuse in 30 minutes that was started at 6:15 PM. Determine the completion time.

- Add the 30-minutes infusion time to the 6:15 PM start time.

$$
\begin{array}{r}
6:15 \text{ PM} \\
+\ 30 \text{ min} \\
\hline
\end{array}
$$

**Completion time:** 6:45 PM

**Example 2:** An IV with an infusion time of 12 hours is started at 2:00 AM. Determine the completion time.

- Add the 12-hour infusion time to the 2:00 AM start time.

$$
\begin{array}{r}
2:00 \text{ AM} \\
+\ 12:00 \\
\hline
14:00
\end{array}
$$

$$
\begin{array}{r}
14:00 \\
-\ 12:00 \text{ (subtract 12 hours)} \\
\hline
\end{array}
$$

**Completion time:** 2:00 PM

## ▦ PRACTICE **PROBLEMS**

Calculate the following completion times in military (international) time.

56. An IV started at 0215 to infuse in 2 hr 30 min _____

57. An IV started at 0250 to infuse in 5 hr 10 min _____

58. An IV started at 0900 is to infuse in 6 hr 30 min _____

Calculate the following completion times in traditional time.

59. An IV started at 6:30 AM that has an infusion time of 45 min _____

60. An IV started at 7:05 PM that has an infusion time of 8 hr _____

**Answers on p. 120**

---

**POINTS TO REMEMBER**

Use these formulas to convert between Fahrenheit and Celsius temperature.

- To convert from °C to °F: $°F = 1.8 \,(°C) + 32$ $or \dfrac{9}{5}(°C) + 32$.

- To convert from °F to °C: $°C = \dfrac{°F - 32}{1.8}$ $or \,(°F - 32) \div \dfrac{9}{5}$.

- When converting between Fahrenheit and Celsius, carry math to hundredths and round to tenths.

**Conversions Relating to Length**

- Conversions can be made by using any of the methods presented in the chapter on conversions; however, moving of decimals is limited to converting between metric measures.

$$1 \text{ cm} = 10 \text{ mm}$$
$$1 \text{ inch} = 2.5 \text{ cm}$$

**Conversions Relating to Weight**

$$2.2 \text{ lb} = 1 \text{ kg}$$
$$16 \text{ oz} = 1 \text{ lb}$$

- Weight conversion of pounds to kilograms is done most often because many medications are based on kilograms of body weight.
- Body weight is **essential** for determining dosages in infants and neonates.
- To convert pounds to kilograms, divide by 2.2. Round answer to the nearest tenth.
- To convert pounds and ounces to kilograms, convert the ounces to the nearest tenth of a pound; add this to the total pounds. Convert the total pounds to kilograms and round answer to the nearest tenth.
- To convert kilograms to pounds, multiply by 2.2. Round answer to the nearest tenth.

**Conversions Relating to Time**

- The 24-hour clock is also referred to as military time, international time, or 24-hour time.
- To change traditional AM time to military time, omit the colon and AM and make sure that a 4-digit number is written, adding a zero in the beginning as needed.
- To change traditional PM time to military time, omit the colon and PM and add 1200 to the time.
- To convert military time to traditional AM time, insert a colon and add AM. Delete any zero in front of numbers.
- To convert military time to traditional PM time, subtract 1200, insert the colon, and add PM.
- When calculating completion times in military (international time):
  - If the added infusion time exceeds 2400, subtract 2400 from the total. There are only 24 hours in a day, and the day ends at 2400. Subtracting 2400 will give you the correct completion time, which would be the next day.
  - When calculating the completion time, if the minutes are equal to or greater than 60 minutes, subtract 60 from the number of minutes and then add the equivalent 1 hour (60 minutes = 1 hour) to the hours.

## ⊙ CHAPTER **REVIEW**

For each of the following statements, change the given temperature to its corresponding equivalent in °C or °F. (Round to the nearest tenth.)

1. Notify health care provider for temperature greater than 101.4°F. _____ °C

2. Store medication at room temperature, 77°F. _____ °C

3. Store medication within temperature range of 15°C to 30°C. _____ °F

4. An infant has a body temperature of 36.5°C. _____ °F

5. Store vaccine at 6°C. _____ °F

6. A nurse reports a temperature of 37.8°C. _____ °F

7. Do not expose a medication to temperatures greater than 84°F. _____ °C

8. A medication contains a crystalline substance with a melting point of about
   186°C. _____ °F

9. Store vaccine at 4°C. _____ °F

10. Do not expose medication to temperatures greater than 88°F. _____ °C

Convert temperatures as indicated. Round your answer to the nearest tenth.

11. −10°C = _____ °F        18. 64.4°F = _____ °C

12. 0°F = _____ °C          19. 35°C = _____ °F

13. 102.8°F = _____ °C      20. 50°F = _____ °C

14. 29°C = _____ °F         21. 39.8°C = _____ °F

15. 106°C = _____ °F        22. 86°F = _____ °C

16. 70°F = _____ °C         23. 41°C = _____ °F

17. 39.6°C = _____ °F

Convert the following to the equivalent indicated. Do NOT round off.

24. 18 in = _____ cm        30. 4 in = _____ cm

25. 31 cm = _____ in        31. 36.6 cm = _____ mm

26. 44.5 cm = _____ mm      32. 6.2 in = _____ cm

27. 32 in = _____ cm        33. 350 mm = _____ in

28. 3 cm = _____ mm         34. $21\frac{1}{2}$ in = _____ cm

29. 7.9 cm = _____ mm       35. 2 in = _____ mm

Convert the following weights in pounds to kilograms (round to the nearest tenth where indicated).

36. 63 lb = _____ kg      39. 81 lb = _____ kg

37. 150 lb = _____ kg      40. 27 lb = _____ kg

38. 78 lb = _____ kg

Convert the following weights in kilograms to pounds (round to the nearest tenth of a pound where indicated).

41. 77.3 kg = _____ lb      44. 9 kg = _____ lb

42. 7 kg = _____ lb      45. 56.1 kg = _____ lb

43. 4.5 kg = _____ lb

46. A child weighs 70 lb during a pediatric clinic visit. How many kilograms does the child weigh? (Round to the nearest tenth.) _____

47. A client's wound measures 41 mm. How many centimeters is this? _____ cm

48. A client weighs 99.2 kg. How many pounds does the client weigh? (Round to the nearest tenth.) _____ lb

49. An infant's head circumference is 40 cm. How many inches is this? _____ in

50. An infant's head circumference is 40.6 cm. How many millimeters is this? _____ mm

Convert the following weights to kilograms. (Round to the nearest tenth as indicated.)

51. 7 lb, 1 oz = _____ kg      54. 8 lb, 10 oz = _____ kg

52. 9 lb, 3 oz = _____ kg      55. 5 lb, 5 oz = _____ kg

53. 10 lb, 12 oz = _____ kg

Convert the following military (international) times to traditional times (AM/PM).

56. 0032 = _____      58. 1345 = _____

57. 0220 = _____      59. 2122 = _____

Convert the following traditional times to military (international) times.

60. 5:20 AM = _____      62. 4:30 PM = _____

61. 12:00 midnight = _____      63. 1:35 PM = _____

State the following completion times as indicated.

64. An IV started at 1905 that has an infusion time of 8 hr _____ (military time).

65. An IV with a start time of 1245 that has an infusion time of 5 hr 30 min _____ (military time).

66. An IV started at 1900 that has an infusion time of 12 hr _____ (military time).

67. An IV started at 0245 to infuse over 5 hours and 30 minutes _____ (military time, and traditional).

68. An IV started at 11:50 PM with an infusion time of 3 hr 30 min _____ (traditional).

69. An IV started at 0025 with an infusion time of 1 hr 15 min _____ (military time and traditional time).

70. An IV started at 4:45 AM that has an infusion time of 9 hr 40 min _____ (traditional time).

**Answers on p. 121**

---

## ⭐ ANSWERS

### Chapter 8
### Answers to Practice Problems

| | | | | |
|---|---|---|---|---|
| 1. 39.2°F | 13. 375 mm | 25. 9.1 kg | 37. 1030 | 49. 2:40 AM |
| 2. 38.3°C | 14. 51.25 cm | 26. 29.1 kg | 38. 2010 | 50. 12:59 PM |
| 3. 100.6°F | 15. 37 cm | 27. 10 kg | 39. 1745 | 51. 5:25 AM |
| 4. 38.5°C | 16. 2.6 in | 28. 55 kg | 40. 0016 | 52. 4:20 PM |
| 5. 99.5°F | 17. 250 cm | 29. 38.6 kg | 41. 0620 | 53. 10:50 AM |
| 6. 68°F to 77°F | 18. 12.8 in | 30. 44 lb | 42. 1330 | 54. 6:30 PM |
| 7. 38.3°C | 19. 15.2 in | 31. 101.2 lb | 43. 1145 | 55. 12:00 PM (noon) |
| 8. −13.9°C | 20. 50 cm | 32. 216 lb | 44. 2358 | 56. 0445 |
| 9. 98.6°F | 21. 2.9 kg | 33. 22.9 lb | 45. 0210 | 57. 0800 |
| 10. 7.8°C | 22. 5.5 kg | 34. 76.8 lb | 46. 2:07 AM | 58. 1530 |
| 11. 4 in | 23. 4.7 kg | 35. 12.8 lb | 47. 5:43 PM | 59. 7:15 AM |
| 12. 4.5 cm | 24. 3.5 kg | 36. 0730 | 48. 12:04 AM | 60. 3:05 AM |

ⓔvolve

For additional information, refer to the Conversions and Equivalents section of the Elsevier's Interactive Drug Calculation Application, Version 1, on Evolve.

## Answers to Chapter Review

| | | | | |
|---|---|---|---|---|
| 1. 38.6°C | 16. 21.1°C | 31. 366 mm | 45. 123.4 lb | 59. 9:22 PM |
| 2. 25°C | 17. 103.3°F | 32. 15.5 cm | 46. 31.8 kg | 60. 0520 |
| 3. 59°F to 86°F | 18. 18°C | 33. 14 in | 47. 4.1 cm | 61. 2400 |
| 4. 97.7°F | 19. 95°F | 34. 53.75 cm | 48. 218.2 lb | (0000 used in military) |
| 5. 42.8°F | 20. 10°C | 35. 50 mm | 49. 16 in | 62. 1630 |
| 6. 100°F | 21. 103.6°F | 36. 28.6 kg | 50. 406 mm | 63. 1335 |
| 7. 28.9°C | 22. 30°C | 37. 68.2 kg | 51. 3.2 kg | 64. 0305 |
| 8. 366.8°F | 23. 105.8°F | 38. 35.5 kg | 52. 4.2 kg | 65. 1815 |
| 9. 39.2°F | 24. 45 cm | 39. 36.8 kg | 53. 4.9 kg | 66. 0700 |
| 10. 31.1°C | 25. 12.4 in | 40. 12.3 kg | 54. 3.9 kg | 67. 0815, 8:15 AM |
| 11. 14°F | 26. 445 mm | 41. 170.1 lb | 55. 2.4 kg | 68. 3:20 AM |
| 12. −17.8°C | 27. 80 cm | 42. 15.4 lb | 56. 12:32 AM | 69. 0140, 1:40 AM |
| 13. 39.3°C | 28. 30 mm | 43. 9.9 lb | 57. 2:20 AM | 70. 2:25 PM |
| 14. 84.2°F | 29. 79 mm | 44. 19.8 lb | 58. 1:45 PM | |
| 15. 222.8°F | 30. 10 cm | | | |

# UNIT THREE

## Methods of Administration and Calculation

Note: The safe and accurate administration of medications to a client is an important and primary responsibility of a nurse. Being able to read and interpret an order correctly and calculate medication dosages is necessary for accurate administration.

# CHAPTER 9
# Medication Administration

## Objectives

*After reviewing this chapter, you should be able to:*

1. State the consequences of medication errors
2. Identify the causes of medication errors
3. Identify the role of the nurse in preventing medication errors
4. Identify the role of the Institute for Safe Medication Practices (ISMP) and The Joint Commission (TJC) in the prevention of medication errors
5. State the basic six "rights" of safe medication administration
6. Identify factors that influence medication dosages
7. Identify the common routes for medication administration
8. Define *critical thinking*
9. Explain the importance of critical thinking in medication administration
10. Identify important critical thinking skills necessary in medication administration
11. Discuss the importance of client teaching
12. Identify special considerations relating to the elderly and medication administration
13. Identify home care considerations in relation to medication administration

## Medication Errors

Medications are therapeutic measures aimed at improving a client's health and are a primary form of treatment for most illnesses. Safe medication administration is not just a nursing responsibility, it requires the collaborative effort of all health care providers, drug manufacturers, health care organizations, clients, and their families. To promote safety in medication administration, everyone must be vigilant in embracing safety as a priority. According to the Emergency Care Research Institute (ECRI), numerous studies show a link between a positive safety culture (where safety is a shared priority) and improved patient safety within a health care organization. A safety culture is viewed as an organization's shared perceptions, beliefs, values, and attitudes that combine to create a commitment to safety and effort to minimize harm (ECRI Institute, 2019). When medication errors occur, the consequences can be harmful and threatening to the life of a client. According to the National Coordinating Council for Medication Error Reporting and Prevention (NCC-MERP), a medication error is defined as follows:

> A medication error is any preventable event that may cause or lead to inappropriate medication use or patient harm while the medication is in the control of the health care professional, patient, or consumer. Such events may be related to professional practice, health care products, procedures, and systems, including prescribing, order communication, product labeling, packaging, and nomenclature, compounding, dispensing, distribution, administration, education, monitoring, and use.

Outcomes from medication errors include increased hospital stay, increased health care costs, acute or chronic disability, and even death. Additional indirect consequences can affect the nurse involved both emotionally and professionally and could result in loss of position, legal consequences, or loss of license to practice.

According to NCCMERP, experts estimate that as many as 98,000 people die in any given year from medical errors that occur in hospitals. A significant number of these deaths are due to medication errors. In addition, NCCMERP believes there is no acceptable incidence rate for medication errors. Every health care organization's goal should be to continually improve systems to prevent harm to patients resulting from medication errors.

With the increased focus on client safety and creating a "culture of safety," it is no surprise that medication safety is linked to a health organization's ability to attract clients, meet the requirements of accreditation, and obtain reimbursement for services. Publications regarding the numerous medication errors have caused astonishment among members of the health care profession, national organizations, and society as a whole. According to current literature, despite considerable effort, technological advances, preventive strategies, and systematic methods of reporting errors, medication errors continue to be one of the most prevailing causes of client harm.

*To Err is Human: Building a Safer Health System,* published by the Institute of Medicine (IOM, 1999), brought awareness to the number of annual deaths ascribed to preventable medical errors, including medication errors. Information concerning medication errors has serious implications for the health and safety of clients and warrants a collaborative approach with numerous strategies to prevent future errors. A focus on safety has implications for those involved in the education of nurses as well, with safety being a central concept. The critical role of nurses in medication safety (prevention of errors) is a primary focus of this text and is based on the knowledge and understanding of careful, correct, and safe medication administration.

Reporting of significant or sentinel events that result in client harm has become an expectation from those involved in health care delivery. Promotion of a "culture of safety" has become a focus and priority to prevent harm to those entrusted to the health care system.

## Organizations Involved in Safe Medication Practices

There are many health care groups, government and nongovernment agencies, and professional organizations that address patient safety issues, establish standards, and make recommendations in health care to advance client safety and create a culture of safety. Discussion of these organizations helps further reinforce the importance of safety in medication administration and the avoidance of harm to clients in our care across health care settings. This text will provide a brief discussion of some of the organizations.

The IOM, affiliated with the National Academies of Science, is a nonprofit organization that serves as a resource on health care issues. Based on research studies, the IOM provides reliable information and makes recommendations for best practices. The IOM became involved in the promotion of client safety and published reports that included data on medication errors and prevention. The IOM (2006) landmark report *Identifying and Preventing Medication Errors* presented an agenda for reduction of medication errors, including collaboration among doctors, nurses, pharmacists, the Food and Drug Administration and other government agencies, hospitals and other health care organizations, and patients. The prevention of patient harm is a priority. The most effective way to reduce errors was identified as the establishment of a partnership between patients and their health care provider. Although *To Err is Human* is more than 20 years old and *Identifying and Preventing Medication Errors* is more than 10 years old, they are still relevant today. Efforts to increase awareness of and reduce medication errors and improve client safety continue, but there is more work needed.

The Institute for Safe Medication Practices (ISMP) is a nonprofit organization devoted to the causes of medication errors and strategies for their prevention. ISMP serves as a resource for medication safety information for health care professionals, hospitals, and other health care entities. Many initiatives by ISMP have changed medication practices in health care settings. ISMP published a list of abbreviations, symbols, and dose designations that were prone to cause medication errors if misread or misinterpreted, and therefore should not be used. This list has become well known, supported by patient safety organizations, and has become standard practice. The list can be found on ISMP's website: http://www.ismp.org. It is included in Appendix D of this text and will be referred to in later chapters.

Among its many initiatives, ISMP runs a National Medication Errors Reporting Program (ISMP MERP), which is a voluntary confidential practitioner medication error reporting program. Other initiatives include publication of newsletters with real-time error information, a list of High-Alert Medications (medications that have an increased risk of causing significant harm), and a list of drug names that look alike or sound alike (Confused Drug Names). All of the resources mentioned can be found on ISMP's website.

The Joint Commission (TJC) is an independent, not-for-profit organization. TJC provides accreditation to U.S. hospitals and health care facilities and has worked to achieve high standards in the U.S. health care system. One of its goals has been in the area of medication errors. TJC implemented National Patient Safety Goals, one of which is aimed at assisting health care facilities in the prevention of devastating medication errors. In 2002, TJC launched a *Speak Up* campaign to urge patients to take a larger role in preventing errors by becoming active participants in their care. This includes posters and brochures that are displayed in health care facilities that provide patients with questions and strategies to use to avoid medication errors in hospitals or clinics. Information regarding *Speak Up* can be found on TJC's website, https://www.jointcommission.org/speakup.aspx. TJC also developed a "Do Not Use" list of abbreviations as a national safety patient goal, which emphasizes the importance of not using several abbreviations that can cause misinterpretation and lead to medication errors. The list also includes some abbreviations that are found on ISMP's list of Error-Prone Abbreviations, Symbols, and Dose Designations. The TJC official list can be found on TJC's website, https://www.jointcommission.org/assets/1/18/Do_Not_Use_List_6_28_19.pdf, and in Appendix C of this text. TJC addressed the practice of medication reconciliation in a National Patient Safety Goal (NPSG) (#8). Reconciling medications continues to be important in medication safety and is addressed in the 2020 NPSG Goal #3-Hospital 2020 NPSG (NPSG.03.06.01) (https://www.jointcommission.org/standards/national-patient-safety-goals/). This process requires verification of clients' medications beginning on admission and following the client through transfers within the health-care facility and from one institution to another. Adherence to this prevents medication errors that include omission and drug interactions. In addition to reconciling medications, other aspects related to improving medication safety are included in Goal #3 (e.g., labeling of medications, reduction of harm for clients receiving anticoagulant therapy).

The U.S. Food and Drug Administration (FDA) recognized the potential of barcoding to improve client safety. In 2004, the FDA issued a regulation that required all new pharmaceuticals to be barcoded upon launch into the market (FDA, 2004). The barcodes are used with a barcode-scanning system and computerized database. Some hospitals have barcode scanners that are linked to the hospital's electronic medical records. The barcoding allows the health care provider to scan the client's barcode prior to administering medications, which allows access to the client's medication record. The FDA is also responsible for the placement of the "black box" warning on certain medications. A black box warning appears on the label of a prescription medication to alert consumers and health care providers to safety concerns, such as serious adverse effects or life-threatening risks. In addition, the ISMP and FDA suggested the use of "Tall Man" lettering to differentiate drugs with look-alike names. To prevent errors the drug name is highlighted by various methods, which include uppercase letters and boldface to call attention to differences between look-alike drug names. This list is included in Appendix B of this text.

A Risk Evaluation and Mitigation Strategy (REMS) is a drug safety program that the FDA can require for certain medications with serious safety concerns to help ensure the benefits of the medication outweigh its risks. The purpose of REMS is to reinforce medication use behaviors and actions that support the safe use of that medication. Part of the program also includes the provision of a medication guide or package insert each time the medication is dispensed.

National Quality Forum (NQF) is a nonprofit, voluntary, consensus standard-setting organization established in 1999. To ensure that all patients are protected from injury while receiving care, NQF developed and endorsed a set of Serious Reportable Events (SREs). According to NQF, SREs are a compilation of serious, largely preventable, and harmful clinical events; this compilation is designed to help the health care field assess, measure, and report performance in providing safe care. According to NQF the purpose of the SREs is to facilitate uniform and comparable public reporting to enable systematic learning across health care organizations and systems and to drive systematic national improvements in patient safety based on what is learned both about the events and about how to prevent recurrence. SREs go beyond the hospital setting and address patient safety across a range of settings in which patients receive care, including office-based settings and ambulatory surgery centers. An SRE that has particular reference to this text is listed under the area of Care Management Events. It is indicated as 4A, patient death or serious injury associated with a medication error (e.g., errors involving the wrong drug, wrong dose, wrong patient, wrong time, wrong rate, wrong preparations, or wrong route of administration). Notice this SRE includes the "rights" of medication administration, which has been cited as one of the reasons for medication error when they are not consistently followed by nurses in medication administration.

The Quality and Safety Education for Nurses (QSEN) project has the goal of preparing student nurses with the knowledge, skills, and attitudes (KSAs) that are needed to improve the quality and safety of client care. QSEN looks at six (6) competencies (patient-centered care, teamwork and collaboration, evidence-based practice quality improvement, safety, and informatics). Relevant to medication administration is safety and informatics, which relates to technology to mitigate errors, and teamwork and collaboration, since the prevention of medication errors requires collaboration of all members of the health care team to create a culture of safety that also includes active participation of the client in a partnership with health care providers. Reference to QSEN will be referred to in areas in which it is applicable in this text.

## Overview of Medication Errors

Medication errors can occur anywhere in the medication process from the prescribing of the medication by the health care provider to the dispensing of the medication from the pharmacy to the administering of the medication by the nurse. The causes of medication errors can involve multiple factors, including lack of information about the medication and lack of information about the client to whom the medication is being administered to (e.g., allergies, other medications the client is taking, the reason for the medication being administered), and confusing medication names (look-alike or sound-alike). Other causes of medication errors include errors in mathematical calculations of dosages, incomplete orders, failure to observe "rights" of medication administration when administering medications, and miscommunication of orders. Miscommunication of medication orders can involve poor handwriting, misuse of zeros and decimal points, confusion of metric and other dosing units, use of inappropriate abbreviations and errors in computer order entry. Other contributing factors to medication errors include failure to educate clients properly about medications they are taking, administration of medications without critical thought, and failure to comply with the required policy or procedure related to medication administration. With the shortage of nursing personnel, factors such as shift changes, floating staff, double shifts, and workload increases have contributed to errors. A nurse who is chronically overworked can make errors because of exhaustion. Adaptations to the demands of new technology in health care can also contribute to errors. Distractions and interruptions as contributory factors to medication errors have been found to be plausible in the literature. Systemic errors (e.g., medications that are not properly labeled, medications with similar names placed in close proximity to one another) can lead to medication errors.

> **⚠ SAFETY ALERT!**
> Focus solely on the task at hand, medication administration (when the actual act of medication occurs). Distractions can result in error during medication administration, jeopardize the client's safety, and may cause harm.

Certain medications, referred to as high-alert medications, have also been identified as contributing to harmful errors. Medications on this list include concentrated electrolyte solutions (such as potassium chloride), insulin, heparin, and chemotherapy drugs. These medications require double verification before administering. Failure to conduct double verification can result in errors.

## Preventing Medication Errors

The best solution to the problem of medication errors is prevention. To prevent medication errors, personnel involved in the administration of medications must do meticulous planning and implement the task properly, paying close attention to detail. Technological advances in terms of medication (e.g., use of barcode medication administration, automated dispensing cabinets [ADC], computer prescriber order entry [CPOE]) have been instituted in many facilities as a means of preventing and decreasing medication errors; however, computer technology cannot replace human intellect or negate the need to follow various steps in medication administration to ensure client safety. These advances are useful only if the systems are effective and efficient.

Medication administration is more than just giving the medication because it is ordered. The nurse should be knowledgeable about the action, uses, side effects, expected response, contraindications, and range of dosage for the medication being administered. Consult a valid and current drug reference about any medication that is unfamiliar.

It is not possible to completely eliminate distractions and interruptions in health care facilities, however; safety is essential during the preparation of medications. Best practice strategies include the preparation of medications in a designated "No Interruption Zone" and educating staff on the importance of avoiding interruption of the nurse administering medications. The nurse can also ensure safety when administering medications to clients by attending to the "rights" of medication administration. The rights of medication administration are essential safety checks that should be performed each time with the administration of each and every medication. These rights include administering the right medication to the right client, in the right dosage, by the right route, at the right time, followed by the right documentation. We will discuss these rights and additional rights in this chapter that enhance client safety.

High-alert medications can have devastating consequences if not administered properly. Double-check high-alert medications with another nurse to prevent errors that could result in overdose or other errors that can cause fatal harm to a client. Avoid workarounds, or shortcuts; these are signs of errors waiting to happen.

Medication administration involves using the nursing process, which includes assessment, nursing diagnosis/nursing problem, planning, implementation, and evaluation. The nursing process is a systematic, rational method of planning individualized nursing care, which begins with the assessment of the client.

> **(!) SAFETY ALERT!**
> Failure to think about what you are doing and why you are doing it and failure to assess a client can result in errors. You are accountable for your actions.

In the 2018-2019 *Targeted Medication Safety Best Practices for Hospitals* (TMSBP), ISMP identified the following new best practice (#14) in terms of preventing medication errors: Seek out and use information about medication safety risks and errors that have occurred in other organizations outside of your facility and take action to prevent similar errors. According to ISMP, errors that occur in an institution can be a learning process for another to identify risks or practices in their institution to prevent the occurrence of similar errors. According to ISMP, the TMSBP was developed to identify, inspire, and mobilize widespread, national adoption of best practices for specific medication safety issues that continue to cause fatal and harmful errors in patients, despite repeated warnings in ISMP publications. The best practices were set forth in 2016-2017. The 2018-2019 has revisions of two previous practices and the addition of three new best practices, which include the previous one discussed here.

The prevention of medication errors and decreasing their rate of occurrence require adherence to medication administration policies and guidelines at your institution and adherence to standards and guidelines developed by organizations that include ISMP and TJC.

### The Nurse's Role in Medication Error Prevention

In addition to the consistent use of the basic six rights of medication administration, nurses are essential to reducing medication errors and improving client outcomes. An effective way to reduce medication errors as identified in a report by the IOM's *Identifying and Preventing Medication Errors*, is a partnership between clients and their health care providers. Emphasis is placed on open communication between nurses and clients, which included not only talking to clients but also listening. As noted previously, TJC's *Speak Up* campaign also urged clients to take an active role in preventing errors by becoming more active in their care. When a nurse is administering medications, clients should be encouraged to ask questions about their medications, and they should receive clear and complete responses to the questions. Questions raised by the client in regard to the medication keep the client informed and can sometimes be a warning to the nurse regarding medications the client is receiving, or alert the nurse to a possible error. Always stop and listen; do not disregard questions. This may prevent an error from occurring and may require further questioning of the client. When questions are encouraged, it maintains open communication between the client and nurse and can prevent medication errors.

By way of brochures and posters displayed in health care facilities, clients are encouraged to use strategies to avoid medication mistakes. These include tips such as check your medications; ask questions; and make sure your doctors, nurses, and other caregivers check your wristband and ask your name before giving you medicine (Figure 9.1). Nurses can reduce errors by making more use of information technologies when administering medications. Using reference information provided by a reliable source or downloaded content on personal digital assistants (PDAs), smartphones, or iPads will enhance the nurse's ability to apply critical thinking when making judgments related to medication administration. With the increasing technology in health care, nurses must be able to identify safety risks and prevent adverse events when using it.

When medication errors occur, they should be reported following the organization's procedure for reporting. Not reporting an error violates the ethical principle of beneficence, which is the moral obligation to prevent harm. Not reporting an error also does not prioritize the client's safety. When an error occurs, after the safety of the client is ensured, the next step should be reporting the error. Nurses need to use information sources that provide vital information related to medication errors and prevent their occurrence (e.g., ISMP, TJC). The prevention of medication errors, the use of technology in prevention, and the education of nurses with an emphasis on maintaining the safety of the client coincide with the Quality and Safe Education for Nurses (QSEN) goal to improve the quality and safety of client care. Medication administration and strategies to prevent errors (e.g., consistent use of the six basic rights, analyzing the causes of medication errors, discouraging

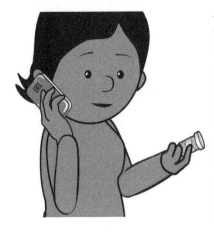

**Julie says:**

**"Read the label on your medicine to make sure it's yours. If something doesn't seem right or if you don't understand, Speak Up!"**

Watch the Speak Up™ videos online at www.jointcommission.org/speakup.

The Joint Commission

**Figure 9.1** Sample of Speak Up poster. (Copyright © The Joint Commission, 2013.)

the use of unsafe abbreviations, and the benefits of safety-enhancing technologies such as barcoding) can be placed under competency 5, which is Safety. Also relevant here is the use of Informatics under competency 6, to mitigate errors. Note, only some strategies are presented here for the prevention of medication errors. Throughout the text there will be further discussion regarding the prevention of medication errors and recommendations to prevent their occurrence based on safety standards established by organizations that include TJC, ISMP, and the FDA.

## Critical Thinking and Medication Administration

There are numerous definitions for *critical thinking*. The best way to define critical thinking is as a process of purposeful, intentional thinking that includes being reasonable and rational. Thinking is based on reason. Critical thinking is important to all phases of nursing but is particularly relevant in the discussion of medication administration. Critical thinking is necessary to the development of clinical reasoning skills and clinical judgment.

Critical thinking encompasses several skills relevant to medication administration. One such skill is the ability to identify an organized approach to the task at hand. For example, in medication administration, calculating dosages in an organized, systematic manner (formula, ratio and proportion, dimensional analysis) decreases the likelihood of errors.

A second skill characteristic of critical thinking is the ability to be an autonomous thinker—for example, challenging a medication order that is written incorrectly rather than passively accepting the order. Critical thinking also involves the ability to distinguish irrelevant information from that which is relevant. For example, when reading a medication label, the nurse is able to decipher from the label the information necessary for calculating the correct dosage. Critical thinking involves reasoning and the application of concepts—for example, choosing the correct type of syringe to administer a dosage and using concepts learned to decide the appropriateness of a dosage. Critical thinking also involves asking for clarification of what is not understood and not making assumptions. Clarifying a medication order and dosage indicates critical thinking. Checking the accuracy and reliability of information decreases the chance of medication errors. The ability to validate information requires a high level of thinking and decreases the chance of medication errors that could be harmful to the client.

Critical thinking is essential to the safe administration of medications. This process allows a nurse to think before doing, translate knowledge into practice, and make appropriate judgments. To safely administer medication, the nurse must base decisions on rational thinking and thorough knowledge of medication administration. Proper medication administration involves evaluation of the client and the medication's effects, which requires critical thinking and skills of assessment. A nurse who administers medication in a routine manner, rather than with thought and reasoning, is not using critical thinking skills.

> **! SAFETY ALERT!**
> Remember that the nurse who administers a medication is legally liable for the medication error regardless of the reason for the error occurrence.

## Factors That Influence Medication Dosages and Action

Several factors influence medication dosages and the way they act, including the following:
1. Route of administration
2. Time of administration
3. Age of the client
4. Nutritional status of the client
5. Absorption and excretion of the medication
6. Health status of the client
7. Gender of the client
8. Ethnicity and culture of the client
9. Genetics

All these factors affect how clients react to a medication and the dosage they receive, and all must be considered when medications are prescribed and administered. Because of differences in the actions and types of medications, clients respond in various ways, and therefore dosages must be individualized. No two clients will respond to a medication in the same manner. Nurses must keep these factors in mind when administering medications. These factors can account for individuals responding differently to the same medication.

## Special Considerations for the Elderly

Elderly individuals can be considered high-risk medication consumers. Approximately two-thirds of older adults use both prescription and nonprescription medications, and one-third of all prescriptions are written for older adults. The growing older population represents a special challenge for health care professionals. With the number of individuals over the age of 65 rapidly increasing, the use of medications in this age group will also increase. According to the Administration on Aging (AOA) *2018 Profile of Older Americans,* over the past 10 years, the population age 65 and over increased from 37.8 million in 2007 to 50.9 million in 2017 (a 34% increase) and is projected to reach 94.7 million in 2060. Between 2007 and 2017 the population age 60 and over increased 35% from 52.5 million to 70.8 million. The 85 and over population is projected to more than double from 6.5 million in 2017 to 14.4 million in 2040 (a 123% increase). According to the U.S. Census Bureau, older Americans will make up more than 20% of the U.S. population starting in 2030.

Because of medical advances and focus on healthier lifestyles, people are now living longer. As with children (see Chapter 24), special considerations should be given to the client who is older. The elderly population experiences more chronic conditions and co-morbidities (including degenerative diseases, physical disabilities); consequently there is more use of and demand for health care services, which include specialty care in some cases and increased use of medications. With the aging process come physiological changes that have a direct effect on medications and their action in the elderly individual. Aging causes the slowing down of the body's functions. Other physiological changes include a decrease in circulation, slower absorption, slower metabolism, a decrease in excretory functions, and a decrease in the ability to respond to stress, such as the stress of medications on the system. Other changes with aging include a decrease in body weight, which can affect the dosage of medications, and changes in mental status, possibly caused by the effects of physical illness or physiological changes in the neurological system that can occur with aging. These physiological changes can cause unexpected medication reactions and make the elderly person more sensitive to the effects of many medications.

According to Willihnganz, Gurevitz, and Clayton (2020), although people who are more than 65 years old represent about 14% of the U.S. population, they consume more than 25% of all prescription medicines and 33% of all nonprescription medicines sold. A recent study of the U.S. noninstitutionalized adult population has indicated that more than 90% of persons 65 years old or older use at least one medication per week. More than 40% use five or more medications, and 12% use 10 or more different medications per week. Because the elderly are often taking more than one medication (polypharmacy), problems such as medication interactions, severe adverse reactions, medication and food interactions, and an increase in medication errors occur. The Beers criteria is a list of medications that are used to evaluate quality and safety in nursing homes. According to Willihnganz, Gurevitz, and Clayton (2020), these medications are considered to be potentially inappropriate for older patients. It is thought that the medications on this list cause adverse effects more commonly and should be avoided in older adult patients unless treatment with other medicines has failed. It is recommended that practitioners be aware of the medications on this list and educate clients regarding prescription and nonprescription medications. The 2019 updated Beers Criteria can be found on the American Geriatrics website: https://www.americangeriatrics.org. The Centers for Medicare and Medicaid Services has incorporated the Beers criteria into federal safety regulations for long-term care facilities. As the senior population continues to increase, there is a need to focus on reducing medication errors in this group.

As a rule, the elderly client will require smaller dosages of medications (as dosage size increases, the number of adverse effects and their severity increase), and the dosages should be given farther apart to prevent accumulation of medications and toxic effects.

With aging, visual and hearing problems may develop. Special attention must be given when teaching clients about their medications to help prevent medication errors. Develop a relationship with the client; building rapport and trust is important for the elderly. Take time and talk to the elderly, listen to what they say, and never assume they do not know how much or what medications they are taking. Ascertain that all instructions are written as clearly as possible, choosing fonts that are friendly to older eyes. Make sure the client has appropriate measuring devices to facilitate ease and accuracy when measuring (e.g., a dropper or measuring cup with calibrated lines to indicate small dosages [0.2 mg, 0.4 mg, etc.]). To lessen the chance of taking too much medication or forgetting a dosage, try to establish specific times compatible with the client's routine for taking medications.

Omission of medications is a common cause of error for the elderly at home. This may be due to the cost of medication or forgetfulness. Establishing medication times when possible to coincide with the client's routine and engaging a family member or friend if possible in the teaching process may help in preventing omission of medications. Help the client recognize tablets by the name on the bottle, not by color. If the print on medications is too small for the client to read, encourage the use of a magnifying glass. Other measures might include providing a simple chart that outlines the medications to be taken, times they are to be taken, and special instructions if needed. Such a chart should be geared to the client's visual ability and comprehension level. Encourage the elderly client to request that childproof containers not be used; some older people will have difficulty opening child-resistant containers. Recommend medication aids for the client, such as special medication containers divided into separate compartments for storing daily or weekly medication dosages. (Figure 9.2 shows examples of medication containers.) As the aging population increases, the need for safer medication administration has become even more of a priority. Currently there are services available through the pharmacy that package medications for the client according to the time of the day they are taken. The pharmacy sorts the medications and places them in an easy-to-open package. A 30-day supply of medications is provided to the client based on the medications ordered by the health care provider. This eliminates the need for clients to pour their medications daily. This service is referred to as multi-dose drug dispensing (MDD). Examples include the services provided by CVS Pharmacy (referred to as multidose medications) (https://www.cvs.com/content/multidose?); Amazon (referred to as Pill Pack) (https://www.pillpack.com/how-itworks); and some community pharmacies.

A careful and complete medication history, including illicit drugs, should be obtained from the elderly client. This should include over-the-counter medications, alternative medicines, and vitamins. The elderly client may think that these products are safe; however,

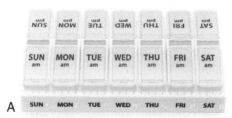

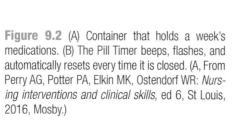

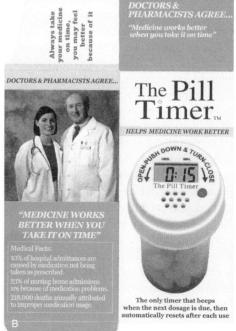

**Figure 9.2** (A) Container that holds a week's medications. (B) The Pill Timer beeps, flashes, and automatically resets every time it is closed. (A, From Perry AG, Potter PA, Elkin MK, Ostendorf WR: *Nursing interventions and clinical skills,* ed 6, St Louis, 2016, Mosby.)

they may cause dangerous interactions with prescribed medications. Encourage clients to check with their health care provider before taking over-the-counter medications.

When teaching the elderly, it is important to remember that they are mature adults who are capable of learning; they may need and deserve additional time for learning to take place. Be patient, use simple language, and maintain the independence of the elderly as much as possible. Always allow ample time for processing, individualize the teaching, and remember to always foster feelings of self-worth. Always have your clients demonstrate back to you what you have taught them. Correct teaching can decrease misunderstandings and errors in medication.

## The Rights of Medication Administration

The "rights" of medication administration can be looked at as being standards. By definition, standards are actions that ensure safe nursing practice. The "rights" of medication administration are a set of safety checks that serve as guidelines for the practitioner to follow when administering medications to prevent errors and ensure client safety. The "rights" must be consistently followed when administering medications to a client. There have been many medication errors linked to inconsistency in following the "rights." Over the years there have been five, then six, and now, in many places, eight or more rights. There are six basic rights of medications administration that are required safety checks that must be performed with the administration of each and every medication to a client. The six basic rights include the right client, right medication, right dose, right route, right time, and right documentation. **A violation of any of the six basic rights constitutes a medication error.** Additional rights include right indication, right to know, and right to refuse. A new right being considered is the right response (Box 9.1).

| BOX 9.1 | The Rights of Medication Administration |
|---|---|
| 1. Right client | 6. Right documentation |
| 2. Right medication | 7. Right indication |
| 3. Right dose | 8. Right to know |
| 4. Right route | 9. Right to refuse |
| 5. Right time | 10. Right response |

1. **The right client**—Always make sure you are administering medications to the right client. Failure to correctly identify the right client has been cited as one of the three most common causes of medication errors. Since 2003, TJC has required that clients be identified with at least two unique client identifiers (e.g., client's full name, birthdate, medical record number, but not the client's room number). This requirement was initiated as a National Patient Safety Goal; it has been a standard since 2004 and applies to both inpatient and outpatient settings. It is permissible to check the two identifiers with the client's armband, medication administration record, or chart and ask the client to state his or her name or parent to state the child's name.

   In institutions that use barcode medication administration (BCMA), the client's identification bracelet is scanned as well as the medication being administered. In basic nursing education programs, emphasis is placed on establishing the correct identification of the client prior to medication administration. Students are required to compare two client-specific identifiers with the client's armband, medication administration record (MAR), or chart and by asking the client to state her or his name (as a third identifier). To avoid administering medications to the wrong client, the steps identified need to be consistently implemented regardless of how familiar the nurse is with the client. Always know and use the unique identifiers recognized and required by the facility. Advanced technology does not eliminate your responsibility to correctly identify a client. Misidentification can result in the wrong client receiving the wrong medication.

**SAFETY ALERT!**

Always verify your client's identity by using the two identifiers designated by your institution each time medications are administered. This will help ensure you have the right client and avoid an error.

2. **The right medication**—When medications are ordered, the nurse should compare the MAR (medication administration record) or computer record with the actual order. When administering medications, the nurse should check the label on the medication container against the order. Medications should be checked three times: before preparing, after preparing, and before administration to the client. With unit dosages (each medication dosage is prepared in the prescribed dosage, packaged, labeled, and ready to use), the label should still be checked three times. Remember, regardless of the medication distribution system, the medication label should be checked three times. Errors frequently occur because of similarity in medication names and similar packaging.

   Many medications have names that sound alike, or have names or packaging that is similar. ISMP and the FDA recommend the use of "Tall Man" lettering to alert health professionals to the potential for error with look-alike names. In the use of this method, the medication name is mixed-case or enlarged, bolded, or in italics to emphasize the differing portions of the two names. Tall Man lettering is being used at many institutions. See Appendix B, which shows a listing of the FDA and ISMP lists of look-alike drug names with recommended Tall Man lettering. The right medication also includes checking the expiration date on the medication label. If the medication has expired, contact the pharmacy for an updated supply and discard according to the institution policy. In institutions that use BCMA, the client's identification band is scanned, and each medication is scanned and electronically checked against the electronic medication administration record (eMAR).

   Administer only medications that you have prepared and that are clearly labeled. Avoid distractions when preparing medications; do not multitask. Some institutions have instituted "no interruption zones" in areas such as the medication room to prevent distractions.

> **! SAFETY ALERT!**
> If the medication name is not clear or the medication does not seem to be appropriate for the client, question the order. Always double-check that you have the correct medication. If you are unfamiliar with a medication, refer to a reference to ensure you have the correct medication and prevent errors.

3. **The right dose**—Always perform and check calculations carefully, without ignoring decimal points. If you misread a decimal point, the client could receive a dose significantly different from the one ordered. Risk of harm from dosage errors in the pediatric population is great. Caution should be taken when administering medications to children. Errors can occur because of the frequency of weight-based calculations, the need for decimal points, and fractional dosages. Many errors have occurred with infusion pumps and calculations involving administration of parenteral fluids and medications. Electronic infusion pumps have reduced medication errors. Although infusion pump technology has increased administration safety, the nurse cannot rely fully on these devices. It is a nursing responsibility to be trained in the use of infusion pumps and to be alert for potential problems.

   To ensure the right dose of medication, interpret abbreviations correctly. Factors such as illegible handwriting, miscalculation of the amount, and use of inappropriate abbreviations can result in administration of the wrong dose. Always have someone else check a dosage that causes concern. In some agencies, certain medication dosages are required to be checked by two nurses (e.g., insulin, heparin). These medications have been a common source of errors in administration. If a dosage or abbreviation in a written order is not clear, call the prescriber for verification; do not assume.

   Computer entry does not eliminate the use of incorrect dosing symbols. Nurses should always consult a reference to confirm the dosage when in doubt. After dosages are calculated, they should be administered using standard measuring devices, such as calibrated medicine droppers and cups. Always double-check a dosage and confirm pump settings. Before administering medications, it is the responsibility of the nurse to question orders thought to be inappropriate. Examples of questionable orders include a single dose to be composed of more than two or three dosage units (e.g., tablets, capsules, vials) and orders for atypically high doses. In order to recognize unusual dosages, the nurse has the responsibility to become familiar with the usual medication dosages for the clients they care for. The same principle of questioning applies to the preparation of IV solutions. If more than two or three dosage units are needed to prepare the solution, this could signal an error. Always ask the question, Does this dose seem reasonable?

In later chapters you will learn to calculate the amount to administer to a client. Thinking what is reasonable and using a common sense approach when calculating dosages is imperative to prevent errors. Full attention to accurate dosage calculation ensures that you avoid error and harm to a client when administering medications.

4. **The right route**—Route refers to how a medication is administered (e.g., by mouth, injection). A medication intended for one route is unsafe if administered by another route. Oral medications (e.g., tablets, capsules, caplets) are administered by mouth. Nurses should always consult a reliable reference to confirm the correct route for a medication that is unfamiliar. Always check that the route, if listed on the medication label, matches the route ordered. If the route is not indicated, use a reference to identify the correct route. The route of the medication should be stated on the order. Do not assume which route is appropriate. Orders to administer medications by a feeding tube that should not be crushed (e.g., enteric coated) require that the nurse seek clarification of the order or have the order changed by the prescriber to ensure safe medication administration.

5. **The right time**—Medications should be given at the correct time of day and interval (e.g., three times a day [t.i.d.] or every 6 hours [q6h]). Judgment should be used as to when medications should be given or not given. If several medications are ordered, set priorities and administer medications that must act at a certain time. For example, insulin should be given at an exact time before meals. The right time should also include the right time sequence! For example, a client may be receiving a diuretic b.i.d., and the institution may have b.i.d. as 9:00 AM and 9:00 PM. The nurse will need to know that the diuretic should not be given in the late evening so that the individual is not going to the bathroom all night. This requires critical thinking. The nurse must know whether a time schedule can be altered or requires judgment in determining the proper time to be administered. Know the institutional policy concerning medication times.

Factors such as the purpose of the medication, medication interactions, absorption of the medication, and side effects must be considered when medication times are scheduled. Administer medications at the right time. In most cases, this means the medication must be administered within 30 minutes of the scheduled time. (Up to 30 minutes before or after the scheduled time.) This is referred to as the "30-minute rule."

The "30-minute rule" for medication administration, enacted by the Centers for Medicare & Medical Services (CMS), required that medications be given within 30 minutes before or 30 minutes after their scheduled time. According to the ISMP, who conducted a survey of nurses in response to the 30-minute rule, many nurses developed unsafe practices and workarounds that threatened client safety and increased the potential for medication errors. Some of the unsafe practices that resulted from time pressures included taking risky shortcuts including deception (e.g., medication documented as being given at a certain time when it was delayed or given beforehand); administering medications without performing assessments and/or checking vital signs, lab values, weight and allergy status; skipping barcode scanning; and skipping important double checks to save time.

As a result of the survey findings, CMS provided hospitals the flexibility to establish policies and procedures for the timing of medication, which includes establishing policies for identification of medications that require exact or precise timing for administration and are not eligible for scheduled dosing times. CMS defines time-critical scheduled medications as those in which early or late administration longer than 30 minutes may cause harm or have a significant impact on the intended therapeutic or pharmacological effect. Non–time-critical scheduled medications are those in which a longer or shorter interval of time since the prior dose does not significantly alter the medication's therapeutic effect or otherwise cause harm, and therefore the hospitals may establish, as appropriate, either a 1- or 2-hour window of administration.

ISMP, in collaboration with a panel and organizations including TJC and the American Nurses Association (ANA), developed Acute Care Guidelines for Timely Administration of Scheduled Medications. These guidelines can be reviewed on the ISMP website: https://www.ismp.org/node/361. Currently, this is the most well-vetted set of guidelines on the ISMP website. Hospitals are recommended to use the ISMP guidelines as a resource and to develop their own medication administration policies. Nurses are therefore expected to be familiar with and competent in their agency's policy regarding medication administration.

Before administering prn (when required, whenever necessary) medications, check to ascertain that adequate time has passed since the previous dose, or severe consequences may occur because the medication was administered to the client too soon.

All medication orders should include the frequency that a medication is to be administered. Administration of a medication at the prescribed time or right time is important to maximize the therapeutic effect and maintain therapeutic blood levels. Errors have occurred in medication administration because of misinterpretation of time and frequency in medication orders. TJC has taken steps to prevent errors by prohibiting the use of certain abbreviations related to dosing frequency (e.g., qod and qd have been mistaken for each other; instead of qod, write "every other day" and instead of qd write "daily" or "every day"). These abbreviations are included on TJC's "Do Not Use" list (see Appendix C).

6. **The right documentation**—Correct documentation is referred to as the sixth right of medication administration. Medications should be charted accurately as soon as they are given—on the right client's medication record, under the right date, and next to the right time. If a medication is refused, it should be documented as such with a notation on the medication record or in the nurse's notes. Never chart a medication as given before administering it or without documentation as to why it was not given. Follow the policy of the institution when documenting. All documentation should be legible. Unintentional overmedication of a client could result if a nurse fails to document a medication that was given and a nurse on a following shift also gives the medication to the client.

Documentation of medications administered is done on the client's medication administration record (MAR), which is a paper form or electronic record that tracks the medications a client receives. A computerized record is used as a working document that records medications as they are administered and is referred to as an electronic medication administration record (eMAR). This system allows electronic tracking of medications administered to help reduce errors. With some of the electronic medication systems, the medication barcode and the client's identification band is scanned, and the information is documented into the client's eMAR. **Remember: "If it's not documented, it's not done."**

The six basic rights that have been discussed should always be consistently followed when administering medications. In addition to the six rights, the nurse should always view the client receiving medications as an important and valuable asset in the prevention of medication errors. Always listen to concerns verbalized by the client when administering medications regardless of the checks that you have performed before administration (e.g., "The other nurse just gave me medication," "I have never taken this medication before"). Statements such as these by a client should not be ignored. Always listen carefully and be attentive to the concerns of a client. Consider what the client verbalizes as correct and investigate concerns before administering the medication; this can be valuable in preventing medication errors.

---

**(!) SAFETY ALERT!**

When a client questions a medication, **STOP** and **LISTEN**. This may be the opportunity to identify an error before a client is harmed.

7. **The right indication**—This is also referred to as the right reason. The nurse has the responsibility for knowing the reason a medication is being administered to ensure it is being given for the right reason. If the nurse understands the reason for a medication that is ordered, it will help in the identification of when to hold or not give a medication that may cause harm if administered. Knowing why prevents errors. If in doubt about the reason for a medication that is ordered, verify the order with the prescriber before administering.

8. **The right to know—All clients have a right to be educated regarding the medication they are taking.** Clients are more likely to be compliant if they understand why they are taking a medication, and education allows them to make an informed decision. Information that clients should receive includes dose, reason, effect, and side effects of the medication. Clients should also be provided information regarding drug-drug interactions, drug-food interactions, and the use of herbal medications, dietary supplements, and drug interactions. Clients knowing about their medication helps to foster medication safety.

9. **The right to refuse**—In addition to the six basic rights of medication administration, another right is **a client has the right to refuse medications.** When this occurs, the nurse needs to document the refusal correctly and make appropriate persons aware of the refusal. The right to refuse may be denied to the client who has a mental illness. A client deemed to be dangerous to self or others can be taken to court and mandated to take medication. Though the client has the right to refuse medication or treatment, the law referred to as Kendra's Law in New York state may provide some exception to a client's right to refuse treatment (e.g., medication). Kendra's Law is legislation designed to protect the public and individuals living with mental illness by ensuring that potentially dangerous mentally ill outpatients are safely and effectively treated.

   Kendra's Law is court-ordered assisted outpatient treatment (AOT). It authorizes the courts to issue orders that would require mentally ill persons who are unlikely to survive safely in the community without supervision to accept medications and other needed mental health services. In other words, if a client is in the community and noncompliant with the treatment regimen (e.g., medication), the client can be petitioned to court by an individual (e.g., spouse, parent, adult roommate).

   Nurses should always be aware of the state laws, policies, and procedures for their jurisdiction relative to the administration of medications to refusing clients. It is extremely important for nurses to check frequently for side effects related to medications and to listen carefully to client complaints. The reason for the refusal of medications should be carefully analyzed and documented in all cases. Education of the client and a reassuring therapeutic relationship can assist in diminishing a client's refusal.

10. **The right response**—This is a new right that is being considered by some facilities. This right applies to making certain the medication has the effect intended and includes monitoring the client and documenting. For example, if a sleep medication is ordered, is the client able to sleep?

According to *Fundamentals of Nursing* (Potter, Perry, Stockert, & Hall, 2017), in accordance with The Patient Care Partnership (American Hospital Association, 2003) and because of the potential risks related to medication administration, a patient has the following rights, which include: to refuse a medication regardless of the consequences; to not receive unnecessary medications; to have qualified nurses or physicians assess a medication history, including allergies and use of herbs; and to receive labeled medications safely without discomfort in accordance with the six rights of medication administration.

In addition to some specific mandates mentioned by TJC to ensure client safety and prevent the occurrence of medication errors, another National Patient Safety Goal focused on medications that clients may be taking, including herbals, vitamins, and nonprescription products. Patients and families may not accurately report all their medications and dosages, as well as home remedies. This can lead to errors in medication administration and adverse effects. Nurses need to get a thorough history of medications being taken by a client to prevent medication interactions that may be fatal to the client.

## Medication Reconciliation

According to TJC, communication is vital, and it is the root cause of many sentinel events, including medication errors. In response to this, TJC focused on medication reconciliation as a National Patient Safety Goal to reduce the risk of errors during transition points. This National Patient Safety Goal requires hospitals to reconcile medications across the continuum of care. This also includes transfer within the institution (i.e., from one unit to another unit). Medication reconciliation is a requirement for ambulatory care, assisted living, behavioral health, home care, and long-term organizations. Medication reconciliation is to be applied in any setting or service where medications are to be used or the client's response to treatment or service could be affected by medications that the client has been taking.

In the context of the goal, reconciliation is the process of comparing the medications that the client/patient/resident has been taking before the time of admission or entry into a new setting with the medications that the organization is about to provide. The purpose of the reconciliation is to avoid errors of transcription, omission, duplication of therapy, or drug-drug and drug-disease interactions.

Medication reconciliation is an important step in the prevention of medication errors and can assist in obtaining accurate medication histories and ensure continuity of appropriate therapy. This process should begin on admission; discharge orders should be compared and reconciled with the most recent inpatient medication orders and the original list of medications taken at home. Nurses can play a major role in the reconciliation process. This must become an important focus to prevent errors and misunderstanding regarding medications that a client may be taking, especially when discharged. Ensuring client knowledge regarding prehospital medications and posthospital medications may be a step in preventing errors and medication interactions. For additional information about medication reconciliation, refer to TJC's National Patient Safety Goals (http://www.jointcommission.org).

## Client Education

One of the most important nursing functions is educating the client. Educating clients about their medications is imperative in preventing errors and improving the quality of health care. Educating clients regarding medications plays a role in preventing adverse reactions and achieving adherence to prescribed therapy; taking the correct dosage of the right medication at the right time helps prevent problems with medication administration. Remember that clients cannot be expected to follow a medication regimen—taking the correct dosage of the right medication at the right time—if they have not been taught. Not knowing what to do results in noncompliance, inaccurate dosages, and other problems. Nurses are in a unique position to teach clients, and this has been a traditional activity of nursing practice. Education should begin in the hospital and be a major part of discharge planning because, once discharged, clients need to have been educated about their medications to continue taking them safely and correctly at home. With today's emphasis on outpatient treatment and early discharge, thorough client education regarding medications is necessary.

When the nurse is teaching a client, it is important to thoroughly assess the needs of the client. Determine what the client knows about the medication prescribed; how to take the medication; and the frequency, time, and dosage. Identify the client's learning needs, including literacy level and language most easily and clearly understood. Identify relevant ethnic, cultural, and socioeconomic factors that may influence medication use; consider factors such as age and physical capabilities. A variety of teaching strategies may have to be used to facilitate and enhance learning. Return demonstrations on proper use of medication equipment and reading dosages, in addition to repeated instructions and directions, may be necessary, especially regarding management at home.

What a client needs to know about a medication varies with the medication. There may be numerous pieces of information clients should learn regarding their medications. The items discussed here relate particularly to dosage administration. To ensure that the client takes the right medication in the right dosage, by the right route at the right time, client education should include the following:

- Both the brand and generic names of the medication or medications being taken
- Clear explanation of the amount of the medication to be taken (e.g., one tablet, 1/2 tablet)
- Clear explanation of when to take the medication (Prepare a chart created with the client's lifestyle in mind. For example, if the medication is to be taken with meals, perhaps the chart can indicate the client's mealtime and the medication scheduled accordingly.)
- Clear demonstration of measuring oral dosages, such as liquids (encourage the use of appropriate measuring devices)
- Clear explanation of the route of administration (e.g., place under the tongue)

In addition to teaching clients about prescription medications they are taking, it is imperative that nurses question clients about any other over-the-counter medications they might be taking at home, including herbal medications and dietary supplements. Some herbal medications might interact with medications they are taking (e.g., ephedra can accelerate heart rate, ginkgo and garlic may inhibit blood clotting). Nurses must be alert to any factors that may interfere with client safety.

Though nurses cannot ensure that clients will act on or retain everything they are taught, nurses are responsible for providing information to the client that will prevent error-prone situations and enable safe medication administration. Nurses evaluate retention by providing follow-up, and, if necessary, finding alternative ways of dealing with a client who has a "no way" attitude.

## Home Care Considerations

Home health nursing has become a large part of the health care delivery system and continues to grow. This is due to factors such as the promotion of cost-effective health care and early discharge. Home care nursing may involve many activities, such as providing treatments, dressing changes, hospice care, client/family teaching, and medication administration. Medication administration involves administration of medications in various ways (e.g., IV, p.o., injection). The increased movement of nursing into the home of the client, which is not a controlled setting, has some important nursing implications. Home health nursing increases the autonomy of practice. The nurse must conduct a thorough assessment, communicate effectively, problem solve, and use expert critical thinking skills. Thinking must be rational, reasonable, and based on knowledge.

The principles regarding medication administration are the same as in a structured setting (e.g., hospital, acute care facility, nursing home). The six basic rights are still guidelines for the nurse to follow to ensure safe administration. It is imperative that the client be well educated about safe administration. Depending on the client's condition, home nursing services may be provided on a scheduled or intermittent basis to monitor the status of a client. Not all clients have a health aide, family member, or continuous nursing services in the home (around the clock). It is essential that the nurse calculate medication administration in a systematic, organized manner and adhere to the six rights of medication administration. For example, according to TJC, in all initial visits in the home care setting, two identifiers should occur. The correct address is an acceptable identifier when used in conjunction with another person-specific indicator. Thereafter, direct facial recognition is acceptable if there is continuing one-on-one care in which the nurse "knows" the individual. The sixth right—documentation—is essential everywhere, including home health care. Documentation of medications is not just for legal purposes; it plays a significant role in cost reimbursement and payments. Correct interpretation of medication orders and validation are imperative. Proper education of the client concerning the medication, dosage, and route of administration is crucial in order for the client to manage in the home environment. Some may look at it as "the client being totally at your mercy." Clients depend on the nurse to provide direction for them to ensure safe medication administration at home. The nurse must be able to teach the client to use appropriate measuring devices for measuring prescribed dosages and determining the accuracy of the dosage.

When possible, encourage clients to use devices that are readily available in many pharmacies, such as calibrated oral syringes or plastic cups with measurements. Use of these devices can help prevent errors that often occur when clients measure their medication with household utensils. (As discussed in the chapters on systems of measure, the nurse must be able to convert dosages among the various systems.) The nurse providing services to the client in the home must be innovative and knowledgeable and demonstrate excellent critical thinking skills. Open communication with the client is essential. It is crucial to know what clients are taking and how. Remember that clients have to be taught. They may not know that they cannot resume previously taken medications or herbal remedies.

## The Nurse's Role in Medication Error Prevention

In addition to the consistent use of the basic six rights of medication administration, nurses are essential to reducing medication errors and improving client outcomes. An effective way to reduce medication errors as identified in the IOM report *Identifying and Preventing Medication Errors*, is a partnership between clients and their health care providers. Emphasis was placed on open communication between nurses and clients, which included not only talking to clients but also listening. In response to this, TJC launched a *Speak Up* campaign that urged clients to take an active role in preventing errors by becoming more active in their care. When administering medications, client questions should be encouraged, and the nurse should be prepared to answer them.

## Routes of Medication Administration

Route refers to how a medication is administered or the method of delivery by which the medication enters into the body. The nurse is responsible for ensuring that the client receives the medication by the right route. Medications can be administered by several routes.

Oral (p.o.). Oral medications are administered by mouth (e.g., tablets, capsules, caplets, liquid solutions). The information contained on a medication label for (e.g., tablets, capsules) will not specify oral as the route of administration; however, unless another route is specified on the label, tablets and capsules are administered by the oral route. Liquid solutions for oral use will specify the route oral.

Sublingual (SL). Sublingual medications are placed under the tongue and are designed to be readily absorbed through the blood vessels in this area. Medications designed to be administered by the sublingual route should not be swallowed. Nitroglycerin used for relief of angina (chest pain) is a medication commonly administered by the sublingual route (tablet, or metered spray referred to as nitroglycerin lingual aerosol, which can be sprayed onto or under the tongue). Another medication administered sublingually is Suboxone, which is used for opioid dependence.

Buccal. Buccal tablets are placed in the mouth between the gums and inner lining of cheek (buccal pouch) absorbed by buccal mucosa. Clients should be instructed not to chew, swallow, or take with liquids. Fentora (fentanyl buccal tablet), used in the management of breakthrough pain in cancer patients already receiving opioid therapy for persistent cancer pain, is an example of a medication administered by the buccal route.

Other forms of medications administered by the oral route will be discussed in more detail in Chapter 16, Calculation of Oral Medications.

Parenteral. Parenteral medications are administered by a route other than by mouth or gastrointestinal tract. Parenteral medications are administered by injection. Parenteral routes include intravenous (IV), intramuscular (IM), subcutaneous (subcut), and intradermal (ID). Labels on parenteral medications specify the route, (e.g., IM and IV use).

Insertion. Medication is placed into a body cavity, where the medication dissolves at body temperature (e.g., suppositories). Vaginal medications, creams, and tablets may also be inserted by using special applicators provided by the manufacturer.

Instillation. Medication is introduced in liquid form into a body cavity. It can also include placing an ointment into a body cavity, such as erythromycin eye ointment, which is placed in the conjunctiva of the eye. Nose drops and ear drops are also instillation medications.

Inhalation. Medication is inhaled through the mouth or nose into the respiratory tract (e.g., through nebulizers used by clients for asthma). Bronchodilators and corticosteroids may be administered by inhalation through the mouth using an aerosolized, pressurized metered-dose inhaler (MDI). In some institutions, these medications are administered to the client with special equipment, such as positive pressure breathing equipment or the aerosol mask. Other medications in inhalation form include pentamidine isethionate, which is used to treat *Pneumocystis jiroveci*, (previously classified as *Pneumocystis carinii*) a type of pneumonia found in clients with acquired immunodeficiency syndrome (AIDS). Another example is Trelegy Ellipta (inhalation powder) used to treat chronic obstructive pulmonary disease (COPD). Devices such as "spacers" or "extenders" have been designed for use with inhalers to allow all of the metered dose to be inhaled, particularly in clients who have difficulty using inhalers.

Intranasal. A medicated solution is instilled into the nostrils. This route is used to administer medications that include the antidiuretic hormone vasopressin and a nasal mist influenza vaccine. Another example is a new medication, Onzetra Xsail (nasal powder), used for the acute treatment of migraines.

Topical. The medication is applied to the external surface of the skin. It can be in the form of lotion, ointment, or paste.

*Percutaneous.* Medications are applied to the skin or mucous membranes for absorption. This includes ointments, powders, and lotions for the skin; instillation of solutions onto the mucous membranes of the mouth, ear, nose, or vagina; and inhalation of aerosolized liquids for absorption through the lungs. The primary advantage is that the action of the medication, in general, is localized to the site of application.

*Transdermal.* Transdermal medication, which is becoming more popular, is contained in a patch or disk and applied topically. The medication is slowly released and absorbed through the skin and enters the systemic circulation. These topical applications may be applied for 24 hours or for as long as 7 days and have systemic effects. Examples include nitroglycerin for angina, nicotine transdermal (Nicoderm) for smoking cessation, clonidine for hypertension, Duragesic (fentanyl) for moderate to severe chronic pain in opioid-tolerant patients, and birth control patches.

Forms of oral medications (tablets, capsules), oral solutions, and routes for parenteral medications are discussed in more detail in later chapters.

Some medications are supplied in multiple forms and therefore can be administered by several routes. For example, Zofran (ondansetron hydrochloride is used to prevent nausea and vomiting associated with cancer chemotherapyand radiation therapy and to prevent and treat nausea and vomiting after surgery. Zofran is supplied as film-coated tablets, orally disintegrating tablets, oral solution, and solution for injection.

## Equipment Used for Medication Administration

Medicine Cup. Equipment used for oral administration includes a 30-mL or 1-oz medication cup made of plastic, used to measure most liquid medications. The cup has measurements in all three systems of measure (Figure 9.3). By looking at the medicine cup, you can see that 30 mL = 1 oz, 5 mL = 1 tsp, and so forth. Remember that any volume less than 1 tsp (5 mL) should be measured with a more accurate device, such as an oral syringe, dropper, or calibrated spoon.

Although the medicine cup is commonly used for administering liquid medications, many facilities still use medicine cups that have measures such as drams (dr), cubic centimeter (cc), and household measures. It is important to note that units of measure such as dr and cc are no longer used in clinical practice. There have been medication errors made because of confusion with different dosing scales on the medication cup. To avoid dosing errors, the recommendations that have been made include that health care institutions purchase cups that have printed, rather than embossed, measurements so that they are easier to read, and ideally the measuring cups should be printed with milliliters (mL) only. To avoid confusion with different measurement systems, organizations such as the American Academy of Pediatrics (AAP), the Institute for Safe Medication Practices (ISMP), and the Centers for Disease Control and Prevention (CDC) have called for adoption of the metric system (mL) as the standard for prescribing and measuring doses of liquid medications.

Soufflé Cup. A soufflé cup is a small paper or translucent plastic cup used for solid forms of medication, such as tablets and capsules (Figure 9.4).

Calibrated Dropper. A calibrated dropper may be used to administer small amounts of medication to an adult or child (Figure 9.5). The calibrations are usually in milliliters but can be in drops. Droppers are also used to dispense eye, nose, and ear medications

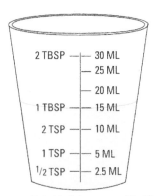

**Figure 9.3** Medicine cup. (Modified from Turner SJ: *Mulholland's the nurse, the math, the meds: drug calculations using dimensional analysis,* ed 4, St Louis, 2019, Elsevier.)

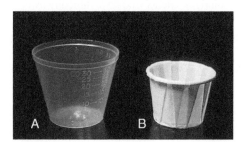

**Figure 9.4** (A) Plastic medicine cup. (B) Soufflé cup. (Courtesy of Chuck Dresner. From Willihnganz M, Gurevitz S, Clayton BD: *Clayton's basic pharmacology for nurses,* ed 18, St Louis, 2020, Elsevier.)

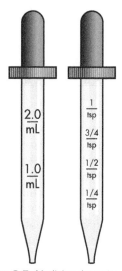

**Figure 9.5** Medicine droppers.

in a squeeze drop bottle and designed for that purpose. The amount of the drop, abbreviated gtt, and size vary according to the diameter of the opening at the tip of the dropper. For this reason, it is important to remember that droppers should not be used as a medication measure unless they are calibrated. Also, because of variation, a properly calibrated dropper is often packaged with the medication (see Figure 9.5) and calibrated for the specified dose. Examples include children's vitamins; nystatin oral solution; and furosemide oral solution. Use the calibrated dropper only with the medicine for which it is designed or packaged with.

> **CRITICAL THINKING**
>
> **BE SAFE. THINK:** Drops from a dropper with a large opening provide more medication than drops from a smaller opening.

> **SAFETY ALERT!**
>
> Droppers are accurate when used to measure the specific medication they are calibrated to, not for measuring other medications. Do not interchange droppers that are packaged with medications. Using a dropper for the wrong medication could result in a serious medication error.

**Nipple.** An infant feeding nipple with additional holes may be used for administering oral medications to infants (Figure 9.6).

**Oral Syringe.** An oral syringe may be used to administer liquid medications orally to adults and children. No needle is attached (Figure 9.7A). An oral syringe is often in color and has an eccentric (off-center) tip to differentiate it from a parenteral syringe. In addition, it usually indicates for oral use on the barrel.

**Calibrated Spoon.** A device that is calibrated usually holds up to 10 mL. Often household and metric units are indicated on the spoon. Designed with a spoon-end shape to make it easier to administer oral medications. Many of the calibrated spoons designed for pediatrics are often in color and may be in the shape of animals (Figure 9.7B).

**Parenteral Syringe.** A parenteral syringe is used for IM, subcut, ID, and IV medications. These syringes come in various sizes and are marked in milliliters or units. The specific types of syringes are discussed in more detail in Chapter 17. **The barrel** of the syringe holds the medication and has calibrations on it that indicate the capacity of the syringe. The

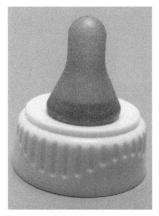

**Figure 9.6** Nipple. (Modified from Willihnganz M, Gurevitz S, Clayton BD: *Clayton's basic pharmacology for nurses,* ed 18, St Louis, 2020, Elsevier.)

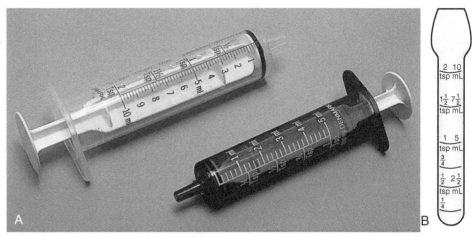

**Figure 9.7** A, Oral syringes. B, Calibrated spoon. (Courtesy of Chuck Dresner. From Willihnganz M, Gurevitz S, Clayton BD: *Clayton's basic pharmacology for nurses,* ed 18, St Louis, 2020, Elsevier.)

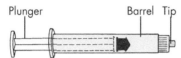

**Figure 9.8** Parts of a syringe. (From Potter PA, Perry AG, Stockert P, Hall A: *Fundamentals of nursing,* ed 9, St Louis, 2017, Mosby.)

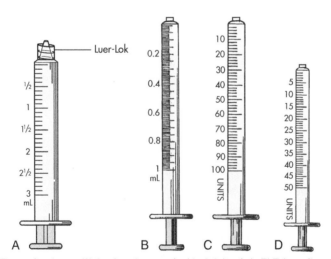

**Figure 9.9** Types of syringes. (A) 3-mL syringe marked in 0.1 (tenths). (B) Tuberculin syringe marked in 0.01 (hundredths) and 0.1 (tenths) of a mL. (C) Insulin syringe marked in units (100). (D) Lo-Dose Insulin syringe marked in units (50). (From Potter PA, Perry AG, Stockert P, Hall A: *Fundamentals of nursing,* ed 9, St Louis, 2017, Mosby.)

**plunger** is used to pull medication into the syringe or to inject medication out of the syringe (Figure 9.8). The needle is attached to the **tip** of the syringe. The size of the needle depends on how the medication is given (e.g., subcut or IM), the viscosity of the medication, and the size of the client. See Figure 9.9 for samples of the types of syringes.

## Equipment for Administering Oral Medications to a Child

Various types of calibrated equipment are on the market for administering medications to children. Most of the available equipment is for oral use. Caregivers should be instructed to always use calibrated measuring devices that are appropriate for measuring prescribed dosages when administering medications to a child. Household spoons vary in size and are

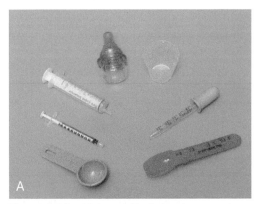 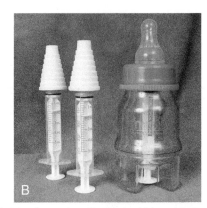

**Figure 9.10** (A) Acceptable devices for measuring and administering oral medication to children *(clockwise)*: measuring spoon, plastic syringes, calibrated nipple, plastic medicine cup, calibrated dropper, hollow-handled medicine spoon. (B) Medibottle used to deliver oral medication via a syringe. (A, From Hockenberry MJ, Wilson D: *Wong's nursing care of infants and children,* ed 9, St Louis, 2011, Mosby. B, Courtesy Paul Vincent Kuntz, Texas Children's Hospital, Houston.)

not reliable devices for accurate dosing. Figure 9.10 presents samples of equipment used to administer oral medications to a child.

> ⚠ **SAFETY ALERT!**
> Remember, to prevent errors in medication administration, the device or equipment you use must be calibrated for the dose you need to administer in order to accurately measure the dose.

> ⚙ **POINTS TO REMEMBER**
> - The basic six rights of medication administration serve as guidelines for nurses when administering medications (the right client, the right medication, the right dose, the right route, the right time, and the right documentation). Additional rights include the right indication, the right to know, the right to refuse, and the right response.
> - Medication administration includes using critical thinking and the nursing process.
> - There are numerous reasons for medication errors.
> - Medication errors can harm clients physically and economically and can be fatal.
> - Nurses are accountable for medications administered regardless of the reason for the error.
> - Nurses are responsible for ensuring the client's safety when administering medications. This includes ensuring that the right client receives the right medication in the right dose, by the right route, at the right time, followed by the right documentation.
> - Nurses play a critical role in the prevention of medication errors.
> - Talking to clients and listening to them can prevent errors. Encourage client questions.
> - Know the policy of the institution regarding timely administration of medications.
> - QSEN (The Quality and Safety Education for Nurses) goal is to improve the quality and safety of client care.
> - Technology to prevent errors and medication safety is relevant to the QSEN safety competency and informatics.
> - The elderly and children require special considerations with medication administration.
> - Medication errors should be reported immediately.
> - A calibrated dropper should be used when administering medications with a dropper.
> - Dosages less than 1 teaspoon should be measured with a device such as an oral syringe, dropper, or calibrated spoon.
> - A medication cup has the capacity of 30 mL. A soufflé cup is used to dispense solid forms of medications.
> - Medications are administered by various routes.

## ▦ PRACTICE **PROBLEMS**

Answer the following questions by filling in the correct word or words to complete the sentence.

1. A dose for oral use that is less than 5 mL should not be measured in a

   _____ .

2. The _____ and _____ need special considerations regarding medication dosages.

3. _____ refers to the way in which a medication is administered.

4. _____ medications have an increased risk of causing significant client harm.

5. A _____ cup is used for dispensing solid forms of medication.

6. Application of medication to the external surface of the skin is referred to as the

   _____ route.

7. Medication administration is a process that requires critical thinking and the nursing process, which includes:

   a. _____   d. _____

   b. _____   e. _____

   c. _____

8. Being an autonomous thinker is an example of _____ .

9. _____ droppers should be used for medication administration.

10. When medications are placed between the gums and inner lining of the cheek, they are administered by the _____ route.

**Answers on p. 147**

## ◉ CHAPTER **REVIEW**

1. Name the six basic rights of medication administration.

   Right _____   Right _____

   Right _____   Right _____

   Right _____   Right _____

2. The Joint Commission requires that clients be identified using _____ client identifiers, neither of which can be the _____ .

3. A medication label should be read _____ times.

4. Medications should be charted _____ you have administered them.

5. Name three routes of medication administration. _____

_____

6. The medicine cup has a (an) _____ capacity.

7. Droppers are calibrated to administer standardized drops regardless of what type of

dropper is used. True or False? _____

8. The syringe used to administer a dosage by mouth is referred to as a (an)

_____ .

9. Parenteral syringes are marked in _____ or
units.

10. The medicine cup indicates that 2 tablespoons are approximately _____ mL.

11. The _____ _____ lists medications
that should be avoided in elderly clients.

12. ISMP is an abbreviation for _____ .

13. TJC is an abbreviation for _____ .

14. The route by which medicated solutions are instilled into the nostrils is _____ .

15. REMS is an abbreviation for _____ .

16. QSEN is an abbreviation for _____ .

17. True or False. Black box warnings are placed on all prescription medications.
_____

18. True or False. Medication errors should be reported immediately.

_____

19. True or False. Establishing a partnership between the client and the health care provider can help in the prevention of medication errors. _____

20. True or False. Clients do not have the right to refuse medications. _____

For questions 21-25, read the statements carefully and indicate which right of medication
administration has been violated.

21. The medication label indicated for optic use, and the medication was instilled into

the client's ears. The right _____ .

22. The prescriber ordered Glipizide and the client received Glyburide. The right

    _____ .

23. The nurse charted all her medications on the medication record before she

    administered them. The right _____ .

24. The nurse administers a medication at 10 PM that was scheduled for 10 AM. The

    right _____ .

25. The dosage to be administered was $1\frac{1}{2}$ tsp. The client received 15 mL. The right

    _____ .

For questions 26-27, identify the right that is violated.

26. A client asks why she is receiving a medication. The nurse knows why, does not tell
    the client, and administers the medication. The right _____

27. A client with a history of low blood pressure (hypotension) has an order for an anti-
    hypertensive medication. The right _____

28. An organization's shared perceptions, beliefs, values, and attitudes that combine to
    create a commitment to safety and effort to minimize harm is referred to as

    _____ .

29. When a nurse is unfamiliar with a medication that has been ordered, the nurse

    should consult a _____ .

30. SREs is an abbreviation for_____ , which are

    endorsed by NQF. NQF is an abbreviation for_____ .

**Answers on p. 148**

---

## ⭐ ANSWERS

## Chapter 9
### Answers to Practice Problems

1. medicine cup
2. elderly and children
3. route
4. High-alert

5. soufflé
6. topical
7. assessment, nursing diagnosis/
   nursing problem, planning, implementation, evaluation

8. critical thinking
9. calibrated
10. buccal

## Answers to Chapter Review

1. medication, dose, client, route, time, documentation
2. two unique, client's (patient's) room number
3. three
4. after
5. parenteral, oral, inhalation, insertion, topical, percutaneous, intranasal, instillation, sublingual, buccal, transdermal
6. 30 mL or 1 oz
7. False
8. oral syringe
9. milliliters (mL)
10. 30 mL
11. Beers criteria
12. Institute for Safe Medication Practices
13. The Joint Commission
14. intranasal
15. Risk Evaluation and Mitigation Strategy
16. Quality and Safety Education for Nurses
17. False
18. True
19. True
20. False
21. Route
22. Medication
23. Documentation
24. Time
25. Dose
26. Right to know
27. Right indication or right reason
28. Safety culture
29. Reputable drug reference
30. Serious Reportable Events, National Quality Forum

# Understanding and Interpreting Medication Orders

## Objectives

*After reviewing this chapter, you should be able to:*

1. Identify the components of a medication order
2. Identify the meanings of standard abbreviations used in medication administration
3. Interpret a given medication order
4. Identify abbreviations, acronyms, and symbols recommended by TJC's "Do Not Use" List and ISMP's List of Error-Prone Abbreviations, Symbols, and Dose Designations
5. Read and write correct medical notations

Medication administration begins with a medication order. Before the nurse can administer any medication, there must be a written legal order written by a licensed health care professional who is authorized to prescribe medication, granted by the state in which they are licensed. Health care professionals authorized to prescribe medications include physicians, physician's assistants, dentists, nurse midwives, and nurse practitioners, depending on state law. Health care providers use medication orders to convey the therapeutic plan for a client, which includes medications. Medication orders communicate to the nurse or designated health care worker which medication or medications to administer to a client. Health care agency policies can vary regarding medication orders. Nurses must be aware of and follow the policies.

In the acute care setting, there are different types of medication orders that can be written:

- **Standing order.** Sometimes referred to as a routine order, a standing order may be written to indicate a medication is to be given for a specified number of doses. For example, ampicillin 1 g IV q6h for 4 doses. A standing order can also indicate that a medication should be administered until it is discontinued or is replaced by another order. For example, Colace 100 mg po tid. Most health care facilities have policies relating to automatic cancellation of an order after a certain time period. For example, 72 hours for narcotics; 30 days for standing orders.
- **prn order.** This order is administered as needed. This type of order allows for the client to receive the medication at their request and allows for the use of nursing judgment on when a medication should be administered based on the client's need and safety. Medications that are ordered on a prn basis need a time interval and reason included in the order, such as "q6h prn for pain." This means a medication can be administered every 6 hours as needed for pain. Examples of prn orders, Tylenol 650 mg po q4h prn for temperature greater than 101°F, Zofran (ondansetron hydrochloride) 4 mg po q6h prn for nausea and vomiting.
- **Stat order.** This means a medication is to be given immediately but only once unless it is re-ordered. For example, Ativan 2 mg IM stat.
- **Single (one-time) order.** This order specifies a medication to be given only once at a specified time. For example, Demerol 50 mg IM and atropine 0.4 mg IM on call to the operating room.

Medication orders are written as prescriptions in private practice or in clinics. The medication the health care provider is ordering in these settings is written on a prescription form that usually comes as a pad and is filled by a pharmacist at a drugstore (pharmacy) or the hospital. Medication orders can be oral (verbal) or written.

Regardless of the mechanism used for a medication order, the nurse has responsibilities relating to the order to ensure safe administration. The nursing responsibilities include the interpretation of common medication abbreviations, identification of the components of a medication order, selecting the correct medication and dosage, administering the medication by the correct route at the right time to the right client, educating the client regarding the medication, monitoring the client's response to the medication, and documenting the medication administered. **Although the nurse is not the originator of the medication order, it is important to remember the nurse is the point person before the client receives the medication ordered. If a calculation or double check of an order is not done, the nurse who administers the medication shares the liability for the injury, even if the order was incorrect, and is responsible for the medication error.**

## Verbal Orders

Usually, medication orders must be written and signed by the prescribing practitioner or directly entered into the computer by the prescriber. Verbal orders are discouraged as a routine policy. Most health care agencies have policies regarding who may accept verbal orders and under what circumstances they can be accepted. Nurses must know the policy of the institution and follow it. However, certain situations or emergencies may require a verbal order that is stated directly in person or by telephone from a licensed physician or another qualified practitioner who is licensed to prescribe. In most health care institutions, the nurse or other authorized personnel can receive a verbal order. Such orders, however, are usually received by the nurse. Verbal orders can be particularly error prone for several reasons, including the order being misheard, poor phone reception, sound-alike drug names, and the nurse assuming the intended order when the order given is incomplete.

Recognizing the errors that can occur with verbal orders and wanting to decrease the potential errors when an oral or telephone order is taken, The Joint Commission (TJC) requires that only "designated qualified staff" may accept verbal or telephone orders. TJC requires that the authorized individual receiving a verbal or telephone order first **write it down** in the patient's chart or enter it into the computer record; second, **read it back** to the prescriber; and then third, **receive confirmation** from the prescriber who gave the order that it is correct. For the nurse to only repeat back the order is not sufficient to prevent errors and is not allowed by TJC. Any questions or concerns relating to the order should be clarified with the prescriber during the conversation. A verbal order must contain the same elements as a written order and be accurate: the date of the order, name and dosage of the medication, route, frequency, any special instructions, and the name of the individual giving the order. TJC advises that in emergency situations, such as a code, doing a formal "read-back" is not feasible, and a "repeat-back" is acceptable to avoid compromising client safety.

It must be noted that it was a verbal or telephone order, and the signature of the nurse taking the order is required. Many institutions require that the order must be signed by the prescriber within 24 hours. Some institutions may require that medication orders written by a person other than a physician be countersigned by designated personnel.

> *i* **TIPS FOR CLINICAL PRACTICE**
>
> It is important to be familiar with specific policies regarding verbal or telephone medication orders and responsibilities in this regard because they vary according to the institution or health care facility.

> *!* **SAFETY ALERT!**
>
> Acceptance of a verbal order is a major responsibility and can lead to medication errors. Accept a verbal order only in an emergency situation. If you accept a verbal order, follow the policy of TJC. Always clarify questions about the order during the conversation. If you are unsure of the medication or the spelling, spell it back to the prescriber and get confirmation. NEVER ASSUME.

Depending on the institution, the medication order may be written on a sheet labeled "physician's order sheet" or "order sheet." After the medication order has been written, the nurse or, in some institutions, a trained unit clerk transcribes the order. This means the order is written on the medication administration record (MAR). In an instance in which the nurse does not transcribe the order, the nurse is accountable for what is written and for verifying the order, initialing it, and checking it before administering.

At some institutions, computers are used for processing medication orders. Medication orders are either electronically transmitted or manually entered directly into the computer from an order form. Computerized provider order entry (CPOE) is also referred to as computerized physician order entry, computerized practitioner order entry, and computerized provider order management (CPOM). CPOE systems are used in many institutions to transmit orders electronically. The use of CPOE has decreased the number of medication order errors and has decreased the problems that have been identified from handwritten orders, which has been repeatedly identified as a contributing factor in medication errors. The use of the computer allows immediate transmission of the order to the pharmacy. The computerized medication record can be seen directly on the computer screen or on a printed copy. Medication orders done by computer entry allow the prescriber to make changes if indicated, and the orders are signed by the prescriber with an assigned electronic code. Once the medication is received on the unit, the medication order is implemented and the client receives the medication.

## Transcription of Medication Orders

Incorrect transcription of medication orders, misinterpretation of medical abbreviations and symbols, and illegible handwriting have been well documented in the literature as contributing factors to medication errors. The advent of technology for prescribing medications has resulted in medication orders being more legible and a decrease in medication errors. However, there are still some institutions that still have handwritten orders.

Whether a medication order is electronically transmitted or handwritten, the order must be clearly understood to ensure safe administration and prevent errors. Before transcribing an order or preparing a dosage for administration, the nurse must be familiar with reading and interpreting an order. To interpret a medication order, the nurse must know the components of a medication order, the standard abbreviations and symbols used in writing a medication order, as well as those abbreviations and symbols that should not be used. In an effort to prevent errors that occur as a result of misinterpretation of abbreviations and symbols, organizations such as The Joint Commission (TJC) and the Institute for Safe Medication Practices (ISMP) developed a list of abbreviations, symbols, and dose designations that should not be used because they can cause misinterpretation, which results in medication errors. TJC developed a list called the "Do Not Use" List (https://www.jointcommission.org/-/media/tjc/documents/resources/patient-safety-topics/do_not_use_list_6_28_19.pdf? and also Appendix C), and ISMP published a list of Error-Prone Abbreviations, Symbols and Dosage Designations (see Appendix D), which includes the abbreviations and symbols on TJC's "Do Not Use" List. ISMP has recommended that these abbreviations, symbols, and dose designations be strictly prohibited when communicating medication information, including medication orders. The nurse must have knowledge of error-prone abbreviations, symbols, and dose designations in addition to abbreviations that should not be used to prevent misinterpretation, promote safe medication administration, and prevent errors with medication orders that can be fatal to the client (QSEN Competency 5-Safety). The nurse therefore must recognize those abbreviations that are error prone and memorize the abbreviations and symbols commonly used in medication administration. The abbreviations include units of measure, route, and frequency for the medication ordered. The common abbreviations and symbols used in medication administration are listed in Tables 10.1 and 10.2.

### TIPS FOR CLINICAL PRACTICE

The use of abbreviations, acronyms, and symbols in the writing of medication orders can have safety implications, and certain abbreviations can mean more than one thing. Care must be taken to use only abbreviations, acronyms, and symbols that have been approved.

| TABLE 10.1 | Symbols and Abbreviations for Units of Measure Used in Medication Administration | | | |
|---|---|---|---|---|
| **Abbreviation/Symbol** | **Meaning** | | **Abbreviation/Symbol** | **Meaning** |
| c, C | cup | | mg | milligram |
| g | gram | | mL | milliliter |
| gtt | drop | | oz | ounce |
| kg | kilogram | | pt | pint |
| L | liter | | qt | quart |
| mcg | microgram | | T, tbs | tablespoon |
| mEq* | milliequivalent | | t, tsp | teaspoon |

*mEq (milliequivalent) is a drug measure in which electrolytes are measured; it expresses the ionic activity of a medication.

| TABLE 10.2 | Commonly Used Medication Abbreviations | | |
|---|---|---|---|
| **Abbreviation** | **Meaning** | **Abbreviation** | **Meaning** |
| $\bar{a}$ | before | ODT | orally disintegrating tablet |
| aa, $\overline{aa}$ | of each | | |
| a.c., ac | before meals | $\bar{p}$ | after |
| ad lib. | as desired, freely | p.c., pc | after meals |
| am, AM | morning, before noon | per | through or by |
| amp | ampule | pm, PM | evening, before midnight |
| aq | aqueous, water | | |
| b.i.d., bid | twice a day | p.o. | by mouth, oral |
| b.i.w. | twice a week | p.r. | by rectum |
| $\bar{c}$ | with | p.r.n., prn | when necessary/ required, as needed |
| c, C | cup | | |
| cap, caps | capsule | q. | every |
| CD | controlled dose | q.a.m. | every morning |
| CR | controlled release | q.h., qh | every hour |
| dil. | dilute | q2h, q4h, q6h, q8h, q12h | every 2 hours, every 4 hours, every 6 hours, every 8 hours, every 12 hours |
| DS | double strength | | |
| EC | enteric coated | | |
| elix. | elixir | | |
| ER | extended release | | |
| fl, fld. | fluid | q.i.d., qid | four times a day |
| GT | gastrostomy tube | q.s. | a sufficient amount/ as much as needed |
| gtt | drop | | |
| h, hr | hour | rect | rectum |
| ID | intradermal | $\bar{s}$ | without |
| IM | intramuscular | sl, SL | sublingual |
| IV | intravenous | sol, soln | solution |
| IVPB | intravenous piggyback | s.o.s., SOS | may be repeated once if necessary |
| IVSS | intravenous Soluset | SR | sustained release |
| KVO | keep vein open (a very slow infusion rate) | S&S | swish and swallow |
| | | stat, STAT | immediately, at once |
| | | subcut | subcutaneous |
| LA | long acting | supp | suppository |
| LOS | length of stay | susp | suspension |
| min | minute | syp, syr | syrup |
| mix | mixture | tab | tablet |
| NAS | intranasal | t.i.d., tid | three times a day |
| NG, NGT | nasogastric tube | tr., tinct | tincture |
| noc, noct | at night | ung., oint | ointment |
| n.p.o., NPO | nothing by mouth | vag, v | vaginally |
| NS, N/S | normal saline | XL | long acting |
| | | XR | extended release |

*Note:* Abbreviations may be written with or without the use of periods; this does not alter the meaning.

## CLINICAL **REASONING**

It is important for you to concentrate on understanding what abbreviations or symbols mean in the context of the order.

## Writing a Medication Order

The health care provider writes a medication order on a form called the *physician's order sheet*. Order sheets vary from institution to institution. The order sheet should have the client's name on it. A prescription blank is used to write medication orders for clients who are being discharged from the hospital or are seeing the health care provider in an outpatient facility. Nurses often have to explain these orders to clients so that they understand the dosages and other relevant information relating to their medications to ensure safety.

## Components of a Medication Order

When a medication order is written, it must contain the following seven important parts or it is considered invalid or incomplete: (1) client's full name, (2) date and time the order was written, (3) name of the medication, (4) dosage of the medication, (5) route of administration, (6) frequency of administration, and (7) signature of the person writing the order. These parts of the medication order are discussed in detail in the following sections.

> **! SAFETY ALERT!**
> If any of the components of a medication order are missing, the order is not complete and not a legal medication order. When in doubt, clarify the order with the prescriber.

Client's Full Name. Using the client's full name helps prevent confusion between one client and another, thereby preventing administration of the wrong medication to a client. Many institutions use a nameplate to imprint the client's name and record number on the order sheet; in addition, there is usually a place to indicate allergies. In institutions that use computers, the computer screen may also show identifying information for the client, such as age and known medication allergies.

Date and Time the Order Was Written. The date and time of the order include the month, day, year, and the time the order was written. This will help in determining the start and stop of the medication order. A record of the time the order was written is preferred in many institutions, but omission does not invalidate the order. This same information is required in computer entry of medication orders. In many institutions, the health care provider (or person legally authorized to write a medication order) is required to include the length of time the medication is to be given (e.g., 7 days); or he or she may use the abbreviation LOS (length of stay), which means the client is to receive the medication during the entire stay in the hospital. Even when not written as part of the order, LOS is implied unless stated otherwise. The policy of indicating the length of time a medication is to be given varies from institution to institution. At some institutions, if there is no specified time period for particular medications, it is assumed to be continued until otherwise stopped by the health care provider or a protocol in place for certain medications, such as controlled substances (narcotics). Some medications have automatic stop times according to the facility (e.g., narcotics, certain antibiotics).

Name of the Medication. The medication may be ordered by the generic or brand name (Figure 10.1). To avoid confusion with another medication, the name of the medication should be written clearly and spelled correctly.

Trade name—The brand name or proprietary name is the name under which a manufacturer markets the medication. The brand or trade name is followed by the registration symbol, ®. The name may be written all in capital letters or may have a combination of capital and lowercase letters. It is generally the largest printed information on the label. The same medication may be made by different drug manufacturers, which assign a trade name to that drug. Therefore a medication can have several trade names. It is important to note that some medications may not have trade names.

**Generic name**—The proper name, chemical name, or nonproprietary name of the medication. It is a name given by the manufacturer that first created the medication. It is usually designated in lowercase letters or a different typeface. Sometimes the generic name is also placed in parentheses. When a medication label has both the trade name and generic name on the label, the generic name is usually found under the trade name (Figure 10.1). Occasionally, only the generic name will appear on the label (Figure 10.2). Each medication has only one generic name. A medication is licensed under its generic name. **By law, the generic name must appear on all medication labels**. The generic name is also registered with the United States Pharmacopeia (USP). USP is an organization that promotes public health by establishing standards to ensure the quality of medicines and other health care technologies. The name is also recorded with a national listing of medications: the United States Pharmacopeia-National Formulary (USP-NF), a book that includes standards for medications, dosage forms, and drug substances. The letters USP after a generic name on a medication label indicates that the medication complies with the USP standards (see Figure 10.2). This name is not specific to the manufacturer. Therefore a medication label **must** indicate the generic name, and some labels may include a trade name. The prescriber may order medications using the generic name. Information found on a medication label with examples of labels is further discussed in Chapter 12, Reading Medication Labels.

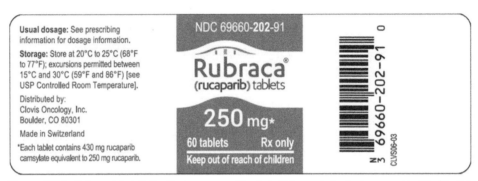

**Figure 10.1** Rubraca label. Notice the two names. The first, *Rubraca*, is the trade name, identified by the registration symbol®. The name in smaller and different print is *rucaparib*, the generic or official name.

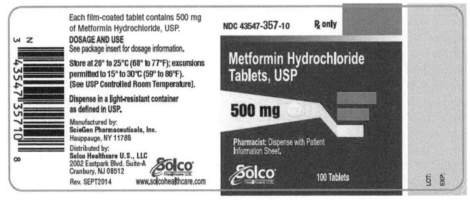

**Figure 10.2** Metformin hydrochloride is the generic name on the label. Notice the abbreviation USP that appears after the generic name on the label.

---

**TIPS FOR CLINICAL PRACTICE**

Nurses must be familiar with both the generic name and the trade name for a medication. To ensure correct medication identification, nurses should crosscheck trade and generic names as needed with a medication reference.

Checking the names of medications even when they are generic is essential in preventing errors. Some very different medications have similar generic names, such as pyridostigmine bromide (Mestinon), which is used to treat myasthenia gravis, and pyrimethamine (Daraprim), which is used to treat parasitic disorders, such as toxoplasmosis.

When reading the name of a medication, never assume. Sometimes orders may be written with abbreviated medication names. This has been discouraged unless the abbreviation is common and approved. Some abbreviations used for medications can cause confusion with another medication; for example, $MgSO_4$ (intended use: magnesium sulfate) and $MSO_4$ (intended use: morphine sulfate). These two are cited on TJC's "Do Not Use" List because they have often been mistaken for each other.

For example, the acronym AZT may be used. "AZT 100 mg p.o." (intended medication order zidovudine [Retrovir], 100 mg, which is used for HIV) can be misread as azathioprine (Imuran), an immunosuppressant. The use of acronyms in writing medication orders is not recommended by TJC; the prescriber must write the complete medication name to avoid misinterpretation.

There are many medications on the market that have names that are similar, that look alike, and sound alike but have very different actions. To minimize confusion and the risk of medication errors ISMP published a list of look-alike, sound-alike (LASA) medication names and instituted the use of "tall man" lettering to decrease the confusion between medication names. Both the FDA-approved and the ISMP-recommended tall man (mixed case) letters have been included in this list. "Tall-man" lettering uses mixed-case (capital and lowercase) or enlarged letters, and bolding of sections of the medication name to emphasize differing portions of the medication name from other similar medication names. The list can be viewed on the ISMP website (https://www.ismp.org/sites/default/files/attachments/2017-11/tallmanletters.pdf) and is included in Appendix B of this text.

> **SAFETY ALERT!**
> A case of mistaken identity with medications can have tragic results.

**Dosage of the Medication.** The amount and strength of the medication should be written clearly to avoid confusion. Dosage indicates the amount or weight provided in the form (e.g., per tablet, per milliliter). The dosage includes the strength of the medication with the unit of measurement (e.g., 40 mg).

To avoid misinterpretation, "U," which stands for units, should not be used when insulin, heparin, or any other medication order that uses units is written. The word *units* should be written out. This would also include "mU" (milliunits). Errors have occurred as a result of confusion of "U" with an "O" in a handwritten order. The abbreviation "U" for units is on TJC's Official "Do Not Use" List and on ISMP's List of Error-Prone Abbreviations, Symbols, and Dose Designations.

**Example:**    6U subcut stat of Humulin Regular Insulin. The U is almost completely closed and could be misread as 60 units. The word *units* should be written out. The handwritten letters "q.d.," when used in prescription writing, can be misinterpreted as "q.i.d." if the period is raised and the tail of the "q" interferes. Example: Lasix 40 mg q.i.d.

**Route of Administration.** The route of administration is a very important part of a medication order because medications can be administered by several routes. As already stated, route refers to how a medication is administered or the method of delivery by which the medication enters into the body. Never assume that you know which route is appropriate. Standard and acceptable abbreviations should be used to indicate the route.

**Examples:**    p.o. (oral, by mouth)    IM (intramuscular)

    ID (intradermal)    IV (intravenous)

> **SAFETY ALERT!**
> Administering a medication by a route other than what the form indicates constitutes a medication error. Regardless of the source of an error, if you administer the wrong dosage, or give a medication by a route other than what it is intended for, you have made a medication error and are legally responsible for it.

**Time and Frequency of Administration.** Standard abbreviations should be used to indicate when and what times a medication is to be administered.

**Examples:** q.i.d. (four times a day), stat (immediately)

The time intervals at which a medication is administered are determined by the institution, and most health care facilities have routine times for administering medications.

**Example:** t.i.d. (three times a day) may be 9 AM, 1 PM, and 5 PM, or 10 AM, 2 PM, and 6 PM

Factors such as the purpose of the medication, medication interactions, absorption of the medication, and side effects should be considered when medication times are scheduled. It is important to realize that when abbreviations such as b.i.d. and t.i.d. are used, the amount you calculate is for one dosage and not for the day's total. The frequency indicates the dosage (amount) of medication given at a single time.

**Signature of the Person Writing the Order.** For a medication order to be legal, it must be signed by the health care provider. The health care provider writing the order must include his or her signature on the order, and it should be legible. At some institutions, in addition to the signature of the physician or other person licensed to write orders, to ensure legibility the prescriber must stamp the order with a rubber stamp that has his or her name clearly printed on it after an order has been written. Orders that are done by computer entry require a signature created by using an assigned electronic code or electronic signature. In some institutions, depending on the rank of the physician or the person writing the order, an order may have to be co-signed by a senior physician.

**Example:** Residents or interns and persons other than a physician writing an order must secure the signature of an attending physician.

In addition to the seven required components of a medication order already discussed, any special instructions or parameters for certain medications need to be clearly written.

**Examples:** 1. Hold if blood pressure (BP) is below 100 systolic.
2. Administer a half-hour before meals ($\frac{1}{2}$ hour a.c.).

Medications ordered as needed or whenever necessary (p.r.n.) should indicate the purpose of administration as well. In addition, a frequency must be written to state the minimum time allowed between dosages. Example: q4h prn.

**Examples:** 1. For chest pain
2. Temperature above 101°F
3. For blood pressure (BP) greater than 140 systolic and 90 diastolic

In instances in which specific instructions are not stated, nursing judgment must be used to determine whether it is appropriate to administer a medication.

For dosage calculations, the nurse is usually concerned with the medication name, dosage of the medication, route, and time or frequency of administration. This information is necessary in determining a safe and reasonable dosage for a client.

> **! SAFETY ALERT!**
> Never assume what an order states! Clarify an order when in doubt. If an order is not clear, or if essential components are omitted, it is not a legal order and should not be implemented. The nurse is accountable!

## Interpreting a Medication Order

Medication orders should be written following a specific sequence:
1. Name of the medication
2. The dosage, expressed in standard abbreviations or symbols
3. Route
4. Frequency

Example:     Colace       100 mg       p.o.       t.i.d.
               ↓             ↓            ↓           ↓
             name        dosage        route    frequency
          of medication

This order means the prescriber wants the client to receive Colace (name of medication), which is a stool softener, 100 milligrams (dosage) by mouth (route), three times a day (frequency). The use of abbreviations in a medication order is a form of shorthand. For the purpose of interpreting orders, it is important for nurses to commit to memory common medical abbreviations, abbreviations related to the systems of measure, as well as recognizing error-prone abbreviations, symbols, and dosage designations that should not be used. Refer to Tables 10.1 and 10.2 for medical abbreviations and symbols used in medication administration. Be systematic when interpreting the order to avoid an error. The medication order follows a specific sequence when it is written correctly (the name of the medication first, followed by the dosage, route, and frequency); interpret the order in this manner as well; avoid "scrambling the order."

Let's look at some medication orders for practice reading and interpreting.

**Example 1:**   Buspar 15 mg po b.i.d.

This order means: Give Buspar 15 milligrams orally (by mouth) two times a day.

**Example 2:**   Procaine Penicillin G 250,000 units IV q6h.

This order means: Give Procaine Penicillin G 250,000 units by intravenous injection every 6 hours.

**Example 3:**   Motrin 400 mg po q6h prn for pain.

This order means: Give Motrin 400 milligrams orally (by mouth) every 6 hours whenever necessary (as required) for pain.

**SAFETY ALERT!**
p.r.n. must have a frequency that designates the minimum time allowed between doses.

Orders are transcribed in some institutions where unit dose (a system that uses single-unit packages of medications that are dispersed to fill each dose requirement) is used. In some institutions, more transcribing may be necessary because the MAR may have the capacity to be used for only a limited period (e.g., 3 days, 5 days). It is therefore necessary to transcribe orders again at the end of the designated period.

In facilities in which computers are used, the medication order is entered into the computer, and a printout lists the currently ordered medications. The computer is able to scan for information such as medication incompatibilities, safe dosage ranges, recommended administration times, and allergies; it can also indicate when a new order for a medication is required.

Computerized order entry and charting do not eliminate the nurse's responsibility for double-checking medication orders before administering. Nurses need to be aware that the use of certain abbreviations, acronyms, and symbols can cause misinterpretation that may result in the potential for or actual error and cause significant harm to clients.

For the safety of clients and to prevent errors in misinterpretation, prescribers responsible for writing medication orders **must** pay attention to what they write; it could save a life. In addition to knowing correct medication notations, those who administer medications must know the safe dosage and be able to recognize discrepancies in a dosage that can sometimes be caused by misinterpretation of an order.

### SAFETY ALERT!

Acceptable abbreviations and medical notations are subject to change. Stay abreast of the guidelines and recommendations of TJC, ISMP, and your health care institution regarding acceptable abbreviations and medical notations.

When writing orders, prescribers should avoid nonstandard abbreviations and avoid abbreviations and symbols that have been identified as error prone. It is important to note that CPOE can still result in errors in medication orders. Therefore all forms of communicating medical information, whether a written order or CPOE according to organizations that include ISMP, TJC, and the National Coordinating Council for Medication Error Reporting and Prevention (NCCMERP), should avoid the use of error-prone abbreviations, symbols, and dose designations that have led to medication errors.

### SAFETY ALERT!

The consequences of misinterpreting abbreviations, symbols, and dosages may be fatal.

### POINTS TO REMEMBER

- A primary responsibility of the nurse is the safe administration of medications to a client.
- Interpret medication orders systematically, the way in which they are written (the name of the medication, the dosage, the route, and frequency).
- The seven components of a medication order are as follows:
  1. The full name of the client
  2. Date and time the order was written
  3. Name of the medication to be administered
  4. Dosage of the medication
  5. Route of administration
  6. Time or frequency of administration
  7. Signature of the person writing the order
- All medication orders must be legible, and standard abbreviations and symbols must be used.
- Memorize the meaning of common abbreviations and symbols.
- The nurse needs to be aware of acronyms, symbols, and abbreviations that should not be used. Their use can increase the potential for errors in medication administration.
- Oral (verbal) orders must be written down, read back to the prescriber, and confirmed with the prescriber that the order is correct.
- If any of the seven components of a medication order are missing or seem incorrect, the medication order is not legal. Do not assume—clarify the order!
- If you are in doubt as to the meaning of an order, clarify it with the prescriber before administering.
- Always crosscheck medications; misidentification can result in a medication error.

## PRACTICE **PROBLEMS**

Interpret the following abbreviations.

1. p.c. _____     4. b.i.d. _____

2. h _____     5. p.r.n. _____

3. q12h _____

Interpret the following orders. Use either *administer* or *give* at the beginning of the sentence.

6. Zidovudine 200 mg p.o. q4h. _____

   _____

7. Procaine Penicillin G 400,000 units IV q8h. _____

   _____

8. Gentamicin sulfate 45 mg IVPB q12h. _____

   _____

9. Regular Humulin insulin 5 units subcut, a.c. at 7:30 AM and at bedtime. _____

   _____

10. Vitamin $B_{12}$ 1,000 mcg IM, every other day. _____

    _____

11. Prilosec 20 mg p.o. bid. _____

    _____

12. Tofranil 75 mg p.o. at bedtime. _____

    _____

13. Restoril 30 mg p.o. at bedtime. _____

    _____

14. Mylanta 30 mL p.o. q4h p.r.n. _____

    _____

15. Synthroid 200 mcg p.o. daily. _____

    _____

**Answers on p. 163**

## ⊙ CHAPTER **REVIEW**

List the seven components of a medication order.

1. _____    5. _____

2. _____    6. _____

3. _____    7. _____

4. _____

Write the meaning of the following abbreviations.

8. ODT _____    14. b.i.w. _____

9. ad. lib. _____    15. SR _____

10. subcut _____    16. syr _____

11. c̄ _____    17. n.p.o. _____

12. a.c. _____    18. sl _____

13. q.i.d. _____

Write the abbreviations for the following:

19. after meals _____    25. may be repeated once if necessary ___

20. three times a day _____    26. without _____

21. intramuscular _____    27. immediately _____

22. every eight hours _____    28. ointment _____

23. suppository _____    29. milliequivalent _____

24. intravenous _____    30. by rectum _____

Interpret the following orders. Use either *administer* or *give* at the beginning of the sentence.

31. Methergine 0.2 mg p.o. q4h for 6 doses. _____

_____

32. Digoxin 0.125 mg p.o. once a day. _____

_____

33. Regular Humulin insulin 14 units subcut daily at 7:30 AM. _____

_____

34. Demerol 50 mg IM and atropine 0.4 mg IM on call to the operating room.

_____

35. Ampicillin 500 mg p.o. stat, and then 250 mg p.o. q.i.d. thereafter. _____

_____

36. Lasix 40 mg IM stat. _____

_____

37. Librium 50 mg p.o. q4h p.r.n. for agitation. _____

_____

38. Tylenol 650 mg p.o. q4h p.r.n. for pain. _____

_____

39. Mylicon 80 mg p.o. p.c. and bedtime. _____

_____

40. Otezla 30 mg p.o. b.i.d. _____

_____

41. Nembutal 100 mg p.o. at bedtime p.r.n. _____

_____

42. Flomax 0.4 mg p.o. daily. _____

_____

43. Dilantin 100 mg p.o. t.i.d. _____

_____

44. Minipress 2 mg p.o. b.i.d.; hold for systolic BP less than 120. _____

_____

45. Aimovig 70 mg subcut once a month. _____

_____

46. Ampicillin 1 g IVPB q6h for 4 doses. _____

_____

47. Heparin 5,000 units subcut q12h. _____

_____

48. Dilantin susp 200 mg by NGT q AM and 300 mg by NGT at bedtime. _____

_____

49. Benadryl 50 mg p.o. stat. _____

_____

50. Epogen 3,500 units subcut three times a week. _____

_____

51. Zofran 8 mg p.o. q12h for 2 days following chemotherapy. _____

_____

52. Septra DS 1 tab p.o. daily. _____

_____

53. Neomycin ophthalmic ointment 1% in the right eye t.i.d. _____

_____

Indicate whether the statement is True or False.

54. The trade name will always be indicated on the medication label. _____

_____

55. A medication can have several trade names. _____

_____

56. Tall man lettering is used for all medications. _____

_____

57. Some medication labels only indicate the generic name on the label. _____

_____

Identify the missing part from the following medication orders. Assume that the date, time, and signature are included on the orders.

58. Dicloxacillin 250 mg q.i.d. _____

59. Synthroid 0.05 mg p.o. _____

60. Nitrofurantoin p.o. q6h for 10 days. _____

61. 25 mg p.o. q12h, hold if BP less than 100 systolic. _____

62. Solu-Cortef 100 q6h. _____

63. Describe what your action would be if the following order was written:

Prilosec 20 mg daily. _____

Using the discussion on medication abbreviations, symbols, and acronyms that should not be used, identify the mistake in the following orders and correct each order.

64. Inderal20mg p.o. daily. _____

65. Lasix 10.0 mg p.o. b.i.d. _____

66. Humulin Regular insulin 4U IV stat. _____

67. Haldol .5 mg p.o. t.i.d. _____

**Answers below and on p. 164**

## ⭐ ANSWERS

### Chapter 10
#### Answers to Practice Problems

1. after meals
2. hour
3. every 12 hours
4. twice daily, twice a day
5. when necessary/required, as needed
6. Give or administer zidovudine 200 milligrams orally (by mouth) every 4 hours.
7. Give or administer Procaine Penicillin G 400,000 units by intravenous injection every 8 hours.
8. Give or administer gentamicin sulfate 45 milligrams by intravenous piggyback injection every 12 hours.
9. Give or administer regular Humulin insulin 5 units by subcutaneous injection before the morning meal at 7:30 AM and at bedtime.
10. Give or administer vitamin $B_{12}$ 1,000 micrograms by intramuscular injection every other day.
11. Give or administer Prilosec 20 milligrams orally (by mouth) twice a day (two times a day).
12. Give or administer Tofranil 75 milligrams orally (by mouth) at bedtime.
13. Give or administer Restoril 30 milligrams orally (by mouth) at bedtime.
14. Give or administer Mylanta 30 milliliters orally (by mouth) every 4 hours when necessary (when required).
15. Give or administer Synthroid 200 micrograms orally (by mouth) daily.

#### Answers to Chapter Review

1. name of the client
2. date and time the order was written
3. name of the medication
4. dosage of medication
5. route by which medication is to be administered
6. time and/or frequency of administration
7. signature of the person writing the order
8. orally disintegrating tablet
9. as desired
10. subcutaneous
11. with
12. before meals
13. four times a day
14. twice a week
15. sustained release
16. syrup
17. nothing by mouth
18. sublingual
19. p.c. *or* pc
20. t.i.d. *or* tid
21. I.M. *or* IM
22. q.8.h. *or* q8h
23. supp
24. I.V. *or* IV
25. s.o.s. *or* sos
26. s̄
27. stat *or* STAT
28. ung *or* oint
29. mEq
30. p.r. *or* pr

31. Give or administer Methergine 0.2 milligrams orally (by mouth) every 4 hours for 6 doses.
32. Give or administer digoxin 0.125 milligrams orally (by mouth) once a day.
33. Give or administer regular Humulin insulin 14 units by subcutaneous injection daily at 7:30 AM.
34. Give or administer Demerol 50 milligrams by intramuscular injection and atropine 0.4 milligrams by intramuscular injection on call to the operating room.
35. Give or administer ampicillin 500 milligrams orally (by mouth) immediately (at once) and then 250 milligrams orally (by mouth) four times a day thereafter.
36. Give or administer Lasix 40 milligrams by intramuscular injection immediately (at once).
37. Give or administer Librium 50 milligrams orally (by mouth) every 4 hours when necessary (when required) for agitation.
38. Give or administer Tylenol 650 milligrams orally (by mouth) every 4 hours when necessary (when required) for pain.
39. Give or administer Mylicon 80 milligrams orally (by mouth) after meals and at bedtime.
40. Give or administer Otezla 30 milligrams orally (by mouth) twice a day (two times a day).

41. Give or administer Nembutal 100 milligrams orally (by mouth) at bedtime when necessary (when required).

42. Give or administer Flomax 0.4 milligrams orally (by mouth) daily.

43. Give or administer Dilantin 100 milligrams orally (by mouth) three times a day.

44. Give or administer Minipress 2 milligrams orally (by mouth) two times a day (twice a day). Hold for systolic blood pressure less than 120.

45. Give or administer Aimovig 70 milligrams by subcutaneous injection once a month.

46. Give or administer ampicillin 1 gram by intravenous piggyback injection every 6 hours for 4 doses.

47. Give or administer heparin 5,000 units by subcutaneous injection every 12 hours.

48. Give or administer Dilantin suspension 200 milligrams by nasogastric tube every morning and 300 milligrams by nasogastric tube at bedtime.

49. Give or administer Benadryl 50 milligrams orally (by mouth) immediately (at once).

50. Give or administer Epogen 3,500 units by subcutaneous injection three times a week.

51. Give or administer Zofran 8 milligrams orally (by mouth) every 12 hours for 2 days following chemotherapy.

52. Give or administer Septra double-strength 1 tablet orally (by mouth) daily.

53. Give or administer neomycin ophthalmic ointment 1% to the right eye three times a day.

54. False

55. True

56. False

57. True

58. route of administration

59. frequency of administration

60. dosage of medication (drug)

61. name of medication (drug)

62. dosage of medication (drug) and route of administration

63. Notify the prescriber that the order is incomplete; route is missing from the order; do not administer, order not legal. Never assume.

64. Inderal 20 mg p.o. daily. There should be adequate spacing between the medication name, dosage, and unit of measure. Could be misread as 120 mg, which is 6 times the dosage ordered.

65. Lasix 10 mg p.o. bid. Trailing zeros could cause dosage to be interpreted as 100 mg, which is 10 times the intended dose.

66. Humulin Regular Insulin 4 units IV stat. The abbreviation for units here could be misread as a zero, which could result in 10 times the dose being administered. Write out units.

67. Haldol 0.5 mg p.o. tid. Omission of the leading zero before the decimal point could result in the dosage being read as 5 mg, which would be 10 times the dosage ordered.

# CHAPTER 11
# Medication Administration Records and Drug Distribution Systems

## Objectives

*After reviewing the chapter, you should be able to:*

1. State the components of a medication order
2. Identify the necessary components of a medication administration record (MAR)
3. Read an MAR and identify medications that are to be administered on a routine basis, including the name of the medication, the dosage, the route of administration, and the time of administration
4. Read an MAR and identify medications that are administered, including the name of the medication, the dosage, the route of administration, and the time of administration
5. Identify the various medication distribution systems used

## Medication Orders

As already discussed, before any medication can be administered or transcribed there must be an order. Health care facilities usually have a special form for recording medication orders. The terms *medication orders* and *doctor's orders* are used interchangeably, and the forms vary from institution to institution. As technology becomes a central component of health care and health care facilities transition to the electronic medical record, handwritten medication order forms are gradually being replaced by computerized provider order entry (CPOE), which is also referred to as computerized physician/practitioner/prescriber order entry. CPOE relates to the process in which the prescriber enters and sends orders (medications and treatments) electronically using a computer application. A medication order, whether handwritten or electronically generated (computer), must have the following components:

- Client identification information, which includes information such as the client's full name, the client's date of birth, allergies, and other identifying information
- Name of the medication
- Dosage of medication
- Route of administration
- Frequency of administration and any special instructions related to administration if needed: for example, for moderate pain, hold for apical pulse less than 60
- Date and time the order was written
- Signature of the prescriber

## Medication Administration Record

Medication administration records (MARs) are legal documents that contain a record of medications a client has received and is currently receiving. MARs may be handwritten (Figure 11.1) or electronically generated (Figure 11.2). In institutions in which handwritten orders are still used, after the medication order has been verified, the order is transcribed to an MAR in a paper format according to the institution policy for transcription of medication orders. The person responsible for transcription of orders to a handwritten MAR depends on the institution. If the order is not transcribed by the nurse, the nurse is still responsible for double-checking the transcription against the prescriber's order to make certain the order is complete and that there are no discrepancies. In institutions where orders are generated electronically, the orders are transcribed to the electronic medication administration record (eMAR) by the computer. Medication orders are viewed and charted on the computer. Even though the system is computerized, the nurse still has the responsibility of verifying the order before administering medications.

DEPARTMENT OF NURSING
MEDICATION ADMINISTRATION RECORD

Identifying Client Information (Name, Room Number, Date of Birth, Medical Record Number)

| Diagnosis: | |
|---|---|
| **ALLERGIES:** NKDA | Date: 4/2/2020 |

| Order Date | Exp. Date | RN Initial | Medication-Dosage, Frequency, Route | Date 2020 | 4/2 | 4/3 | 4/4 | 4/5 | 4/6 | 4/7 | 4/8 |
|---|---|---|---|---|---|---|---|---|---|---|---|
| | | | | Time | Initial | Initial | Initial | Initial | Initial | Initial | Initial |
| 4/2/20 | 5/2/20 | DG | Colace 100 mg po bid | 0900 | DG | JN | | | | | |
| | | | | 1700 | NN | NN | | | | | |
| | | | | | | | | | | | |
| | | | | | | | | | | | |
| | | | | | | | | | | | |
| 4/2/20 | 5/2/20 | DG | Furosemide 40 mg po daily | 0900 | DG | | | | | | |
| | | | | | | | | | | | |
| | | | | | | | | | | | |
| | | | | | | | | | | | |
| 4/2/20 | 5/2/20 | DG | Digoxin 0.125 mg po daily | 0900 | DG | JN | | | | | |
| | | | check apical pulse (AP) | AP | 76 | 80 | | | | | |
| | | | Hold if less than 60 or above 100 beats per minute (bpm) | | | | | | | | |

| | Initial | Print Name/Title | | Initial | Print Name/Title | | Initial | Print Name/Title |
|---|---|---|---|---|---|---|---|---|
| 1 | DG | Deborah Gray RN | 5 | | | 9 | | |
| 2 | NN | Nancy Nurse RN | 6 | | | 10 | | |
| 3 | JN | Jane Nightingale RN | 7 | | | 11 | | |
| 4 | | | 8 | | | 12 | | |

**Figure 11.1** Handwritten medication administration record (MAR). Note: This MAR is intended to show the basic information that would be included on an MAR.

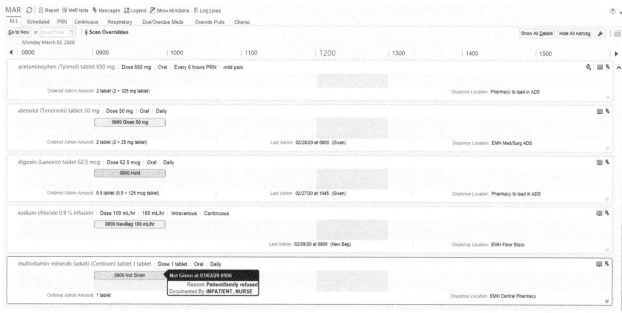

© 2020 Epic Systems Corporation. Used with permission.

**Figure 11.2** Electronic medication administration record (eMAR). (Used with permission of Epic Systems Corporation.)

There is no standard form for MARs, and they vary from institution to institution. The various MAR forms used at different institutions represent differences in form only. Whether the MAR is electronic or handwritten, it contains the same information indicated on a medication order and specifies the actual time to administer the medication or the actual time of administration, as well as the essential information (the name of each medication, the dosage, route, and frequency) that is common to all and to their purpose. The MAR is used to determine what medications are ordered and the dosage, route, and time at which each is to be given and is also verified with the prescriber's orders.

Different forms may be used in the home care setting for the charting of medications that are administered. Sample MARs are included in this chapter. As you look at the sample MARs, it is important to locate and identify the information common to all MARs. Your clinical instructor will orient you to actual MARs used in the clinical setting for your clinical experience.

> ### TIPS FOR CLINICAL PRACTICE
> Regardless of whether the MAR is handwritten or electronic, the nurse or health care provider uses the record to check the medication order, prepare the correct dosage, and record the medication administered to a client.

## Essential Components on a Medication Administration Record

If a handwritten MAR is used, the information on the medication record must be legible and transcribed carefully to avoid errors. In addition to client information (name, date of birth, medical record number, allergies), the following information is necessary on all MARs regardless of the format:

1. **Dates.** This information usually includes the date the order was written, the date the medication is to be started (if different from the order date), and when to discontinue it.

2. **Medication information.** This includes the medication's full name, the dosage, the route, and the frequency. Abbreviations used on the medication record should be standard abbreviations and follow the guidelines and restrictions of The Joint Commission (TJC), ISMP, and the health care institution.

3. **Time of administration.** This will be based on the desired administration ordered by the prescriber, such as t.i.d. and the institution's standard times for scheduled or routine medications. (Thus t.i.d. may mean 9 AM, 1 PM, and 5 PM at one institution and 10 AM, 2 PM, and 6 PM at another.) A nurse should always become familiar with the hours for medication administration designated by a specific institution as well as the type of time being used (traditional or military time). Many clinical facilities use military time. Medications that are ordered for p.r.n. and one-time dosages are recorded at the time they are administered. Abbreviations for time and frequency should adhere to TJC and ISMP guidelines.

4. **Identification of health care professional administering medications.** Most handwritten MARs have a place for initials of the person transcribing the medications to the MAR, and the person administering the medication. The initials are then written under the signature section to identify who gave the medication. Some MARs may request the title as well as the signature of the person. The policy regarding initialing after each administration varies by institution and by the charting system used. See Figure 11.1 for an example. In institutions that use a computerized eMAR, the person uses their own specific code to log into the system, scans the medication, and administers the medication. It is documented as given, and the name is automatically entered.

5. **Special instructions (parameters).** Any special instructions relating to a medication should be indicated on the MAR. For example, "Hold if systolic blood pressure is less than 100" or "p.r.n. for moderate pain."

> **TIPS FOR CLINICAL PRACTICE**
>
> The nurse must stay alert to the guidelines of TJC and ISMP regarding abbreviations and medical notations.

## Documentation of Medications

Documentation is the sixth "right of medication administration." Regardless of the format used to document the administration of medications, the documentation must be accurate, and legally all medications administered must be documented. Regardless of whether the handwritten MAR or eMAR is used, documentation should be done immediately after medications are given. Remember, this practice will prevent forgetting to document, which can result in the administration of the medication by another nurse or health care provider who thought the medication was not administered. No documentation can be interpreted as not being administered. Documentation should include not only medications administered but also documentation regarding refusals, delays in administration, and responses to medication administration (including adverse effects). It is important to remember that the type of notation used and where the notation is done for handwritten MARs can vary from one institution to the other. In institutions that use the eMAR, the documentation is done in the computer. The computerized MAR allows the documentation of comments regarding the medication administration at the computer terminal.

> **SAFETY ALERT!**
>
> Document properly and accurately any medications administered to prevent medication errors caused by overmedicating or undermedicating.

## Use of Technology in Medication Administration

In an effort to minimize medication errors, many health care facilities have instituted some form of computer-based medication administration. Some of the technology used has already been discussed. Additional technology designed to prevent medication errors includes computer-based drug administration (CBDA), a technological software system. The purpose of the software is to automate the medication administration process and improve accuracy and efficiency in documentation. This system comprises the computerized prescriber order system, the barcode administration system, and the electronic medication administration record (eMAR), and the pharmacy information systems.

Many institutions have moved to CPOE. The CPOE systems are used to transmit orders electronically. Depending on the institution and the sophistication of the software, information such as medication incompatibilities, medication allergies, range of dosages, and recommended medication times may be part of the system. With the computer used to process medication orders, they can be viewed on the computer screen or on a printout. A corresponding MAR is available at some institutions based on the computerized order entry. Software has also been developed that allows for the use of CPOE and clinical decision-making support systems (CDSSs).

A clinical decision support system is also known as a clinical decision support program (CDS program). The CDS systems may be standalone software programs, or they may be integrated into parts of other systems. A definition of the clinical decision support system according to Robert Hayward of the Centre for Health Evidence is: "Clinical decision support systems link health observations with health knowledge to influence health choices by clinicians for improved health care." In other words, the CDS health information technology provides the physician and other health professions with support to assist in clinical decision-making.

Despite the fact that use of technology such as CPOE has reduced errors associated with medication errors, according to a news release by ISMP (January 24, 2019), "If the conventions used to communicate medication information electronically are not carefully considered, these technologies may contribute to medication errors rather than mitigate risks. Examples of issues with electronic communication that have resulted in medication errors include misinterpretation of symbols, dose designations, and abbreviations; unsafe defaults used to prepopulate fields with missing data (for example, default to number of teaspoons to administer rather than mL); and restricted character spaces or truncated listings that make it impossible to communicate the full name and dose of a medication." As a result, to improve safety in communicating about medications when working with electronic formats ISMP developed Guidelines for Safe Electronic Communication of Medication Information. These guidelines can be found on the ISMP website: https://www.ismp.org/node/1322 (ISMP Guidelines for Safe Electronic Communication of Medication Information, 2019). The guidelines developed provide specific recommendations relating to the safe presentation of information electronically regarding medications that include medication names, dosages, and weights and measures.

There are many information technology applications for medication safety, and some of them have been discussed in this text (they include computerized physician order entry, automated dispensing cabinets, and barcoding medication system). Technology will continue to grow, and its use will vary from institution to institution. Technology is only one of many tools that can be used to enhance client safety.

## Medication Distribution Systems

The medication distribution system varies from one institution to the next. The various distribution systems are discussed in the following sections.

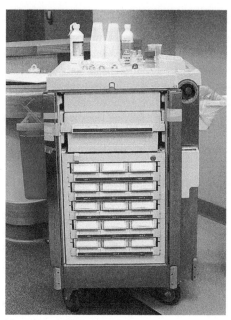

**Figure 11.3** Unit-dose cabinet. (From Willihnganz M, Gurevitz S, Clayton BD: *Clayton's basic pharmacology for nurses,* ed 18, St Louis, 2020, Elsevier.)

## Unit-Dose System

Many institutions use a system of medication administration referred to as a *unit-dose drug dispensing system* (UDDS). This system has decreased medication preparation time because the medications are prepared daily in the pharmacy and sent to the unit. Medications are dispensed by the pharmacy in individual dosages as prescribed. Packages provide a single dosage of medication. The package is labeled with generic and trade names (and sometimes manufacturer, lot number, and expiration date). Depending on the distribution system, the individual packages may be labeled with the client's name and barcode. The medications are placed in a client-identified drawer in a large unit-dose cabinet at the nurse's station.

Unit dose is also used as part of another medication system in some institutions (e.g., a computerized unit-dose medication cart). In the computerized unit-dose system, each dosage for the client is released individually and recorded automatically. This system is used for monitoring controlled substances and other items used in the unit (e.g., medications used by the unit in large volumes). The type of medication form used for this system varies from one institution to another. In some instances, this system has decreased the amount of time spent transcribing orders or eliminated the need for transcription. In some institutions, however, transcription of medication orders to the MAR is still required. The prescriber's orders are therefore written on a separate order sheet and sent to the pharmacy. Figure 11.1 illustrates the transcription of orders to the MAR.

At some institutions the prescriber's order is done by computer entry, eliminating the need for transcription. Figure 11.3 shows a unit-dose cabinet.

## Computer-Controlled Dispensing System

The use of automated dispensing cabinets (ADCs) is on the rise in health care facilities. This system is gaining increased popularity in many institutions and health care facilities. The computer-controlled dispensing system is supplied by the pharmacy daily with stock medications. Controlled substances are also kept in the cart, and the system provides a detailed record indicating which controlled substances were used and by whom. The medication order is received by the pharmacy for the client and then entered into the system. To access medications in this system, the nurse uses a security code and password or biometric fingerprint scan.

The three most common dispensing systems include the Pyxis Med Station system (Figure 11.4), the Omnicell Omni Rx, and the AcuDose-Rx.

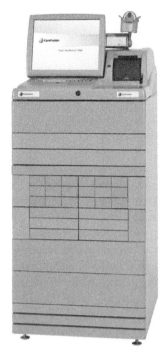

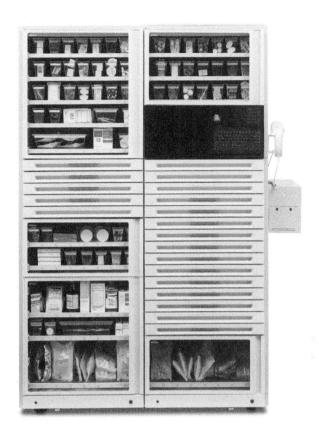

**Figure 11.4** Pyxis Med Station. (Courtesy and © Becton, Dickinson and Company, Franklin Lakes, NJ.)

**Figure 11.5** Omnicell XT Automated Dispensing Cabinet. (Used with permission of Omnicell, Inc.)

The Omnicell system shown in Figure 11.5 is an automated dispesding cabinet (ADC) that assists in providing for a safer process to get the medication to the client as well as in safer medication management. The ADC includes features such as an integrated medication label printer with barcoded labels, the ability to integrate with major advanced electronic health record (EHR) systems, and management of controlled substances (eliminating the need for count-backs at the ADC). The ADC is enhanced by data intelligence; Omnicell Essentials, the cloud-based Essential dashboard, reveals medication inventory and drug diversion issues and points to areas that need attention.

These systems allow storage of items such as vials and premixed IVs and allow nurses to obtain any medications stored in the device for any client and even to override the system in an emergency. However, overrides eliminate verification of medications by the pharmacy, which could result in an error. Currently, almost 90% of all automated dispensing cabinets are linked to pharmacy information systems, thereby decreasing errors by ensuring that the nurse can only access medications for a specific client.

Some institutions have added barcoding to this process during the administration phase of the medication process. At the client's bedside, the nurse uses a handheld scanner that records the barcode on the client's wristband and the unit-dose medication packet, linking this information to the client database. If there is an error, the administration process is halted; if the information is correct, the medication is administered and documentation in the MAR occurs automatically. Literature supports that use of ADCs has reduced medication errors by dispensing the correct medication.

Recognizing the need to guide health care organizations in the safest use of ADCs, ISMP first issued guidelines for the safe use of ADCs in 2009. Following the review of reported errors occurring with the use of ADCs, the guidelines were revised in 2019. The updated guidelines for the safe use of ADCs can be viewed on the ISMP website at https://www. ismp.org/news/ismp-issues-updated-guidelines-safe-use-automated-dispensing-cabinets. The health care provider must still remember the importance of client safety and follow the "Six Rights of Medication Administration" when using technology.

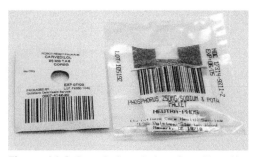

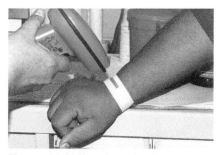

**Figure 11.6** Barcode for unit drug dose. (From Kee JL, Marshall SM, Woods K, Forrester MC: *Clinical calculations: With applications to general and speciality areas,* ed 8, St Louis, 2017, Elsevier.)

**Figure 11.7** Barcode reader. (From Kee JL, Marshall SM, Woods K, Forrester MC: *Clinical calculations: With applications to general and speciality areas,* ed 8, St Louis, 2017, Elsevier.)

## Barcode Medication Delivery

Barcode medication delivery use is increasing in some health care facilities. The basic system of barcoding verifies that a client receives the right dosage of the right medication by the right route at the right time. This system requires that each client wear an ID with a unique barcode to identify the individual. Each medication must therefore have a barcode. Computers installed at the client's bedside and/or handheld devices enable the nurse to scan the barcode on the client's identification band and the medication to be administered. Once the information has been validated to the client and the client's medication profile, the medication given is documented on an online MAR (see Figure 11.6 showing a barcode for unit medication dose, and Figure 11.7 showing a barcode reader). Barcoding is being added to some medication distribution systems as mentioned in the discussions of automated dispensing systems and unit-dose systems. Many pharmacists are using the barcode system to prepare unit-dose medications. Like other systems, barcode systems with additional features are also available. The complexity or simplicity of the barcode system depends on the institution. The barcode medication administration system allows overrides in cases where medications need to be administered in an emergency. However, literature points out that an override bypasses the important step of order verification by the pharmacist.

## Role of the Nurse When Using Technology

The use of computer-based technology in medication administration has been identified as one of the best practices to minimize medication errors. The use of computerized systems as a tool for reducing medication errors speaks to two Quality and Safety Education for Nurses (QSEN) competencies: safety to reduce risk of harm to clients and informatics and the use of technology to mitigate errors.

Even though the use of technology in the health care system has proliferated as stated, it is one tool of many that can be used to decrease medication errors. The use of technology tools such as CPOE, eMAR, and the various medication administration systems are not a total safeguard to the elimination of medication errors, and no system is completely without fault. Regardless of the medication system used, the nurse must recognize the importance of safety first and realize that no system eliminates the need for the nurse to follow the standard administration procedures for medication administration, such as verifying all aspects of the medication order and consistent use of the rights of medication administration when administering medications—the right client, right medication, right dosage, right time, right route, and right documentation. When we lose sight of the importance of checks or omit them, errors can occur from skipping steps.

Literature relating to the use of technology in the health care system reinforces the need for proper education of nurses and other health care providers to its proper use to avoid compromising client safety. The institution of technology into medication administration requires a collaborative approach and commitment by all health care providers involved to client safety as the main focus. Any technology implemented in the health care setting should not substitute for knowledge of the health care provider, eliminate critical thinking, nor eliminate the taking of basic safety precautions. With the influx of new medications, varied medication distribution systems, and increasing technology in the health care system, nurses will be presented with new challenges and different types of errors; therefore nurses must be knowledgeable and prepared to meet their responsibilities, remembering client safety is the main focus to prevent harm to the client. The role and responsibilities of the nurse cannot be negated with the use of technology; the role of the nurse is more enhanced by its use.

## Scheduling Medication Times

Many health care facilities have routine schedules for administering medications, which vary from one institution to another. Common abbreviations are used for scheduling and prescribing medications. As previously mentioned in this chapter, the nurse must become familiar with the administration schedule used at a specific institution. Table 11.1 shows some examples of commonly used abbreviations in scheduling of medications. The nurse must be knowledgeable about abbreviations prohibited for use by TJC and ISMP related to dosing frequency (QSEN Competency 5, Safety).

## Military Time

Many hospitals and health care agencies use military time (international time). Medication orders may include the time of administration in military time when documenting the administration of medications on the MAR. The FDA recommends the use of military time. The nurse therefore needs to be familiar with how to convert traditional time to military time. Review content relating to converting time between traditional and military in Chapter 8 if necessary.

| TABLE 11.1 | Commonly Used Abbreviations for Scheduling Medications |
|---|---|
| **Abbreviation** | **Meaning** |
| a.c.* | before meals |
| b.i.d | twice a day |
| p.c.* | after meals |
| p.r.n. | as needed (when necessary/required) |
| q | every |
| q.h. | every hour |
| q2h, q3h, q4h | every 2 hours, 3 hours, 4 hours |
| q6h, q8h, q12h, q24h | every 6 hours, 8 hours, 12 hours, 24 hours |
| q.i.d. | four times a day |
| stat | immediately (at once), now |
| t.i.d. | three times a day |

*Based on mealtimes.

**POINTS TO REMEMBER**

- The system used for medication administration plays a role in determining the type of medication record used and whether transcription of orders is necessary.
- Regardless of the type of medication record used at an institution, the nurse should know the data that are essential for the medication record and understand the importance of accuracy and clarity on medication orders.
- Persons transcribing orders should transcribe them in ink and write legibly to avoid medication errors. All essential notations or instructions should be clearly written on the medication record. Notations used should follow TJC and ISMP regulations.
- Documentation of medications administered should be done promptly, accurately, and only by the person administering them.
- To avoid errors in administration, always check transcribed orders against the prescriber's orders.
- The use of technology has reduced medication errors.
- Nurses need to be aware of the different distribution systems in use.
- Regardless of the system used, safety is the priority, and the nurse must still use the process in medication administration of verifying the order, administering the medication to the right client, right dosage, right route, right time, and right documentation.
- A facility may use traditional or military (international) time to designate administration times. The FDA recommends the use of military time.
- Technology is only one tool of many that can be used for medication safety.

---

## ▦ PRACTICE **PROBLEMS**

1. True or False? Illegible prescribers' handwriting is the most common reason for medication errors on handwritten MARs (medication administration records).

   _____

2. True or False? The use of technology is a foolproof method to prevent medication errors. _____

3. True or False? Medication administration forms have information that is common to all, regardless of the form used. _____

4. "The right _____ must receive the right _____ in the right _____ by the right _____ at the right _____ followed by the right _____."

5. The _____ is responsible for the medication administered, regardless of the reason for the error.

6. The Pyxis is an example of _____ .

7. The ability to _____ a system eliminates _____ by the pharmacy, which increases the likelihood of a medication error.

8. True or False? All health care institutions document medications using traditional time. _____

9. What is the last step in medication administration? _____

10. CPOE is an abbreviation for _____ .

Refer to the handwritten MAR (Figure 11.1) to answer the following questions.

11. How many times a day is furosemide ordered? _____

12. Identify the medications and their doses administered at 0900 _____

13. K-Dur 10 mEq is ordered. What does mEq mean? _____

14. What action must you take before administering Digoxin? _____

15. What is the equivalent of the scheduled administration time for K-Dur in traditional time? _____

16. True or False? ADC is an abbreviation for Automated Dispensing Cabinets.

    _____

17. The use of technology eliminates the need to use the rights of medication administration. _____

**Answers on p. 178**

## NGN Case Study

**Learning Outcomes:**

1. Identify the necessary components of a medication administration record (MAR)
2. Read an MAR and identify medications that are to be administered on a routine basis, including the name of the medication, the dosage, the route of administration, and the time of administration

**Case Scenario:** The nurse is working on the medical surgical unit, and the computerized charting system goes down unexpectedly. The hospital has the ability to print out important information from each client's chart during unexpected downtime. The charge nurse hands you a paper copy of the MAR for each of your clients. The nurse checks the MARs to ensure correctness and prepares to administer the morning medications. **Using the MAR provided below, please complete the statements by choosing the *most likely* options for the missing information from the list of options provided.**

Client Name:

Date of Birth:

Medical Record Number:

Allergies:

| Date | Medication Dosage, Frequency, and Route | Time Due | Nurse's Initials |
|------|------------------------------------------|----------|------------------|
| 10/24/20 | Furosemide 40 mg po daily | 0900 | |
| | Atorvastatin 10 mg po daily | 2100 | |
| | Lisinopril 20 mg po b.i.d.<br><br>**Hold if SBP less than 90 mm Hg. | 0900<br>B/P<br>2100<br>B/P | |
| | Lantus Insulin 20 units subcut daily | 2100 | |
| | Docusate Sodium 100 mg po b.i.d. | 0900<br><br>2100 | |

| Nurse's Initials | Printed Name | Nurse's Signature |
|------------------|--------------|-------------------|
| | | |
| | | |

The nurse will give the client the _____1_____ . Before giving the Lisinopril the nurse needs to check the client's____2_____ . After administering the medications, the nurse would _____3_____ . The nurse should make certain to also _____4_____ .

| 1 | 2 | 3 | 4 |
|---|---|---|---|
| Furosemide, Atorvastatin, Lisinopril, Lantus Insulin, Docusate Sodium | Heart rate to make sure it is greater than 90 beats per minute | Throw the MAR away | Put initials, printed name, and signature at the bottom of the MAR |
| Furosemide, Lisinopril, Docusate Sodium | Blood pressure to make sure the SBP is less than 90 mm Hg | Document by initialing in the box next to the time for each medication that was administered | Put name on the bottom of the page without initials |
| Atorvastatin, Lisinopril, Lantus Insulin, Docusate Sodium | Blood pressure to make sure the SBP is greater than 90 mm Hg | Cross off the medication to indicate it was given | Ask the client to initial the form |

**Reference:** Morris D: *Calculate with confidence,* ed 8, St Louis, Elsevier, copyright 2022.
*Case Study answers and rationales can be found on Evolve.*

---

## ◎ CHAPTER **REVIEW**

1. Who determines the medication administration times? _____

2. Do b.i.d. and q2h have the same meaning? _____ Explain: _____

   _____

   _____

3. What is the purpose of barcoding? _____

4. The abbreviation *eMAR* stands for _____.

5. Times for medication administration can be indicated in _____ or _____.

Refer to the portion of the transcribed MAR provided to answer questions 6-10.

| | | Time | 5/2/20 | 5/3/20 | 5/4/20 | 5/5/20 | 5/6/20 | 5/7/20 | 5/8/20 |
|---|---|---|---|---|---|---|---|---|---|
| 5/2/17 | Vasotec po qd | 1000 | | | | | | | |
| | Hold for SBP less than 100 | B/P | | | | | | | |
| | | | | | | | | | |
| | | | | | | | | | |
| | | | | | | | | | |
| | | | | | | | | | |
| | | | | | | | | | |
| 5/2/17 | Neurontin 400 mg po tid | 1000 | | | | | | | |
| | | 1400 | | | | | | | |
| | | 1800 | | | | | | | |
| | | | | | | | | | |
| | | | | | | | | | |
| | | | | | | | | | |
| | | | | | | | | | |
| 5/2/17 | Heparin 5,000 U daily | 1000 | | | | | | | |
| | | | | | | | | | |
| | | | | | | | | | |
| | | | | | | | | | |
| | | | | | | | | | |
| | | | | | | | | | |
| 5/2/17 | Benadryl 50 mg po q6h prn | | | | | | | | |
| | for itching | | | | | | | | |
| | | | | | | | | | |
| | | | | | | | | | |
| | | | | | | | | | |
| | | | | | | | | | |
| | | | | | | | | | |
| | | | | | | | | | |

6. What dosage of Neurontin should be administered? _____

7. Are any of the medication orders incomplete? If so, which medication and what

   information is missing? _____

8. Indicate the time of day in traditional time that each medication should be given.

   _____

9. Which order(s) contain(s) error-prone abbreviations? How should the order be

   corrected? _____

10. Why are no times listed for Benadryl? _____

**Answers on p. 178**

# ⭐ ANSWERS

## Chapter 11

### Answers to Practice Problems

1. True
2. False
3. True
4. client, medication (drug), dosage (dose), route, time, documentation
5. nurse
6. automated dispensing cabinet (ADC). Sometimes referred to as computer-controlled dispensing system
7. override, verification
8. False
9. documentation
10. Computerized prescriber order entry, computerized provider entry, computerized practitioner order entry
11. Once a day
12. Colace 100 mg, furosemide 40 mg, K-Dur 10 mEq, Digoxin 0.125 mg
13. Milliequivalent
14. Check the client's apical pulse
15. 9:00 AM, 5:00 PM
16. True
17. False

### Answers to Chapter Review

1. hospital, institution, or health care facility
2. No; b.i.d. means the order will be given two times in 24 hours, whereas a q2h order would be given 12 times in 24 hours.
3. to ensure dispensing and administration of the correct medication to the right client
4. electronic medication administration record
5. traditional time, military time (international time)
6. 400 mg
7. Yes. For Vasotec, the dosage is missing; for heparin, the route is missing.
8. Vasotec 10:00 AM; Neurontin 10:00 AM, 2:00 PM, 6:00 PM; Heparin 10:00 AM.
9. Vasotec frequency should be stated as every day or daily. Heparin units should be written out and not abbreviated.
10. Benadryl is ordered whenever necessary or required (prn). It is not given on a routine schedule and is charted each time it is given, spaced at 6-hour intervals.

# CHAPTER **12**
# Reading Medication Labels

## Objectives

*After reviewing this chapter, you should be able to identify:*

1. The trade and generic names of medications
2. The dosage strength of medications
3. The form in which a medication is supplied
4. The total volume of a medication container where indicated
5. Directions for mixing or preparing a medication where necessary
6. Information on combined-medication labels

The safe administration of medications to a client includes the nurse accurately reading and identifying key information found on a medication label. The medication label contains information such as the dosage strength that is necessary to perform dosage calculations, as well as information that is essential to clinical practice. The design of a medication label is unique to the drug manufacturer; however, the essential information on a medication label includes the medication name, form, total volume, total amount in container (for solid forms of medication such as tablets and capsules), route of administration, warnings, storage requirements, and manufacturing information. Additional information includes expiration dates, National Drug Code (NDC) number, and, if applicable, reconstitution information and Control Substance Schedule. Some medication labels make reference to a package insert for additional information relating to a medication, which includes information such as contraindications, dosage and administration, and other information that may not be indicated on the label. It is important to read a medication label carefully and recognize essential information to ensure that the client receives the *right medication in the right dosage by the right route.*

> **(!) SAFETY ALERT!**
>
> Always read the label carefully. Reading the label three (3) times will prevent an error in administration of the wrong medication.

## Reading Medication Labels

The nurse should be able to recognize the following pertinent information on a medication label.

### Generic Name

Every medication has an official name, referred to as the generic name. Medications have only one generic name. A medication is licensed under its generic name. **By law, the generic name must appear on all medication labels.** If there is only one name on the medication label, it is the generic name. The generic name is given by the manufacturer that first develops the medication, but the name is not specific to the manufacturer. It is also recorded with a national listing of medications: the United States Pharmacopeia (USP) and the National Formulary (NF). Prescribers are ordering medications more often by generic name. In many institutions, pharmacists are dispensing medications by generic name to decrease costs. Nurses therefore need to know the generic name as well as the trade name for medications and crosscheck medications to prevent inaccurate medication identification.

On a medication label that has both the trade name and generic name, the generic name is usually found directly under the brand name and sometimes is enclosed in parentheses. Sometimes only the generic name may appear on the medication label or package. This is common for medications that have been used for many years, are well established, and do not require marketing under a different trade name. Examples include atropine and morphine (Figure 12.1A and B). Another example of a medication commonly used in the clinical setting and often seen only with the generic name on the label is Lasix. Lasix is the trade or brand name; however, it is often seen with the generic name only, furosemide (Figure 12.2). Notice on the labels shown in Figures 12.1 and 12.2 the letters *USP* after the generic name. As stated, this is one of the two official listings of medications. The other is *NF*. *USP* after the generic name indicates the medication complies with the USP standards. Do not confuse these abbreviations (letters) with other initials (letters, abbreviations) that designate a special form of a medication, such as CR, which means controlled release.

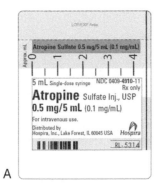 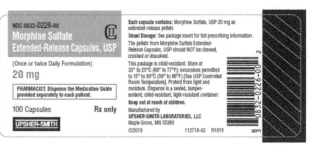

A B

**Figure 12.1** (A) Atropine label (injectable solution). Dosage strength 0.5 mg per 5 mL or 0.1 mg per mL. (B) Morphine sulfate label. Extended-release capsules. The dosage strength is 20 mg per extended-release capsule.

**Figure 12.2** Furosemide label. The dosage strength is 20 mg per 2 mL or 10 mg per mL.

**SAFETY ALERT!**

It is important to avoid confusing official listings (USP or NF) with other initials (letters) or abbreviations on a medication label, which may serve to identify additional medications or specific actions or reactions to a medication. Use caution with medications that have similar spellings.

## Trade Name

The trade name is also referred to as the *brand name* or *proprietary name*; it is the manufacturer's name for the medication. The same medication may be made by different manufacturers, which assign a trade name to that medication. Therefore a medication can have multiple trade names. It is important to note that some medications may not have trade names. The trade name is generally the largest printed information on the label, which makes it very prominent. The name may be written all in capital letters or may have a combination of capital and lowercase letters. The trade name is followed by the ®, which is the registration symbol, or ™ for trademark. The registered mark ® means the trade name has been legally registered with the U.S. Patent and Trademark Office (USPTO) by the manufacturer and cannot be used by another company. ™ indicates the name is the trademark for that company. Once the USPTO formally registers the trademark, the symbol ® then appears on the medication label. In Figures 12.3 and 12.4 notice the trade name is listed before the generic name.

Figure 12.3 shows the label for Xarelto. Xarelto is the trade name identified by the ® registration symbol. The name underneath in smaller print and enclosed in parentheses, rivaroxaban, is the generic, or official, name of the medication.

Figure 12.4 shows the label for Verzenio. Notice the ™ symbol after the trade name Verzenio. The name underneath in smaller print and enclosed in parentheses, abemaciclib, is the generic or official name.

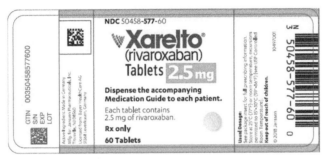

**Figure 12.3** Xarelto label.

> **SAFETY ALERT!**
> It is important for the nurse to crosscheck all medications, whether just the generic name or both the trade and generic names are indicated on the label to accurately identify a medication. Failure to crosscheck medications could lead to choosing the wrong medication to administer, a violation of the rights of medication administration (the "right" medication).

## The Medication Name and Tall Man Lettering

As already stated (in Chapter 10), there are several medications that have names that look alike and sound alike. Remember that even medications with similar names may have markedly different chemical structures and actions. For example, buspirone (BuSpar) is an antianxiety medication, and bupropion (Wellbutrin) is used to treat major depressive disorders. Although the generic names are similar, the action, composition of the medications, and their use are different.

To minimize confusion and the risk of medication errors, the Food and Drug Administration (FDA) requires the "Tall Man" letters be used in generic name pairs that are associated with errors. ISMP also published a recommended list of additional medication names using "Tall Man" lettering. "Tall Man" uses mixed-case (lower- and uppercase) and bolding to emphasize differing portions of the medication name. For example, the two medications discussed using "Tall Man" letters are shown as: bus**PIR**one and bu**PROP**ion. Notice the letters are bolded and capitalized to indicate the differing portions of the name. The FDA and ISMP Lists of Look-Alike Drug Names with Recommended Tall Man Letters can be found in Appendix B. A complete listing of medications written with Tall Man lettering can be found at https://www.ismp.org/sites/default/files/attachments/2017-11/tallmanletters.pdf. There are also some medication labels that indicate the medication name in Tall Man

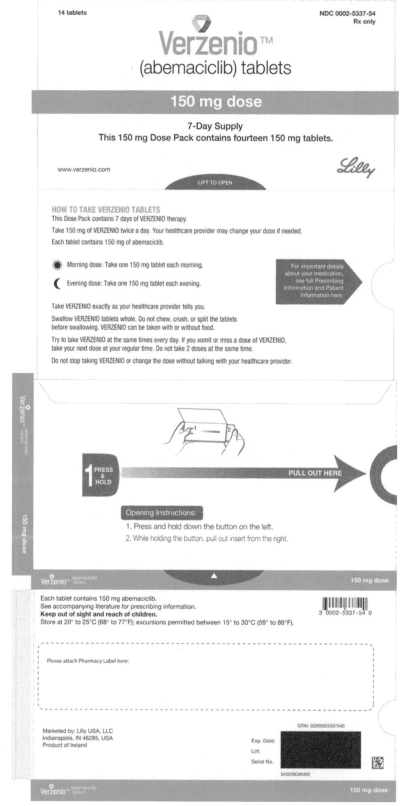

**Figure 12.4** Verzenio label.

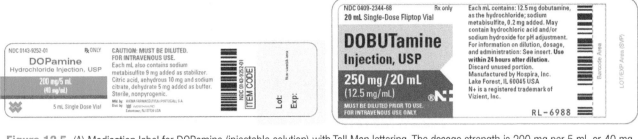

**Figure 12.5** (A) Medication label for DOPamine (injectable solution) with Tall Man lettering. The dosage strength is 200 mg per 5 mL or 40 mg per mL. (B) Medication label for DOBUTamine (injectable solution) label with Tall Man lettering. The dosage strength is 250 mg per 20 mL or 12.5 mg per mL.

lettering on the label that are found on the Tall Man list, which provides another safety alert for the health care provider. See Figure 12.5A, Dopamine, 12.5B, Dobutamine. These two medications are indicated on the Tall Man list. (**DOP**amine confused with **DOBUT**amine): Notice the use of uppercase lettering and lowercase with the highlighting of a section of the medication names to help distinguish the names from each other.

## Dosage Strength

Dosage strength refers to the weight or amount of the medication provided in a specific unit of measure (e.g., the weight per tablet, capsule, milliliter). The dosage strength is made up of the strength of the medication with the unit of measurement and the dosage form. For solid forms of medications, the dosage strength is the amount of medication per tablet, capsule, etc. For liquid medications (oral and parenteral) the dosage strength is the amount of medication present in a certain amount of solution. See Figure 12.6, Namenda (oral solution), and Figure 12.7, Penicillin V Potassium (oral solution).

A medication label may identify more than one dosage strength, which allows the nurse to choose any one of the dosage strengths for calculation purposes. (See Figure 12.1A for Atropine; Figure 12.2 for Furosemide; Figure 12.5A for **DOP**amine and 12.5B for **DOBUT**amine.) There are also medication labels that indicate the equivalent unit of measurement on a label such as mcg and mg, which eliminates the need for conversion when calculating a dosage. See Figure 12.8 for Lanoxin and 12.7 for Penicillin V Potassium, which have two different but equivalent dosage strengths shown on the label as well. Sometimes you may see solutions expressed (dosage) as a ratio or percentage. Refer to labels in Figures 12.9 and 12.10. Notice the labels also express the dosage strength in milligrams per milliliters.

Refer to the sample labels, which identify the dosage strengths for the medications.

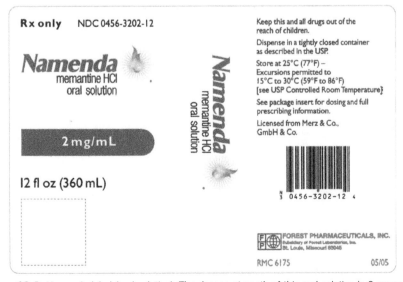

**Figure 12.6** Namenda label (oral solution). The dosage strength of this oral solution is 2 mg per mL.

Usual Dosage - 250 or 500 mg every 6 to 8 hours.
See package insert.

Dispensing Directions - Prepare solution at the time of
dispensing by adding a total of **65 mL** water in two
portions to the bottle as follows: Loosen powder by
tapping the bottle, add about half the water, and shake
well. Add the remaining water and shake well to
complete solution. This provides 100 mL of solution.

Manufactured for:
**DAVA Pharmaceuticals, Inc.**
Fort Lee, NJ 07024, USA
by:
**Suir Pharma Ireland Ltd.,**
Clonmel, Ireland
03/2014

NDC 67253-203-10

**PENICILLIN V
POTASSIUM for
ORAL SOLUTION, USP**

RECONSTITUTE w/65 mL WATER

Equivalent to
**250 mg** (400,000 units)

Penicillin V per 5mL when
reconstituted according to directions

**100 mL bottle**          **Rx only**

**DAVA**

**Figure 12.7** Penicillin V Potassium label (oral solution). The dosage strength of this oral solution is 250 mg (per 5 mL) or 400,000 units (per 5 mL).

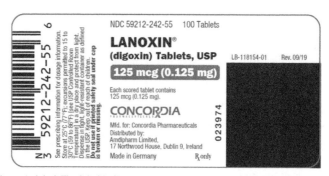

**Figure 12.8** Lanoxin label. The label indicates 125 mcg (0.125 mg), which means 125 mcg is equivalent to 0.125 mg. The dosage strength is 125 mcg per tablet or 0.125 mg per tablet.

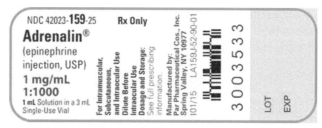

**Figure 12.9** Adrenalin label (injectable solution). Adrenalin contains 1 g of medication per 1,000 mL solution (1 : 1,000) and 1 mg per mL.

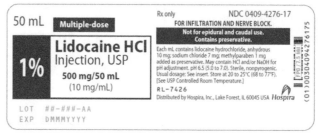

**Figure 12.10** Lidocaine label (injectable solution). Lidocaine 1% contains 1 g of medication per 100 mL of solution and 500 mg per 50 mL or 10 mg per mL.

> **⚠ SAFETY ALERT!**
> The Institute for Safe Medication Practices (ISMP) recommends that the slash mark (/) not be used to separate two doses to indicate "per" because it can be misread and mistaken as the number 1. Use *per* rather than the slash mark. Example: Use 10 mg *per* 5 mL rather than 10 mg/5 mL, which could be misread as 10 mg and 15 mL. This practice will be followed in this text.

> **⚠ SAFETY ALERT!**
> Always read a medication label carefully to avoid errors and administration of the wrong medication. Medication names can be deceptively similar. Similarity in name does not mean similarity in action. For example, *Inderal* and *Inderide* are similar names, but the action and the contents of the medication are different. Inderal delivers a certain dose of propranolol hydrochloride. Inderide combines two antihypertensive agents (propranolol hydrochloride and hydrochlorothiazide, a diuretic antihypertensive).

## Form

The form specifies the type of preparation contained in the package that contains the strength of the medication. Medications are available in a variety of forms.

- Examples of forms include solid forms such as tablets, capsules, caplets, and suppositories. There are also liquid forms, which include oral solutions and injectable solutions. Solutions may be indicated by milliliters (mL). Some medications are available in powder or as patches. Other forms include inhalants, drops, creams, and ointments.
- Labels may also indicate abbreviations or words that describe the form of the medication. Examples include *CR* (controlled release), *LA* (long acting), *DS* (double strength), *SR* (sustained release), *XL* (long acting), *ES* (extra strength), and *XR* (extended release). Some labels may use abbreviations such as *EC* (enteric coated) or just indicate enteric coated. These medications should not be crushed. See the label in Figure 12.11A for Ery tablets.
- Abbreviations that describe the form of a medication indicate the medication has been prepared in a way that allows extended action, or slow release, of the active ingredient. Often these medications are given less frequently. Examples include Procardia XL, Inderal LA, Calan SR, and Metformin extended release. These special forms should be swallowed whole and never crushed unless otherwise indicated. Always read labels carefully. Refer to labels in Figure 12.11A–C for samples of medication labels indicating special forms. Notice Figure 12.11B, the label for Rabeprazole Sodium Delayed Release Sprinkle Capsules, indicates they are delayed release and states, "Open capsule and sprinkle contents on liquid or soft food. Do Not crush or chew capsule contents." Also notice label for Ery Tab; the tablets are enteric coated as well as delayed release.

> **⚠ SAFETY ALERT!**
> Administering the incorrect form of medication is a medication error!

> **⚠ SAFETY ALERT!**
> Certain forms should not be crushed nor dissolved for use through a nasogastric, gastrostomy, or jejunostomy tube without first consulting a pharmacist or medication guide for information regarding whether a medication can be crushed or altered. Altering oral medications by crushing may result in an alteration of the medication's action and cause unintended outcomes.

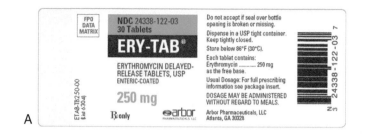

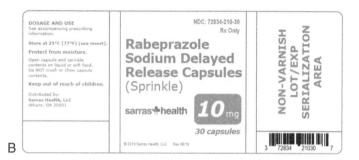

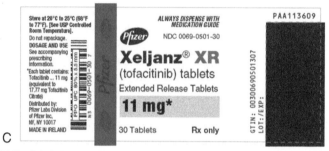

**Figure 12.11** (A) Ery Tab Delayed Release Tablet and Enteric Coated. (B) Rabeprazole Sodium Delayed Release Sprinkle Capsules. (C) Xeljanz XR Extended Release Tablets.

## Route of Administration

The route of administration describes how the medication is to be administered, or the method of delivery by which the medication enters the body. Common routes include oral, injection (IV, IM, subcut). Examples of other routes include enteral (into the gastrointestinal tract through a tube), ophthalmic, topical (transdermal patches), inhalation, sublingual, and others. When looking at labels for tablets or capsules, the route of administration is not specified on the medication label. It is understood that such solid forms as tablets, capsules, and caplets are administered orally, unless otherwise specified. Any form intended for oral use should be administered orally.

Because all tablets, capsules, and liquids are not always given orally and swallowed, read the label carefully because any variation from oral administration is indicated on the label. Examples include sublingual tablets, otic suspension for use in ears; some capsules are placed in an inhaler and not swallowed. For example, the label for Nitrostat indicates it is administered sublingually (under the tongue) (Figure 12.12A). Another form for sublingual use is sublingual film. For example, Suboxone, which is used to treat opioid dependence, is a sublingual film. The form allows for rapid absorption of medication, which is desired in the treatment of these clients. See Figure 12.12B.

Liquid medications may be administered orally or by injection. Labels for oral liquid medications as well as for injection will indicate the route. Oral liquids may indicate oral solution, oral suspension. The route may be indicated on the label for injectable medications such as "for IM, subcut or IV" use. See Figures 12.13 to 12.15. Labels will indicate routes for others as well.

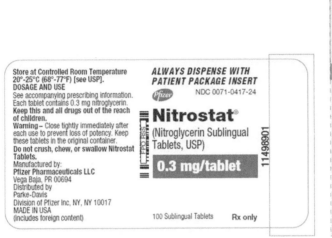

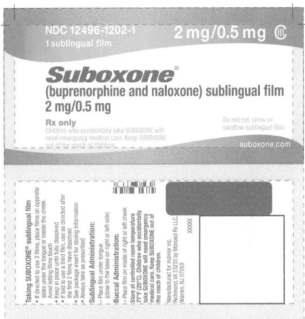

**Figure 12.12** (A) Nitrostat label (sublingual). (B) Suboxone (sublingual film).

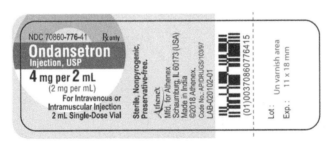

**Figure 12.13** Ondansetron label (IV and IM).

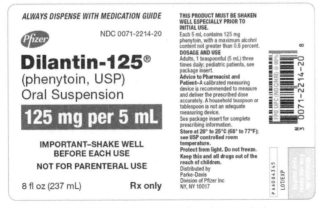

**Figure 12.14** Dilantin-125 label (oral suspension).

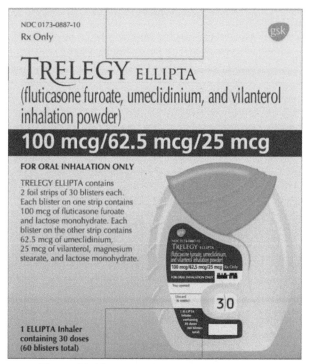

**Figure 12.15** Trelegy Ellipta label (oral inhalation).

## Barcoding Symbols

Dating back to 2004, the U.S. Department of Health and Human Services (HHS) required that barcodes be placed on the medication label (human and biological agents). Barcode symbols appear on medication labels as thin and heavy lines arranged in a group. Barcodes are particularly important at institutions where barcoding is used as part of the medication distribution system. Refer to the barcodes indicated on the labels in Figures 12.1 to 12.9. Barcodes can also be used for stock reorder.

## Total Volume

On labels of solutions for injections or oral liquids, total volume, as well as dosage strength, is stated. Total volume refers to the quantity contained in a bottle, vial, or ampule. For liquids, total volume refers to the total fluid volume.

There have been documented medication errors caused by misinterpretation of dosage strength and total volume. In 2009 the Food and Drug Administration (FDA) required that single and multidose injectable product labels indicate the dosage strength of a medication per total volume be prominent on the label, followed in close proximity by the dosage strength per mL enclosed in parentheses. Notice the clindamycin label shown in Figure 12.16 indicates 2 mL is the vial size (total volume). The dosage strength is stated for the entire vial (300 mg per 2 mL) and per mL (150 mg per mL). The ondansetron label shown in Figure 12.17 indicates 20 mL is the vial size (total volume). The dosage strength is stated for the entire vial (40 mg per 20 mL) and per mL (2 mg per mL). In Figure 12.18, Namenda, the total volume is 12 fluid ounces (360 mL), and the solution or liquid contains 2 mg per mL (dosage strength).

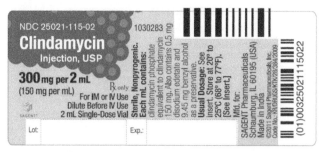

**Figure 12.16** Clindamycin Injectable label.

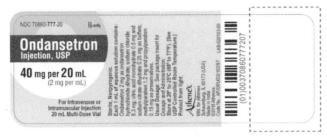

**Figure 12.17** Ondansetron Injectable label.

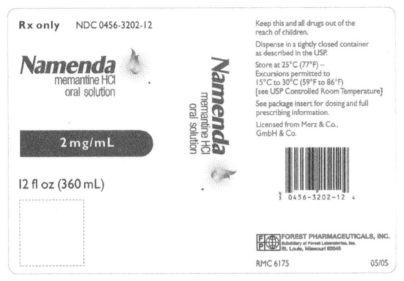

**Figure 12.18** Namenda Oral Solution label.

## Total Amount in Container

For solid forms of medication, such as tablets, capsules, and the like, the total amount is the total number of tablets or capsules, or other solid form, in the container. The dosage strength, as well as the total amount in the container, is included on labels of solid forms of medication, such as tablets or capsules. With **unit dose** for a client's ordered medication, the package contains one dose of the medication.

Examples:
- In Figure 12.1B (Morphine Sulfate Extended-Release Capsules), the total amount of extended-release capsules in the container is 100 extended-release capsules, whereas the dosage strength is 20 mg per extended-release capsule.
- In Figure 12.3 (Xarelto tablets), the total amount of tablets in the container is 60 tablets, whereas the dosage strength is 2.5 mg per tablet.

---

**SAFETY ALERT!**

It is important to recognize the difference between the amount per milliliter and the total volume to avoid confusion and errors. Do not confuse total volume, total amount in container with dosage strength. Confusion of these items can cause a serious medication error.

## Directions for Mixing or Reconstituting a Medication

When medication comes in a powdered form, the directions for how to mix or reconstitute it and with what solution are found on the label or package insert. The directions for reconstitution should be followed exactly as directed for accuracy in administration. See the label in Figure 12.19 for directions for reconstituting Levothyroxine Sodium. Reconstitution is discussed further in Chapter 18.

## Warnings

Medications may come with warnings, alerts, or precautions that are related to safety, effectiveness, or administration considerations and need to be followed. Storage alerts might also be on the label. These precautions, warnings, and alerts may be printed on the label by the manufacturer or added by the pharmacy that dispenses the medication. Always read precautions or special alerts carefully, and follow the instructions given precisely. Examples of precautions, warnings, or alerts on a label may include the following: shake well, protect from light, may be habit forming. For example, refer to the front of the Famotidine label in Figure 12.20 ("Shake well before using, Not for injection"). Notice on the top right side of the label it states, "Keep container tightly closed." Labels may also carry warnings for specific groups of clients. For example, a label may caution that you should find out which other medications may not be taken with the medication (refer to Norvir label, Figure 12.21). Notice the Norvir label also directs the client to store the medicine at room temperature and take with meals.

## Expiration Date

Medication labels contain information such as the expiration date (which may be indicated with the abbreviation *Exp*). Expiration dates indicate the last date on which a medication should be used. Typically, the date appears as the month/year. This information can be found on the back or side of a label. Medications requiring reconstitution provide specific expiration instructions. Refer to the Famotidine label in Figure 12.20. Discard unused portion of reconstituted suspension after 30 days (upper right side of label). In the hospital setting, medications that have expired should be returned to the pharmacy. *Note:* Expiration dates must always be checked on medications, and expiration dates are always present on actual prescriptions. The labels shown in this text may not all have expiration dates because they are used solely for educational purposes.

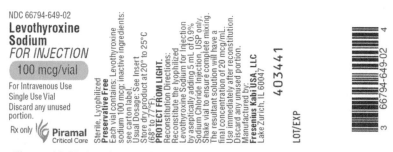

**Figure 12.19**  Levothyroxine Sodium label (see directions for reconstituting).

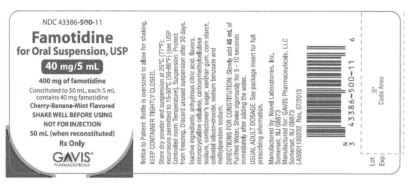

**Figure 12.20**  Famotidine label. (Shake well before using. Not for Injection. Keep container tightly closed.) Discard unused suspension after 30 days.

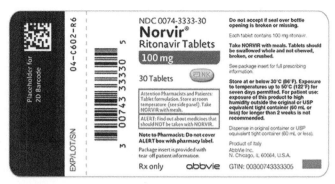

**Figure 12.21** Norvir label. (Store at room temperature, take Norvir with meals, find out about medicines that should not be taken with Norvir.)

---

**TIPS FOR CLINICAL PRACTICE**

It is imperative that nurses check the expiration dates on medications as a routine habit.

---

**SAFETY ALERT!**

Remember to always read the expiration date. After the expiration date, the medication may lose its potency or cause adverse or different effects from the intended. Discard expired medications according to agency policy. For some medications, such as narcotics, disposal must be witnessed. Never give expired medications to a client! Clients must be educated in *all* aspects of medication administration, so teach them to check medications for expiration dates, and discard medications that have expired properly. Teach clients about community medication disposal days or days in some communities when they can take unused or expired medications to the police department. Encourage clients not to flush medications down the drainage system.

## Dosage and Administration

The dosage and administration portion on a medication label may state wording such as "usual dosage," "dosage and use," or "dosage and administration." This information may be indicated on the label, or it may state to see the package insert for full prescribing information (see Figure 12.1B, Morphine Sulfate Extended-Release Capsules label, " package insert for prescribing information;" and Figure 12.7, Penicillin V Potassium label (oral solution) label, "Usual Dosage: 250 or 500 mg every 6 to 8 hours. See package insert").

## Single-Dose and Multi-Dose Packaging

This information is indicated on the label for medications used for injection. The label will indicate single-dose or multi-dose vial. See Figure 12.5A, DOPamine label; 12.5B, DOBUTamine label; and Figure 12.13, Ondansetron label. A single-dose container (vial) holds enough medication for a typical single dose. If the single-dose container holds more than the ordered dose, the excess medication is discarded regardless of the volume remaining. A **single-dose** vial does not contain antimicrobial preservatives to minimize bacterial growth once the vial has been used. A **multi-dose** container (vial) contains enough medication for more than one dose and contains a preservative. Single-dose and multi-dose packaging is discussed further in Chapter 17, Parenteral Medications.

*Storage Directions*—This section of the medication label provides information as to how a medication should be stored to prevent the medication from losing its potency or effectiveness. Usually, information is given on the label relating to temperature for storing the medication. Refer to the Morphine Sulfate Extended-Release Capsules label, Figure 12.1B, and the Dilantin-125 label, Figure 12.14. When medications come in a powdered form and must be reconstituted, storage information is usually indicated on the label telling how long the medication is effective once it has been reconstituted. Refer to the Levothyroxine Sodium label, Figure 12.19, and the Famotidine label, Figure 12.20.

*Lot/Control Numbers*—Federal law requires that all medication packages be identified by a lot/control number. This number is important in the event that medications have to be recalled.

*National Drug Code (NDC) Number*—This is a number required by federal law to be given to all medications. Each medication has a unique NDC number. The NDC number consists of NDC followed by three discrete groups of numbers (example: NDC 0074-3333-30 for Norvir, Figure 12.21).

*Manufacturer's Name*—All medication labels will indicate the name of the company that manufactured the medication (examples: Pfizer, Parke-Davis, or Teva). Abbvie is the manufacturer's name on the Norvir label in Figure 12.21. This information can be valuable if you have questions about the medication. Refer to the various medication labels provided in the chapter. It is important to not confuse the manufacturer's name with the name of the medication.

*Abbreviations such as USP (United States Pharmacopoeia) and NF (National Formulary)*—USP and NF are the two official national lists of approved medications. Special guidelines are given to the manufacturer related to use and placement of these initials on medication labels. On the Adrenalin label in Figure 12.9, notice that USP follows Epinephrine Injection. Notice the placement of USP on the lidocaine label (see Figure 12.10).

## Controlled Substance Schedule

Controlled substances are medications or therapeutic agents with the potential for abuse and addiction and are regulated by state and federal laws. Controlled substances are regulated under the Controlled Substance Act (CSA). Medications considered controlled substances are classified into schedules that rank them according to their abuse potential and physical and psychological dependence. They are ranked from Schedule I to Schedule V. Medications that have the highest abuse potential are Schedule I, and medications with the lowest or limited abuse potential are Schedule V. Controlled substances are indicated on a medication label with a large "C," indicating the medication is a controlled substance, and a Roman numeral (uppercase) to identify the schedule number (I-V) the medication is classified under, inserted in the center of the letter "C." Refer to the label for Morphine Sulfate Extended-Release capsules in Figure 12.1B, which indicates morphine is Schedule II (notice the letter "C" with II).

## Combination Medications

A combination medication is a combination of two or more medications that are in one form. The label indicates the dosage strength for each medication. Combination medications are sometimes ordered by the number of tablets, capsules, or milliliters to be administered rather than by the dosage strength. Combined medications such as Sinemet (trade name) are used in the treatment of Parkinson's disease, come in several dosage strengths, and cannot be ordered without a specific dosage; the number of tablets alone is insufficient to fill the order. **It must include the dosage strength!** Example: Sinemet 25 mg/100 mg 1 tab po t.i.d.

**Example 1:** The label for Sinemet indicates that the medication contains carbidopa and levodopa. The first number specifies the amount of carbidopa, and the second number represents the amount of levodopa. This is further indicated on the label. See the label for Sinemet in Figure 12.22.

**Example 2:** Percocet, which is used to treat moderate to severe pain, is a combination of oxycodone (narcotic pain reliever) and acetaminophen (Tylenol, non-narcotic pain reliever). The medication comes in varying strengths of oxycodone (2.5 mg to 10 mg) and acetaminophen (325 mg to 650 mg). Orders for this medication must specify the dosage strength. Example: Percocet 2.5 mg/325 mg 1-2 tabs po q6h prn for pain. See the label for Percocet in Figure 12.23.

**Example 3:** Septra, an antibacterial, is also manufactured under the trade name Bactrim, which is a combination of trimethoprim and sulfamethoxazole. For example, a Septra (Bactrim) tablet contains 80 mg of trimethoprim and 400 mg of sulfamethoxazole. DS (double-strength) Septra (Bactrim) contains 160 mg of trimethoprim and 800 mg of sulfamethoxazole. See the label for

Bactrim DS in Figure 12.24. Since Bactrim DS is available in one strength, it can be ordered by the number of tablets. **Example:** Bactrim DS 1 tab po q12h for 14 days. See label for Bactrim in Figure 12.24. Note this same order written with medications in their generic name would specify the dosage strength for each medication: for example, sulfamethoxazole/trimethoprim 800 mg/160 mg 1 tab po q12h for 14 days.

**Example 4:** Biktarvy is a fixed combination of three (3) medications used to treat HIV type-1 (HIV-1). Biktarvy contains ictegravir, emtricitabine, and tenofovir alafenamide. The first number specifies the amount of bictegravir, the second number represents the amount of emtricitabine, and the third number represents the amount of tenofovir alafenamide. This is also indicated on the label. The medication is ordered by the number of tablets. Example: Biktarvy 1 tab po daily. See the label for Biktarvy in Figure 12.25.

Although tablets and capsules that contain more than one medication are often ordered by the brand name and the number of tablets or capsules to be given (e.g., Bactrim DS 1 tab po q12h), the health care provider may order this medication by another route (e.g., intravenous [IV]). The injectable form, which is for IV infusion, is available in the generic name (see the IV label in Figure 12.26). With the IV order, the nurse calculates the dosage to be given based on the dosage strength of the trimethoprim. The nurse would learn such information described by using appropriate resources, such as a reference medication book (*Physician's Desk Reference [PDR]*), pharmacist, hospital formulary, and available information technology.

> **⚠ SAFETY ALERT!**
> The numbers following a medication name may be used to identify the dosage strengths of more than one medication in a preparation, and initials may be used to identify a special medication action. Read labels carefully to validate that you have the right medication and dosage for combined medications.

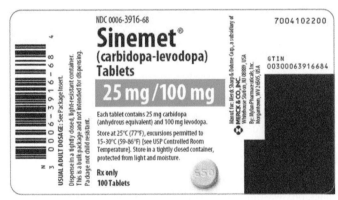

**Figure 12.22** Sinemet 25 mg/100 mg label. The dosage strength of carbidopa is 25 mg, and levodopa is 100 mg.

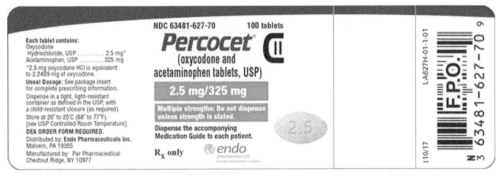

**Figure 12.23** Percocet 2.5 mg/325 mg label. The label indicates the dosage strength of oxycodone hydrochloride as 2.5 mg and acetaminophen (Tylenol) is 325 mg.

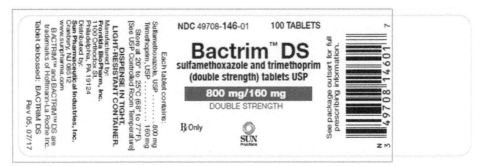

**Figure 12.24** Bactrim DS 800 mg/160 mg label. The label indicates the dosage strength of sulfamethoxazole as 800 mg and trimethoprim is 160 mg.

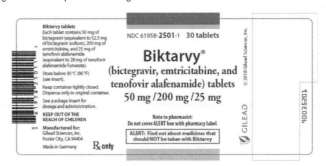

**Figure 12.25** Biktarvy 50 mg/200 mg/25 mg label. The dosage strength of bictegravir is 50 mg, 200 mg is the dosage strength of emtricitabine, and 25 mg is the dosage strength of tenofovir alafenamide.

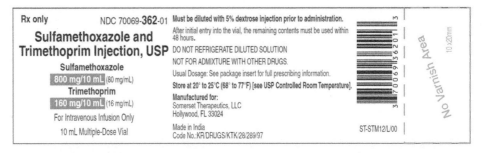

**Figure 12.26** IV label for Sulfamethoxazole and Trimethoprim. Notice the dosage strength is stated for both medications per total volume of the vial, and directly next to it is the dosage strength for each medication per mL. (Calculation of ordered dosages is based on the Trimethoprim).

## Black Box Warning

The Food and Drug Administration (FDA) mandates that certain prescription medications contain a black box warning. This warning is designed to call attention to serious adverse effects that may cause serious injury or death. The alert or warning is outlined with a black box on the medication label with the text inside describing the serious adverse effects. In order for the FDA to require a black box warning label, the confirmation of the potential adverse effects of the medication is done through research and/or clinical data. In addition to the black box warning appearing on the prescription medication's label, it can also be found on the medication package insert, the FDA website, and on the web page of the drug company, if they have a website. Figure 12.27 shows the black box warning for Vraylar (used to treat schizophrenia and bipolar disorder). Refer to the Latuda label in Figure 12.28; notice the statement that refers to giving the patient the accompanying medication guide each time Latuda is dispensed. The guide being referred to provides more information regarding the adverse effects of the medication. Notice Figure 12.30 on p. 195, an excerpt of the prescribing information for Zyprexa, which also shows a black box warning.

## Unit-Dose Packaging

Unit-dose packaging is a method by which the pharmacist prepares and packages a client's ordered medication into a single-unit package that provides enough medication for one dose. The unit-dose system decreases errors associated with administration of medications and decreases the need for large amounts of medications on the unit. Figure 12.29 shows examples of unit-dose packaging.

## Medication Information

To decrease errors and manage the risks of medications and adverse medication effects, the U.S. Food and Drug Administration (FDA) mandates the format in which medication information is provided on Prescription Medication Package Inserts. Since 2016, the FDA has mandated the new format for package inserts, which includes categories such as the highlights of prescribing information, boxed warning, recent major changes, indications and usage, and adverse reactions, which includes the following statement under the section, "To report SUSPECTED ADVERSE REACTIONS, contact (Manufacturer) at (phone # and Web address) or FDA at 1-800-FDA-1088 or www.fda.gov/medwatch." See Figure for an excerpt from the prescribing information for the medication Zyprexa (olanzapine).

---

**Warning: Increased mortality in elderly patients with dementia-related psychosis; and suicidal thoughts and behaviors**

Increased mortality in elderly patients with dementia-related psychosis
Elderly patients with dementia-related psychosis treated with antipsychotic drugs are at an increased risk of death. VRAYLAR is not approved for the treatment of patients with dementia-related psychosis *[see warnings and precautions (5.1)]*.
Suicidal thoughts and behaviors
Antidepressants increased the risk of suicidal thoughts and behaviors in pediatric and young adult patients in short-term studies. Closely monitor all antidepressant-treated patients for clinical worsening, and for the emergence of suicidal thoughts and behaviors *[see warnings and precautions (5.2)]*. The safety and effectiveness of VRAYLAR have not been established in pediatric patients *[see use in specific populations (8.4)]*.

---

**Figure 12.27** Black box warning for Vraylar.

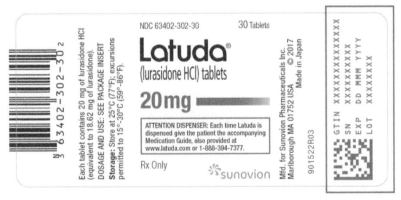

**Figure 12.28** Latuda label.

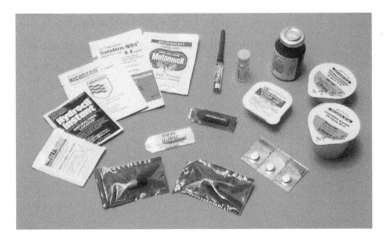

**Figure 12.29** Unit-dose packages. (From Willihnganz, M, Gurevitz SL, Clayton BD: *Clayton's basic pharmacology for nurses,* ed 18, St Louis, 2020, Elsevier.)

**HIGHLIGHTS OF PRESCRIBING INFORMATION**
**These highlights do not include all the information needed to use ZYPREXA RELPREVV safely and effectively. See full prescribing information for ZYPREXA RELPREVV.**

**ZYPREXA RELPREVV (olanzapine) For Extended Release Injectable Suspension**
**Initial U.S. Approval: 1996**

---

**WARNING: POST-INJECTION DELIRIUM/SEDATION SYNDROME and INCREASED MORTALITY IN ELDERLY PATIENTS WITH DEMENTIA-RELATED PSYCHOSIS**

*See full prescribing information for complete boxed warning.*

- Patients are at risk for severe sedation (including coma) and/or delirium after each injection and must be observed for at least 3 hours in a registered facility with ready access to emergency response services. Because of this risk, ZYPREXA RELPREVV is available only through a restricted distribution program called ZYPREXA RELPREVV Patient Care Program and requires prescriber, healthcare facility, patient, and pharmacy enrollment. (2.1, 5.1, 5.2, 10.2, 17)

- Elderly patients with dementia-related psychosis treated with antipsychotic drugs are at an increased risk of death. ZYPREXA RELPREVV is not approved for the treatment of patients with dementia-related psychosis. (5.3, 5.16, 17)

---

------------------ **RECENT MAJOR CHANGES** ------------------

Warnings and Precautions (5.8)                    10/2019

------------------ **INDICATIONS AND USAGE** ------------------

ZYPREXA® RELPREVV™ is a long-acting atypical antipsychotic for intramuscular injection indicated for the treatment of schizophrenia. (1.1)

Efficacy was established in two clinical trials in patients with schizophrenia: one 8-week trial in adults and one maintenance trial in adults. (14.1)

------------------ **DOSAGE AND ADMINISTRATION** ------------------

150 mg/2 wks, 300 mg/4 wks, 210 mg/2 wks, 405 mg/4 wks, or 300 mg/2 wks. See Table 1 for dosing recommendations. (2.1)

**ZYPREXA RELPREVV is intended for deep intramuscular gluteal injection only.**
- Do not administer intravenously or subcutaneously. (2.1)
- Be aware that there are two ZYPREXA intramuscular formulations with different dosing schedules. ZYPREXA IntraMuscular (10 mg/vial) is a short-acting formulation and should not be confused with ZYPREXA RELPREVV. (2.1)
- Establish tolerability with oral olanzapine prior to initiating treatment. (2.1)
- ZYPREXA RELPREVV doses above 405 mg every 4 weeks or 300 mg every 2 weeks have not been evaluated in clinical trials. (2.1)
- Use in specific populations (including renal and hepatic impaired, and pediatric population) has not been studied. (2.1)
- Must be suspended using only the diluent for ZYPREXA RELPREVV provided in the convenience kit. (2.2)

------------------ **DOSAGE FORMS AND STRENGTHS** ------------------

Powder for suspension for intramuscular use only: 210 mg/vial, 300 mg/vial, and 405 mg/vial. (3, 11, 16)

------------------ **CONTRAINDICATIONS** ------------------

None.

------------------ **WARNINGS AND PRECAUTIONS** ------------------

- *Elderly Patients with Dementia-Related Psychosis:* Increased risk of death and increased incidence of cerebrovascular adverse events (e.g. stroke, transient ischemic attack). (5.3)
- *Suicide:* The possibility of a suicide attempt is inherent in schizophrenia, and close supervision of high-risk patients should accompany drug therapy. (5.4)
- *Neuroleptic Malignant Syndrome:* Manage with immediate discontinuation and close monitoring. (5.5)
- *Drug Reaction with Eosinophilia and Systemic Symptoms (DRESS):* Discontinue if DRESS is suspected. (5.6)

- *Metabolic Changes:* Atypical antipsychotic drugs have been associated with metabolic changes including hyperglycemia, dyslipidemia, and weight gain. (5.7)
  - *Hyperglycemia and Diabetes Mellitus:* In some cases extreme and associated with ketoacidosis or hyperosmolar coma or death, has been reported in patients taking olanzapine. Patients taking olanzapine should be monitored for symptoms of hyperglycemia and undergo fasting blood glucose testing at the beginning of, and periodically during, treatment. (5.7)
  - *Dyslipidemia:* Undesirable alterations in lipids have been observed. Appropriate clinical monitoring is recommended, including fasting blood lipid testing at the beginning of, and periodically during, treatment. (5.7)
  - *Weight Gain:* Potential consequences of weight gain should be considered. Patients should receive regular monitoring of weight. (5.7)
- *Tardive Dyskinesia:* Discontinue if clinically appropriate. (5.8)
- *Orthostatic Hypotension:* Orthostatic hypotension associated with dizziness, tachycardia, bradycardia and, in some patients, syncope, may occur especially during initial dose titration. Use caution in patients with cardiovascular disease, cerebrovascular disease, and those conditions that could affect hemodynamic responses. (5.9)
- *Leukopenia, Neutropenia, and Agranulocytosis:* Has been reported with antipsychotics, including ZYPREXA. Patients with a history of a clinically significant low white blood cell count (WBC) or drug induced leukopenia/neutropenia should have their complete blood count (CBC) monitored frequently during the first few months of therapy and discontinuation of ZYPREXA RELPREVV should be considered at the first sign of a clinically significant decline in WBC in the absence of other causative factors. (5.11)
- *Seizures:* Use cautiously in patients with a history of seizures or with conditions that potentially lower the seizure threshold. (5.13)
- *Potential for Cognitive and Motor Impairment:* Has potential to impair judgment, thinking, and motor skills. Use caution when operating machinery. (5.14)
- *Hyperprolactinemia:* May elevate prolactin levels. (5.17)
- *Laboratory Tests:* Monitor fasting blood glucose and lipid profiles at the beginning of, and periodically during, treatment. (5.18)

------------------ **ADVERSE REACTIONS** ------------------

Most common adverse reactions (≥5% in at least one of the treatment groups and greater than placebo) associated with ZYPREXA RELPREVV treatment: headache, sedation, weight gain, cough, diarrhea, back pain, nausea, somnolence, dry mouth, nasopharyngitis, increased appetite, and vomiting. (6.1)

**To report SUSPECTED ADVERSE REACTIONS, contact Eli Lilly and Company at 1-800-LillyRx (1-800-545-5979) or FDA at 1-800-FDA-1088 or www.fda.gov/medwatch**

------------------ **DRUG INTERACTIONS** ------------------

- *CNS Acting Drugs:* Caution should be used when used in combination with other centrally acting drugs and alcohol. (7.2)
- *Antihypertensive Agents:* Enhanced antihypertensive effect. (7.2)
- *Levodopa and Dopamine Agonists:* May antagonize levodopa/dopamine agonists. (7.2)
- *Diazepam:* May potentiate orthostatic hypotension. (7.1, 7.2)
- *Alcohol:* May potentiate orthostatic hypotension. (7.1)
- *Carbamazepine:* Increased clearance of olanzapine. (7.1)
- *Fluvoxamine:* May increase olanzapine levels. (7.1)

------------------ **USE IN SPECIFIC POPULATIONS** ------------------

- *Pregnancy:* May cause extrapyramidal and/or withdrawal symptoms in neonates with third trimester exposure. (8.1)
- *Pediatric Use:* Safety and effectiveness of ZYPREXA RELPREVV in children <18 years of age have not been established. (8.4)

**See 17 for PATIENT COUNSELING INFORMATION and Medication Guide.**

**Revised: 10/2019**

**Figure 12.30** Prescribing information for Zyprexa, including a black box warning.

**FULL PRESCRIBING INFORMATION: CONTENTS***

**WARNING: POST-INJECTION DELIRIUM/SEDATION SYNDROME
and INCREASED MORTALITY IN ELDERLY PATIENTS WITH
DEMENTIA-RELATED PSYCHOSIS**

*Sections or subsections omitted from the full prescribing information
are not listed.

Figure 13.30, cont'd

## Over-the-Counter (OTC) Labels

Over-the-Counter (OTC) medicines are medications that a client can purchase without a prescription. The FDA requirements regarding the format for OTC include Medication Facts (the name of the medication and its purpose), uses of the medication, warnings, and directions of how to take the medication. The information is found on the packaging itself (Figure 12.31, OTC label for Aleve). The OTC label is presented in a simpler format than the format for prescription medications.

To safely administer medications, it is critical that the nurse be able to identify information on the medication label that is required for calculations and administration of the right medication in the right dosage. Remember that cross-checking medication names prevents errors. Use appropriate resources to verify needed information, and question discrepancies before administering.

The amount of information found on a medication label varies; however, some information is consistent on all labels and includes name of medication, dosage, amount in the package, manufacturer's name, expiration date, and lot/control number.

Encourage clients to carefully read the information relating to medications they are taking. Prescription drug information is accessible on DailyMed, an interagency online health information clearinghouse created cooperatively by the FDA and the National Library of Medicine (NLM), available at http://dailymed.nlm.nih.gov. Clients should be made aware of this resource.

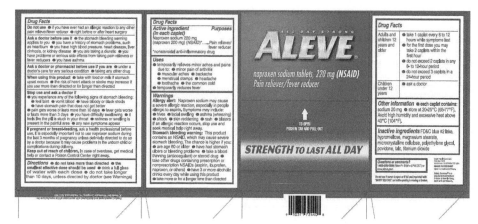

**Figure 12.31** OTC label for Aleve.

**POINTS TO REMEMBER**

- Read medication labels three times.
- Identify directions for mixing when indicated.
- Read labels carefully, and do not confuse medication names; they are often deceptively similar. When in doubt, check appropriate resources, such as a reference book or the hospital pharmacist. Always cross-reference medication names to avoid administering the wrong medication.
- Read the label on combined medications carefully to ascertain whether you are administering the correct medication dosage.
- Extra abbreviations or initials after a medication name may identify additional medications in the preparation or a special action.
- Read labels carefully to identify trade and generic names, dosage strength, form, total amount in container, total volume, and route of administration.
- Do not confuse special forms such as SR (sustained release) and XL (extended release) with USP and NF official listing for medications.
- A **single-dose** vial typically holds one medication dose and does not have a preservative. A vial labeled "single dose" indicates the vial should be discarded after the ordered dose of medication is withdrawn, regardless of the volume remaining.
- A **multi-dose** vial contains a preservative and may be used to administer multiple doses of a medication.
- The black box warning is required by the FDA on certain medications. The black box warning that appears on a prescription medication's label is designed to alert the consumer to the adverse effects of a medication that carry a risk for serious injury or death.
- Dosage and administration may be stated on a label or indicate refer to package insert.
- Unit dose packages for a client's ordered medication contains enough medication for one dose.
- Tall Man lettering is used to distinguish the name of a medication from another medication with a similar name.
- Read directions relating to storage.
- Carefully read alerts on medication labels.
- Do not administer expired medications.
- Controlled medication labels indicate the potential for abuse and are ranked Schedule I to Schedule V.
- When writing dosages, ISMP recommends using *per* instead of a slash (/) because of misinterpretation and being mistaken as the number *1*.
- Administering the incorrect form of a medication is a medication error.
- Be certain that you administer the right medication.

## PRACTICE **PROBLEMS**

Use the labels to identify the information requested.

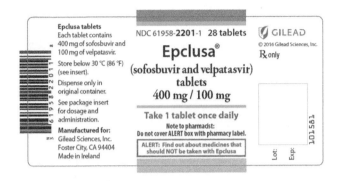

1. The label shown is an example of a label for _____

2. The medication name on the label is generic and/or trade name _____

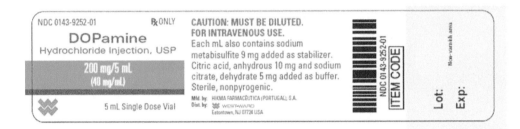

3. Choose the information that is listed on the label.

   a. Multi-dose vial

   b. Tall Man lettering

   c. IV use

   d. Trade name

   e. Controlled substance schedule

   f. Dosage strength 200 mg per 5 mL, 40 mg per mL

   g. Total volume is 5 mL

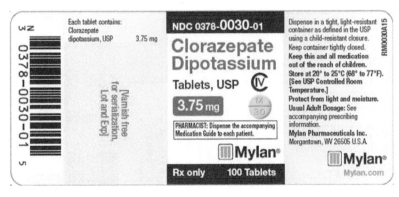

4. Trade name _____        Total amount in container _____

   Generic name _____        Controlled substance schedule _____

   Form _____        Pharmacist directions _____

   Dosage strength _____

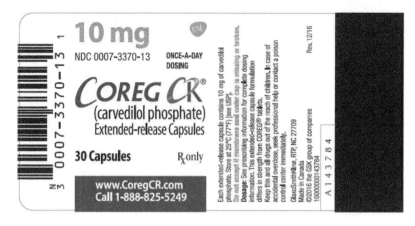

5. Trade name _____     Dosage strength _____

   Generic name _____     Total amount in container _____

   Form _____

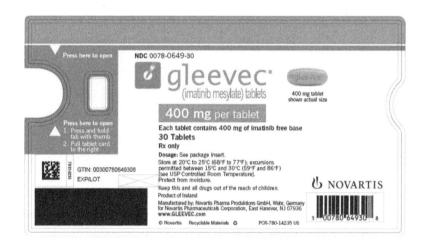

6. Trade name _____     Dosage strength _____

   Generic name _____     Total amount in container _____

                                        Storage _____

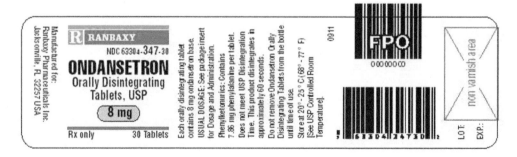

7. Trade name _____     NDC number _____

   Generic name _____     Form _____

NDC 65862-218-60

Rx only

**Cefdinir for Oral Suspension, USP**

**125 mg/5 mL**

SHAKE WELL BEFORE USING.
Keep bottle tightly closed.

Any unused portion must be discarded
10 days after mixing.

RECONSTITUTE WITH 38 mL WATER

60 mL
when reconstituted

AUROBINDO

Each 5 mL of reconstituted suspension
contains 125 mg cefdinir USP.

Usual Dosage: Children-14 mg/kg/day in a single dose or
in two divided doses, depending on age, weight, and type
of infection. See package enclosure for full prescribing
information. This bottle contains 1.5 g cefdinir.

Do not accept if seal over bottle opening is broken or
missing.

DIRECTIONS FOR RECONSTITUTION

Prepare suspension at time of dispensing by adding a
total of 38 mL water to the bottle. Tap bottle to loosen the
powder, then add about half the water, and shake. Add the
remaining water and shake to complete suspension. This
provides 60 mL of suspension.

Keep this and all drugs out of the reach of children.

Store dry powder and reconstituted suspension at 20° to
25°C (68° to 77°F); excursions permitted to 15° to 30°C
(59° to 86°F) [see USP Controlled Room Temperature].
Use within 10 days. SHAKE WELL BEFORE EACH USE.
Keep bottle tightly closed.

Distributed by:
Aurobindo Pharma USA, Inc.
279 Princeton-Hightstown Road
East Windsor, NJ 08520

Made in India

Code: TS/DRUGS/78/1996

P1421420

* Over Printing Zone

**Coding Area**
(45 x 20 mm)
Dotted lines not to be printed

8. Trade name _____

   Generic name _____

   Form _____

   Dosage strength when
   constituted _____

   Directions before use _____

**Answers on p. 213**

---

## ◉ CHAPTER **REVIEW**

Read the label, and identify the information requested.

NDC 65162-**822**-09

**Paricalcitol Capsules**

**1 mcg**

Rx only
90 Capsules

amneal

Each capsule contains:
1 mcg Paricalcitol, USP, and 1.2% v/v (1.0% wt/wt)
alcohol, USP dehydrated.

See package insert for full prescribing information.

Store at 20° to 25°C (68° to 77°F); excursions permitted to
15° to 30°C (59° to 86°F) [see USP Controlled Room
Temperature].

Dispense in a USP tight container. Do not accept if seal over
bottle opening is broken or missing.

Distributed by:     **Amneal Pharmaceuticals**
                    Bridgewater, NJ 08807

Rev. 01-2016-00

Non-Varnish Area

1. Trade name _____

   Generic name _____

   Total amount in container _____

   Form _____

   Dosage strength _____

Non-varnish area

NDC 0641-6184-01    2 mL Ampul  **Rx ONLY**

# Digoxin Injection, USP

## 500 mcg/2 mL

### 0.5 mg/2 mL (250 mcg/mL)

FOR SLOW IV OR DEEP IM USE

**NOVAPLUS**®

Distributed by: ❀ WEST-WARD

(01)00306416184014

PLB935-NOV/1

Lot:

Non-varnish area

Exp:

2. Trade name _____    Form _____

   Generic name _____    Dosage strength _____

   NDC number _____    Total volume _____

NDC 69238-1831-1

**amneal**

**LEVOTHYROXINE SODIUM TABLETS, USP**

**50 mcg (0.05 mg)**

**Rx ONLY**
**100 TABLETS**

Mfd. by Rev. 2/17    Mfd. for Rev. 09-2018-00

Dispense in a tight, light-resistant container.

**Storage Conditions:** 20-25°C (68-77°F) with excursions between 15-30°C (59-86°F).

**Dosage:** For complete prescribing information see insert.

Keep this and all medication out of reach of children.

MFD FOR: AMNEAL PHARMACEUTICALS LLC BRIDGEWATER, NJ 08807

MFD BY: JEROME STEVENS PHARMACEUTICALS, INC. BOHEMIA, NY 11716

Made in the USA

No Varnish

3 N 69238 18311 5

3. Trade name _____    Form _____

   Generic name _____    Dosage strength _____

   Storage conditions _____    Total amount in container _____

FPO    FPO    FPO

NDC 70428-011-11
Rx Only

1 Single-use
Cloth

## Qbrexza™
(glycopyrronium) cloth

**2.4%**

For Topical Use Only

Each pouch contains 1 cloth
with 2.8 grams of solution

95012345678903 000123

**CAUTION:** Flammable, keep away from heat or flame. Keep out of reach of children. Wash hands right away after application. Avoid contact with eyes.

**Directions for Use:** Wipe cloth across one entire underarm one time. Using the same cloth, wipe the other underarm one time. A single cloth should be used to apply Qbrexza to both underarms. See package insert for more information.

**Usual Dosage:** See package insert.

Each pouch contains:
glycopyrronium.....................................................66 mg
(equivalent to 105 mg of glycopyrronium tosylate) in a solution of citric acid, dehydrated alcohol, purified water, and sodium citrate.

Store at room temperature, 20°C–25°C (68°F–77°F); excursions permitted to 15°C–30°C (59°F–86°F) [See USP Controlled Room Temperature].

Manufactured for: Dermira, Inc.
Menlo Park, CA 94025
877-337-5553

LOT
EXP    FPO

4. Trade name _____    Form _____

   Generic name _____    Dosage strength _____

   Directions for use _____

---

**DOSAGE AND USE**
See accompanying prescribing information.

Store at 25°C (77°F) (see insert).

**Protect from moisture.**

Open capsule and sprinkle contents on liquid or soft food. Do NOT crush or chew capsule contents.

**Keep out of reach of children.**

Distributed by:
**Sarras Health, LLC**
Athens, GA 30601

NDC: 72834-210-30
Rx Only

## Rabeprazole Sodium Delayed Release Capsules
(Sprinkle)

sarras✚health

**10**mg

**30 capsules**

© 2019 Sarras Health, LLC    Rev 06/19

NON-VARNISH
LOT/EXP
SERIALIZATION
AREA

3  72834  21030  7

5. Generic name _____    Total amount in container _____

   Form _____    Can this medication be crushed? _____
                                          _____
   Dosage strength _____

Store at 20°C to 25°C (68°F to 77°F); excursions permitted to 15°C to 30°C (59°F to 86°F) [see USP Controlled Room Temperature].

Dispense in tight (USP), child-resistant containers.

**DOSAGE AND USE**
See accompanying prescribing information.

*Each tablet contains 103.40 mg of bosutinib monohydrate equivalent to 100 mg of bosutinib.

Distributed by Pfizer Labs
Division of Pfizer Inc
NY, NY 10017
MADE IN SPAIN

*Pfizer*   NDC 0069-0135-01

GTIN:
00300690135014

PAA073112

**Bosulif®**
**(bosutinib) tablets**

**100 mg***

Do not crush or cut tablet
For Oncology Use Only

120 Tablets    **Rx only**

Exp.
Lot
SN

6. Trade name _____       Total amount in container _____

   Generic name _____      Administration directions _____

   Form _____              Directions for use _____

   Dosage strength _____

Truvada tablets
Each tablet contains 200 mg of emtricitabine and 300 mg of tenofovir disoproxil fumarate, which is equivalent to 245 mg of tenofovir disoproxil.

Store at 25 °C (77 °F) (see insert).

Keep container tightly closed. Dispense only in original container.

See package insert for dosage and administration.

**Manufactured for:**
Gilead Sciences, Inc.
Foster City, CA 94404
Made in Canada

GILEAD

NDC 61958-0701-1

**Truvada®**
**(emtricitabine and tenofovir disoproxil fumarate) tablets**

**200 mg/300 mg**

30 tablets    ℞ only

DISPENSER: Each time Truvada is dispensed give the patient the attached Medication Guide.

101661

7. Trade name _____       Dosage strength _____

   Generic name _____      Directions to dispenser _____

   Form _____

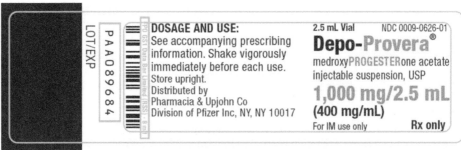

**DOSAGE AND USE:**
See accompanying prescribing information. Shake vigorously immediately before each use. Store upright.
Distributed by
Pharmacia & Upjohn Co
Division of Pfizer Inc, NY, NY 10017

LOT/EXP   PAA089684

2.5 mL Vial    NDC 0009-0626-01

**Depo-Provera®**
medroxyPROGESTERone acetate injectable suspension, USP

**1,000 mg/2.5 mL**
**(400 mg/mL)**

For IM use only    **Rx only**

8. Trade name _____       Directions for use _____

   Generic name _____      Total volume _____

   Dosage strength _____   Is Tall Man lettering used on the label?

   _____

NDC 72152-547-20    Rx ONLY    Single-dose vial

20 mL

**Zulresso™**
(brexanolone) injection

**100 mg/20 mL**
**(5 mg/mL)** CIV

FOR INTRAVENOUS INFUSION
AFTER DILUTION.

**STORAGE:** Refrigerate at 2° to 8°C
(36° to 46°F). **DO NOT FREEZE.**
**STORE PROTECTED FROM LIGHT.**
Discard unused portion.
**DOSAGE & ADMINISTRATION:**
See Full Prescribing Information.
Manufactured for:
Sage Therapeutics, Inc.,
Cambridge, MA 02142

**Sage**
Therapeutics™

54701-4

LOT X123456
EXP MMMYYYY

9. Trade name _____        Type of vial _____

   Generic name _____       Dosage and administration _____

   Form _____               Directions for use _____

   Dosage strength _____

—22 mL*
—20 mL
—18 mL
—16 mL
—14 mL
—12 mL
—10 mL
—8 mL
—6 mL

*Approximate volume of solution when empty dropper cap is attached to the bottle. For inventory purposes only.

**NURSE/PATIENT:** Fill dropper to the
level of the prescribed dose. For ease
of administration, add dose to
approximately 30 mL (1 fl oz) or more
of juice or other liquid. May also be
added to applesauce, pudding or other
semi-solid foods. The drug-food
mixture should be used immediately
and not stored for future use.
Return dropper to bottle after use.
PROTECT FROM LIGHT.
**Discard opened bottle after 90 days.**
Dispense only in this bottle and only
with the calibrated dropper provided.
Rev. 09-2019-02

Distributed by: **Amneal Pharmaceuticals LLC**
Glasgow, KY 42141

NDC 65162-**687**-84    CIV
**Lorazepam Oral**
**Concentrate, USP**

**2 mg/mL**

Each mL contains 2 mg lorazepam, USP

**Usual Dosage:** See Package Insert
for Complete Prescribing Information.

**Store at cold temperature.**
**Refrigerate at 2° to 8°C (36° to 46°F).**

**Rx only**                    **30 mL**

✦amneal

0.85" x 0.57"
unvarnished area
for Lot & Exp

10. Generic name _____        Directions for dispensing _____

    Form _____                How long is the opened bottle good
                                          for? _____

    Dosage strength _____

                                          Directions for administration _____
    Total volume _____

    Controlled substance schedule _____

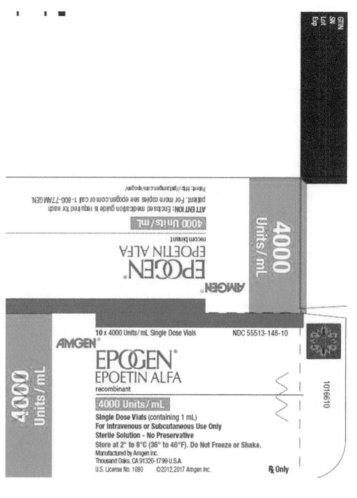

11. Trade name _____     Total volume _____

    Generic name _____     Directions for use _____

    Dosage strength _____

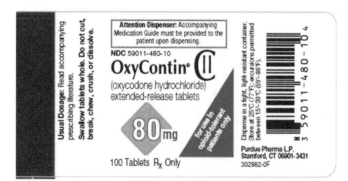

12. Trade name _____     Total amount in container _____

    Generic name _____     Directions for use _____

    Form _____     Controlled substance schedule _____

    Dosage strength _____

NDC 68682-652-20                    Rx only ℞

## Diazepam Rectal Gel

**10 mg** Delivery System

For Rectal Administration Only

LOT:

EXP:

Refer to package
insert for prescribing
information.

Store at 25°C (77°F);
excursions permitted to
15° to 30°C (59° to 86°F).
**KEEP OUT OF REACH
OF CHILDREN.**

Dose →

9570200

**FPO**

Do not cover
the window with
prescription label.

Manufactured for:
Oceanside Pharmaceuticals,
a division of
Valeant Pharmaceuticals
North America LLC
Bridgewater, NJ 08807 USA

Manufactured by:
DPT Laboratories, Ltd.
San Antonio, TX 78215 USA

OCEANSIDE
PHARMACEUTICALS

(01)00368682652208

---

13. Form _____          Directions for use _____

    NDC number _____          Controlled substance schedule _____

---

Store at 20° - 25° C (68° - 77° F);
excursions permitted to 15° - 30° C
(59° - 86° F).
[See USP Controlled Room
Temperature.]
Dispense in light - resistant container.

Code No. : MH/DRUGS/25/KD/638

LOT

EXP.

NDC 75834-500-01                    **100 tablets**

## Metformin Hydrochloride
### Extended Release Tablets USP

**500 mg**

**PHARMACIST :** Dispense with a patient
information leaflet.

NIVAGEN
PHARMACEUTICALS

℞ only

Each tablet contains 500 mg of
metformin hydrochloride USP.
See enclosed package insert for
dosage information.

Manufactured by:
Inventia Healthcare Private Limited
Additional Ambernath M.I.D.C.,
Ambernath (East) - 421506, INDIA.

Distributed by:
Nivagen Pharmaceuticals Inc.
Sacramento, CA 95827

AT2118E-01

0   75834 50001   9

---

14. Trade name _____          Dosage strength _____

    Generic name _____          Total amount in container _____

    Form _____          Directions to pharmacist _____

Store at 20°C to 25°C (68°F to 77°F); excursions permitted to 15°C to 30°C (59°F to 86°F) [See USP Controlled Room Temperature].

**DOSAGE AND USE**
See accompanying prescribing information.

\* Each tablet contains 28.0 mg sertraline hydrochloride equivalent to 25 mg sertraline.

Distributed by Roerig
Division of Pfizer Inc.,
NY, NY 10017

FPO UPC (80%)

N 3   0049-4960-30   0

PAA085191

ALWAYS DISPENSE WITH MEDICATION GUIDE

NDC 0049-4960-30

**Zoloft**®
(sertraline hydrochloride)
tablets

**25 mg\***

30 Tablets          **Rx only**

GTIN: 00300494960300
LOT:/EXP:

15. Generic name _____     Dosage strength _____

    Form _____     Directions for dispensing _____

**4 mL**     NDC 0409-1412-34     Sterile Injection
Single-dose Vial     **Rx only**     **Usual Dosage:** See insert. Store at 20 to 25°C (68 to 77°F). [See USP Controlled Room Temperature.] Contains Benzyl Alcohol

**Bumetanide**
Injection, USP
**1 mg/4 mL** (0.25 mg/mL)
**INTRAVENOUS or
INTRAMUSCULAR USE**

Dist. by Hospira, Inc.
Lake Forest, IL
60045 USA     Hospira

PAA118728     LOT/EXP     ###AA     DMMMYYYY

16. Generic name _____     Total volume _____

    Form _____     Directions for use _____

    Dosage strength _____

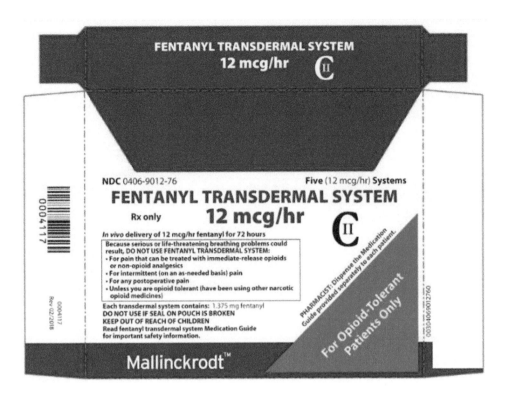

17. Form _____

    Dosage of fentanyl in each transdermal
system _____

    For what time period is 12 mcg per
hour of fentanyl delivered? _____

Directions for use _____

Is there a black box warning on the
label? _____

Controlled substance schedule _____

18. Trade name _____

    Generic name _____

    Form _____

Dosage strength _____

Directions for use _____

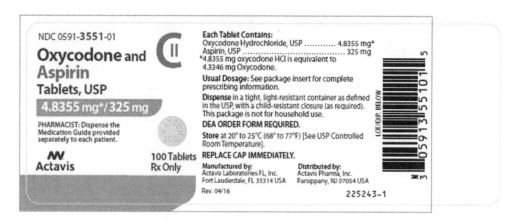

19. This medication is an example of _____ _____

    This medicine contains

    _____ of oxycodone and _____ of

    _____

    Controlled substance schedule _____

    Usual dosage _____

    Directions to pharmacist _____

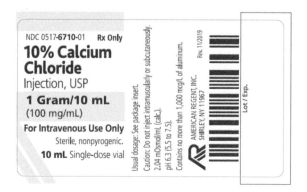

20. The dosage strength of this medication expressed as a percentage is _____

21. The dosage strength of this medication in mg per mL is _____

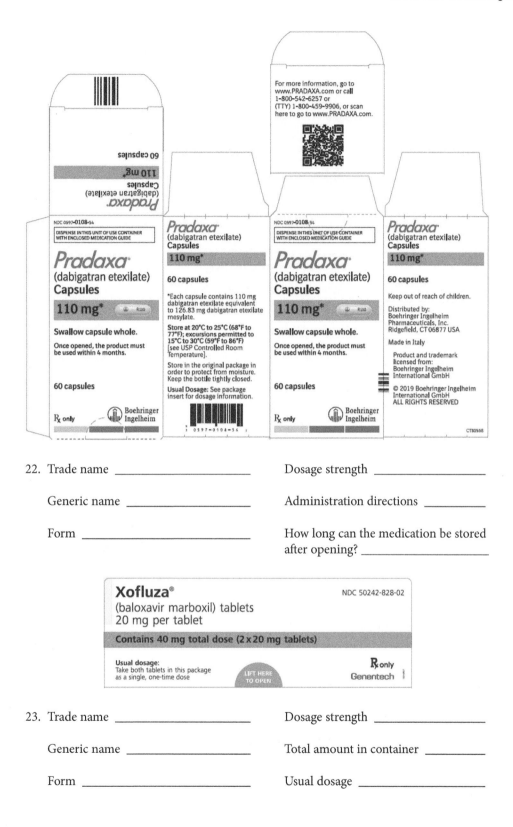

22. Trade name _____    Dosage strength _____

    Generic name _____    Administration directions _____

    Form _____    How long can the medication be stored
    after opening? _____

**Xofluza®**
(baloxavir marboxil) tablets
20 mg per tablet                    NDC 50242-828-02

**Contains 40 mg total dose (2 x 20 mg tablets)**

Usual dosage:
Take both tablets in this package          ℞ only
as a single, one-time dose      LIFT HERE    Genentech
                                  TO OPEN

23. Trade name _____    Dosage strength _____

    Generic name _____    Total amount in container _____

    Form _____    Usual dosage _____

NDC 64406-006-02     60 capsules

# Tecfidera.
## (dimethyl fumarate)
## delayed-release capsules

### 240 mg

Dispense in Original Package.
**Swallow capsule whole.**

Rx only

24. Generic name _____     Dosage strength _____

    Form _____     Directions for administration _____

1 x 60 mg Single-Dose Prefilled Syringe          NDC 55513-710-01

**AMGEN®**

## prolia®
### (denosumab)

60 mg/mL

60 mg/mL.   Injection – **For Subcutaneous Use Only.**
Single-dose Prefilled Syringe. Discard unused portion.

Sterile Solution – No Preservative.                                **Rx Only**
Refrigerate at 2° to 8°C (36° to 46°F). Do not freeze. Avoid excessive shaking. Protect from direct light and heat.
**This Product Contains Dry Natural Rubber.**
Manufactured by: Amgen Inc., Thousand Oaks, CA 91320-1799                    Product of Singapore

25. Generic name _____     Directions for use _____

    Dosage strength _____     Drug manufacturer _____

    Form _____

**Answers on pp. 213-215**

## ⭐ ANSWERS

### Chapter 12
### Answers to Practice Problems

1. Combination medication

2. Generic and trade name

3. b. Tall Man lettering

   c. IV use

   f. Dosage strength 200 mg per 5 mL; 40 mg per mL

   g. Total volume is 5 mL

4. Trade name: no trade name stated
   Generic name: clorazepate dipotassium
   Form: tablets
   Dosage strength: 3.75 mg per tablet (tab)
   Total amount in container: 100 tablets
   Controlled substance schedule: 4, IV
   Pharmacist instructions: Dispense the accompanying
      medication guide to each patient.

5. Trade name: Coreg CR
   Generic name: carvedilol phosphate
   Form: extended-release capsules
   Dosage strength: 10 mg per extended-release capsule
   Total amount in container: 30 extended-release capsules

6. Trade name:  Gleevec
   Generic name: imatinib mesylate
   Dosage strength: 400 mg per tablet (tab)
   Total amount in container: 30 tablets (tabs)
   Storage: Store at 25°C (77°F) excursions permitted to
      15°C–30°C (59°F–86°F).
   Controlled room temperature. Protect from moisture.

7. Trade name: none stated
    Generic name: ondansetron
    NDC number: 63304-347-30
    Form: orally disintegrating tablets (tabs)

8. Trade name: none stated
   Generic name: cefdinir
   Form: powder; oral suspension when reconstituted
   Dosage strength when reconstituted: 125 mg per 5 mL
   Total volume when mixed: 60 mL
   Directions before use: shake well

### Answers to Chapter Review

1. Trade name: no trade name stated
   Generic name: paricalcitol
   Total amount in container 90 capsules (caps)
   Form: capsules (caps)
   Dosage strength: 1 mcg per capsule (cap)

2. Trade name: no trade name stated
   Generic name: digoxin
   NDC number: 0641-6184-01
   Form: Injectable solution (liquid)
   Dosage strength: 500 mcg per 2 mL, 0.5 mg per 2 mL,
      250 mcg per mL
   Total volume: 2 mL

3. Trade name: no trade name stated
   Generic name: levothyroxine sodium
   Storage conditions: 20-25°C (68-77°F) with excur-
      sions between 15-30°C (59-86°F)
   Form: tablets (tabs)
   Dosage strength: 50 mcg per tablet (tab), 0.05 mg per
      tablet (tab)
   Total amount in container: 100 tablets (tabs)

4. Trade name: Qbrexza
   Generic name: glycopyrronium
   Directions for use:  For Topical Use Only. Wipe cloth
      across one entire underarm one time. A single
      cloth should be used to apply Qbrexza to both un-
      derarms. See package insert for more information.
   Form: cloth
   Dosage strength: 2.8 g of solution per cloth

5. Generic name: rabeprazole sodium
   Form: Delayed release sprinkle capsules
   Dosage strength: 10 mg per delayed release sprinkle
      capsule (cap)
   Total amount in container: 30 delayed release sprinkle
      capsules (caps)
   Can this medication be crushed? No (label indicates
      do not crush or chew capsule contents)

6. Trade name: Bosulif
   Generic name: bosutinib
   Form: tablet (tab)
   Dosage strength: 100 mg per tablet (tab)
   Total amount in container: 120 tablets (tabs)
   Administration directions: Do not crush or cut tablet.
   Directions for use: For oncology use only

7. Trade name: Truvada
   Generic name: emtricitabine and tenofovir disoproxil
      fumarate
   Form: tablets (tabs)
   Dosage strength: 200 mg of emtricitabine and 300 mg
      of tenofovir disoproxil fumarate
   Directions to dispenser: Each time Truvada is dis-
      pensed, give the patient the attached medication
      guide.

8. Trade name: Depo-Provera
   Generic name: medroxyprogesterone acetate
   Dosage strength: 1,000 mg per 2.5 mL, 400 mg
   per mL
   Directions for use: For IM use only
   Total volume: 2.5 mL
   Is Tall Man lettering used on the label? Yes, it is used
   in the generic name (medroxyPROGESTERone
   acetate)

9. Trade name: Zulresso
   Generic name: brexanolone
   Form: injectable solution (liquid)
   Dosage strength: 100 mg per 20 mL, 5 mg per mL
   Type of vial: Single-dose vial
   Dosage and administration: See full Prescribing
   Information
   Directions for use: For intravenous infusion after
   dilution

10. Generic name: lorazepam
    Form: Oral concentrate
    Dosage strength: 2 mg per mL
    Total volume: 30 mL
    Controlled substance schedule: 4, IV
    Directions for dispensing: Dispense only in this bottle
    and only with the calibrated dropper provided.
    How long is the opened bottle good for? 90 days
    Directions for administration: Fill dropper to the
    level of the prescribed dose. For ease of adminis-
    tration, add dose to approximately 30 mL (1 fl oz)
    or more of juice or other liquid. May also be added
    to applesauce, pudding, or other semi-solid foods.
    The drug-food mixture should be used immedi-
    ately and not stored for future use. Return dropper
    to bottle after use.

11. Trade name: Epogen
    Generic name: epoetin alfa
    Dosage strength: 4,000 units per mL
    Total volume: 1 mL
    Directions for use: For intravenous or subcutaneous
    use only

12. Trade name: Oxycontin
    Generic name: oxycodone hydrochloride
    Form: extended-release tablets (tabs)
    Dosage strength: 80 mg per extended-release tablet
    (tab)
    Total amount in container: 100 extended-release tab-
    lets (tabs)
    Directions for use: For use in opioid-tolerant patients
    only
    Controlled substance schedule: 2, II

13. Form: Rectal gel
    NDC number: 68682-652-20
    Directions for use: For rectal administration only
    Controlled substance schedule: 4, IV

14. Trade name: no trade name stated
    Generic name: metformin hydrochloride
    Form: extended-release tablets (tabs)
    Dosage strength: 500 mg per extended-release tablet
    (tab)
    Total amount in container: 100 extended-release tab-
    lets (tabs)
    Directions to pharmacist: Dispense with a patient in-
    formation leaflet.

15. Generic name: sertraline hydrochloride
    Form: tablets (tabs)
    Dosage strength: 25 mg per tablet (tab)
    Directions for dispensing: Always dispense with med-
    ication guide

16. Generic name: bumetanide
    Form: injectable solution (liquid)
    Dosage strength: 1 mg per 4 mL, 0.25 mg per mL
    Total volume: 4 mL
    Directions for use: Intravenous or intramuscular use

17. Form: Transdermal patch
    Dosage of fentanyl in each transdermal system: 1.375
    mg of fentanyl per transdermal system
    For what time period is 12 mcg per hour of fentanyl
    delivered? 72 hours
    Directions for use: For opioid-tolerant patients only
    Is there a black box warning on the label? Yes
    Controlled substance schedule: 2, II

18. Trade name: Ilumya
    Generic name: tildrakizumab-asmn
    Form: injectable solution (liquid)
    Dosage strength: 100 mg per mL
    Directions for use: For subcutaneous use only

19. This medication is an example of a combined
    medication.
    This medication contains 4.8355 mg of oxycodone
    and 325 mg Aspirin
    Controlled substance schedule: 2, II
    Usual dosage: See package insert for complete pre-
    scribing information.
    Directions to pharmacist: Dispense the medication
    guide provided separately to each patient.

20. The dosage strength of this medication expressed as a
    percentage is: 10%

21. The dosage strength of this medication in mg per mL
    is: 100 mg per mL

22. Trade name: Pradaxa
    Generic name: dabigatran etexilate
    Form: capsule (cap)
    Dosage strength: 110 mg per capsule (cap)
    Administration directions: Swallow capsule whole.
    How long can the medication be stored after
    opening? 4 months

23. Trade name: Xofluza
    Generic name: baloxavir marboxil
    Form: tablets (tabs)
    Dosage strength: 20 mg per tablet (tab)
    Total amount in container: 2 tablets (tabs)
    Usual dosage: Take both tablets in this package as a single, one-time dose.

24. Generic name: dimethyl fumarate
    Form: delayed-release capsules (caps)
    Dosage strength: 240 mg per delayed-release capsule (cap)
    Directions for administration: Swallow capsule whole.

25. Generic name: denosumab
    Dosage strength: 60 mg per mL
    Form: injectable solution (liquid)
    Directions for use: For subcutaneous use only
    Drug manufacturer: Amgen

# CHAPTER 13
## Dosage Calculation Using the Ratio and Proportion Method

### Objectives

*After reviewing this chapter, you should be able to:*

1. Set up a ratio proportion in the *linear format*
2. Set up a ratio and proportion in the *fraction format*
3. Solve simple calculation problems using the linear format and the fraction format

Several methods are used for calculating dosages. The most common methods are *ratio and proportion* and use of the *formula*. Regardless of the method used the nurse **must** be able to calculate a dose correctly when required to administer medications safely. For the nurse to safely and accurately calculate a dosage, the nurse must demonstrate the ability to utilize a mathematical method that enables the logical set-up of the calculation; solve the problem; and identify whether an answer is rational, applying the principles learned for medication administration. This text covers the various calculation methods (*ratio and proportion, formula, and dimensional analysis*) over the next three (3) chapters. After the various methods have been presented, students can choose the method they find easiest and most logical to use. First, let's discuss calculating using the method of ratio and proportion. If necessary, review Chapter 3 on ratio and proportion.

### Use of Ratio and Proportion in Dosage Calculation

When you know three of the four values of a proportion, you can solve the proportion to determine the unknown quantity. In dosage calculation, it is often necessary to find only one unknown quantity. As you recall from Chapter 3 (*ratio and proportion*), the proportion can be set up using colons (ratio format). A ratio set up using colons (:) is referred to as the linear format. The colons are used to show the relationship between two numbers. The fraction method can also be used. The fractional ratio and proportion method compares two equivalent fractions. Recall that a proportion is a relationship comparing two ratios. In addition to solving for the unknown quantity, it is essential to also be competent in setting up the proportion correctly.

> ! **SAFETY ALERT!**
> If you set up the proportion incorrectly, you could calculate the dose incorrectly and administer the wrong dose, which could have serious consequences for the client.

Let's look at using ratio and proportion to calculate dosages using the linear format and the fraction format. For example, suppose you had a medication with a dosage strength of 50 mg per 1 mL, and the prescriber ordered a dosage of 25 mg. A ratio and proportion may be used to determine how many milliliters to administer. Remember to include units of measure when writing a ratio and proportion to avoid errors.

## Linear Format

When the ratio and proportion are written using colons (ratio format), this can be written in a linear format. The first ratio is termed the *known ratio*; this information is what you have available, or the information from the medication label, and is stated first. The second ratio is the *unknown ratio* and is stated second. It contains the ordered dose and the unknown quantity, which is represented by $x$.

Example 1:
$$50 \text{ mg} : 1 \text{ mL} = 25 \text{ mg} : x \text{ mL}$$
(*known ratio*) (*unknown ratio*)

Solution:
$$50 \text{ mg} : 1 \text{ mL} = 25 \text{ mg} : x \text{ mL}$$
(known)     (unknown)

$50x = $ product of extremes

$25 = $ product of means

$50x = 25$ is the equation

$\dfrac{50x}{50} = \dfrac{25}{50}$ (Divide both sides by 50, the number in front of $x$.)

$x = 0.5 \text{ mL}$

## Fraction Format

When you are setting up the ratio and proportion using the fraction format, the *known ratio* is what you have available, or the information from the medication label, and is stated first (placed on the left side of the proportion). The desired, or what is ordered to be administered, is the *unknown ratio* (placed on the right side). The ordered dose and the unknown quantity is represented by $x$. Therefore, using the example, the ratio and proportion would be stated as follows:

Example 1:
$$\frac{50 \text{ mg}}{1 \text{ mL}} = \frac{25 \text{ mg}}{x \text{ mL}}$$
(*known ratio*) (*unknown ratio*)

Solution: To solve for $x$, use the principles presented in Chapter 3 on ratio and (fraction format) proportion. (The fraction format is solved by cross-multiplication.)

$$\frac{50 \text{ mg}}{1 \text{ mL}} = \frac{25 \text{ mg}}{x \text{ mL}}$$
(known) (unknown)

$$\frac{50x}{50} = \frac{25}{50}$$

$x = 0.5 \text{ mL}$

**SAFETY ALERT!**

It is important to remember when stating ratios that the units of measure should be stated in the same sequence (in the examples, mg : mL = mg : mL or $\frac{mg}{mL} = \frac{mg}{mL}$). Labeling the terms in the ratios, including $x$, is also essential. These pointers are crucial to preventing calculation errors.

**Example 2:** Order: 40 mg p.o. of a medication.

Available: 20-mg tablets (tab, tabs). How many tabs will you administer?

**Fraction Format With Solution:**

$$\frac{20 \text{ mg}}{1 \text{ tab}} = \frac{40 \text{ mg}}{x \text{ tab}}$$

(known)  (unknown)

$$\frac{20x}{20} = \frac{40}{20}$$

$$x = 2 \text{ tabs}$$

*or*

**Linear Format With Solution:**

20 mg : 1 tab = 40 mg : $x$ tab
(known)   (unknown)

$$\frac{20x}{20} = \frac{40}{20}$$

$$x = 2 \text{ tabs}$$

**Example 3:** Order: 1 g p.o. of an antibiotic.

Available: 500-mg capsules (cap, caps). How many caps will you administer?

**Solution:** Notice that the dosage ordered is in a different unit from what is available. Proceed first by changing the units of measure so that they are the same. As shown in Chapter 7, ratio and proportion can be used for conversion.

After making the conversion, set up the problem and calculate the dosage to be given. In this example, the conversion required is within the same system (metric).

In this example, grams are converted to milligrams by using the equivalent 1,000 mg = 1 g. After making the conversion of 1 g to 1,000 mg, the ratio is stated as follows:

$$\frac{500 \text{ mg}}{1 \text{ cap}} = \frac{1,000 \text{ mg}}{x \text{ caps}} \qquad or \qquad 500 \text{ mg} : 1 \text{ cap} = 1,000 \text{ mg} : x \text{ caps}$$

(known)  (unknown)                    (known)                (unknown)

$$x = 2 \text{ caps} \qquad\qquad\qquad x = 2 \text{ caps}$$

An alternate method of solving might be to convert milligrams to grams. In doing this, 500 mg would be converted to grams by using the same equivalent: 1,000 mg = 1 g. However, decimals are common when measures are changed from smaller to larger in the metric system: 500 mg = 0.5 g. Even though converting the milligrams to grams would net the same final answer, *conversions that net decimals are often the source of calculation errors.* Therefore, if possible, avoid conversions that require their use. As a rule, it is best to convert to the measure stated on the medication label. Doing this consistently can prevent confusion. As with the other examples, this proportion could be stated as a fraction as well.

For the purpose of learning to calculate dosages by using ratio and proportion, this chapter emphasizes the mathematics used to calculate the answer. Determining whether an answer is logical is essential and necessary in the calculation of medication. An answer *must make sense.* Determining whether an answer is logical will be discussed further in later chapters covering the calculation of dosages by various routes.

**POINTS TO REMEMBER**

**Important Points When Calculating Dosages Using Ratio and Proportion**

- Make sure all terms are in the same unit and system of measure before calculating. If they are not, a conversion will be necessary before calculating the dosage.
- When conversion of units is required, conversions can be made by converting what is ordered to the units in which the medication is available or by changing what is available to the units in which the medication is ordered. Be consistent as to how you make conversions. It is usual to convert what is ordered to the same unit and system of measure you have the medication available in.
- When stating ratios, the known is stated first. The known ratio is what is available or on hand or the information obtained from the medication label.
- The unknown ratio is stated second. The unknown ratio is the dosage desired, or what the prescriber has ordered.
- The terms of the ratios in a proportion must be written in the same sequence.

  Example: $mg:mL = mg:mL$ or $\dfrac{mg}{mL} = \dfrac{mg}{mL}$.

- Label all terms of the ratios in the proportion, including $x$.
- Before calculating the dosage, make a mental estimate of the approximate and reasonable answer.
- Label the value you obtain for $x$ (e.g., mL, tabs). Double-check the label for $x$ by referring back to the label of $x$ in the original ratio and proportion; it should be the same.
- A proportion can be stated in a linear format using colons (ratio format) or as a fraction.
- Double-check all work.
- Be consistent in how ratios are stated and conversions are done.
- An error in the setup of the ratio and proportion can cause an error in calculation.

## 🖩 PRACTICE **PROBLEMS**

Answer the following questions by indicating whether you need less than 1 tab or more than 1 tab. Refer to Chapter 3 if you have difficulty in answering the questions in this area.

1. A client is to receive 0.2 mg of a medication. The tablets available are 0.4 mg.

   How many tablets do you need? _____

2. A client is to receive 1.25 mg of a medication. The tablets available are 0.625 mg.

   How many tablets do you need? _____

3. A client is to receive 7.5 mg of a medication. The tablets available are 15 mg.

   How many tablets do you need? _____

4. A client is to receive 10 mg of a medication. The tablets available are 20 mg.

   How many tablets do you need? _____

5. A client is to receive 100 mg of a medication. The tablets available are 50 mg.

   How many tablets do you need? _____

For questions 6-25, solve the problems using ratio and proportion. Express your answer in mL to the nearest tenth where indicated. Indicate whether less or more of the medication is needed to administer the dosage ordered.

6. Order: 7.5 mg p.o. of a medication.

   Available: Tablets labeled 5 mg _____

7. Order: 45 mg p.o. of a medication.

   Available: Tablets labeled 30 mg _____

8. Order: 0.09 g p.o. of a medication.

   Available: Capsules labeled 45 mg _____

9. Order: 0.25 mg IM of a medication.

   Available: 0.5 mg per mL _____

10. Order: 100 mg p.o. of a liquid medication.

    Available: 125 mg per 5 mL _____

11. Order: 20 mEq IV of a medication.

    Available: 40 mEq per 10 mL _____

12. Order: 5,000 units subcut of a medication.

    Available: 10,000 units per mL _____

13. Order: 50 mg IM of a medication.

    Available: 80 mg per 2 mL _____

14. Order: 0.5 g p.o. of an antibiotic.

    Available: Capsules labeled 250 mg _____

15. Order: 400 mg p.o. of a liquid medication.

    Available: 125 mg per 5 mL _____

16. Order: 50 mg IM of a medication.

    Available: 80 mg per mL _____

17. Order: 60 mg IM of a medication.

    Available: 30 mg per mL _____

18. Order: 15 mg of a medication.

    Available: Tablets labeled 5 mg _____

19. Order: 0.24 g p.o. of a liquid medication.

    Available: 80 mg per 7.5 mL _____

20. Order: 20 g p.o. of a liquid medication.

    Available: 10 g per 15 mL _____

21. Order: 0.125 mg IM of a medication.

    Available: 0.5 mg per 2 mL _____

22. Order: 0.75 mg IM of a medication.

    Available: 0.25 mg per mL _____

23. Order: 375 mg p.o. of a liquid medication.

    Available: 125 mg per 5 mL _____

24. Order: 10,000 units subcut of a medication.

    Available: 7,500 units per mL _____

25. Order: 0.45 mg p.o. of a medication.

    Available: Tablets labeled 0.3 mg _____

26. Order: 20 mg IM of a medication.

    Available: 25 mg per 1.5 mL _____

27. Order: 150 mg IV of a medication.

    Available: 80 mg per mL _____

28. Order: 2 mg IM of a medication.

    Available: 1.5 mg per 0.5 mL _____

29. Order: 500 mcg IV of a medication.

    Available: 750 mcg per 3 mL _____

30. Order: 0.15 mg IM of a medication.

    Available: 0.2 mg per 1.5 mL _____

31. Order: 1,100 units subcut of a medication.

    Available: 1,000 units per 1.5 mL _____

32. Order: 0.6 g IV of a medication.

    Available: 1 g per 3.6 mL _____

33. Order: 3 g IV of a medication.

    Available: 1.5 g per mL _____

34. Order: 35 mg IM of a medication.

    Available: 40 mg per 2.5 mL _____

35. Order: 0.3 mg subcut of a medication.

    Available: 1,000 mcg per 2 mL _____

36. Order: 200 mg IM of a medication.

    Available: 0.5 g per 2 mL _____

37. Order: 10 mEq IV of a medication.

    Available: 20 mEq per 10 mL _____

38. Order: 165 mg IV of a medication.

    Available: 55 mg per 1.1 mL _____

39. Order: 35 mg subcut of a medication.

    Available: 45 mg per 1.2 mL _____

40. Order: 700 mg IM of a medication.

    Available: 1,000 mg per 2.3 mL _____

Write a proportion and solve for the following unknown quantity.

41. If 15 mL of solution contains 75 mg of medication, how many mg of medication are in 60 mL of solution?

42. A client must take three tablets per day for 28 days. How many tablets should the pharmacy supply to fill this order?

43. A health care provider is instructed to administer 700 mL of a solution every 8 hours. How many hours will be needed to administer 2,100 mL?

44. Two tablets contain a total of 6.25 mg of a medication. How many milligrams of medication are in 10 tablets?

45. If 80 mg of medication is in 480 mL of solution, how many milliliters of solution contain 60 milligrams?

**Answers on pp. 233-237**

## ⊙ CHAPTER **REVIEW**

### Part I

Read the medication labels where available, and calculate the number of tablets or capsules necessary to provide the dosage ordered.

1. Order: Phenobarbital 15 mg p.o. t.i.d.

   Available: Phenobarbital tablets labeled 15 mg _____

2. Order: Erythromycin (delayed-release capsules) 0.5 g p.o. q12h for 10 days.

   Available:

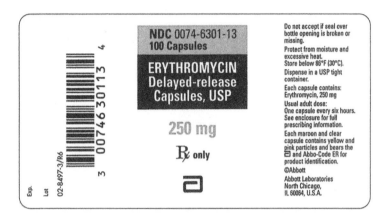

   _____

3. Order: Brilinta 180 mg p.o. stat.

   Available:

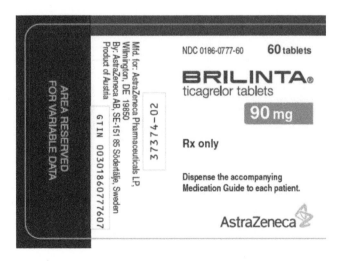

   _____

4. Order: Dilatrate-SR 80 mg p.o. q12h.

Available:

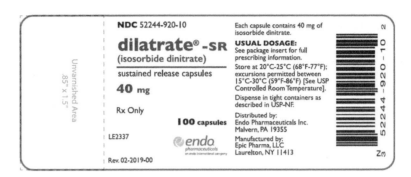

5. Order: Dexamethasone 4 mg p.o. q8h.

Available:

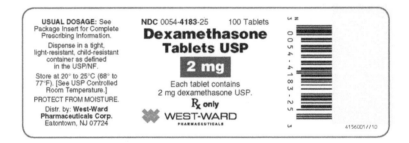

6. Order: Digoxin 125 mcg p.o. daily.

Available:

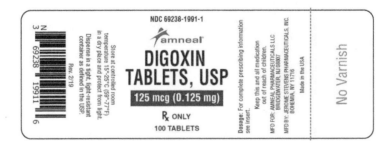

7. Order: Ibrance 125 mg p.o. daily for 21 days.

   Available:

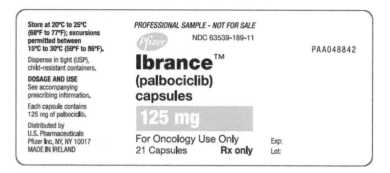

8. Order: Cephalexin 0.5 g p.o. q.i.d.

   Available:

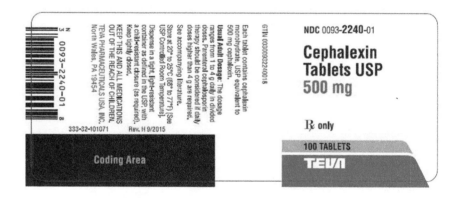

9. Order: Nuplazid 34 mg p.o. daily.

   Available:

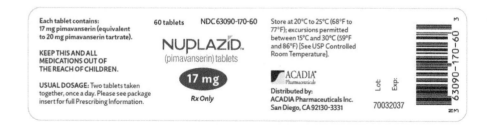

10. Order: Rifampin 0.6 g p.o. daily.

    Available: Rifampin capsules labeled 300 mg

    _____

11. Order: Xanax 0.5 mg p.o. b.i.d.

    Available: Scored tablets (can be broken in half)

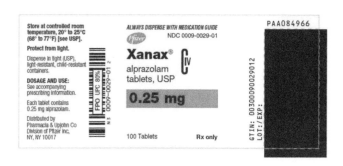

    _____

12. Order: Rubraca 600 mg p.o. bid.

    Available:

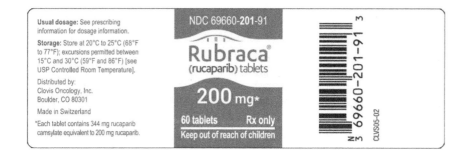

    _____

13. Order: Prandin 2 mg p.o. tid before meals.

    Available:

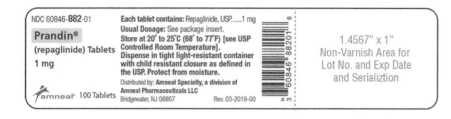

    _____

14. Order: Risperdal 8 mg p.o. daily.

    Available:

    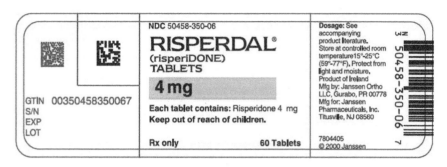

    _____

15. Order: Lasix 60 mg p.o. daily.

    Available:

    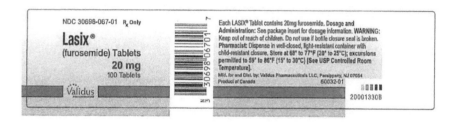

    _____

16. Order: Latuda 80 mg p.o. daily.

    Available:

    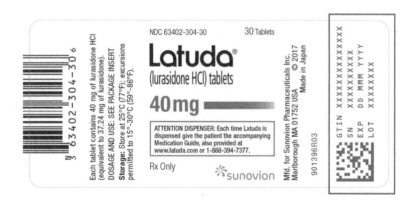

    _____

17. Order: Calcitrol 0.5 mcg p.o. daily.

    Available:

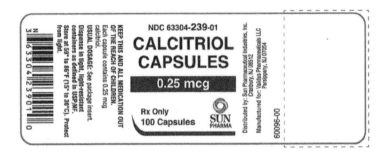

_____

**Answers on p. 237**

## Part II

Calculate the volume necessary (in milliliters) to provide the dosage ordered, using medication labels where available. Express your answer as a decimal fraction to the nearest tenth where indicated.

18. Order: Dilantin 100 mg by gastrostomy tube t.i.d.

    Available: Dilantin 125 mg per 5 mL        _____

19. Order: Benadryl 50 mg p.o. at bedtime.

    Available: Benadryl oral solution labeled 12.5 mg per 5 mL

20. Order: Gentamicin 50 mg IM q8h.        _____

    Available:

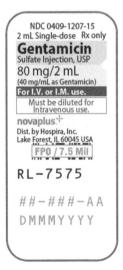

_____

21. Order: Vibramycin 100 mg p.o. q12h.

    Available:

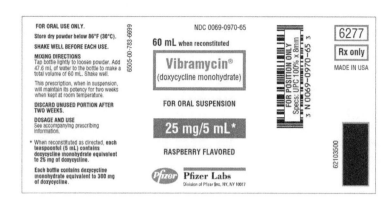

_____

22. Order: Morphine 1.5 mg IM q4h prn for pain.

    Available:

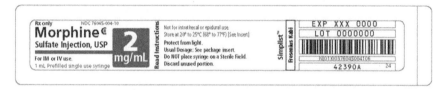

_____

23. Order: Ondansetron 8 mg p.o. q12h for 2 days following chemotherapy.

    Available:

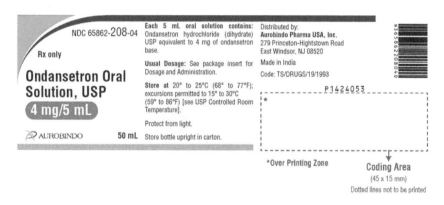

_____

24. Order: Nystatin oral suspension 100,000 units swish and swallow q6h.

    Available: Nystatin oral suspension labeled 100,000 units per mL

_____

25. Order: Heparin 5,000 units subcut daily.

    Available:

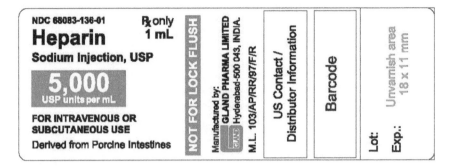

26. Order: Atropine 0.2 mg subcut stat.

    Available:

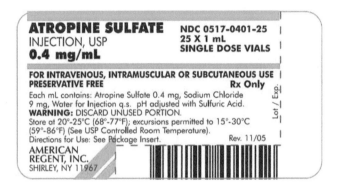

27. Order: Heparin 7,500 units subcut daily. Express answer in hundredths.

    Available:

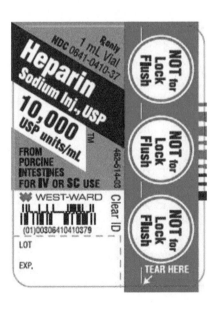

28. Order: Lorazepam 2 mg IM q4h p.r.n. for agitation.

    Available:

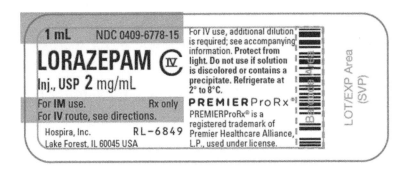

_____

29. Order: Octreotide Acetate 200 mcg subcut q12h.

    Available:

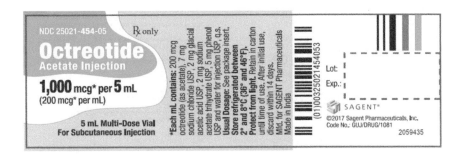

_____

30. Order: Oxcarbazepine 0.6 g p.o. bid.

    Available:

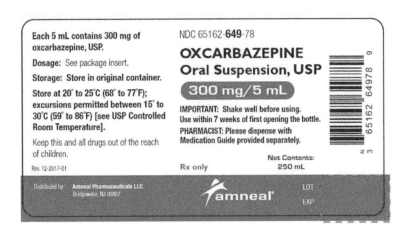

_____

31. Order: Depo-Provera 0.4 g IM at bedtime once a week on Thursday.

Available:

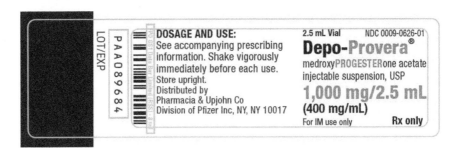

32. Order: Lactulose 30 g p.o. t.i.d.

Available:

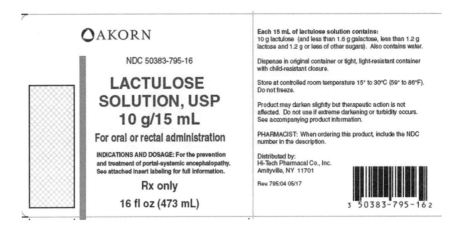

33. Order: Dilantin suspension 200 mg per nasogastric tube every day.

Available:

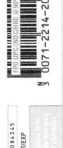

ALWAYS DISPENSE WITH MEDICATION GUIDE

*Pfizer*    NDC 0071-2214-20

# Dilantin-125®
(phenytoin, USP)
Oral Suspension

## 125 mg per 5 mL

IMPORTANT–SHAKE WELL
BEFORE EACH USE

NOT FOR PARENTERAL USE

8 fl oz (237 mL)          **Rx only**

THIS PRODUCT MUST BE SHAKEN WELL ESPECIALLY PRIOR TO INITIAL USE.
Each 5 mL contains 125 mg phenytoin, with a maximum alcohol content not greater than 0.6 percent.
**DOSAGE AND USE**
Adults, 1 teaspoonful (5 mL) three times daily; pediatric patients, see package insert.
**Advice to Pharmacist and Patient**–A calibrated measuring device is recommended to measure and deliver the prescribed dose accurately. A household teaspoon or tablespoon is not an adequate measuring device.
See package insert for complete prescribing information.
Store at 20° to 25°C (68° to 77°F); see USP controlled room temperature.
Protect from light. Do not freeze.
Keep this and all drugs out of the reach of children.
Distributed by
Parke-Davis
Division of Pfizer Inc
NY, NY 10017

PAA084345
LOT/EXP

**Answers on p. 237**

---

## ☆ ANSWERS

## Chapter 13
### Answers to Practice Problems

1. Less than 1 tab
2. More than 1 tab
3. Less than 1 tab
4. Less than 1 tab
5. More than 1 tab
6.
$$\frac{5 \text{ mg}}{1 \text{ tab}} = \frac{7.5 \text{ mg}}{x \text{ tab}}$$
$$\frac{5x}{5} = \frac{7.5}{5}$$
*or*
$$5 \text{ mg} : 1 \text{ tab} = 7.5 \text{ mg} : x \text{ tab}$$
$$\frac{5x}{5} = \frac{7.5}{5}$$
$$x = \frac{7.5}{5}$$

$x = 1.5$ tabs or $1\frac{1}{2}$ tabs. 5 mg is less than 7.5 mg; therefore you will need more than 1 tab to administer the dosage.

7.
$$\frac{30 \text{ mg}}{1 \text{ tab}} = \frac{45 \text{ mg}}{x \text{ tab}}$$
$$\frac{30x}{30} = \frac{45}{30}$$
$$x = \frac{45}{30}$$
*or*
$$30 \text{ mg} : 1 \text{ tab} = 45 \text{ mg} : x \text{ tab}$$
$$\frac{30x}{30} = \frac{45}{30}$$
$$x = \frac{45}{30}$$

$x = 1.5$ tabs or $1\frac{1}{2}$ tabs. 45 mg is more than 30 mg; therefore you need more than 1 tab to administer the dosage.

8. Equivalent: 1,000 mg = 1 g (0.09 g = 90 mg)

$$\frac{45 \text{ mg}}{1 \text{ cap}} = \frac{90 \text{ mg}}{x \text{ cap}}$$

$$\frac{45x}{45} = \frac{90}{45}$$

$$x = \frac{90}{45}$$

$x = 2$ caps. 90 mg is more than 45 mg; therefore you will need more than 1 cap to administer the dosage.

9.

$$\frac{0.5 \text{ mg}}{1 \text{ mL}} = \frac{0.25 \text{ mg}}{x \text{ mL}}$$

$$\frac{0.5x}{0.5} = \frac{0.25}{0.5}$$

$$x = \frac{0.25}{0.5}$$

*or*

0.5 mg : 1 mL = 0.25 mg : $x$ mL

$$\frac{0.5x}{0.5} = \frac{0.25}{0.5}$$

$$x = \frac{0.25}{0.5}$$

$x = 0.5$ mL, 0.25 mg is less than 0.5 mg; you will need less than 1 mL to administer the dosage.

10.

$$\frac{125 \text{ mg}}{5 \text{ mL}} = \frac{100 \text{ mg}}{x \text{ mL}}$$

$$\frac{125x}{125} = \frac{500}{125}$$

$$x = \frac{500}{125}$$

*or*

125 mg : 5 mL = 100 mg : $x$ mL

$$\frac{125x}{125} = \frac{500}{125}$$

$$x = \frac{500}{125}$$

$x = 4$ mL. 100 mg is less than 125 mg; therefore you will need less than 5 mL to administer the dosage.

11.

$$\frac{40 \text{ mEq}}{10 \text{ mL}} = \frac{20 \text{ mEq}}{x \text{ mL}}$$

$$\frac{40x}{40} = \frac{200}{40}$$

40 mEq : 10 mL = 20 mEq : $x$ mL

$$\frac{40x}{40} = \frac{200}{40}$$

$$x = \frac{200}{40}$$

$x = 5$ mL. 20 mEq is less than 40 mEq; you will need less than 10 mL to administer the dosage.

12.

$$\frac{10,000 \text{ units}}{1 \text{ mL}} = \frac{5,000 \text{ units}}{x \text{ mL}}$$

$$\frac{10,000x}{10,000} = \frac{5,000}{10,000}$$

$$x = \frac{5,000}{10,000}$$

*or*

10,000 units : 1 mL = 5,000 units : $x$ mL

$$\frac{10,000x}{10,000} = \frac{5,000}{10,000}$$

$$x = \frac{5,000}{10,000}$$

$x = 0.5$ mL, 10,000 units is more than 5,000 units; therefore you will need less than 1 mL to administer the dosage.

13.

$$\frac{80 \text{ mg}}{2 \text{ mL}} = \frac{50 \text{ mg}}{x \text{ mL}}$$

$$\frac{80x}{80} = \frac{100}{80}$$

$$x = \frac{100}{80}$$

*or*

80 mg : 2 mL = 50 mg : $x$ mL

$$\frac{80x}{80} = \frac{100}{80}$$

$$x = \frac{100}{80}$$

$x = 1.25 = 1.3$ mL. 50 mg is less than 80 mg; therefore you will need less than 2 mL to administer the dosage.

14. Equivalent: 1,000 mg = 1 g (0.5 g = 500 mg)

$$\frac{250 \text{ mg}}{1 \text{ cap}} = \frac{500 \text{ mg}}{x \text{ cap}}$$

$$\frac{250x}{250} = \frac{500}{250}$$

*or*

$$250 \text{ mg} : 1 \text{ cap} = 500 \text{ mg} : x \text{ cap}$$

$$\frac{250x}{250} = \frac{500}{250}$$

$$x = \frac{500}{250}$$

$x = 2$ caps. 500 mg is more than 250 mg; therefore you will need more than 1 cap to administer the dosage.

15.
$$\frac{125 \text{ mg}}{5 \text{ mL}} = \frac{400 \text{ mg}}{x \text{ mL}}$$

$$\frac{125x}{125} = \frac{2,000}{125}$$

$$x = \frac{2,000}{125}$$

*or*

$$125 \text{ mg} : 5 \text{ mL} = 400 \text{ mg} : x \text{ mL}$$

$$\frac{125x}{125} = \frac{2,000}{125}$$

$$x = \frac{2,000}{125}$$

$x = 16$ mL. 400 mg is larger than 125 mg; therefore you will need more than 5 mL to administer the dosage.

16.
$$\frac{80 \text{ mg}}{1 \text{ mL}} = \frac{50 \text{ mg}}{x \text{ mL}}$$

$$\frac{80x}{80} = \frac{50}{80}$$

$$x = \frac{50}{80}$$

*or*

$$80 \text{ mg} : 1 \text{ mL} = 50 \text{ mg} : x \text{ mL}$$

$$\frac{80x}{80} = \frac{50}{80}$$

$$x = \frac{50}{80}$$

$x = 0.62 = 0.6$ mL. 50 mg is less than 80 mg; therefore you will need less than 1 mL to administer the dosage.

17.
$$\frac{30 \text{ mg}}{1 \text{ mL}} = \frac{60 \text{ mg}}{x \text{ mL}}$$

$$\frac{30x}{30} = \frac{60}{30}$$

$$x = \frac{60}{30}$$

*or*

$$30 \text{ mg} : 1 \text{ mL} = 60 \text{ mg} : x \text{ mL}$$

$$\frac{30x}{30} = \frac{60}{30}$$

$$x = \frac{60}{30}$$

$x = 2$ mL. 60 mg is more than 30 mg; therefore you will need more than 1 mL to administer the dosage.

18.
$$\frac{5 \text{ mg}}{1 \text{ tab}} = \frac{15 \text{ mg}}{x \text{ tab}}$$

$$\frac{5x}{5} = \frac{15}{5}$$

*or*

$$5 \text{ mg} : 1 \text{ tab} = 15 \text{ mg} : x \text{ tab}$$

$$\frac{5x}{5} = \frac{15}{5}$$

$$x = \frac{15}{5}$$

$x = 3$ tabs. 15 mg is more than 5 mg; therefore you will need more than 1 tab to administer the dosage.

19. Equivalent: 1,000 mg = 1 g (0.24 g = 240 mg)

$$\frac{80 \text{ mg}}{7.5 \text{ mL}} = \frac{240 \text{ mg}}{x \text{ mL}}$$

$$\frac{80x}{80} = \frac{1,800}{80}$$

$$x = \frac{1,800}{80}$$

*or*

$$80 \text{ mg} : 7.5 \text{ mL} = 240 \text{ mg} : x \text{ mL}$$

$$\frac{80x}{80} = \frac{1,800}{80}$$

$$x = \frac{1,800}{80}$$

$x = 22.5$ mL. 240 mg is more than 80 mg; therefore you would need more than 7.5 mL to administer the dosage.

20.

$$\frac{10 \text{ g}}{15 \text{ mL}} = \frac{20 \text{ g}}{x \text{ mL}}$$

$$\frac{10\,x}{10} = \frac{300}{10}$$

$$x = \frac{300}{10}$$

*or*

$$10 \text{ g} : 15 \text{ mL} = 20 \text{ g} : x \text{ mL}$$

$$\frac{10x}{10} = \frac{300}{10}$$

$$x = \frac{300}{10}$$

$x = 30$ mL. 20 g is more than 10 g; therefore you would need more than 15 mL to administer the dosage.

21.

$$\frac{0.5 \text{ mg}}{2 \text{ mL}} = \frac{0.125 \text{ mg}}{x \text{ mL}}$$

$$\frac{0.5\,x}{0.5} = \frac{0.25}{0.5}$$

*or*

$$0.5 \text{ mg} : 2 \text{ mL} = 0.125 \text{ mg} : x \text{ mL}$$

$$\frac{0.5x}{0.5} = \frac{0.25}{0.5}$$

$$x = \frac{0.25}{0.5}$$

$x = 0.5$ mL. 0.125 mg is less than 0.5 mg; therefore you will need less than 2 mL to administer the dosage.

22.

$$\frac{0.25 \text{ mg}}{1 \text{ mL}} = \frac{0.75 \text{ mg}}{x \text{ mL}}$$

$$\frac{0.25\,x}{0.25} = \frac{0.75}{0.25}$$

*or*

$$0.25 \text{ mg} : 1 \text{ mL} = 0.75 \text{ mg} : x \text{ mL}$$

$$\frac{0.25x}{0.25} = \frac{0.75}{0.25}$$

$$x = \frac{0.75}{0.25}$$

$x = 3$ mL. 0.75 mg is more than 0.25 mg; therefore you will need more than 1 mL to administer the dosage.

23.

$$\frac{125 \text{ mg}}{5 \text{ mL}} = \frac{375 \text{ mg}}{x \text{ mL}}$$

$$\frac{125x}{125} = \frac{1,875}{125}$$

*or*

$$125 \text{ mg} : 5 \text{ mL} = 375 \text{ mg} : x \text{ mL}$$

$$\frac{125x}{125} = \frac{1,875}{125}$$

$$x = \frac{1,875}{125}$$

$x = 15$ mL. 375 mg is more than 125 mg; therefore you will need more than 5 mL to administer the dosage.

24.

$$\frac{7,500 \text{ units}}{1 \text{ mL}} = \frac{10,000 \text{ units}}{x \text{ mL}}$$

$$\frac{7,500x}{7,500} = \frac{10,000}{7,500}$$

*or*

$$7,500 \text{ units} : 1 \text{ mL} = 10,000 \text{ units} : x \text{ mL}$$

$$\frac{7,500x}{7,500} = \frac{10,000}{7,500}$$

$$x = \frac{10,000}{7,500}$$

$x = 1.33 = 1.3$ mL. 10,000 units is more than 7,500 units; therefore you will need more than 1 mL to administer the dosage.

25.

$$\frac{0.3 \text{ mg}}{1 \text{ tab}} = \frac{0.45 \text{ mg}}{x \text{ tab}}$$

$$\frac{0.3x}{0.3} = \frac{0.45}{0.3}$$

*or*

$$0.3 \text{ mg} : 1 \text{ tab} = 0.45 \text{ mg} : x \text{ tab}$$

$$\frac{0.3x}{0.3} = \frac{0.45}{0.3}$$

$$x = \frac{0.45}{0.3}$$

$x = 1.5$ tabs or $1\frac{1}{2}$ tabs. 0.45 mg is more than 0.3 mg; therefore you will need more than 1 tab to administer the dosage.

---

**NOTE**

For questions 26-40 and Chapter Review Parts I and II, answers only are provided. Refer to setup for problems 1-25 and 41-45 for Practice Problems as needed.

26. 1.2 mL
27. 1.9 mL
28. 0.7 mL

29. 2 mL
30. 1.1 mL
31. 1.7 mL

32. 2.2 mL
33. 2 mL
34. 2.2 mL

35. 0.6 mL
36. 0.8 mL
37. 5 mL

38. 3.3 mL
39. 0.9 mL
40. 1.6 mL

41. $\dfrac{75 \text{ mg}}{15 \text{ mL}} = \dfrac{x \text{ mg}}{60 \text{ mL}}$

*or*

$75 \text{ mg} : 15 \text{ mL} = x \text{ mg} : 60 \text{ mL}$

$x = 300 \text{ mg}$

42. $\dfrac{3 \text{ tab}}{1 \text{ day}} = \dfrac{x \text{ tab}}{28 \text{ days}}$

*or*

$3 \text{ tab} : 1 \text{ day} = x \text{ tab} : 28 \text{ days}$

$x = 84 \text{ tab}$

43. $\dfrac{700 \text{ mL}}{8 \text{ hr}} = \dfrac{2{,}100 \text{ mL}}{x \text{ hr}}$

*or*

$700 \text{ mL} : 8 \text{ hr} = 2{,}100 \text{ mL} : x \text{ hr}$

$x = 24 \text{ hr}$

44. $\dfrac{6.25 \text{ mg}}{2 \text{ tab}} = \dfrac{x \text{ mg}}{10 \text{ tab}}$

*or*

$6.25 \text{ mg} : 2 \text{ tab} = x \text{ mg} : 10 \text{ tab}$

$x = 31.25 \text{ mg}$

45. $\dfrac{80 \text{ mg}}{480 \text{ mL}} = \dfrac{60 \text{ mg}}{x \text{ mL}}$

*or*

$80 \text{ mg} : 480 \text{ mL} = 60 \text{ mg} : x \text{ mL}$

$x = 360 \text{ mL}$

## Answers to Chapter Review Part I

1. 1 tab
2. 2 delayed-release caps
3. 2 tabs
4. 2 sustained-release (SR) tabs
5. 2 tabs
6. 1 tab
7. 1 cap
8. 1 tab
9. 2 tabs
10. 2 caps
11. 2 tabs
12. 3 tabs
13. 2 tabs
14. 2 tabs
15. 3 tabs
16. 2 tabs
17. 2 caps

## Answers to Chapter Review Part II

18. 4 mL
19. 20 mL
20. 1.3 mL
21. 20 mL
22. 0.8 mL
23. 10 mL
24. 1 mL
25. 1 mL
26. 0.5 mL
27. 0.75 mL
28. 1 mL
29. 1 mL
30. 10 mL
31. 1 mL
32. 45 mL
33. 8 mL

# CHAPTER 14

# Dosage Calculation Using the Formula Method

## Objectives

*After reviewing this chapter, you should be able to:*

1. Define the components of the formula
2. Identify the information from a calculation problem to place into the formula
3. Calculate medication dosages for the number of tablets or capsules, and the volume to administer for medications in solution using the formula $\frac{D}{H} \times Q = x$

This chapter shows how to use a commonly used *formula method* to calculate a dosage. Using a *formula method* to calculate requires identifying the components of the formula from the calculation problem and inserting the information from the problem into the formula. With the *formula method*, the dose ordered (by the prescriber), the available dose (what is on hand, indicated on the medication label), the dosage form (tablet, capsule, volume of solution), and the amount of the dosage form is inserted into the formula to determine what to administer.

Total reliance on a formula without thinking and asking yourself whether an answer is reasonable can result in errors in calculation and an administration error.

**When using a formula, always use it consistently and in its entirety to avoid calculation errors. Always ask, "Is the answer obtained reasonable?"**

You will learn, for example, that the maximum number of tablets or capsules for a single dosage is usually three. Anything exceeding that should be a red flag to you, even if the answer is obtained from the use of a formula. Use formulas to validate the dosage you think is reasonable, not the reverse. **Think** before you calculate. Always estimate **before** applying a formula. Thinking first will allow you to detect errors and alert you to try again and question the results you obtained.

> **! SAFETY ALERT!**
>
> **Avoid Dosage Calculation Errors**
>
> Do not rely solely on formulas when calculating dosages to be administered. Use critical thinking skills such as considering what the answer should be, reasoning, problem solving, and finding rational justification for your answer. Formulas should be used as tools for validating the dosage you THINK should be given.

## Formula for Calculating Dosages

The formula method can be used when calculating dosages in the same system of measurement. When the dosage desired and the dosage on hand are in different systems, convert them to the same system using one of the methods learned for conversion, before using the formula. It is important to learn and memorize the following formula and its components:

$$\frac{D}{H} \times Q = x$$

Let's examine the terms in the formula before using it.

- D = The dosage desired, or what the prescriber has ordered, including the units of measurement. Examples: mg, g, etc.
- H = The dosage strength available, what is on hand, or the weight of the medication on the label, including the unit of measurement. Examples: mg, g, etc.
- Q = The quantity or the unit of measure that contains the dosage that is available, in other words, the number of tablets, capsules, milliliters, etc. that contains the available dosage. "Q" is labeled accordingly as tablet, capsule, milliliter, etc.
- $x$ = The unknown, the dosage you are looking for, the dosage you are going to administer, how many milliliters, tablets, etc. you will give.

---

- Always get into the habit of inserting the quantity value for **"Q"** into the formula, even though when solving problems that involve solid forms of medication (tabs, caps), **"Q"** is always 1. This will prevent errors when calculating dosages for medications in solution (oral liquids or injectables) in which the solution quantity can be more or less than 1 (such as per 10 mL). When solving problems for medications in solution, include the amount for **"Q,"** which varies and must always be included.
- The available dosage on the label for medications in solution may indicate the quantity of medication per 1 milliliter or per multiple milliliters of solution, such as 80 mg per 2 mL, 125 mg per 5 mL. Some liquid medications may also express the quantity in amounts less than a milliliter, such as 2 mg per 0.5 mL.
- When setting up the formula, notice that **"D,"** which is the dosage desired, is in the numerator, and **"H,"** which is the dosage strength available, is placed in the denominator of the fraction.
- All terms of the formula, including "$x$," must be labeled to ensure accuracy.

> **NOTE**
> The unknown "$x$" and "Q" are always labeled the same (e.g., tabs, mL).

> **! SAFETY ALERT!**
> Omission of the amount for **"Q"** can render an error in dosage calculation. Labeling of all terms of the formula, including "$x$," is a safeguard to prevent errors in calculation. Always think first, what is a reasonable amount to administer, and calculate the dosage using the formula.

## Using the Formula Method

Let's review the steps for using the formula (Box 14.1) before beginning to calculate dosages.

| **BOX 14.1    Steps for Using the Formula** |
| --- |
| 1. Memorize the formula, or verify the formula from a resource. |
| 2. Place the information from the problem into the formula in the correct position, with all terms in the formula labeled correctly, including "$x$." |
| 3. Make sure that all measures are in the same units and system of measure; if not, a conversion must be done *before* calculating the dosage. |
| 4. Think logically, and consider what a reasonable amount to administer would be. |
| 5. Calculate your answer, using the formula $\frac{D}{H} \times Q = x$. |
| 6. Label all answers—tabs, caps, mL, etc. |

Now we will look at sample problems illustrating the use of the formula.

**Example 1:** Order: 0.375 mg p.o. of a medication.

Available: Tablets labeled 0.25 mg

**Solution:** The dosage 0.375 mg is desired; the dosage strength available is 0.25 mg per tablet. No conversion is necessary. What is desired is in the same system and unit of measure as what you have on hand.

## ✓ FORMULA SETUP

$$\frac{D}{H} \times Q = x$$

The desired (D) is 0.375 mg. You have on hand (H) 0.25 mg per (Q) 1 tablet. The label on x is tablet. Notice that the label on x is always the same as Q.

$$\frac{(D) \ 0.375 \ \text{mg}}{(H) \ 0.25 \ \text{mg}} \times (Q) \ 1 \ \text{tab} = x \ \text{tab}$$

$$x = \frac{0.375}{0.25} \times 1$$

$$x = \frac{0.375}{0.25}$$

$$x = 1.5 = 1\frac{1}{2} \ \text{tabs}$$

Therefore x = 1.5 tabs, or $1\frac{1}{2}$ tabs. (Because 0.375 mg is larger than 0.25 mg, you will need more than 1 tab to administer 0.375 mg.) *Note:* Although 1.5 tabs is the same as $1\frac{1}{2}$ tabs, for administration purposes, it would be best to state it as $1\frac{1}{2}$ tabs.

**Example 2:** Order: 7,000 units IM of a medication.

Available: 10,000 units in 2 mL

Solution:
$$\frac{(D) \ 7,000 \ \text{units}}{(H) \ 10,000 \ \text{units}} \times (Q) \ 2 \ \text{mL} = x \ \text{mL}$$

$$x = \frac{7,\cancel{000}}{10,\cancel{000}} \times 2$$

$$x = \frac{14}{10}$$

$$x = 1.4 \ \text{mL}$$

> ⚠ **SAFETY ALERT!**
> Omitting Q here could result in an error. A liquid form of medication is involved; Q must be included because the amount varies and is not always per 1 mL.

> → **RULE**
> **Rule for Different Units or Systems of Measure**
> Whenever the desired amount and the dosage on hand are in different units or systems of measure, follow these steps:
> 1. Choose the identified equivalent (the conversion factor needed to make the conversion).
> 2. Convert what is ordered to the same units or system of measure as what is available by using one of the conversion methods presented in the chapter on converting.
> 3. Use the formula $\frac{D}{H} \times Q = x$ to calculate the dosage to administer.

> ⓘ **TIPS FOR CLINICAL PRACTICE**
> The metric system is the principal system used for medications. When converting is required before calculating a dosage, convert measures to their metric equivalent when possible to decrease the chance of error in calculation.

**Example 3:** Order: 0.1 mg p.o. of a medication daily.

Available: Tablets labeled 50 mcg

**Solution:** Convert 0.1 mg to mcg. The equivalent to use is 1 mg = 1,000 mcg. Therefore 0.1 mg = 100 mcg.

Now that you have everything in the same system and units of measure, use the formula presented to calculate the dosage to be administered.

**Solution:**
$$\frac{(D)\ 100\ mcg}{(H)\ 50\ mcg} \times (Q)\ 1\ tab = x\ tab$$

$$x = \frac{100}{50} \times 1$$

$$x = \frac{100}{50}$$

$$x = 2\ tabs$$

Therefore $x = 2$ tabs. (Because 100 mcg is a larger dosage than 50 mcg, it will take more than 1 tab to administer the desired dosage.)

**Example 4:** Order: 0.2 g p.o. of a liquid medication.

Available: 125 mg per 5 mL

**Solution:** Convert 0.2 g to mg. The equivalent to use is 1,000 mg = 1 g. Therefore 0.2 g = 200 mg.

Now that everything is in the same system and units of measure, use the formula presented to calculate the dosage to be administered.

$$\frac{(D)\ 200\ mg}{(H)\ 125\ mg} \times (Q)\ 5\ mL = x\ mL$$

$$x = \frac{200 \times 5}{125}$$

$$x = \frac{1,000}{125}$$

$$x = 8\ mL$$

Therefore $x = 8$ mL. (Because 200 mg is a larger dose than 125 mg, it will take more than 5 mL to administer the desired dosage.)

**Example 5:** Order: 10 mg subcutaneous of a medication.

Available: 30 mg per mL (Express the answer to the nearest tenth.)

**Solution:** No conversion is required; the dosage ordered is in the same system and unit of measurement as the available.

$$\frac{\text{(D) 10 mg}}{\text{(H) 30 mg}} \times \text{(Q) 1 mL} = x \text{ mL}$$

$$x = \frac{10}{30} \times 1$$

$$x = \frac{10}{30}$$

$$x = \frac{1}{3} = 3\overline{)1.00}^{\,0.33} = 0.33 = 0.3 \text{ mL}$$

Therefore $x = 0.33 = 0.3$ mL rounded to the nearest tenth. (Because 30 mg is larger than 10 mg, it will take less than 1 mL to administer the required dosage.) Milliliter is a metric measure expressed as a decimal number.

---

**CRITICAL THINKING**

Use critical thinking before and after formulaic calculating. It is an essential step in estimating what is reasonable and logical in terms of a dosage. This will help prevent errors in calculation caused by setting up the problem incorrectly or careless math and will remind you to double-check your calculation and identify any error.

---

Remember to memorize the formula presented and follow the steps sequentially.
- Check **first** to see if a conversion is required; if so, **convert** so that everything is in the same units and system of measure.
- **Think** critically as to a reasonable answer.
- Set up terms in the formula and **calculate** to validate the dosage you anticipated was reasonable using the formula.

---

**SAFETY ALERT!**

Always double-check your math. Errors can be made in simple calculations because of lack of caution. Always ask yourself whether the answer you have obtained is reasonable and correct.

---

**POINTS TO REMEMBER**

- The formula $\frac{D}{H} \times Q = x$ can be used to calculate the dosage to be administered.
- The Q is always 1 for solid forms of medications (tabs, caps, etc.) but varies when medications are in liquid form. Do not omit "Q" even when 1.
- Before the dosage to be given is calculated, the dosage desired must be in the same units and system of measure as the dosage available or a conversion is necessary.
- Set up the terms in the formula labeled correctly, including "Q" and "x."
- Think about what a reasonable answer would be.
- Calculate the dosage to administer using the formula to validate your answer as to what was reasonable.
- Double-check all your math, and think logically about the answer obtained.
- Label all answers obtained (e.g., tabs, caps, mL).
- The use of a formula does not eliminate the need to think critically.
- Always systematically follow these steps: **Convert** if necessary, **THINK** about what would be a reasonable answer, set up the terms in the formula, **Calculate** the dosage to administer using the formula.

## ![calculator icon] PRACTICE **PROBLEMS**

For questions 1-15, calculate the problems using the formula method presented in this chapter. Label the answers correctly (tabs, caps). Indicate whether less or more of the medication is needed to administer the dosage ordered.

1. Order: 0.4 mg p.o.

   Available: Tablets labeled 0.2 mg _____

2. Order: 0.75 g p.o.

   Available: Capsules labeled 250 mg _____

3. Order: 90 mg p.o.

   Available: Tablets labeled 60 mg _____

4. Order: 7.5 mg p.o.

   Available: Tablets labeled 2.5 mg _____

5. Order: 0.05 mg p.o.

   Available: Tablets labeled 25 mcg _____

6. Order: 0.4 mg p.o.

   Available: Tablets labeled 200 mcg _____

7. Order: 1,000 mg p.o.

   Available: Tablets labeled 500 mg _____

8. Order: 0.6 g p.o.

   Available: Capsules labeled 600 mg _____

9. Order: 1.25 mg p.o.

   Available: Tablets labeled 625 mcg _____

Calculate the following in milliliters and round to the nearest tenth where indicated. Label answers in mL.

10. Order: 10 mg subcut.

    Available: 15 mg per mL _____

11. Order: 400 mg p.o.

    Available: Oral solution labeled 200 mg per 5 mL _____

12. Order: 15 mEq p.o.

    Available: Oral solution labeled 20 mEq per10 mL _____

13. Order: 125 mg p.o.

    Available: Oral solution labeled 250 mg per 5 mL _____

14. Order: 0.025 mg p.o.

    Available: Oral solution labeled 0.05 mg per 5 mL _____

15. Order: 375 mg p.o.

    Available: Oral solution labeled 125 mg per 5 mL _____

**Answers on pp. 255-256**

## ◎ CHAPTER **REVIEW**

Calculate the following dosages using the medication label or information provided. Label answers correctly: tabs, caps, mL. Answers expressed in milliliters should be rounded to the nearest tenth where indicated.

1. Order: Phenobarbital 30 mg p.o. t.i.d.

    Available:

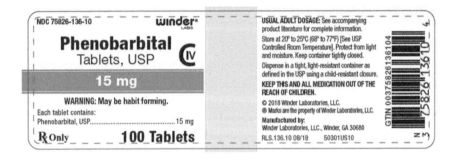

2. Order: Neurontin 0.3 g p.o. bid.

    Available:

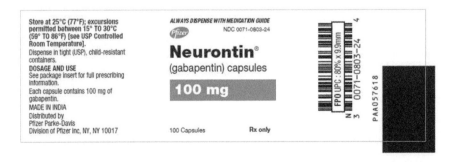

3. Order: Feldene 20 mg p.o. daily.

   Available:

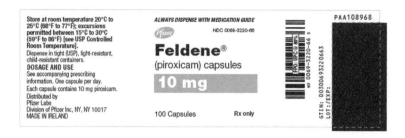

_____

4. Order: Vraylar 3 mg p.o. daily.

   Available:

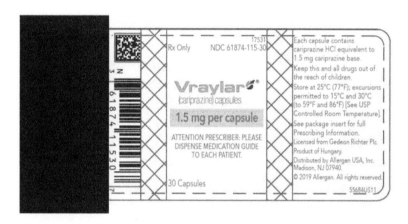

_____

5. Order: Flagyl 0.5 g p.o. b.i.d. for 1 week.

   Available:

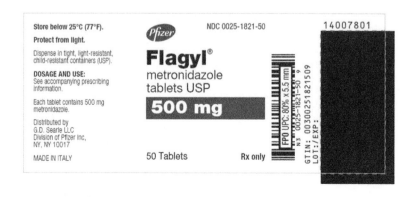

_____

6. Order: Verapamil 5 mg IV stat.

   Available: Verapamil

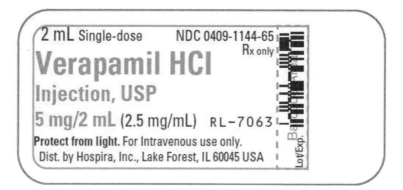

7. Order: Morphine Sulfate (extended-release) 30 mg p.o. q12h.

   Available:

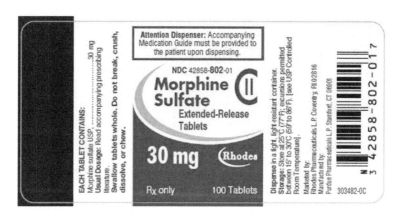

8. Order: Cogentin 1 mg IM at bedtime.

   Available:

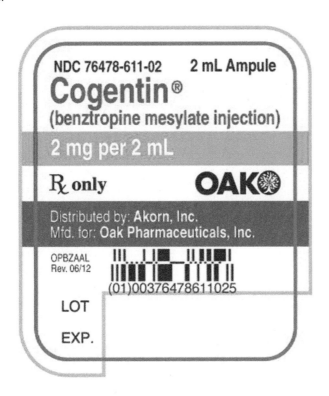

_____

9. Order: Cosentyx 150 mg subcut every 4 weeks.

   Available:

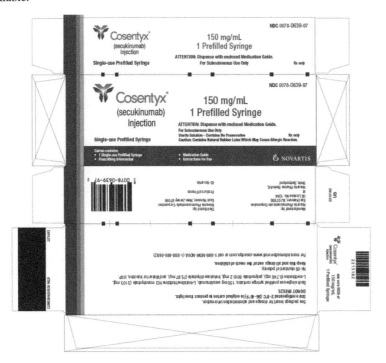

_____

10. Order: Methylprednisolone sodium succinate 35 mg IM daily.

    Available:

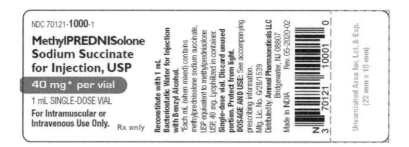

11. Order: Phenobarbital elixir 45 mg p.o. b.i.d.

    Available:

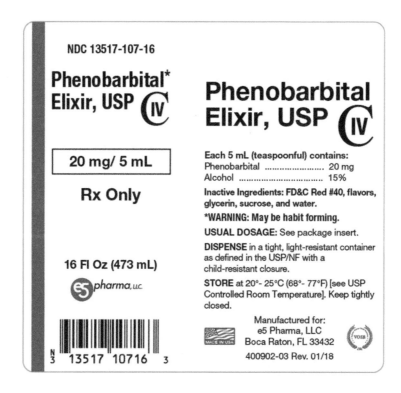

_____

12. Order: Heparin 3,000 units subcut b.i.d.

    Available:

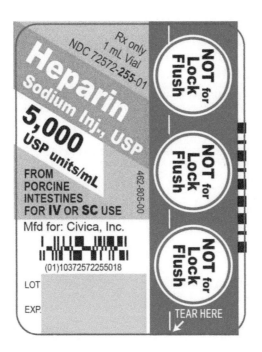

_____

13. Order: Gentamicin 70 mg IV q8h.

    Available:

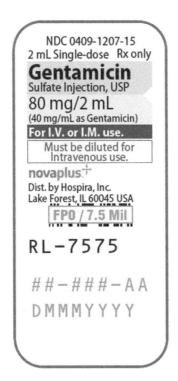

_____

14. Order: Atropine 0.3 mg IM stat.

    Available:

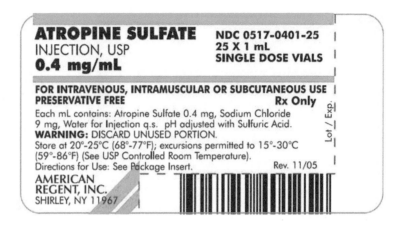

15. Order: Lorazepam 1.5 mg IM stat.

    Available:

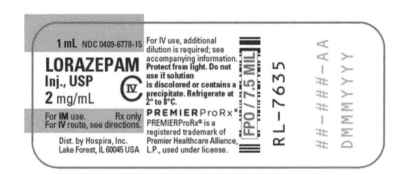

16. Order: Lincocin 0.5 g IM q12h.

    Available:

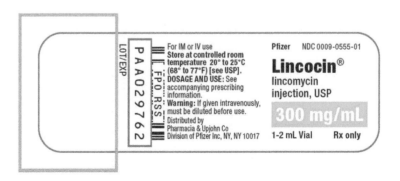

17. Order: Lithium Carbonate (extended-release) 900 mg p.o. q12h.

    Available:

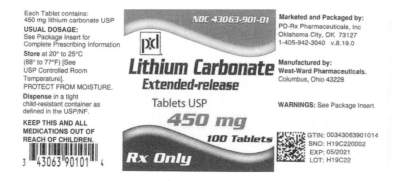

_____

18. Order: Sinemet CR (sustained-release) 50-200 p.o. bid.

    Available:

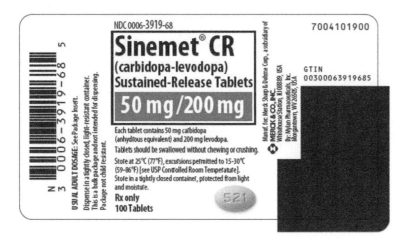

_____

19. Order: Sunosi 37.5 mg p.o. daily for a client with renal impairment.

    Available: Scored tablets (can be broken in half)

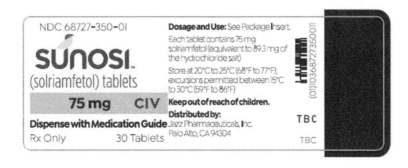

_____

20. Order: Vasotec 5 mg p.o. daily.

    Available:

    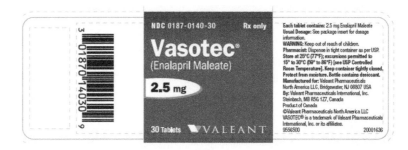

    _____

21. Order: Clozaril 50 mg p.o. b.i.d.

    Available:

    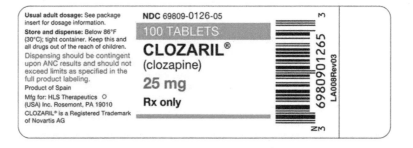

    _____

22. Order: Inderal LA 80 mg p.o. daily.

    Available:

    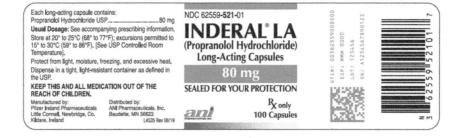

    _____

23.  Order: Targretin 150 mg p.o. daily ac.

Available:

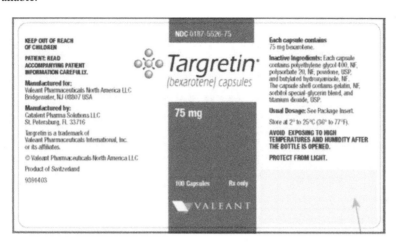

24.  Order: Verzenio 150 mg p.o. bid.

Available:

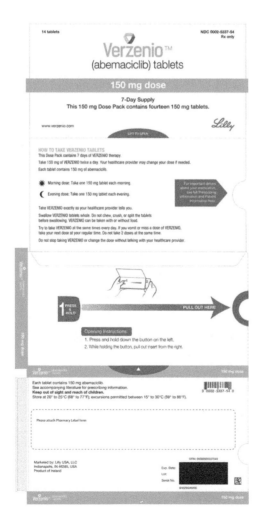

25. Order: Aricept 10 mg p.o. every day at bedtime.

    Available:

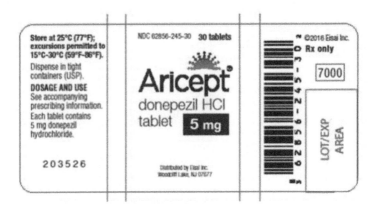

    _____

26. Order: Entresto 49/51 p.o. bid.

    Available:

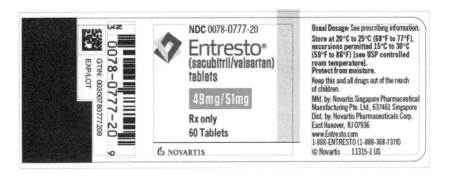

    _____

**Answers on p. 256**

## ★ ANSWERS

<u>**Chapter 14**</u>
**Answers to Practice Problems**

1. $\dfrac{0.4\text{ mg}}{0.2\text{ mg}} \times 1\text{ tab} = x\text{ tab}$

$$x = \dfrac{0.4}{0.2}$$

$x = 2$ tabs. 0.4 mg is greater than 0.2 mg; therefore you will need more than 1 tab to administer the dosage.

2. Equivalent: 1,000 mg = 1 g (0.75 g = 750 mg)

$$\dfrac{750\text{ mg}}{250\text{ mg}} \times 1\text{ cap} = x\text{ cap}$$

$$x = \dfrac{750}{250}$$

$x = 3$ caps. 750 mg is larger than 250 mg; therefore you will need more than 1 cap to administer the dosage.

3. $\dfrac{90\text{ mg}}{60\text{ mg}} \times 1\text{ tab} = x\text{ tab}$

$$x = \dfrac{90}{60}$$

$x = 1.5$ or $1\frac{1}{2}$ tabs. 90 mg is larger than 60 mg; therefore you will need more than 1 tab to administer the dosage.

4. $\dfrac{7.5\text{ mg}}{2.5\text{ mg}} \times 1\text{ tab} = x\text{ tab}$

$$x = \dfrac{7.5}{2.5}$$

$x = 3$ tabs. 7.5 mg is larger than 2.5 mg; therefore you will need more than 1 tab to administer the dosage.

5. Equivalent: 1,000 mcg = 1 mg (0.05 mg = 50 mcg)

$$\dfrac{50\text{ mcg}}{25\text{ mcg}} \times 1\text{ tab} = x\text{ tab}$$

$$x = \dfrac{50}{25}$$

$x = 2$ tabs. 50 mcg is larger than 25 mcg; therefore you will need more than 1 tab to administer the dosage.

6. Equivalent: 1,000 mcg = 1 mg (0.4 mg = 400 mcg)

$$\dfrac{400\text{ mcg}}{200\text{ mcg}} \times 1\text{ tab} = x\text{ tab}$$

$$x = \dfrac{400}{200}$$

$x = 2$ tabs. 400 mcg is larger than 200 mcg; therefore you will need more than 1 tab to administer the dosage.

7. $\dfrac{1,000\text{ mg}}{500\text{ mg}} \times 1\text{ tab} = x\text{ tab}$

$$x = \dfrac{1,000}{500}$$

$x = 2$ tabs. 1,000 mg is more than 500 mg; therefore you will need more than 1 tab to administer the dosage.

8. Equivalent: 1,000 mg = 1 g (0.6 g = 600 mg)

$$\dfrac{600\text{ mg}}{600\text{ mg}} \times 1\text{ cap} = x\text{ cap}$$

$$x = \dfrac{600}{600}$$

$x = 1$ cap. 0.6 g = 600 mg. 600-mg caps are available; therefore give 1 cap to administer the dosage.

9. Equivalent: 1,000 mcg = 1 mg (1.25 mg = 1,250 mcg)

$$\dfrac{1,250\text{ mcg}}{625\text{ mcg}} \times 1\text{ tab} = x\text{ tab}$$

$$x = \dfrac{1,250}{625}$$

$x = 2$ tabs. 1,250 mcg is more than 625 mcg; therefore you will need more than one tab to administer the dosage.

10. $\dfrac{10\text{ mg}}{15\text{ mg}} \times 1\text{ mL} = x\text{ mL}$

$$x = \dfrac{10}{15}$$

$x = 0.66 = 0.7$ mL. 10 mg is less than 15 mg; therefore you will need less than 1 mL to administer the dosage.

11. $\dfrac{400\text{ mg}}{200\text{ mg}} \times 5\text{ mL} = x\text{ mL}$

$$x = \dfrac{2,000}{200}$$

$x = 10$ mL. 400 mg is more than 200 mg; therefore you will need more than 5 mL to administer the dosage.

12. $\dfrac{15 \text{ mEq}}{20 \text{ mEq}} \times 10 \text{ mL} = x \text{ mL}$

$$x = \frac{150}{20}$$

$x = 7.5$ mL. 15 mEq is less than 20 mEq; therefore you will need less than 10 mL to administer the dosage.

13. $\dfrac{125 \text{ mg}}{250 \text{ mg}} \times 5 \text{ mL} = x \text{ mL}$

$$x = \frac{625}{250}$$

$x = 2.5$ mL. 125 mg is less than 250 mg; therefore you will need less than 5 mL to administer the dosage.

14. $\dfrac{0.025 \text{ mg}}{0.05 \text{ mg}} \times 5 \text{ mL} = x \text{ mL}$

$$x = \frac{0.125}{0.05}$$

$x = 2.5$ mL. 0.025 mg is less than 0.05 mg; therefore you will need less than 5 mL to administer the dosage.

15. $\dfrac{375 \text{ mg}}{125 \text{ mg}} \times 5 \text{ mL} = x \text{ mL}$

$$x = \frac{1,875}{125}$$

$x = 15$ mL. 375 mg is more than 125 mg; therefore you will need more than 5 mL to administer the dosage.

## Answers to Chapter Review

 **NOTE**

For Chapter Review problems, only answers are shown. If needed, review the setup of problems in Practice Problems 1 to 15.

1. 2 tabs
2. 3 caps
3. 2 caps
4. 2 caps
5. 1 tab
6. 2 mL
7. 1 extended-release tab
8. 1 mL
9. 1 mL
10. 0.9 mL
11. 11.3 mL
12. 0.6 mL
13. 1.8 mL
14. 0.8 mL
15. 0.8 mL
16. 1.7 mL
17. 2 extended-release tabs
18. 1 sustained-release tab
19. $\frac{1}{2}$ tab or 0.5 tab
20. 2 tabs
21. 2 tabs
22. 1 long-acting caps
23. 2 caps
24. 1 tab
25. 2 tabs
26. 1 tab

# Dosage Calculation Using the Dimensional Analysis Method

## Objectives

*After reviewing this chapter, you should be able to:*
1. Define dimensional analysis
2. Set up a dimensional analysis equation with the appropriate elements for dosage calculation
3. Implement unit cancellation in dimensional analysis
4. Solve dosage calculation problems using dimensional analysis

In this chapter, you will learn how to use *dimensional analysis* (DA) as a method for calculating dosages. It was first introduced as a conversion method in Chapter 7. You may prefer *dimensional analysis to ratio and proportion or formula method.*

Using *dimensional analysis* has advantages, which include the following:
- Applicable to all dosage calculation problems and other required clinical calculations that the nurse may encounter
- No required memorization of a formula
- Setup of one equation to solve a problem even if conversions are required
- Consistent format for setting up the equation

However, as with other methods of calculating dosages (*ratio and proportion or formula method*) previously discussed, memorization of the common equivalents is still a **must**.

*Dimensional analysis* is a method that has been in use in the sciences for many years and is also referred to as the *factor-label method or the unit factor method.* Dimensional analysis can be viewed as a problem-solving method. It involves the process of manipulating units. By manipulating units, you are able to eliminate or cancel unwanted units of measurement, leaving only the desired unit for the answer. Although some may find the formalism of the term *dimensional analysis* intimidating at first, you will find it is simple once you have used it to solve a few problems. As already stated, dimensional analysis can be used for all calculations you may encounter once you become comfortable with the process. One of the primary advantages of dimensional analysis is the reduction in the number of steps in calculations to the use of a single equation. Dimensional analysis will be demonstrated as we proceed through the chapters in this text. *Note*: Remember, as previously stated in the discussion of calculation methods, it is important that you choose a method of calculation you are comfortable with and use it consistently.

## Understanding the Basics of Dimensional Analysis

Let's begin by reviewing making conversions using dimensional analysis before we look at using it to calculate dosages. As you recall from previous chapters, you learned what were referred to as *equivalents* or *conversion factors*: for example, 1 g = 1,000 mg, 1 kg = 1,000 g. In dimensional analysis, the equivalent or conversion factor is written so that the unwanted unit(s) are cancelled (or eliminated) to leave the desired unit.

## Performing Conversions Using Dimensional Analysis

The equivalents (or conversion factors) you learned can be written in a fraction format without changing the value of the unit. This is important to understand when using dimensional analysis. Let's look at the equivalent 1 kg = 1,000 g.

This can be written as:

$$\frac{1\text{ kg}}{1{,}000\text{ g}} \quad or \quad \frac{1{,}000\text{ g}}{1\text{ kg}}$$

Now let's look at the basics in using dimensional analysis for converting units of measure. It is necessary to state the equivalent (conversion factor) in fraction format, maintaining the desired unit in the numerator. In dimensional analysis, how the fraction is written is important. How the fraction is written is based on the unit you want to cancel (or eliminate) to get the unit desired. An equivalent (conversion factor) will give you two fractions:

Examples:     $2.2\text{ lb} = 1\text{ kg} = \dfrac{2.2\text{ lb}}{1\text{ kg}} \quad or \quad \dfrac{1\text{ kg}}{2.2\text{ lb}}$

$1{,}000\text{ mcg} = 1\text{ mg} = \dfrac{1{,}000\text{ mcg}}{1\text{ mg}} \quad or \quad \dfrac{1\text{ mg}}{1{,}000\text{ mcg}}$

## To Make Conversions Using Dimensional Analysis

1. Identify the desired unit.
2. Identify the equivalent (conversion factor) needed.
3. Write the equivalent (conversion factor) in fraction format, keeping the desired unit in the numerator of the fraction. This is written first in the equation. (Notice the unit in the numerator is the same as the unit you desire.)
4. Label all factors in the equation, and label what you desire $x$ (unit desired).
5. Identify unwanted or undesired units, and cancel them. Reduce to lowest terms if possible.
6. If all the labels except the answer label (unit desired) are not eliminated, recheck the equation.
7. Perform the mathematical process indicated.

> **! SAFETY ALERT!**
> Stating the equivalent correctly is crucial. If the equivalent is stated incorrectly, it will not allow you to cancel unit(s) to get the unit desired. Knowing when the equation is set up correctly is an important part of the concept of dimensional analysis.

Let's look at conversion examples to demonstrate the dimensional analysis process.

**Example 1:**  1.5 g = _____ mg
1. The desired unit is mg.
2. Equivalent (conversion factor): 1,000 mg = 1 g
3. Write the equivalent (conversion factor), keeping mg in the numerator to allow you to cancel the unwanted unit, g. (Notice the unit in the numerator of the first fraction is the same as the unit you are looking for.)
4. Write the equivalent (conversion factor) first stated as a fraction, followed by a multiplication sign ($\times$).
5. Perform the indicated mathematical operations.

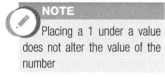
**NOTE**
Placing a 1 under a value does not alter the value of the number

Setup:

$$x\text{ mg} = \frac{1{,}000\text{ mg}}{1\ \cancel{g}} \times 1.5\ \cancel{g}$$

$$or$$

$$x\text{ mg} = \frac{1{,}000\text{ mg}}{1\ \cancel{g}} \times \frac{1.5\ \cancel{g}}{1}$$

$$1{,}000 \times 1.5 = 1{,}500$$

$$x = 1{,}500\text{ mg}$$

**Example 2:**  110 lb = _____ kg

1. The desired unit is kg.
2. Equivalent (conversion factor): 2.2 lb = 1 kg
3. Proceed to set up the problem as outlined.

Setup:

$$x \, kg = \frac{1 \, kg}{2.2 \, \cancel{lb}} \times 110 \, \cancel{lb}$$

*or*

$$x \, kg = \frac{1 \, kg}{2.2 \, \cancel{lb}} \times \frac{110 \, \cancel{lb}}{1}$$

$$x = \frac{110}{2.2}$$

$$x = 50 \, kg$$

---

> **RULE**
>
> All factors entered in the equation must always include the quantity and unit of measure. What you desire or are looking for is "$x$" and is labeled with the unit desired. State all answers following the rules of the system. When there is more than one equivalent (conversion factor) for a unit of measure, use the equivalent (conversion factor) used most often.

---

## PRACTICE **PROBLEMS**

Set up the following problems using the dimensional analysis format; cancel the units. Do not solve.

1. $8\frac{1}{2}$ tsp = _____ mL    6. 0.5 L = _____ mL

2. 15 mg = _____ g    7. 529 mg = _____ g

3. 400 mcg = _____ mg    8. 1,600 mL = _____ L

4. 2 tbs = _____ mL    9. 46.4 kg = _____ lb

5. 0.007 g = _____ mg    10. 5 cm = _____ in

**Answers on pp. 272-273**

---

> **POINTS TO REMEMBER**
>
> - State the equivalent (conversion factor) in fraction format with the desired unit in the numerator.
> - Label all factors in the equation, including "$x$."
> - State the equivalent first in the equation, followed by a multiplication sign ($\times$).
> - Remember the rules relating to conversions.
> - Cancel the undesired units to obtain the unit desired for the answer.

---

## Dosage Calculation Using Dimensional Analysis

As stated, dimensional analysis can be used to calculate dosages with the use of a single equation. A single equation can also be used to calculate the dosage when the dosage desired is in units that differ from what is available (or on hand). When using dimensional analysis to calculate dosages, extract the essential information. To set up a dosage calculation problem using dimensional analysis, you need to know the following information:

- *What is ordered*. This comes from the prescriber's order and contains the strength of the medication and a unit of measurement.
- *The available dosage strength* or what is on hand. This information comes from the medication label. As you recall the dosage strength refers to the weight or amount of the medication provided in a specific unit of measure. The dosage strength is made up of the strength of the medication with the unit of measurement and the dosage form. For solid forms of medications, the dosage strength is the amount per tablet, capsule, etc. **Examples:** 100 mg per tablet (tab), 500 mg per capsule (cap)
- For liquid medications (oral and parenteral) the dosage strength is the amount of medication present in a certain amount of solution. **Examples:** 40 mg per 1 mL, 125 mg per 5 mL
- The desired unit of measure being calculated, which contains the unknown quantity represented by "*x*" with the unit of measurement. **Examples:** *x* tab, *x* mL

When dimensional analysis is used to calculate dosages, the above information become crucial factors in the equation. Dosage strengths, for example, are entered as fractions with a numerator and denominator.

## Steps in Calculating Dosages Using Dimensional Analysis

1. Identify the unit of measure desired in the calculation. With solid forms, the unit will be tab or cap. For parenteral and oral liquids, the unit is milliliter.
2. On the left side of the equation, place the name or appropriate abbreviation for *x*, what you desire or are looking for (e.g., tab, cap, mL).
3. On the right side of the equation, place the available information from the problem in a fraction format. The abbreviation or unit matching the desired unit must be placed in the numerator.
4. Enter the additional factors from the problem, usually what is ordered. Set up the numerator so that it matches the unit in the previous denominator.
5. Cancel out the like units of measurement on the right side of the equation. The remaining unit should match the unit on the left side of the equation and be the unit desired. Reduce to lowest terms if possible.
6. Solve for the unknown *x*.

Let's look at examples using these steps.

**Example 1:**  Order: Lasix 40 mg p.o. daily.

Available: Tablets labeled 20 mg

1. Place the unit of measure desired in the calculation on the left side of the equation, and label it *x*.

$$x \text{ tab} =$$

2. Place the information from the problem on the right side of the equation in a fraction format with the unit matching the desired unit in the numerator. (In this problem each tab contains 20 mg.) You must always think about what is a reasonable answer.

$$x \text{ tab} = \frac{1 \text{ tab}}{20 \text{ mg}}$$

3. Enter the additional factors from the problem, what is ordered, matching the numerator in the previous denominator (in the problem the order is 40 mg). Placing a 1 under it does not change the value.

$$x \text{ tab} = \underset{\substack{\uparrow \\ \text{Amount to} \\ \text{administer}}}{} \frac{1 \text{ tab}}{20 \text{ mg}} \underset{\substack{\uparrow \\ \text{Available} \\ \text{dosage}}}{\times} \frac{40 \text{ mg}}{1} \underset{\substack{\uparrow \\ \text{Ordered} \\ \text{dosage}}}{}$$

4. Cancel the like units of measurement on the right side of the equation. The remaining unit of measurement should be what is desired. Match the unit of measurement on the left side. Proceed with the mathematical process. Notice that after cancellation of units (mg), the desired unit of measure to be administered remains (e.g., tabs in this problem).

$$x \text{ tab} = \frac{1 \text{ tab}}{20 \text{ mg}} \times \frac{40 \text{ mg}}{1}$$

$$x = \frac{1 \times 40}{20}$$

$$x = \frac{40}{20}$$

$$x = 2 \text{ tabs}$$

Now let's look at an example with parenteral medications. You would follow the same steps illustrated in Example 1.

**Example 2:** Order: Gentamicin 55 mg IM q8h.

Available: Gentamicin 80 mg per 2 mL (round answer to the nearest tenth)

1. On the left side of the equation, place the unit desired in this problem (mL).

$$x \text{ mL} =$$

2. On the right side, place the available information from the problem in fraction format, placing the unit matching the unit desired in the numerator. Think what is reasonable to administer.

$$x \text{ mL} = \frac{2 \text{ mL}}{80 \text{ mg}}$$

3. Enter the additional factors from the problem, what is ordered matching the numerator in the previous denominator (in this problem, the order is 55 mg).

$$x \text{ mL} = \underset{\substack{\uparrow \\ \text{Amount to} \\ \text{administer}}}{} \frac{\overset{\substack{\text{Available} \\ \text{dosage} \\ \downarrow}}{2 \text{ mL}}}{80 \text{ mg}} \times \frac{\overset{\substack{\text{Ordered} \\ \text{dosage} \\ \downarrow}}{55 \text{ mg}}}{1}$$

4. Cancel out the like units of measurement on the right side of the equation. The remaining unit of measurement should match the unit on the left side of the equation and be the unit desired.

$$x \text{ mL} = \frac{2 \text{ mL}}{80 \text{ mg}} \times \frac{55 \text{ mg}}{1}$$

$$x = \frac{2 \times 55}{80}$$

$$x = \frac{110}{80}$$

$$x = 1.37 = 1.4 \text{ mL (rounded to the nearest tenth)}$$

### Setting up the Dimensional Analysis Equation When a Conversion Is Required

As already mentioned, dimensional analysis can be used when a medication is ordered in one unit of measurement and is available in a different unit of measurement, thereby necessitating a conversion. To solve the dosage calculation when there are different units, an additional conversion factor is incorporated into the equation. One of the major advantages of dimensional analysis is that it allows multiple factors to be entered in one equation. However, you can also perform the conversion before setting up the equation. Let's look at the steps for incorporating the needed conversion factor (equivalent) into the equation.

The same steps for setting up the equation are followed as previously shown, and the needed conversion factor is incorporated into the equation as follows:

- An additional fraction is inserted into the equation as the second fraction. This fraction is the equivalent (or conversion factor) needed. The numerator must match the unit of the previous denominator.
- The last fraction is the medication ordered. This is written so that the numerator of the fraction matches the unit in the denominator of the fraction immediately before.

Let's look at examples:

**Example 3:** Order: Ampicillin 0.5 g p.o. q6h.

Available: Ampicillin capsules labeled 250 mg

1. On the left side of the equation, place the unit of measure desired in the calculation, and label it $x$.

$$x \text{ caps} =$$

2. Place the information from the problem on the right side of the equation in a fraction format, placing the unit matching the unit desired in the numerator. Think about what is a reasonable amount to administer.

$$x \text{ caps} = \frac{1 \text{ cap}}{250 \text{ mg}}$$

3. The order is for 0.5 g, and the medication is available in 250 mg; a conversion is therefore needed.

From previous chapters, we know 1 g = 1,000 mg; this conversion factor is placed next in the form of a fraction (the numerator of the fraction must match the denominator of the immediately previous fraction).

$$x \text{ caps} = \frac{1 \text{ cap}}{250 \text{ mg}} \times \frac{1,000 \text{ mg}}{1 \text{ g}}$$

4. Next, place the amount of medication ordered in the equation. This will match the denominator of the fraction immediately before. In this problem, it is 0.5 g.

$$x \text{ caps} = \underset{\underset{\text{dosage}}{\text{Available}}}{\frac{1 \text{ cap}}{250 \text{ mg}}} \times \underset{\underset{\text{factor}}{\text{Conversion}}}{\frac{1,000 \text{ mg}}{1 \text{ g}}} \times \underset{\underset{\text{ordered}}{\text{Dose}}}{\frac{0.5 \text{ g}}{1}}$$

5. Cancel out like units of measurement on the right side of the equation; the remaining unit of measurement should match the unit on the left side of equation and be the desired unit. Notice that mg and g cancel, leaving the desired unit, caps.

$$x \text{ caps} = \frac{1 \text{ cap}}{250 \text{ mg}} \times \frac{1{,}000 \text{ mg}}{1 \text{ g}} \times \frac{0.5 \text{ g}}{1}$$

$$x = \frac{1{,}000 \times 0.5}{250}$$

$$x = \frac{500}{250}$$

$$x = 2 \text{ caps}$$

**Example 4:** Order: Enalaprilat 625 mcg IV stat.

Available: Enalaprilat 2.5 mg per 2 mL

1. On the left side of the equation, place the unit of measure desired in the calculation, and label it $x$.

$$x \text{ mL} =$$

2. Place the information from the problem on the right side of the equation in a fraction format, placing the unit matching the unit desired in the numerator. Think about what is a reasonable amount to administer.

$$x \text{ mL} = \frac{2 \text{ mL}}{2.5 \text{ mg}}$$

3. The order is for 625 mcg, and the medication available is 2.5 mg per 2 mL; a conversion is therefore needed. From previous chapters, we know 1 mg = 1,000 mcg; this conversion factor is placed next in the form of a fraction (the numerator of the fraction must match the denominator of the immediately previous fraction).

$$x \text{ mL} = \frac{2 \text{ mL}}{2.5 \text{ mg}} \times \frac{1 \text{ mg}}{1{,}000 \text{ mcg}}$$

4. Next, place the amount of medication ordered in the equation. This will match the denominator of the fraction immediately before, in this problem, it is 625 mcg.

$$x \text{ mL} = \underset{\underset{\text{dosage}}{\underset{\downarrow}{\text{Available}}}}{\frac{2 \text{ mL}}{2.5 \text{ mg}}} \times \underset{\underset{\text{factor}}{\underset{\downarrow}{\text{Conversion}}}}{\frac{1 \text{ mg}}{1{,}000 \text{ mcg}}} \times \underset{\underset{\text{ordered}}{\underset{\downarrow}{\text{Dose}}}}{\frac{625 \text{ mcg}}{1}}$$

5. Next cancel out like units of measurement on the right side of the equation; the remaining unit of measurement should match the unit on the left side of the equation and be the desired unit. Notice that mg and mcg cancel, leaving the desired unit, mL.

$$x \text{ mL} = \frac{2 \text{ mL}}{2.5 \text{ mg}} \times \frac{1 \text{ mg}}{1{,}000 \text{ mcg}} \times \frac{625 \text{ mcg}}{1}$$

$$x = \frac{625 \times 2}{1{,}000 \times 2.5}$$

$$x = \frac{1{,}250}{2500}$$

$$x = 0.5 \text{ mL}$$

> **! SAFETY ALERT!**
> Incorrect placement of units of measure into the equation will not allow cancellation of units and can result in an error in calculation. Dimensional analysis does not eliminate thinking about what a reasonable answer should be.

> **⚙ POINTS TO REMEMBER**
> When using dimensional analysis to calculate dosages:
> - First determine units of the medication you want to administer; for example, tabs, caps, mL, and so on. The unit desired is written **FIRST** to the left of the equation followed by an equal sign (=).
> - The units in the numerator on the left of the equal sign are the same units placed in the numerator of the **first fraction** on the right side of the equation.
> - If a conversion is necessary, the conversion factor is also entered into the right side of the equation, as the second fraction.
> - The ordered dosage is added at the end as the final fraction.
> - Cancel the like units. When all the cancellations have been made, only the units desired remain (e.g., tab, caps, mL).
> - Always determine the units and **THINK** about what a reasonable answer is, set up the equation, and cancel the units.
> - All factors entered into the equation must include the quantity and unit of measure.
> - Incorrect placement of units of measurement will not allow you to cancel units and can result in an incorrect answer.
> - Thinking and reasoning are essential even with dimensional analysis.

## ▦ PRACTICE **PROBLEMS**

Set up the following problems using dimensional analysis. Do not solve.

11. A dose strength of 0.3 g has been ordered.

    Available: 0.4 g per 1.5 mL _____

12. A dose strength of 15 mg is ordered.

    Available: 15 mg per mL _____

13. Order: Ampicillin 1 g p.o. stat.

    Available: Ampicillin capsules labeled 500 mg _____

14. Order: Cefaclor 250 mg p.o. t.i.d.

    Available: Cefaclor oral suspension labeled 125 mg per 5 mL

    _____

15. Order: Methyldopa 0.5 g p.o. daily.

    Available:

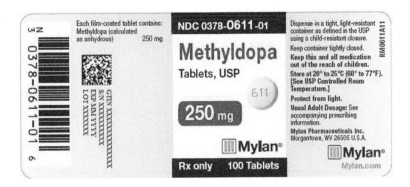

_____

16. Order: Digoxin 0.125 mg p.o. daily.

    Available: Scored tablets (can be broken in half)

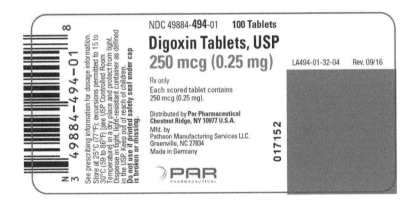

_____

17. Order: Dilantin 300 mg p.o. t.i.d.

    Available:

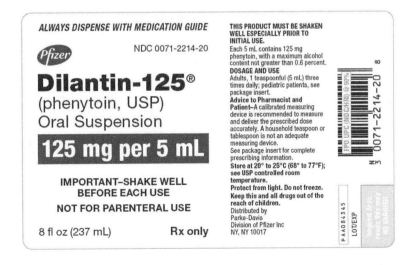

_____

18. Order: Cipro 0.5 g p.o. q12h for 10 days.

    Available: Cipro tablets labeled 250 mg

    _____

19. Order: Clindamycin 0.3 g IV q6h.

    Available: Clindamycin labeled 150 mg per mL

    _____

**Answers on p. 273**

## ◎ CHAPTER REVIEW

Calculate the following medication dosages using the dimensional analysis method. Use medication labels or information provided. Label answers correctly: tab, caps, mL. Answers expressed in milliliters should be expressed to the nearest tenth, except where indicated.

1. Order: Antivert 50 mg p.o. daily.

    Available:

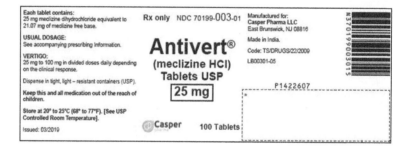

    _____

2. Order: Vibramycin calcium 100 mg p.o. q12h.

    Available:

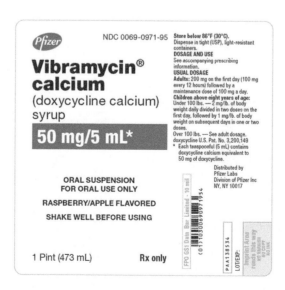

    _____

3. Order: Enalaprilat 0.625 mg IV stat.

   Available:

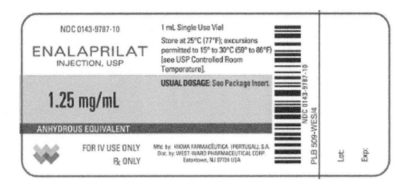

_____

4. Order: Linzess 290 mcg p.o. daily for a client with irritable bowel syndrome with constipation (IBS-C).

   Available:

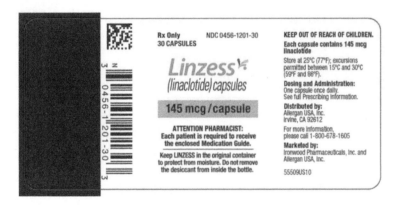

_____

5. Order: Captopril 25 mg p.o. b.i.d.

   Available:

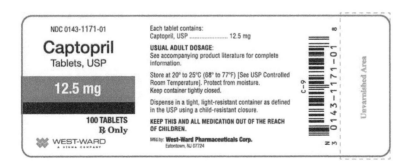

_____

6. Order: Ondansetron 7 mg p.o. q12h for 2 days following chemotherapy.

Available:

_____

7. Order: Heparin 6,500 units subcut q12h.

Available: (Express answer in hundredths)

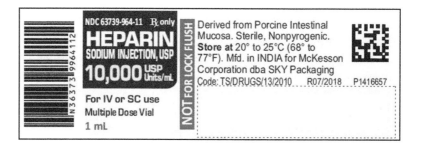

_____

8. Order: Invega 6 mg p.o. daily

Available:

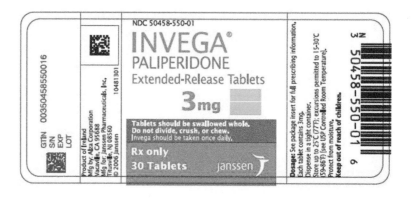

_____

9. Order: Solu-Medrol 175 mg IV daily.

   Available: Solu-Medrol 125 mg per mL

   _____

10. Order: Clarithromycin 0.5 g p.o. q12h for 7 days.

    Available:

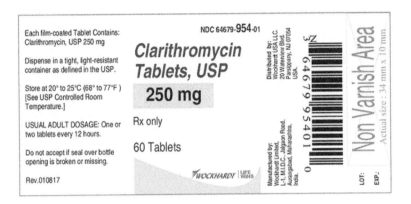

    _____

11. Order: Clonazepam 1 mg p.o. b.i.d.

    Available:

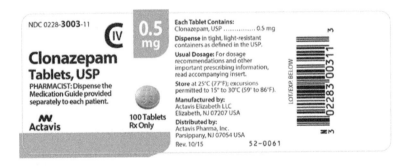

    _____

12. Order: Lyrica CR 165 mg p.o. daily.

    Available:

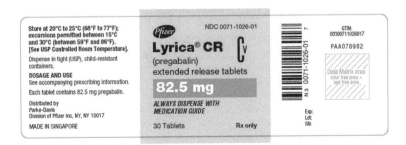

    _____

13. Order: Methotrexate 15 mg IM daily for 5 days.

Available:

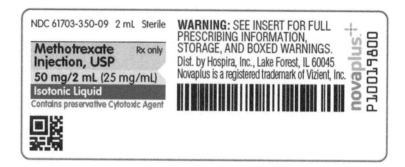

14. Order: Calcitrol 0.5 mcg p.o. daily

Available:

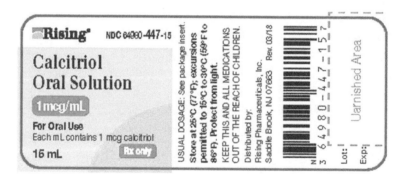

15. Order: Cefaclor 0.4 g p.o. q8h.

Available:

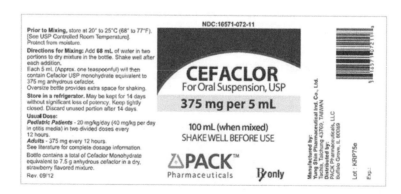

16. Order: Haloperidol decanoate 0.05 g IM every 4 weeks.

    Available:

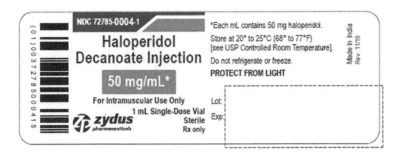

17. Order: Dexamethasone 1.5 mg IV stat.

    Available:

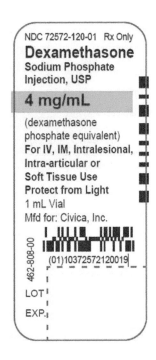

18. Order: Rubraca 500 mg p.o. b.i.d.

    Available:

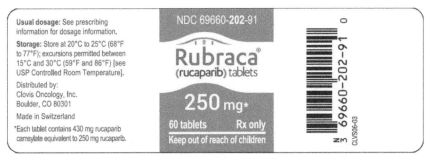

19. Order: Erythromycin Ethylsuccinate oral suspension 0.4 g p.o. q6h.

Available:

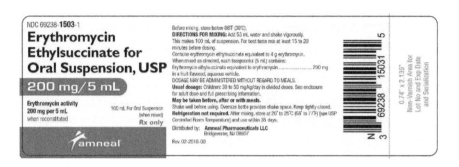

20. Order: Clindamycin 0.6 g IV q12h.

Available:

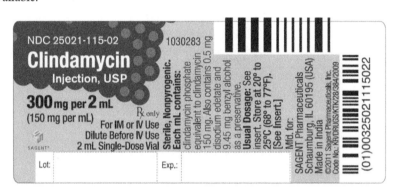

**Answers on pp. 273-274**

## ☆ ANSWERS

### Chapter 15
### Answers to Practice Problems

> **NOTE**
> The following problems could be set up without placing 1 under a value; placing a 1 under the value as shown in the setup for problems 1-19 does not alter the value of the number.

1. $x\,\text{mL} = \dfrac{5\,\text{mL}}{1\,\text{tsp}} \times \dfrac{8\frac{1}{2}\,\text{tsp}}{1}$

2. $x\,\text{g} = \dfrac{1\,\text{g}}{1{,}000\,\text{mg}} \times \dfrac{15\,\text{mg}}{1}$

3. $x\,\text{mg} = \dfrac{1\,\text{mg}}{1{,}000\,\text{mcg}} \times \dfrac{400\,\text{mcg}}{1}$

4. $x\,\text{mL} = \dfrac{15\,\text{mL}}{1\,\text{tbs}} \times \dfrac{2\,\text{tbs}}{1}$

5. $x\,\text{mg} = \dfrac{1{,}000\,\text{mg}}{1\,\text{g}} \times \dfrac{0.007\,\text{g}}{1}$

6. $x\,\text{mL} = \dfrac{1{,}000\,\text{mL}}{1\,\text{L}} \times \dfrac{0.5\,\text{L}}{1}$

7. $x\,\text{g} = \dfrac{1\,\text{g}}{1{,}000\,\text{mg}} \times \dfrac{529\,\text{mg}}{1}$

8. $x\,\text{L} = \dfrac{1\,\text{L}}{1{,}000\,\text{mL}} \times \dfrac{1{,}600\,\text{mL}}{1}$

9. $x\,\text{lb} = \dfrac{2.2\,\text{lb}}{1\,\cancel{kg}} \times \dfrac{46.4\,\cancel{kg}}{1}$

10. $x\,\text{inch} = \dfrac{1\,\text{inch}}{2.5\,\cancel{cm}} \times \dfrac{5\,\cancel{cm}}{1}$

11. $x\,\text{mL} = \dfrac{1.5\,\text{mL}}{0.4\,\cancel{g}} \times \dfrac{0.3\,\cancel{g}}{1}$

12. $x\,\text{mL} = \dfrac{1\,\text{mL}}{15\,\cancel{mg}} \times \dfrac{15\,\cancel{mg}}{1}$

13. $x\,\text{cap} = \dfrac{1\,\text{cap}}{500\,\cancel{mg}} \times \dfrac{1,000\,\cancel{mg}}{1\,\cancel{g}} \times \dfrac{1\,\cancel{g}}{1}$

14. $x\,\text{mL} = \dfrac{5\,\text{mL}}{125\,\cancel{mg}} \times \dfrac{250\,\cancel{mg}}{1}$

15. $x\,\text{tab} = \dfrac{1\,\text{tab}}{250\,\cancel{mg}} \times \dfrac{1,000\,\cancel{mg}}{1\,\cancel{g}} \times \dfrac{0.5\,\cancel{g}}{1}$

16. $x\,\text{tab} = \dfrac{1\,\text{tab}}{0.25\,\cancel{mg}} \times \dfrac{0.125\,\cancel{mg}}{1}$

17. $x\,\text{mL} = \dfrac{5\,\text{mL}}{125\,\cancel{mg}} \times \dfrac{300\,\cancel{mg}}{1}$

18. $x\,\text{tabs} = \dfrac{1\,\text{tab}}{250\,\cancel{mg}} \times \dfrac{1,000\,\cancel{mg}}{1\,\cancel{g}} \times \dfrac{0.5\,\cancel{g}}{1}$

19. $x\,\text{mL} = \dfrac{1\,\text{mL}}{150\,\cancel{mg}} \times \dfrac{1,000\,\cancel{mg}}{1\,\cancel{g}} \times \dfrac{0.3\,\cancel{g}}{1}$

**NOTE**

Placing a 1 under the value does not alter the value of the number.

## Answers to Chapter Review

1. $x\,\text{tab} = \dfrac{1\,\text{tab}}{25\,\cancel{mg}} \times \dfrac{50\,\cancel{mg}}{1}$

$x = \dfrac{50}{25}$

$x = 2\text{ tabs}$

2. $x\,\text{mL} = \dfrac{5\,\text{mL}}{\underset{1}{\cancel{50}}\,\cancel{mg}} \times \dfrac{\overset{2}{\cancel{100}}\,\cancel{mg}}{1}$

$x = \dfrac{5 \times 2}{1}$

$x = \dfrac{10}{1}$

$x = 10\text{ mL}$

3. $x\,\text{mL} = \dfrac{1\,\text{mL}}{1.25\,\cancel{mg}} \times \dfrac{0.625\,\cancel{mg}}{1}$

$x = \dfrac{0.625}{1.25}$

$x = 0.5\text{ mL}$

4. $x\,\text{caps} = \dfrac{1\,\text{cap}}{145\,\cancel{mcg}} \times \dfrac{290\,\cancel{mcg}}{1}$

$x = \dfrac{290}{145}$

$x = 2\text{ caps}$

5. $x\,\text{tab} = \dfrac{1\,\text{tab}}{12.5\,\cancel{mg}} \times \dfrac{25\,\cancel{mg}}{1}$

$x = \dfrac{25}{12.5}$

$x = 2\text{ tabs}$

6. $x\,\text{mL} = \dfrac{5\,\text{mL}}{4\,\cancel{mg}} \times \dfrac{7\,\cancel{mg}}{1}$

$x = \dfrac{35}{4}$

$x = 8.75 = 8.8\text{ mL (to the nearest tenth)}$

7. $x\,\text{mL} = \dfrac{1\,\text{mL}}{10,000\,\cancel{units}} \times \dfrac{6,500\,\cancel{units}}{1}$

$x = \dfrac{6,500}{10,000}$

$x = 0.65\text{ mL}$

8. $x\,\text{tab} = \dfrac{1\,\text{tab}}{3\,\cancel{mg}} \times \dfrac{6\,\cancel{mg}}{1}$

$x = \dfrac{6}{3}$

$x = 2\text{ tabs (extended-release)}$

9. $x\,\text{mL} = \dfrac{1\,\text{mL}}{125\,\cancel{mg}} \times \dfrac{175\,\cancel{mg}}{1}$

$x = \dfrac{175}{125}$

$x = 1.4\text{ mL}$

10. $x\,\text{tab} = \dfrac{1\,\text{tab}}{\underset{1}{\cancel{250}}\,\cancel{mg}} \times \dfrac{\overset{4}{\cancel{1,000}}\,\cancel{mg}}{1\,\cancel{g}} \times \dfrac{0.5\,\cancel{g}}{1}$

$x = \dfrac{4 \times 0.5}{1}$

$x = \dfrac{2}{1}$

$x = 2\text{ tabs (film tabs)}$

11. $x \text{ tab} = \dfrac{1 \text{ tab}}{0.5 \text{ mg}} \times \dfrac{1 \text{ mg}}{1}$

$x = \dfrac{1}{0.5}$

$x = 2 \text{ tabs}$

12. $x \text{ tab} = \dfrac{1 \text{ tab}}{82.5 \text{ mg}} \times \dfrac{165 \text{ mg}}{1}$

$x = \dfrac{165}{82.5}$

$x = 2 \text{ tabs (extended release)}$

13. $x \text{ mL} = \dfrac{1 \text{ mL}}{25 \text{ mg}} \times \dfrac{15 \text{ mg}}{1}$

$x = \dfrac{15}{25}$

$x = 0.6 \text{ mL}$

　　　*or*

$x \text{ mL} = \dfrac{2 \text{ mL}}{50 \text{ mg}} \times \dfrac{15 \text{ mg}}{1}$

$x = \dfrac{2 \times 15}{50}$

$x = \dfrac{30}{50}$

$x = 0.6 \text{ mL}$

14. $x \text{ mL} = \dfrac{1 \text{ mL}}{1 \text{ meg}} \times \dfrac{0.5 \text{ meg}}{1}$

$x = \dfrac{0.5}{1}$

$x = 0.5 \text{ mL}$

15. $x \text{ mL} = \dfrac{5 \text{ mL}}{375 \text{ mg}} \times \dfrac{1,000 \text{ mg}}{1 \text{ g}} \times \dfrac{0.4 \text{ g}}{1}$

$x = \dfrac{5,000 \times 0.4}{375}$

$x = \dfrac{2,000}{375}$

$x = 5.33 \text{ mL} = 5.3 \text{ mL (to the nearest tenth)}$

16. $x \text{ mL} = \dfrac{1 \text{ mL}}{50 \text{ mg}} \times \dfrac{1,000 \text{ mg}}{1 \text{ g}} \times \dfrac{0.05 \text{ g}}{1}$

$x = \dfrac{1,000 \times 0.05}{50}$

$x = \dfrac{50}{50}$

$x = 1 \text{ mL}$

17. $x \text{ mL} = \dfrac{1 \text{ mL}}{4 \text{ mg}} \times \dfrac{1.5 \text{ mg}}{1}$

$x = \dfrac{1.5}{4}$

$x = 0.37 = 0.4 \text{ mL (to the nearest tenth)}$

18. $x \text{ tab} = \dfrac{1 \text{ tab}}{250 \text{ mg}} \times \dfrac{500 \text{ mg}}{1}$

$x = \dfrac{500}{250}$

$x = 2 \text{ tabs}$

19. $x \text{ mL} = \dfrac{5 \text{ mL}}{200 \text{ mg}} \times \dfrac{1,000 \text{ mg}}{1 \text{ g}} \times \dfrac{0.4 \text{ g}}{1}$

$x = \dfrac{5,000 \times 0.4}{200}$

$x = \dfrac{2,000}{200}$

$x = 10 \text{ mL}$

20. $x \text{ mL} = \dfrac{2 \text{ mL}}{300 \text{ mg}} \times \dfrac{1,000 \text{ mg}}{1 \text{ g}} \times \dfrac{0.6 \text{ g}}{1}$

$x = \dfrac{2,000 \times 0.6}{300}$

$x = \dfrac{1,200}{300}$

$x = 4 \text{ mL}$

　　　*or*

$x \text{ mL} = \dfrac{1 \text{ mL}}{150 \text{ mg}} \times \dfrac{1,000 \text{ mg}}{1 \text{ g}} \times \dfrac{0.6 \text{ g}}{1}$

$x = \dfrac{1,000 \times 0.6}{150}$

$x = \dfrac{600}{150}$

$x = 4 \text{ mL}$

## Oral and Parenteral Dosage Forms and Insulin

Oral medications are the easiest, most economical, and most frequently used medications, but sometimes parenteral (nongastrointestinal tract) dosage routes are necessary. Both oral and parenteral medications are available in liquid or powder form. Medications that are available in powdered form must be reconstituted and administered in liquid form. In addition to oral and parenteral dosage forms, this unit examines the varying types of insulin.

# CHAPTER **16**
# Oral Medications

## Objectives

*After reviewing this chapter, you should be able to:*

1. Identify the forms of oral medications
2. Identify information on medication labels used in calculation of dosages
3. Identify equipment used in the administration of oral medications
4. Calculate dosage problems for oral (solid forms) and liquid medications using ratio and proportion, the formula method, or dimensional analysis
5. Apply principles relating to solid forms of medications (tablets and capsules) and oral liquid preparations to determine whether answer obtained is rational

The term *enteral* is used to describe medications that are administered directly into the gastrointestinal tract. With the enteral route, medications can be administered orally, rectally, or, when the oral route is unavailable, through a tube (e.g., nasogastric tube [NGT] or percutaneous endoscopic gastrostomy [PEG]).

Enteral medications are most commonly administered by the oral route (by mouth, or p.o., an abbreviation for the Latin phrase *per os*). Medications that are administered orally come in several forms, including tablets (tab/tabs), capsules (cap/caps), caplets, and liquid preparations. The administration of medications orally is considered to be the easiest, most convenient, and relatively most economical.

In an effort to increase medication safety and reduce errors, safety organizations have recommended that all medications be available in unit-dose packaging. The Joint Commission (TJC) standards require "medications to be dispensed in the most ready-to-administer forms possible to minimize opportunities for error."

A major nursing responsibility in the administration of medications includes engaging in practices that minimize medication errors and promote safe medication administration. To calculate dosages safely, the nurse must read medication labels carefully, identify information relevant to calculation of dosages, and understand and apply principles that apply to administration of medications by the oral route. Calculations involving solid forms (e.g., tablets, capsules) and their preparation for administration are usually simple. Let's begin with discussion of the various forms of solid oral medications.

## Forms of Solid Oral Medications

Solid forms of oral medications come in various forms, which include the most common form, tablets and capsules.

### Tablets

Tablets are preparations of powdered medications that have been compressed into various sizes and shapes and are available in many colors and various types. There are tablets designed for chewing and some that can be dissolved in water, resulting in a liquid that the client drinks. For example, medication guide for Brilinta (ticagrelor), used to decrease the risk of stroke and heart problems after a heart attack, indicates that, if the tablet cannot be swallowed whole, it can be crushed and mixed with water. **Always check** the medication label or a reliable drug reference to verify how a tablet can be administered. Let's discuss the various types of tablets.

Caplets. A caplet is a tablet that has an elongated shape (oval) and a smooth coating for ease of swallowing. Examples: Tylenol and Naproxen (used for pain) are available in caplet form.

Scored Tablets. Scored tablets have indentations, grooves, or markings that allow for ease in breaking the tablet in halves or quarters and sometimes thirds. The medication is evenly distributed throughout the tablet and allows the dose to be divided evenly when the tablet is scored. Figure 16.1 shows an example of a scored tablet. It is not safe practice to break a tablet that is not scored. Splitting or breaking tablets that are not scored have been found to result in inaccurate dosages because of a lack of even distribution of medication. Breaking scored tablets to administer an ordered dosage is allowed but **not optimal**. It is safest and most accurate to administer the least number of whole, undivided tablets possible. Splitting tablets in half, even when scored with a line down the middle, leads to medication errors. Always check to see if the tablet is available in another dosage strength before breaking a scored tablet. Breaking tablets should only be done if no other option exists to administer the dosage. **Safety is always first.** Use practices that promote client safety (Quality and Safety Education for Nurses [QSEN]).

To break tablets evenly, the indentation or groove on the tablet should be used as a guide and be done using a tablet (pill) cutter/splitter, which is readily available in most pharmacies. Figure 16.2 shows a pill/tablet cutter. Clients breaking tablets at home should be encouraged to use a pill or tablet cutter. Ensure that the client fully understands how to use the device and has a clear understanding regarding splitting the tablet. If the client cannot split the tablet, the help of a qualified family member may be needed. Examples of scored tablets include Klonopin (clonazepam [used to treat seizures]), Lanoxin (digoxin [used to treat congestive heart failure and heart rhythm problems]), and Synthroid (levothyroxine [used to treat thyroid deficiency]).

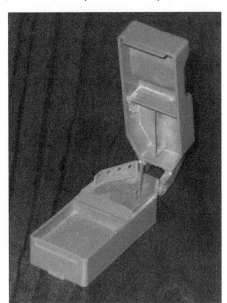

**Figure 16.1** Clonazepam tablet scored.

**Figure 16.2** Pill/tablet cutter. (From Kee JL, Marshall SM: *Clinical calculations: with applications to general and specialty areas,* ed 8, St Louis, 2016, Saunders.)

**SAFETY ALERT!**

Breaking an unscored tablet is risky and dangerous and can lead to administration of an unintended dosage. Question and/or verify any order and any calculation you perform that indicates administering a portion of a tablet that is not scored.

**Enteric-Coated Tablets.** Enteric-coated tablets have a special coating that protects them from the effects of gastric secretions and prevents them from dissolving in the stomach. They are dissolved and absorbed in the small intestines. Enseal is also used to indicate enteric coated.

The enteric coating also prevents the medication from becoming a source of irritation to the gastric mucosa, thereby preventing gastrointestinal upset. Examples include enteric-coated aspirin and iron tablets, such as ferrous gluconate. Enteric-coated tablets should never be crushed, broken, or chewed, because crushing, breaking, and chewing them destroys the special coating and defeats its purpose. They must be swallowed whole with their coating intact.

**Sublingual Tablets.** Sublingual tablets are designed to be placed under the tongue for rapid absorption into the bloodstream by the network of blood vessels in this area. Sublingual tablets should never be swallowed, because this will prevent them from achieving their desired effect. Figure 16.3A shows placement of sublingual tablets. Examples include nitroglycerin, which is used for the relief of acute chest pain, and Abstral (fentanyl), an opioid pain medication used to treat breakthrough cancer pain.

**Buccal Tablets.** Buccal tablets are placed between the gums and cheek for absorption from the blood vessels of the cheek. Clients should be instructed not to chew, swallow, or take liquids. Buccal tablets are designed to be absorbed through the mucous membranes of the mouth. Figure 16.3B shows placement of buccal tablets. Examples include Oravig (miconazole), used to treat oropharyngeal candidiasis (OPC), a oral infection caused by the yeast *Candida* and also referred to as thrush; and Fentora (fentanyl), used to control breakthrough cancer pain not controlled by other medicines.

**Layered Tablets.** Some tablets contain different layers or have cores that separate different medications that may be incompatible with one another; thus incompatible ingredients may be separated and released at different times as the tablet passes through the gastrointestinal tract (Figure 16.4).

Medications in a layered form have become available in which one or more medications can be released immediately from the coating, whereas the same or other medications can be released on a sustained basis from the tablet core. An example of this is Ambien CR. Ambien CR is formulated in a two-layer tablet. The first layer of the tablet dissolves quickly to help in falling asleep, and the second layer dissolves slowly over the night to help the person stay asleep. Another example is Concerta (methylphenidate), a CNS stimulant used in the treatment of attention deficit hyperactivity disorder (ADHD). Concerta has two (2) layers. The first layer dissolves within an hour and releases the initial dose of methylphenidate, and the second layer releases the rest of the medication over a duration of 6 to 7 hours.

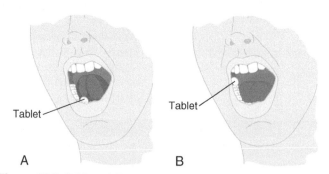

A                    B

**Figure 16.3** Sublingual (A) and buccal (B) tablets. (From Potter PA, Perry AG, Stockert P, Hall A: *Fundamentals of nursing,* ed 9, St Louis, 2016, Mosby.)

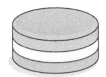

**Figure 16.4** Layered tablet.

Film Tab. A film tab is a tablet sealed with a film. The special coating helps protect the stomach. Some medications that come as film tabs include Biaxin (clarithromycin) and E.E.S. 400 (erythromycin).

Orally Disintegrating Tablets. Orally disintegrating tablets dissolve rapidly, usually within seconds of being placed on the tongue. They are used for their rapid onset of action. Examples of use include treatment of migraine headaches, for clients who have difficulty swallowing, and in clients in whom administration must be ensured because the client often attempts to avoid taking their medications (e.g., the mentally ill). Examples include Klonopin (clonazepam), an anticonvulsant, and Zofran (ondansetron), an antiemetic used for the prevention of nausea and vomiting associated with cancer chemotherapy, radiotherapy, and the prevention of postoperative nausea and vomiting.

A **sublingual film** is now available. The film is placed under the tongue for rapid disintegration. Suboxone (used to manage opiate addiction) is an example of this form. The rapid action of the film is advantageous because the client is unable to retrieve the medication for possible sale on the street and ensures compliance. Suboxone film can be abused in the same manner as other opioids.

Chewable Tablets. Chewable tablets are designed to be chewed, and must be chewed to be effective. Examples of medications that come in chewable form include amoxicillin clavulanate potassium tablets (broad spectrum, anti-infective), Tegretol (carbamazepine), an anticonvulsant, and Dilantin Infatabs (phenytoin) used in the treatment and prevention of seizures.

Timed-Release and Extended-Release Tablets. Look for words and abbreviations that are associated with timed-release and extended-release medications. These include SA, LA, XL, SR, and CR. Medication from these types of tablets is not released immediately but released over a period of time at specific intervals. These types of preparations should not be crushed, chewed, or broken; they should be swallowed whole. If a timed-release or extended-release tablet is crushed, chewed, or broken, all of the medication will be administered at one time and absorbed rapidly causing an unintended effect. Examples include Calan SR, Xeljanz XR, Metformin ER, and Sinemet CR.

## Capsules

A capsule is oval-shaped or round and has a hard or soft gelatinous covering that contains medication in a dry powder, liquid, oil, or miniature pellets. Capsules are available in a variety of sizes and colors. Capsules are not divided or crushed but are administered whole to achieve the desired effect. There are some capsules that may be opened and mixed with food or mixed in water or juice for ease of administration in clients who have difficulty swallowing. For example, Altace (ramipril) used to treat hypertension can be opened and sprinkled on applesauce or mixed in water or juice. Nurses should always check a reliable drug reference to determine which capsules can be opened and mixed with food or in a liquid. Examples of medications that come in capsule form include ampicillin, tetracycline, and Colace. In addition to capsules indicated on a label, some labels may include the term *Kapseals* (e.g., "Kapseals" is seen on some labels for Dilantin extended-release capsules).

Types of Capsules

**Spansules** (timed-release, also known as sustained-release) are capsules that contain many tiny beads (or pellets) of medication that dissolve at spaced intervals for long-acting medications. Spansules may be opened and mixed with food; however, the beads (or pellets) cannot be crushed. The beads (or pellets) delay the release of the medication. An example of a medication that comes in spansule form is Dexedrine spansules sustained-release (dextroamphetamine sulfate), used to treat ADHD and narcolepsy.

**Gelcaps** are soft gelatin shells that contain the medication in a liquid or oil-based form. Gelcaps are not designed to be opened or crushed. Examples include Lanoxicaps (digoxin), used to treat congestive heart failure (CHF) and heart rhythm problems, and PhosLo (calcium acetate), used to prevent phosphate levels from increasing. There are some medications for cold, sinus, and the flu, such as Advil, DayQuil, and NyQuil, which are forms of gelcaps and may use terms that include: "Liquid Gels," "Liqui-Gels," or "Liqui-Caps" on the label.

**Sprinkle capsules** are also available for oral administration and indicate sprinkle capsules on the medication label. Sprinkle capsules can be swallowed whole or opened and sprinkled on food such as applesauce. Examples include Topamax sprinkle capsules (topiramate), used as an anticonvulsant and to treat migraines; Depakote sprinkle capsules (divalproex sodium), used to treat seizure disorders or manic disorders related to bipolar disorder; and Aciphex sprinkle capsules (rabeprazole), which is used to treat symptoms of gastroesophageal reflux disease (GERD).

Medications for oral use are also available as granules (designed to be administered directly into the mouth, taken with food, or liquid) and as powders (designed to be dissolved in a liquid). Other forms of solid preparations for oral administration include lozenges, troches, and pulvules (proprietary capsules containing a dosage of a medication in powdered form). Tablets and capsules are the most common solid forms requiring calculation encountered by the nurse. Figure 16.5 shows various forms of solid oral medications.

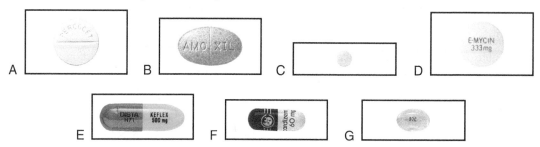

**Figure 16.5** Forms of oral medications. (A) Scored tablet. (B) Chewable tablet. (C) Sublingual. (D) Timed-release tablet. (E) Capsule. (F) Timed-release capsule. (G) Gelatin capsule.

## Crushing Tablets or Opening Capsules

Not all medications can be crushed or opened for administration to clients. The Institute for Safe Medication Practices (ISMP) publishes a list of oral dosage forms that should not be crushed. This list is commonly referred to as the "Do Not Crush" list. The list was first published in July 2007 and updated in 2020. The complete list can be found on ISMP website: https://www.ismp.org/recommendations/do-not-crush Medications may sometimes be ordered for administration into the gastrointestinal tract through a specifically placed tube. For example, a nasogastric tube (NG/NGT) [a tube inserted through the nose into the gastric (stomach) region]. Medications administered by a tube will have to be crushed and dissolved in a small amount of warm water. Determine whether an alternative form of the medication exists if it cannot be crushed, such as oral liquid form.

To maintain safety of the client and prevent an incorrect dose or unintended effect, do not crush or open capsules or tablets that are labeled time-release, sustained-release, delayed release, or extended release. Tablets that are sublingual, buccal, or enteric-coated are never crushed. Capsules are not crushed or opened unless they are designed to be or it is indicated they can be opened. **Always** consult a drug reference, pharmacist, or other reliable resources before crushing a tablet or opening a capsule to ensure that the medication is correctly administered by an approved route, and can be safely administered to avoid harm to a client.

> **⚠ SAFETY ALERT!**
> Medications such as time-release, sustained-release, extended-release, and delayed-release tablets and capsules have special coatings to prevent the medication from being absorbed too quickly. Altering medications that should be administered whole may result in alteration of the medication action (e.g., increasing the rate of absorption or causing the medication to be inactivated) and cause unintended effects.

## Calculating Dosages Involving Tablets and Capsules

When administering solid forms of oral medications (tablets and capsules), the nurse rarely performs complex calculations to determine the number of tablets or capsules needed to administer the dosage ordered. Accurate and safe dosage calculation includes requiring that the nurse understands the medication order, reads the medication label carefully to identify the dosage strength (also referred to as the dosage strength available, what is on hand or available), which is the amount of medication contained in each tablet or capsule, and accurately calculate the dose to administer. To foster clinical reasoning skills and help determine whether the calculated dosage is sensible, accurate, and safe to administer, and to avoid calculation errors, the nurse **must** integrate the following points as an integral part of calculation of dosages involving tablets and capsules.

## POINTS TO REMEMBER

- Converting medication measures from one system to another and one unit to another to determine the dosage to be administered can result in discrepancies, depending on the conversion factor used.
- When the precise number of tablets or capsules is determined and you find that administering the amount calculated is unrealistic or impossible, always use the following rule to avoid an error in administration: *No more than 10% variation should exist between the dosage ordered and the dosage administered.* For example, you may determine that a client should receive 0.9 tablet or 0.9 capsule. Administration of such an amount accurately would be impossible. Following the stated rule, if you determined that 0.9 tablet or 0.9 capsule should be given, you could safely administer 1 tab or 1 cap. This variation usually occurs when conversions are made between apothecary and metric measurements because approximate equivalents are used. There should be no conversion to apothecary. If apothecary measure is indicated, the metric conversion will be beside the apothecary measure, which is often in parenthesis. The 10% variation rule is often applied with adults but not necessarily with the pediatric clients.
- Capsules are not scored and cannot be divided. They are administered in whole amounts only. If a client has difficulty swallowing a capsule, check to see if a liquid preparation of the same medication is available. Never crush or open a timed-release capsule or empty its contents into a liquid or food; this may cause release of all the medication at once. Always use the metric equivalent.
- **Tablets and capsules** may be available in different strengths for administration, and you may have a choice when giving a dosage. For example, 75 mg of a medication may be ordered. When you check what is available, it may be in tablet or capsule form as 10, 25, or 50 mg. In deciding the best combination of tablets or capsules to give, the nurse should always choose the strength that would allow the least number of tablets or capsules to be administered without breaking a tablet, if possible, because breaking is found to result in variations in dosage. In the example given, the best combination for administering 75 mg is one 50-mg tablet or capsule and one 25-mg tablet or capsule.
- Only scored tablets are intended to be divided. It is safest and most accurate not to divide tablets, and give the fewest number of whole, undivided tablets possible.

## RULE

Three (3) tablets or capsules are typically the maximum administered to achieve a single dose. Always **stop, think,** and **recheck** a calculation if a single dose requires more. Question the order before administering if it exceeds three (3).

- It is important to note that although the maximum number of tablets or capsules given to a client is usually three, there may be exceptions, including calcium tablets and some of the solid forms of HIV medications (e.g., tablets, capsules). Example: ritonavir 600 mg p.o. b.i.d. (recommended dosage) (available 100 mg per tab). Although many HIV medications are available in liquid form, many clients have a preference for tablets or capsules.
- **Remember:** Unless the medication is an exception, more than three (3) tablets or capsules to achieve a single dose is unusual and may indicate an error in interpretation of the order, transcription, or calculation. Think! Always question any order that exceeds this amount.
- When calculating dosages using ratio and proportion, the formula method, or dimensional analysis, remember that each tablet or capsule contains a certain amount of medication per tablet or capsule. Example: 325 mg per tablet, 500 mg per capsule. The dosage strength indicated on a label is per tablet or per capsule. This is particularly important when you are reading a medication label on a bottle or single unit-dose package.

*continued*

- In calculating oral dosages, you may encounter measures other than metric measures. For example, electrolytes such as potassium will indicate the number of milliequivalents (mEq) per tablet. Units is another measure you may see for oral antibiotics or vitamins. For example, a vitamin E capsule will indicate 400 units per capsule. Measurements of units and milliequivalents are specific to the medication they are being used for. There is no conversion between these and other systems of measure. (These are discussed in Chapter 17.)
- Always consult a medication reference or pharmacist when in doubt as to whether a capsule may be opened or whether a tablet can be crushed.

> **SAFETY ALERT!**
>
> Regardless of the source of an error, if you administer the wrong dose or give a medication by a route other than that intended, you have committed a medication error and are legally responsible for the error. Always think of the reasonableness of what you have calculated to administer and double-check the dose and route for a medication before administering.

Remembering the points mentioned will be helpful before starting to calculate dosages. Any of the methods presented in Chapters 13, 14, and 15 can be used to determine the dosage to be administered.

To compute dosages accurately, it is necessary to review a few reminders that were presented in previous chapters:

1. Read the order carefully and:
   a. Identify known factors.
   b. Identify unknown factors.
   c. Eliminate unnecessary information that is not relevant.
2. Make sure that what is ordered and what is available are in the same system of measurement and units, or a conversion will be necessary. When a conversion is necessary, it is usual to convert what is ordered into what you have available or what is indicated on the medication label. You can, however, convert the measure in which the medication is available into the same units and system of measure as the dosage ordered. The choice is usually based on whichever is easier to calculate. Use any of the methods presented in Chapters 7, 13, and 15 to make conversions consistent to avoid confusion. If necessary, go back and review these methods.
3. Consider what would be a reasonable answer based on what is ordered.
4. Set up the problem using ratio and proportion, the formula method, or dimensional analysis. Label each component in the setup, including "x."
5. Label the final answer (tablet, capsule).
6. For administration purposes, for oral dosages that are given in fractional dosages (e.g., scored tablets), state answers to problems in fractions. Example: $\frac{1}{2}$ tab or $1\frac{1}{2}$ tabs, instead of 0.5 tabs or 1.5 tabs.

Let's look at some sample problems calculating the number of tablets or capsules to administer.

**Example 1:** Order: Digoxin 0.375 mg p.o. daily

Available: Digoxin (scored tablets) labeled 0.25 mg

### ✓ PROBLEM SETUP

1. No conversion is necessary; the units are in the same system of measure.
   Order: 0.375 mg.
   Available: 0.25-mg tablets
2. Think critically: Tablets are scored; 0.375 mg is larger than 0.25 mg; therefore you will need more than 1 tab to administer the correct dosage.
3. Solve using ratio and proportion, the formula method, or dimensional analysis.

### ✓ Solution Using Ratio and Proportion

Linear Format: 0.25 mg : 1 tab = 0.375 mg : $x$ tab

(known)          (unknown)

(what is available)    (what is ordered)

$$\frac{0.25\,x}{0.25} = \frac{0.375}{0.25}$$

$$x = \frac{0.375}{0.25}$$

$$x = 1.5 = 1\,\tfrac{1}{2}\ \text{tabs}$$

Fraction Format:

$$\frac{0.25\ \text{mg}}{1\ \text{tab}} = \frac{0.375\ \text{mg}}{x\ \text{tab}}$$

$$\frac{0.25\,x}{0.25} = \frac{0.375}{0.25}$$

$$x = \frac{0.375}{0.25}$$

$$x = 1\,\tfrac{1}{2}\ \text{tabs}$$

(It is best to state it as $1\tfrac{1}{2}$ tabs for administration purposes.) You can administer $1\tfrac{1}{2}$ tabs because tablets are scored.

### ✓ Solution Using the Formula Method

$$\frac{\text{(D)}\ 0.375\ \text{mg}}{\text{(H)}\ 0.25\ \text{mg}} \times \text{(Q)}\ 1\ \text{tab} = x\ \text{tab}$$

$$x = \frac{0.375}{0.25}$$

$$x = 1\,\tfrac{1}{2}\ \text{tabs}$$

### ✓ Solution Using Dimensional Analysis

$$x\ \text{tab} = \frac{1\ \text{tab}}{0.25\ \cancel{\text{mg}}} \times \frac{0.375\ \cancel{\text{mg}}}{1}$$

$$x = \frac{0.375}{0.25}$$

$$x = 1\,\tfrac{1}{2}\ \text{tabs}$$

**Example 2:** Order: Flagyl 0.75 g p.o. t.i.d. for 7 days

Available: Flagyl capsules labeled 375 mg per capsule

1. Order: 0.75 g
   Available: 375 mg capsules
2. After making the necessary conversion, think about what is a reasonable amount to administer. (**Note:** Before calculating the dosage to be administered, the ordered dosage and the available dosage must be in the same unit of measure.)

3. Calculate the dosage to be administered using ratio and proportion, the formula method, or dimensional analysis.
4. Label your final answer (capsules).

## ✓ PROBLEM SETUP

1. A conversion is necessary. What the prescriber ordered is in grams and the medication is available in milligrams. Convert g to mg. Equivalent (conversion factor): 1 g = 1,000 mg; 0.75 g = 750 mg. Use any of the methods presented in Chapter 7 for converting. If necessary, review the methods.
   - Notice converting the grams to milligrams eliminated a decimal, which is often the source of calculation errors. Whenever possible, conversions that result in a decimal should be avoided to decrease the chance of error in calculating.
2. After making the conversion, you are now ready to calculate the dosage to be given, using ratio and proportion, the formula method, or dimensional analysis. In this problem we will use the answer obtained from converting what was ordered to what is available (0.75 g = 750 mg). Remember that if dimensional analysis is used, you need only one equation, even if conversion is required. For dimensional analysis, you need the equivalent (conversion factor) in fraction format: $\dfrac{1,000 \text{ mg}}{1 \text{ g}}$.

---

## ✓ Solution Using Ratio and Proportion

Linear Format: 375 mg : 1 cap = 750 mg : $x$ cap

$$\frac{375\,x}{375} = \frac{750}{375}$$

$$x = \frac{750}{375}$$

$$x = 2 \text{ caps}$$

Fraction Format:

$$\frac{375 \text{ mg}}{1 \text{ cap}} = \frac{750 \text{ mg}}{x \text{ cap}}$$

$$\frac{375\,x}{375} = \frac{750}{375}$$

$$x = \frac{750}{375}$$

$$x = 2 \text{ caps}$$

---

## ✓ Solution Using the Formula Method

$$\frac{\text{(D) } 750 \text{ mg}}{\text{(H) } 375 \text{ mg}} \times \text{(Q) } 1 \text{ cap} = x \text{ cap}$$

$$x = \frac{750}{375}$$

$$x = 2 \text{ caps}$$

### ✓ Solution Using Dimensional Analysis

$$x \text{ caps} = \frac{1 \text{ cap}}{375 \text{ mg}} \times \frac{1{,}000 \text{ mg}}{1 \text{ g}} \times \frac{0.75 \text{ g}}{1}$$

$$x = \frac{1{,}000 \times 0.75}{375}$$

$$x = \frac{750}{375}$$

$$x = 2 \text{ caps}$$

Below shows the problem setup in dimensional analysis to calculate the dosage after making conversion:

1. Convert g to mg:

$$x \text{ mg} = \frac{1{,}000 \text{ mg}}{1 \text{ g}} \times 0.75 \text{ g}$$

$$x = \frac{1{,}000 \times 0.75}{1}$$

$$x = \frac{750}{1}$$

$$x = 750 \text{ mg}$$

2. Set up in dimensional analysis after conversion made to calculate dosage:

$$x \text{ caps} = \frac{1 \text{ cap}}{375 \text{ mg}} \times \frac{750 \text{ mg}}{1}$$

$$x = \frac{750}{375}$$

$$x = 2 \text{ caps}$$

*Note:* It is easier to set up the problem in dimensional analysis using one equation that will allow you to convert and calculate the dosage required. This eliminates the need for multiple-step calculations.

**Example 3:** Order: Thorazine 100 mg p.o. t.i.d.
Available: Thorazine tablets labeled 25 mg and 50 mg

### ✓ PROBLEM SETUP

1. No conversion is necessary.
2. Think critically: 100 mg is larger than 25 or 50 mg. Therefore more than 1 tab is needed to administer the dosage. The client should always be given the strength of tablets or capsules that would require the least number to be taken.
3. In this problem, selection of the 50-mg tablets would require the client to receive 2 tabs, whereas using 25-mg tablets would require 4 tabs to be administered.

### ✓ Solution Using Ratio and Proportion

Linear Format: 50 mg : 1 tab = 100 mg : $x$ tab

$$\frac{50\,x}{50} = \frac{100}{50}$$

$$x = \frac{100}{50}$$

$$x = 2 \text{ tabs (50 mg each)}$$

Fraction Format:

$$\frac{50 \text{ mg}}{1 \text{ tab}} = \frac{100 \text{ mg}}{x \text{ tab}}$$

$$\frac{50\,x}{50} = \frac{100}{50}$$

$$x = 100$$

$$x = 2 \text{ tabs (50 mg each)}$$

*Note:* The number of tablets is specified as well as the strength of the tablets.

### ✓ Solution Using the Formula Method

$$\frac{\text{(D) } 100 \text{ mg}}{\text{(H) } 50 \text{ mg}} \times \text{(Q) } 1 \text{ tab} = x \text{ tab}$$

$$x = \frac{100}{50}$$

$$x = 2 \text{ tabs (50 mg each)}$$

### ✓ Solution Using Dimensional Analysis

$$x \text{ tab} = \frac{1 \text{ tab}}{50 \text{ mg}} \times \frac{100 \text{ mg}}{1}$$

$$x = \frac{100}{50}$$

$$x = 2 \text{ tabs (50 mg each)}$$

Example 3 could have been calculated without the use of ratio and proportion, dimensional analysis, or a formula. This is common when problems provide more than one dosage strength. In the case where a conversion is required, you would perform the conversion first, then choose the appropriate dosage strength to administer the least number of tablets or capsules. Add the dosage strengths chosen to ensure that it is equivalent to what is ordered.

## Variation of Tablet and Capsule Problems

You will at times find it necessary to decide how many tablets or capsules are needed. This requires knowing the dosage and frequency. Numerous scenarios could arise, but for the purpose of illustration, let's look at two examples. A client is going out of town on vacation and needs to know whether it is necessary to refill the prescription before leaving.

**Example 1:** A client has an order for Valium 10 mg p.o. q.i.d. and has 5-mg tablets. The client is leaving town for 7 days and asks how many tablets to bring.

**Solution:** To obtain a dosage of 10 mg, the client requires two 5-mg tablets each time. Therefore eight 5-mg tablets are necessary to administer the dosage q.i.d. (four times a day).

Number of tablets needed per day (8) × Number of days needed for (7)
= Total number of tablets needed

$$8 \times 7 = 56$$

Answer:       The total number of tablets needed for 7 days would be 56 tablets.

Example 2:    A client is instructed to take 30 mg of a medication stat as an initial dose and 20 mg tid thereafter. The tablets available are 10-mg tablets. What is the total number of tablets the client will need for 3 days?

Solution:     To obtain a dose of 30 mg, the client will require three 10-mg tablets for the stat dose, and six 10-mg tablets are needed to administer the dose t.i.d. (three times a day).
Number of tablets needed per day (6) × Number of days needed for (3)
= Total number of tablets needed.

$$6 \times 3 = 18 + 3 \text{ (stat dose)} = 21 \text{ tablets}$$

Answer:       The total number of tablets needed for 3 days is 21 tablets.

## Determining the Dosage to Be Given Each Time

Example:      A client is to receive 1 gram of a medication p.o. daily. The medication should be given in four equally divided doses.

How many milligrams should the client receive each time the medication is administered?

Solution:     $\dfrac{\text{Total daily allowance}}{\text{Number of doses per day}} = \text{Dosage to be administered}$

Answer:       $\dfrac{1 \text{ g } (1,000 \text{ mg})}{4} = 250$ mg each time the medication is administered.

### POINTS TO REMEMBER

- The maximum number of tablets and capsules to administer to achieve a single desired dosage is usually three. Question any order for more than this before administering.
- Before calculating a dosage, make sure that the dosage ordered and what is available are in the same system and units of measurement. When a conversion is required, it is usually best to convert the dosage ordered to what is available.
- No more than a 10% variation should exist between the dosage ordered and the dosage administered for adults. Remember, this should only occur when you are converting between apothecary and metric systems because of using approximate equivalents. When possible, always convert to a metric measure or use the metric measure indicated on a label.
- Regardless of the method used to calculate a dosage, it is important to develop the ability to think critically about what is a reasonable amount. Think and question any dosage that seems unreasonable.
- State dosages as you are actually going to administer them. Example: 0.5 tab = ½ tab.
- Tablets that are not scored should not be broken.
- It is safer to administer the least number of whole tablets possible without scoring.
- Read labels carefully and choose the correct medication to administer to match the order and dosage amount.
- When there is a choice of tablets or capsules in varying strengths, choose the strength that allows administration of the least number of tablets or capsules.
- Consult a medication reference or pharmacist when in doubt about a dosage to be administered and whether tablets can be crushed or capsules opened.

## 🔲 PRACTICE **PROBLEMS**

Calculate the correct number of tablets or capsules to be administered in the following problems using the labels or information provided. Use any of the methods presented to calculate the dosage. Remember to label your answers correctly: tabs, caps.

1. Order: Synthroid 0.025 mg p.o. every day.

   Available: Scored tablets

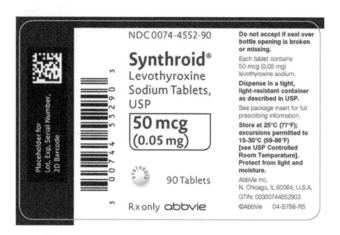

2. Order: Xeljanz 10 mg p.o. b.i.d.

   Available:

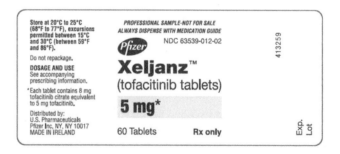

3. Order: Relafen 1 g p.o. daily.

   Available:

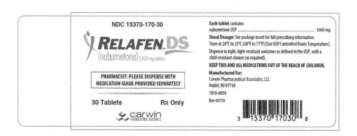

4. Order: Lanoxin 0.125 mg p.o. daily.

   Available: Scored tablets

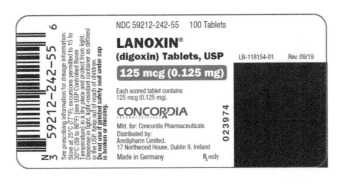

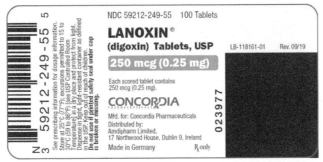

   a. What is the appropriate strength tablet to use?    _____

   b. What will you administer?    _____

5. Order: Ampicillin 1 g p.o. q6h.

   Available: Ampicillin capsules labeled 500 mg and 250 mg

   a. Which strength capsule is appropriate
      to use?    _____

   b. How many capsules are needed for one
      dosage?    _____

   c. What is the total number of capsules needed
      if the medication is ordered for 7 days?    _____

6. Order: Fluconazole 150 mg p.o. daily for 2 weeks.

   Available:

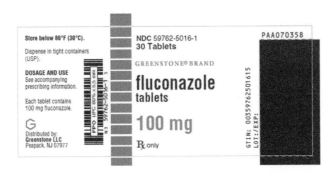

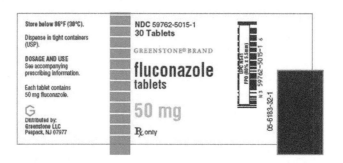

What is the appropriate strength tablet to use? _____

7. Order: Bosulif 0.4 g p.o. daily.

Available:

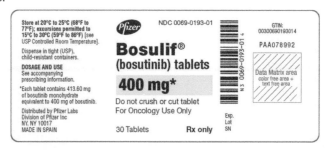

8. Order: Brilinta 180 mg p.o. stat for the initial dose.

Available:

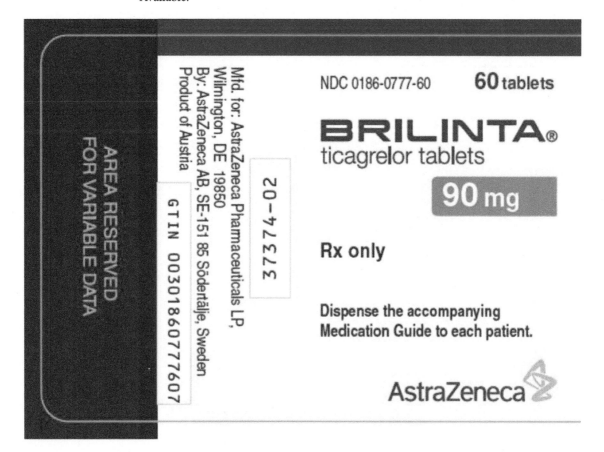

9. Order: Vraylar 3 mg p.o. daily.

   Available:

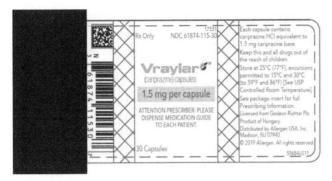

_____

10. Order: Rexulti 2 mg p.o. daily for 3 days for a client with schizophrenia.

    Available:

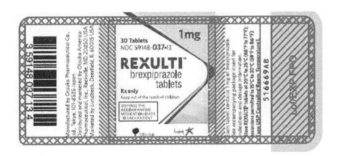

_____

11. Order: Phenobarbital 90 mg p.o. at bedtime.

    Available: Phenobarbital 15-mg tabs and
    30-mg tabs

    a. Which strength tablet is best to administer?    _____

    b. How many tablets of which strength will
       you prepare to administer?    _____

12.  Order: Ziagen 0.6 g p.o. daily.

Available:

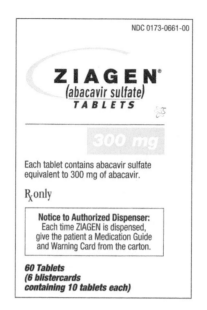

13.  Order: Chlorpromazine Hydrochloride 100 mg p.o. t.i.d.

Available:

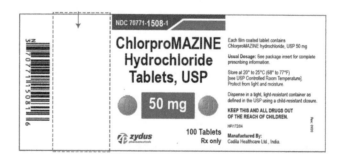

How many tablets are needed for 3 days?

14.  Order: Verapamil 120 mg p.o. t.i.d. Hold for systolic blood pressure less than 100, heart rate less than 55.

Available:

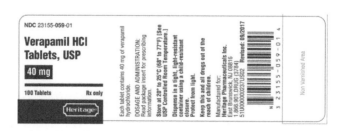

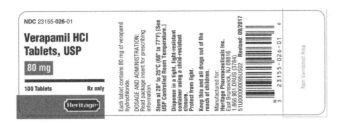

How many tablets of which strength will
you administer?    _____

15. Order: OxyContin (extended release) 20 mg p.o. q12h for pain management.

Available:

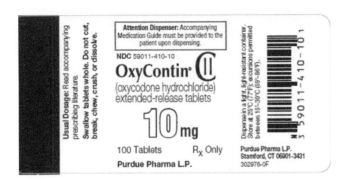

_____

16. Order: Depakote ER 1 g p.o. daily.

Available:

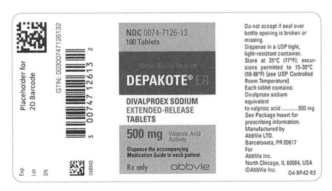

_____

17. Order: Pyridium 0.2 g p.o. t.i.d. after meals.

Available:

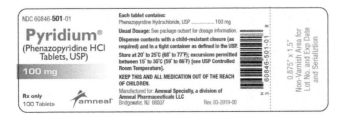

_____

18. Order: Tecfidera DR 240 mg p.o. b.i.d. for a client with multiple sclerosis.

Available:

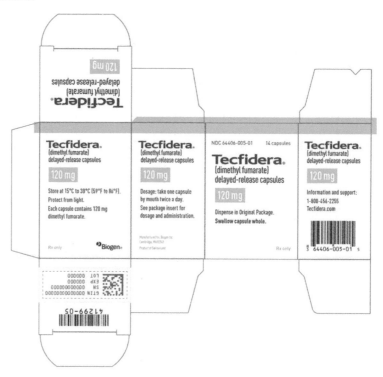

19. Order: Cimetidine 400 mg p.o. b.i.d.

Available:

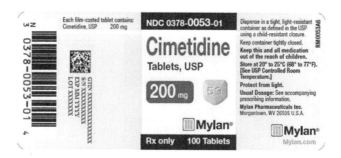

20. Order: Entresto 49/51 mg p.o. b.i.d. as a starting dose for a client with chronic heart failure.

Available:

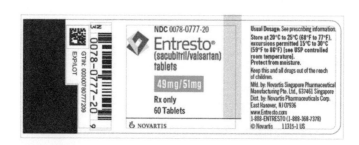

a. How many tablets should the client receive?          _____

b. According to the medication label, Entresto contains
how many medications?          _____

c. Entresto contains _____ mg of sacubitril and _____ mg of valsartan.

21. Order: Cymbalta (delayed-release capsules) 60 mg p.o. daily.

Available:

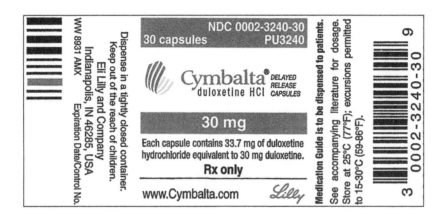

_____

22. Order: Synthroid 75 mcg p.o. daily.

Available: Scored tablets

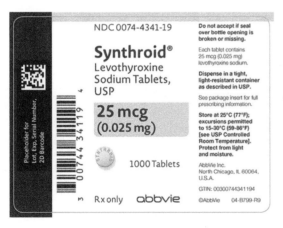
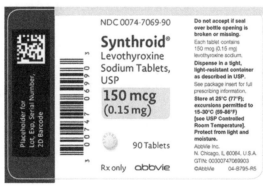

How many tablets of which strength will you
use to administer the dosage?          _____

23. Order: Captopril 25 mg p.o. t.i.d.

    Available:

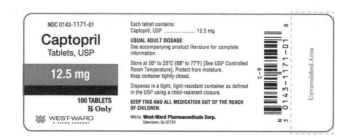

24. Order: Clonazepam 1 mg p.o. b.i.d. and at bedtime.

    Available: Scored tablets

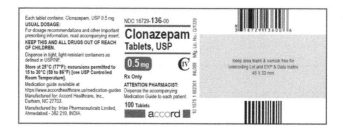

25. Order: Rubraca 500 mg p.o. daily.

    Available:

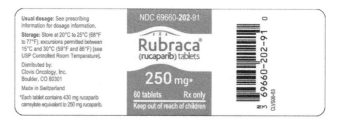

26. Order: Procardia XL 60 mg p.o. daily.

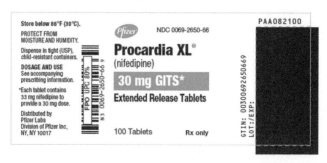

27.  Order: Calcitriol 0.5 mcg p.o. daily.

Available:

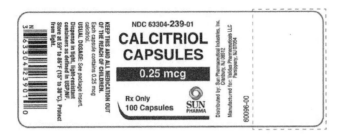

28.  Order: Coreg 6.25 mg p.o. b.i.d. for 2 weeks.

Available:

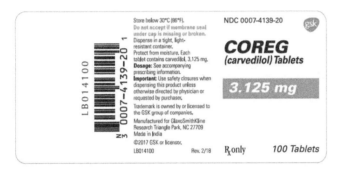

Answers on pp. 326-328

## Calculating Oral Liquids

Enteral medications are also available in liquid form for administration orally or through various types of tubes placed into the stomach or intestines. Examples: nasogastric (tube that is introduced through the nose into the stomach), gastrostomy (tube directly into the stomach), or jejunostomy (tube directly into the jejunum [second part of small intestines]). Liquid medications are also desirable for use in:

- Clients who have dysphagia (difficulty swallowing)
- Young children, infants, and elderly clients
- Instances when medications that cannot be crushed for administration are ordered; then the availability of the medication in liquid form should be investigated.

Liquid medications are prepared in different forms. The most common forms are elixirs, suspensions, and syrups.

1. **Elixir:** The medication is mixed with water, alcohol, and a sweetener, and is aromatic. Example: Phenobarbital elixir.
2. **Suspension**: One or more medications in fine particles in a liquid such as water. The particles cannot be dissolved therefore the suspension must be shaken well before administering for thorough mixing of the particles. Example: Penicillin suspension.
3. **Syrup:** The medication is dissolved in a concentrated sugar (usually sucrose) and water. Example: Colace.

Liquid medications also come as tinctures, emulsions, and extract preparations for oral use. There are also medications for oral use that are available in powder form and must be mixed prior to administering them to a client. The process of mixing the powder with a liquid so that it can be administered is called **reconstitution**. The nurse may reconstitute the medication by following the directions on the medication label or package insert. The process of reconstitution will be discussed in detail in Chapter 18. Although oral liquids may be

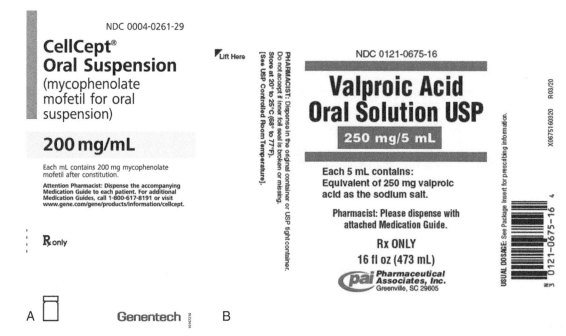

**Figure 16.6** (A) CellCept oral suspension 200 mg per mL. (B) Valproic acid oral solution 250 mg per 5 mL.

administered by means other than by mouth (e.g., nasogastric tube, gastrostomy tube), they should **never** be given by any other route, such as the intravenous (IV) route or by injection.

The labels on medications in liquid form indicate the specific amount or weight of a medication in a given amount of solution. You must calculate the volume or amount of liquid that contains the ordered dosage. The methods presented in Chapters 13 to 15 can be used to calculate the volume or amount to administer the ordered dosage. There are some oral liquid medications that do not require calculation because, when ordered, the specific amount to be administered is stated. Examples: Milk of Magnesia 1 ounce p.o. at bedtime; Robitussin 15 mL p.o. q4h prn; Fer-in-Sol 0.2 mL p.o. daily.

The medication label on oral liquids may indicate the amount of medication per milliliter, ounce, etc. For example, 25 mg per mL, 200 mg per mL (Figure 16.6A). The amount may also be expressed in terms of multiple milliliters of solution, such as 80 mg per 2 mL, 250 mg per 5 mL (Figure 16.6B).

Oral liquids can be measured in small amounts of volume, and a greater range of dosages can be ordered for administration. When you calculate oral liquid medications, the stock, or what you have available, is in liquid form; therefore the label (unit) on your answer will always be expressed in liquid measures such as milliliters.

Like other forms of medications, dosing errors can occur with oral liquids. The reason for dosing errors include inaccurate measurement of oral liquids and the use of improper measuring devices, and non-calibrated devices. The use of calibrated measuring devices (e.g., droppers, calibrated spoons) should be used in the hospital and clients educated on the importance of this at home as opposed to using household measuring devices (e.g., spoons). Household measuring devices vary in size and are inaccurate and may deliver more or less medication than ordered. Clients should be encouraged to use the measuring device that comes with their medication if one does, or ask the pharmacist about an appropriate measuring device.

## Measuring Oral Liquids

The administration of oral liquids requires careful measurement. There can be a greater range of dosages ordered and administered with oral liquids. Several types of equipment are used to administer oral liquid medications. These include medicine cups, droppers, oral syringes, and calibrated spoons.

1. **The standard medicine cup** is usually plastic, has a capacity of 30 milliliters (1 fluid ounce), and is used to measure most liquid medications for oral administration. Most

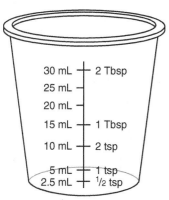

Figure 16.7 Medicine cup.

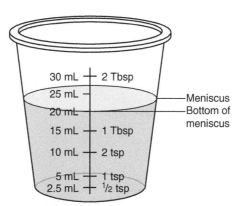

Figure 16.8 Reading meniscus. The meniscus is caused by the surface tension of the solution against the walls of the container. The surface tension causes the formation of a concave or hollowed curvature on the surface of the solution. Read the level at the lowest point of the concave.

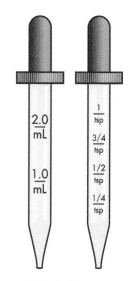

Figure 16.9 Medicine droppers.

medication cups typically indicate metric, household, and apothecary systems of measurement on the cup. Therefore cups include units such as tablespoons (tbs), teaspoons (tsp), milliliters (mL), drams (dr), and ounces (oz).

**Note:** Dram (dr), a unit of measurement in the apothecary system, and cubic centimeter (cc), formerly used interchangeably with milliliters (mL) may still appear on medicine cups in some health care facilities. These units of measurement are no longer used.

Because of the reporting of errors that occurred from nurses confusing dosing scales on a plastic oral liquid dosing cup, a recommendation that was set forth was to move toward medicine cups that allow measurement in milliliters only. Figure 16.7 shows one view of a medication cup.

When measuring liquid medications, place the medication cup on a flat surface, poured at eye level, and read at the bottom of the meniscus (a curvature made by the solution). See Figure 16.8. Always pour liquid medications with the label facing you to avoid covering the label with your hand or obscuring label information if the medication drips down the side of the container.

> **⚠ SAFETY ALERT!**
> To prevent medication errors, take care and do not confuse the dosing scales on a medication cup when pouring medications.

2. **Calibrated droppers** are used for measuring and administering small volumes of liquid medications (Figure 16.9). They may be used to administer certain liquid medications to the eyes, ears, and nose. Another common use is for administration of oral medications especially to children. Droppers have different sized openings that produce different amounts of medication with each drop. Some medications come with a dropper that indicates the dropper is calibrated for the specified dose and can only be used for the medication it is packaged with, to ensure accurate dosing. Some medicine droppers are calibrated in milliliters, drops, teaspoons, or by actual dosage. Clients who are being discharged and taking oral medications at home should **always** be instructed to use only the dropper that comes packaged with the particular medication.

> **⚠ SAFETY ALERT!**
> To avoid medication dosing errors, a **calibrated** dropper should be used **ONLY** for the medication **for which it is intended; droppers are not interchangeable** and drop size varies from one dropper to another.

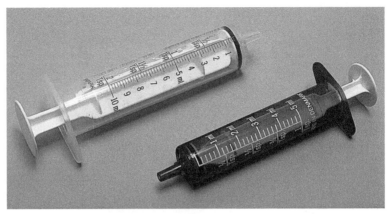

**Figure 16.10** Oral syringes. (Courtesy Chuck Dresner. From Clayton BD, Gurevitz SL, Willihnganz M: *Basic pharmacology for nurses,* ed 18, St Louis, 2020, Elsevier.)

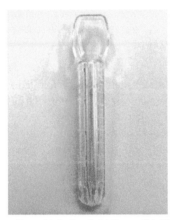

**Figure 16.11** Calibrated spoons. (From Mulholland JM, Turner SJ: *The nurse, the math, the meds: drug calculations using dimensional analysis,* ed 4, St Louis, 2019, Elsevier.)

3. **Oral syringes:** Solutions for oral use should be measured by using a specially calibrated oral syringe (Figure 16.10). Oral syringes are calibrated in tenths of a milliliter and may have teaspoon and tablespoon markings and are used to measure and administer oral liquids to ensure accurate and safe dosages. They come in 1 mL, 3 mL, 5 mL, and 10 mL sizes. Syringes for oral use have unique features that distinguish them from syringes used for injections which include:
   • They are needleless
   • Often come in colors, and are not sterile
   • Some are labeled on the barrel of the syringe, "for oral use only"
   • An eccentric or off-center tip alerts the nurse that a needle should not be attached to this syringe
   • The tip of the oral syringe does not fit adapters and devices made for injectable syringes, such as IV tubing. This prevents medication for oral use from being injected IV or into tissue, which can cause injury or death.

> **(!) SAFETY ALERT!**
> To prevent confusion with the route of administration, **only** use oral syringes to measure and administer oral medications. Oral medications are **never** injected.

4. **Calibrated spoons** are designed with a spoon and a shape for easy administration. They are often used to administer oral liquids to children or elderly clients. Some spoons for children are shaped like animals. They are calibrated in milliliters and equivalent household measures (e.g., teaspoons, tablespoons) (Figure 16.11). Household spoons vary in size and are not reliable for accurate dosing. Always encourage the use of calibrated spoons for measuring medications at home.

Before we proceed to calculate liquid medications, let's review some helpful pointers.
1. The label on the medication container must be read carefully to determine the dosage strength in the volume of solution because it varies.

> **SAFETY ALERT!**
> Do not confuse dosage strength with total volume. Read labels carefully. Confusing dosage strength with total volume can result in errors when performing calculations and lead to the administration of an unintended dose.

For example, the label on a medication may indicate a total volume of 100 mL, but the dosage strength may be 125 mg per 5 mL. It must be noted that dosage strength can be written on solutions in several ways to indicate the same thing. For example, 125 mg per 5 mL may be written as 125 mg/5 mL or 125 mg = 5 mL. Other examples of dosage strength are 20 mg per mL, 20 mg/mL, or 20 mg = 1 mL. It should also be noted that many solutions are also expressing dosage strengths on the label using "per" instead of the slash mark.

> **SAFETY ALERT!**
> The Institute for Safe Medication Practices (ISMP) (https://www.ismp.org/recommendations/error-prone-abbreviations-list) recommends that the "/" (slash mark) not be used to separate doses. The slash mark has been mistaken as the number 1. Use "per" rather than a slash mark to separate doses.

2. Answers are labeled using liquid measures. Example: mL.
3. Calculations can be done by using the same methods (ratio and proportion, the formula method, or dimensional analysis) and the same steps as for solid forms of oral medications.

Now let's look at some sample problems that involve the calculation of oral liquids.

**Example 1:**  Order: Dilantin 200 mg p.o. t.i.d.

Available: Dilantin suspension labeled 125 mg per 5 mL

## ✅ PROBLEM SETUP

1. No conversion is required. Everything is in the same units of measure and the same system.
Order: 200 mg
Available: 125 mg per 5 mL
2. Think critically: What would be a logical answer? Looking at Example 1, you can assume the answer will be greater than 5 mL.
3. Set up the problem using ratio and proportion, the formula method, or dimensional analysis.
4. Label the final answer with the correct unit of measure. In this case the units will be milliliters. Remember: The answer has no meaning if written without the appropriate unit of measure.

---

### ✓ Solution Using Ratio and Proportion

Known          Unknown

Linear Format: 125 mg : 5 mL = 200 mg : $x$ mL

$$125x = 200 \times 5$$

$$\frac{125\,x}{125} = \frac{1{,}000}{125}$$

$$x = \frac{1{,}000}{125}$$

$$x = 8 \text{ mL}$$

Fraction Format:

$$
\begin{array}{cc}
\text{Known} & \text{Unknown} \\
\dfrac{125 \text{ mg}}{5 \text{ mL}} = \dfrac{200 \text{ mg}}{x \text{ mL}}
\end{array}
$$

$$125x = 200 \times 5$$

$$x = \frac{1,000}{125}$$

$$x = 8 \text{ mL}$$

*Note:* Reduction of numbers can be done to make them smaller and easier to deal with.

---

### ✓ Solution Using the Formula Method

$$\frac{\text{(D) } 200 \text{ mg}}{\text{(H) } 125 \text{ mg}} \times \text{(Q) } 5 \text{ mL} = x \text{ mL}$$

$$x = \frac{200}{125} \times 5$$

$$x = \frac{1,000}{125}$$

$$x = 8 \text{ mL}$$

---

### ✓ Solution Using Dimensional Analysis

$$x \text{ mL} = \frac{5 \text{ mL}}{125 \text{ mg}} \times \frac{200 \text{ mg}}{1}$$

$$x = \frac{1,000}{125}$$

$$x = 8 \text{ mL}$$

**Example 2:** Order: Lactulose 30 g p.o. b.i.d.

Available: Lactulose labeled 10 g per 15 mL

---

### ✓ Solution Using Ratio and Proportion

$$
\begin{array}{cc}
\text{Known} & \text{Unknown}
\end{array}
$$

Linear Format: $10 \text{ g} : 15 \text{ mL} = 30 \text{ g} : x \text{ mL}$

$$10x = 30 \times 15$$

$$\frac{10\,x}{10} = \frac{450}{10}$$

$$x = \frac{450}{10}$$

$$x = 45 \text{ mL}$$

Fraction Format:

$$\text{Known} \qquad \text{Unknown}$$

$$\frac{10\text{ g}}{15\text{ mL}} = \frac{30\text{ g}}{x\text{ mL}}$$

$$10x = 30 \times 15$$

$$\frac{10\,x}{10} = \frac{450}{10}$$

$$x = 45\text{ mL}$$

---

## ✓ Solution Using the Formula Method

$$\frac{(D)\ 30\text{ g}}{(H)\ 10\text{ g}} \times (Q)\ 15\text{ mL} = x\text{ mL}$$

$$x = \frac{300 \times 5}{125}$$

$$x = \frac{450}{10}$$

$$x = 45\text{ mL}$$

---

## ✓ Solution Using Dimensional Analysis

$$x\text{ mL} = \frac{15\text{ mL}}{10\ \cancel{g}} \times \frac{30\ \cancel{g}}{1}$$

$$x = \frac{450}{10}$$

$$x = 45\text{ mL}$$

Example 3: Order: Cefdinir 0.3 g p.o. q 12 h.

Available: Cefdinir oral suspension labeled 125 mg per 5 mL

1. A conversion is necessary. What the prescriber ordered is in grams here, and the medication is available in milligrams.
   - Convert grams to milligrams.
   - Equivalent (conversion factor)
     1,000 mg = 1 g
   - Use any of the methods presented for converting
     0.3 g = 300 mg

---

## ✓ Solution Using Ratio and Proportion

$$\text{Known} \qquad \text{Unknown}$$

Linear Format: 125 mg : 5 mL = 300 mg : $x$ mL

$$125x = 300 \times 5$$

$$\frac{125x}{125} = \frac{1,500}{125}$$

$$x = \frac{1,500}{125}$$

$$x = 12\text{ mL}$$

Fraction Format:

$$
\begin{array}{cc}
\text{Known} & \text{Unknown} \\
\dfrac{125 \text{ mg}}{5 \text{ mL}} & = \dfrac{300 \text{ mg}}{x \text{ mL}}
\end{array}
$$

$$125x = 300 \times 5$$

$$x = \frac{1,500}{125}$$

$$x = 12 \text{ mL}$$

## ✓ Solution Using the Formula Method

$$\frac{\text{(D) } 300 \text{ mg}}{\text{(H) } 125 \text{ mg}} \times \text{(Q) } 5 \text{ mL} = x \text{ mL}$$

$$x = \frac{300 \times 5}{125}$$

$$x = \frac{1,500}{125}$$

$$x = 12 \text{ mL}$$

## ✓ Solution Using Dimensional Analysis

$$x \text{ mL} = \frac{5 \text{ mL}}{125 \text{ mg}} \times \frac{1,000 \text{ mg}}{1 \text{ g}} \times \frac{0.3 \text{ g}}{1}$$

$$x = \frac{5,000 \times 0.3}{125}$$

$$x = \frac{1,500}{125}$$

$$x = 12 \text{ mL}$$

### POINTS TO REMEMBER

- Liquid medications can be calculated using the same methods as those used for solid forms (tabs, caps).
- Read labels carefully on medications; identify the dosage strength of the medication contained in a certain amount (volume) of solution.
- Do not confuse dosage strength (amount of medication contained in a certain amount of solution) with total volume (the amount in the container).
- Administration of accurate dosages of liquid medications requires the use of calibrated devices (calibrated droppers, calibrated spoons, and oral syringes).
- Oral syringes are designed for oral use only. Use oral syringes to measure and administer oral liquids.
- When using a medication cup to administer oral liquid medications, pour the medication at eye level and read at eye level at bottom of meniscus on a flat surface.
- The use of ratio and proportion, the formula method, or dimensional analysis is a means of validating an answer; however, it still requires thinking in terms of the dosage you will administer and applying principles learned to calculate dosages that are sensible and safe.
- Use "per" to separate dosages when writing, not a slash mark. Example: 125 mg per 5 mL, not 125 mg/5 mL.
- Do not use the dropper packaged with a particular medication to administer other medications.

## ▦ PRACTICE **PROBLEMS**

Calculate the following dosages for oral liquids in milliliters using the labels or information provided. Do not forget to label your answer. Round answers to the nearest tenth where indicated.

29. Order: Lyrica 75 mg p.o. b.i.d.

    Available:

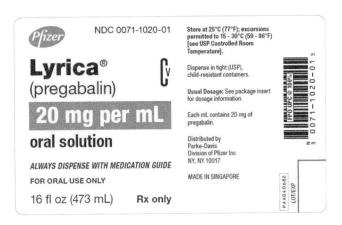

30. Order: Prednisolone sodium phosphate 40 mg p.o. daily.

    Available:

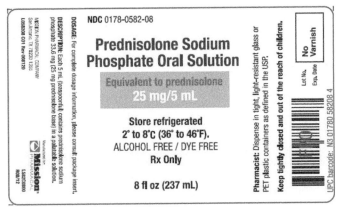

31. Order: Potassium chloride 20 mEq p.o. b.i.d.

    Available:

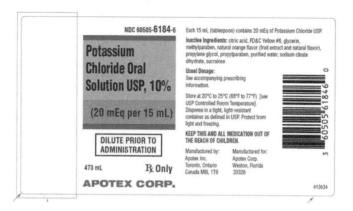

32. Order: Calcitriol 2 mcg p.o. daily.

    Available:

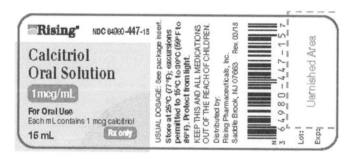

33. Order: Clemastine fumarate syrup 2 mg p.o. q12h.

    Available:

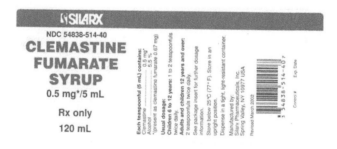

34. Order: Dilantin 100 mg p.o. t.i.d.

    Available:

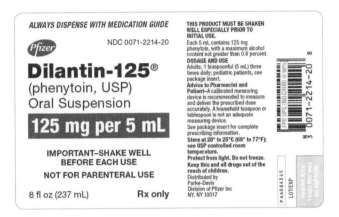

35. Order: Digoxin 125 mcg p.o. every day.

    Available:

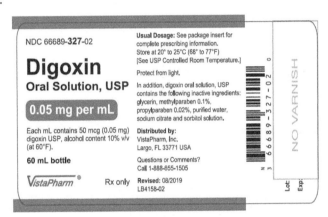

36. Order: Amoxicillin 0.5 g p.o. q6h.

    Available: *Reconstituted medication

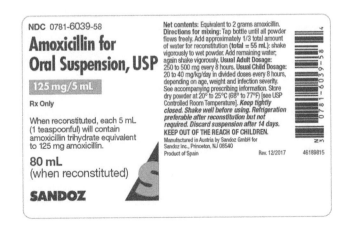

37. Order: Phenobarbital 60 mg p.o. at bedtime.

Available:

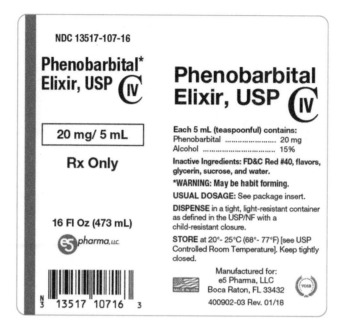

38. Order: Lithium carbonate 600 mg p.o. t.i.d.

Available:

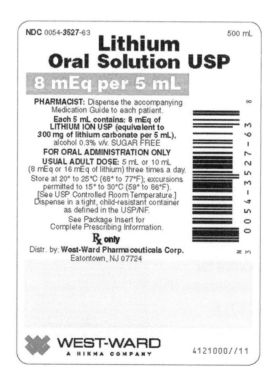

39. Order: Erythromycin ethylsuccinate 0.5 g by gastrostomy tube q6h for 10 days.

    Available: *Reconstituted medication

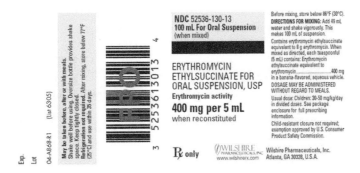

40. Order: Sulfamethoxazole/trimethroprim 200 mg/40 mg 160 mg p.o. q12h for 10 days (calculation based on trimethroprim).

    Available: *Reconstituted medication

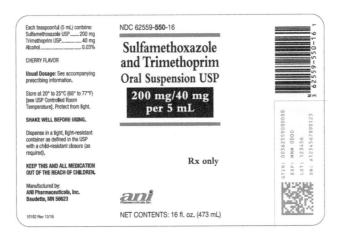

41. Order: Tamiflu 75 mg p.o. b.i.d. for 5 days.

    Available: *Reconstituted medication

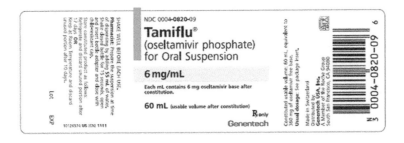

42. Order: Neurontin 0.3 g p.o. t.i.d.

Available:

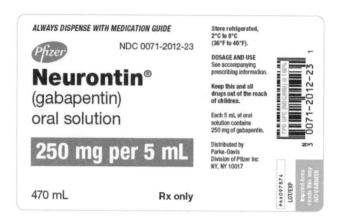

43. Order: Ondansetron 8 mg q12h for 2 days.

Available:

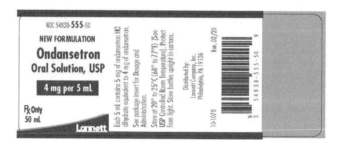

44. Order: Amoxicillin and Clavulanate Potassium 0.25 g p.o. q8h (ordered according to the dose of amoxicillin).

Available: *Reconstituted medication

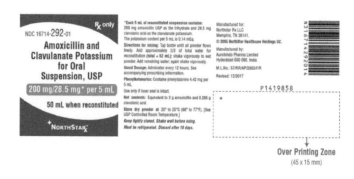

45. Order: Zovirax 200 mg p.o. q4h for 5 days.

    Available:

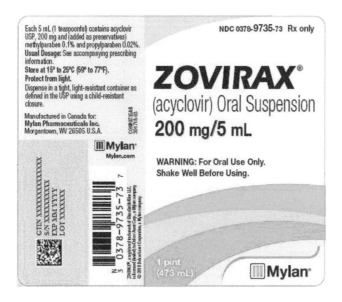

_____

46. Order: Fluoxetine 30 mg p.o. every day in AM.

    Available:

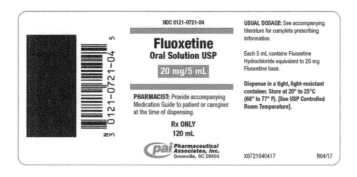

_____

47. Order: Promethazine 12.5 mg p.o. t.i.d.

    Available:

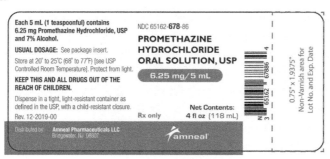

_____

48. Order: Oxycodone Hydrochloride 30 mg p.o. q12h p.r.n. for pain.

    Available:

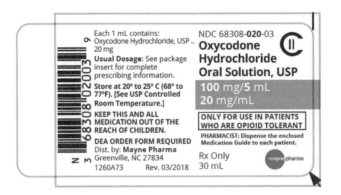

**Answers on pp. 328-330**

## ⚕ CLINICAL **REASONING**

1. **Scenario:** Order: Digoxin 0.75 mg p.o. daily. In preparing to administer medications, you find 0.125-mg tabs (scored) in the medication drawer for the client.
   a. Based on the tablets available, how many would you have to administer? _____
   b. What action should you take? _____
   c. What is the rationale for your action? _____

2. **Scenario:** Order: Diflucan 150 mg p.o. daily. The pharmacy sends two 100-mg un-scored tabs.
   a. What action should you take to administer the dosage ordered? _____
   b. What is the rationale for your action? _____

3. **Scenario:** Order: Percocet 2 tabs p.o. q4h p.r.n. for pain for a client who is allergic to aspirin. The nurse administers Percodan 2 tabs.

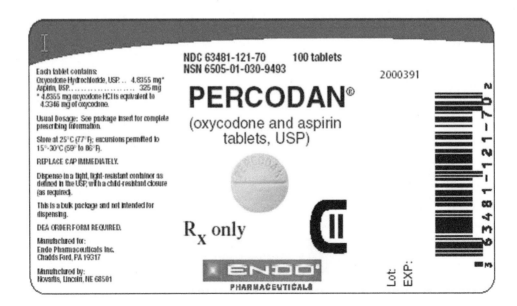

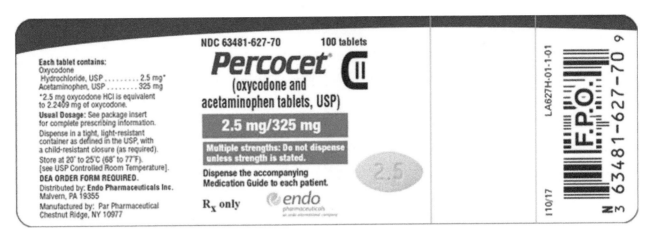

a. What client right was violated? _____

b. What contributed to the error? _____

c. What is the potential outcome of the error? _____

d. What preventive measures could have been taken to prevent the error? _____

**Answers on p. 331**

---

## ⊙ CHAPTER **REVIEW**

Calculate the following dosages using the medication label or information provided. Express volume answers in milliliters; round answers to the nearest tenth as indicated. Remember to label answers: tab, caps, mL.

1. Order: Neurontin 0.6 g p.o. t.i.d.

   Available:

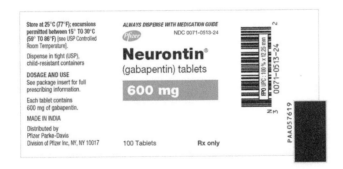

2. Order: Vraylar 4.5 mg p.o. daily.

   Available:

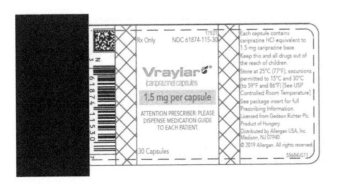

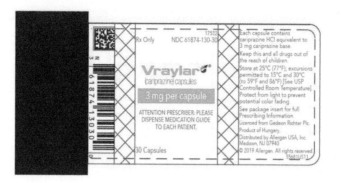

How many capsules of which strength will you administer?

_____

3. Order: Bosulif 0.5 g p.o. daily.

Available:

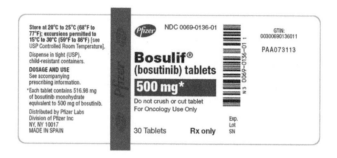

_____

4. Order: Carvedilol 25 mg p.o. b.i.d.

Available:

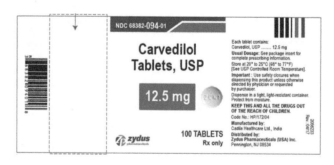

_____

5. Order: Penicillin V Potassium 0.5 g p.o. q6h.

   Available: *Reconstituted medication

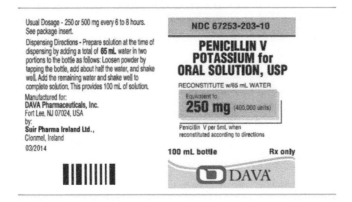

_____

6. Order: Dexamethasone 0.75 mg p.o. daily.

   Available:

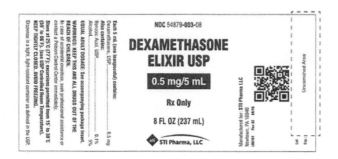

_____

7. Order: Cialis 10 mg p.o. 1 hr before sexual activity for a client with erectile dysfunction.

   Available:

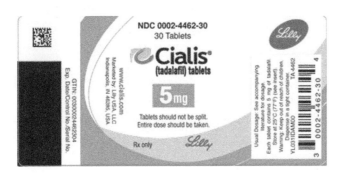

_____

8. Order: Ativan 1 mg p.o. q4h p.r.n. for agitation.

   Available:

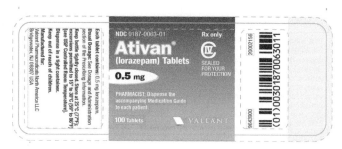

_____

9. Refer to the label for Mavyret to answer the questions.

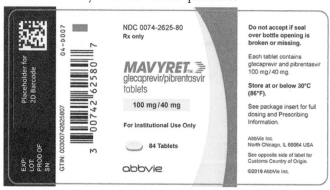

   a. Mavyret is a fixed-dose combination medication that contains _____ mg of glecaprevir and _____ mg of pibrentasvir in each tablet.

   b. If the recommended total daily dosage is 300 mg of glecaprevir and 120 mg of pibrentasvir, how many tablets will the client need to take for the daily dosage?

   _____

10. Order: Aldactone 100 mg p.o. daily.

    Available:

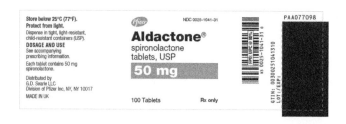

_____

11. Order: Digoxin 0.1 mg p.o. daily.

    Available:

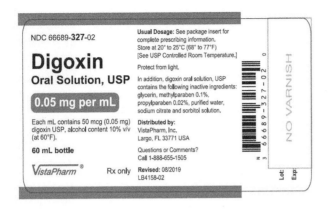

12. Order: Ziagen 0.3 g p.o. b.i.d.

    Available:

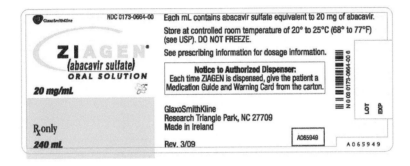

13. Order: Theophylline extended-release 0.6 g p.o. daily.

    Available:

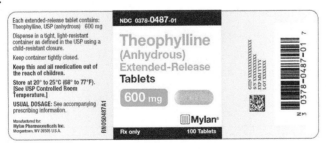

14. Order: Xanax 0.75 mg p.o. t.i.d.

Available:

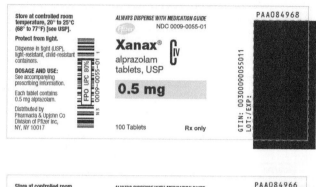

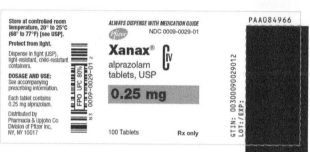

How many tablets of which strength will you administer?

_____

15. Order: Erythromycin (delayed-release) 0.5 g p.o. q12h.

Available:

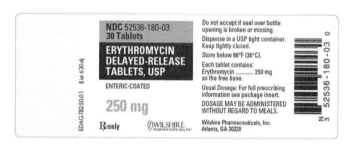

_____

16. Order: Ibrance 125 mg p.o. daily for 21 days.

Available:

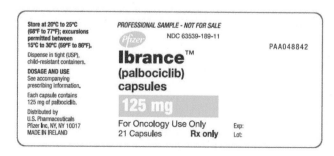

_____

17. Order: Metformin (extended-release) 1 g p.o. daily.

    Available:

    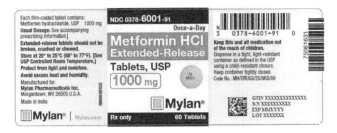

    _____

18. Order: Clozapine 50 mg p.o. daily.

    Available:

    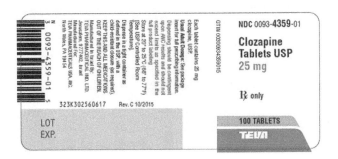

    a.  How many tabs will you administer for
        each dosage?                          _____

    b.  How many tabs will be needed for 7 days?   _____

19. Order: Lipitor 30 mg p.o. daily.

    Available:

    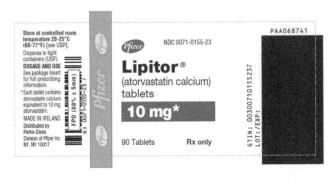

    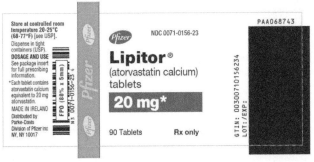

    What will you administer to the client?   _____

20. Order: Eliquis 10 mg p.o. b.i.d. for 7 days.

    Available:

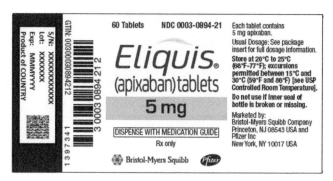

    a. How many tablets will you administer per dose?  _____

    b. How many tablets are needed for 7 days?  _____

21. Order: Prednisolone 25 mg p.o. daily.

    Available:

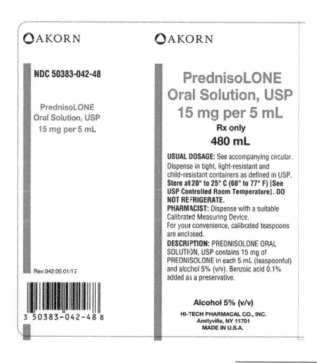

22. Order: Ondansetron 24 mg p.o. 30 minutes before start of chemotherapy.

    Available:

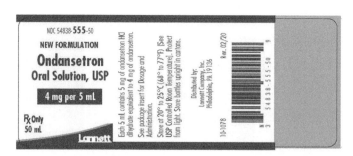

23. Order: Latuda 60 mg p.o. daily.

    Available:

    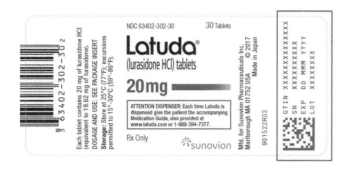

    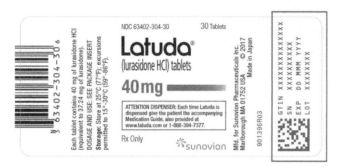

    How many tablets of which strength will you
    administer? _____

24. Order: Lasix 40 mg p.o. daily.

    Available:

    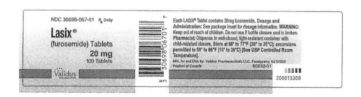

    _____

25. Order: Strattera 0.1 g p.o. daily.

    Available:

    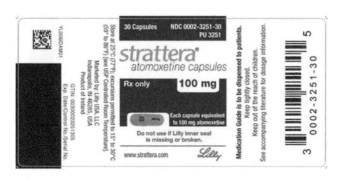

    _____

26. Order: Inderal LA 120 mg p.o. daily.

    Available:

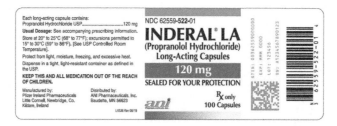

27. Order: Suboxone 16 mg/4 mg sublingual daily.

    Available:

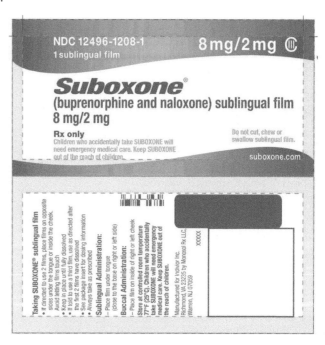

28. Order: Amoxicillin and clavulanate 0.5 g by gastrostomy tube q8h (ordered according to the dose of amoxicillin).

    Available: *Reconstituted medication

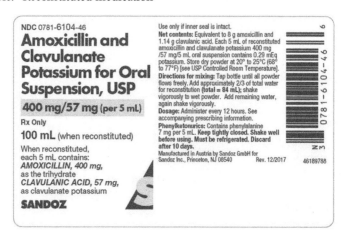

29. Order: Zyprexa 15 mg p.o. daily.

Available:

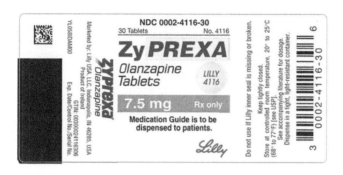

_____

30. Order: Entresto 97/103 p.o. b.i.d.

Available:

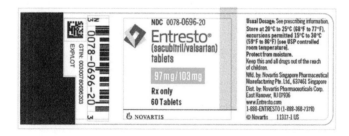

_____

31. Order: Zoloft 175 mg p.o. daily.

Available:

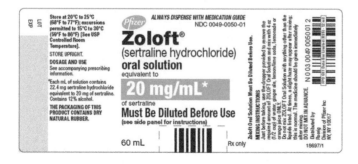

a. How much, and what liquids can this medication
   be mixed with? _____

b. How long after mixing the medication should
   it be administered? _____

c. How many mL will you administer? _____

32. Order: Cytotec 200 mcg p.o. q.i.d.

Available:

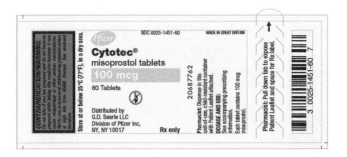

33. Order: Trileptal 0.6 g p.o. b.i.d.

Available:

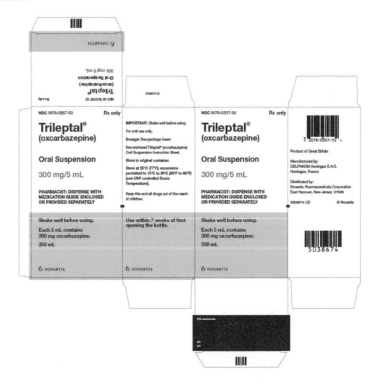

34. Order: Terbutaline 5 mg p.o. q8h.

Available:

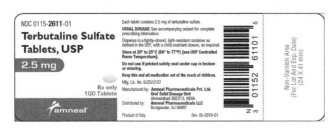

35. Order: Epclusa 400 mg/100 mg p.o. daily.

    Available:

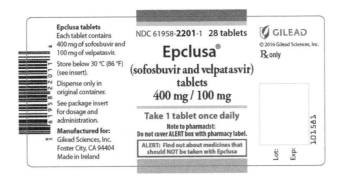

36. Refer to the label for Biktarvy to answer the questions:

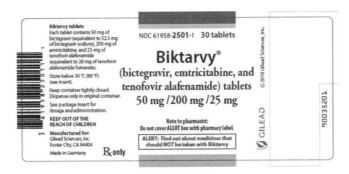

    a. What alert is indicated on the medication?      _____

    b. Biktarvy is a fixed-dose combination medication that contains    _____
       medications. What are the medications contained in Biktarvy per tablet?

    c. Indicate the dosage strength for each medication.     _____

**Answers on p. 331**

Answers on p. 331

For additional practice problems, refer to the Oral Dosages section of the Elsevier's Interactive Drug Calculation Application, Version 1, on Evolve.

# ⭐ ANSWERS

## Chapter 16
### Answers to Practice Problems

The answers to the practice problems include the rationale for the answer where indicated. Where necessary, the methods for calculation of the dosage are shown as well. Although not shown, dimensional analysis can also be used. If necessary, review setup in this chapter and in Chapter 15. Ratio and proportion could also be set up in fraction format; review Chapter 13 if necessary.

> **NOTE**
> Unless stated, no conversion is required to calculate dosage. In problems that required a conversion before calculating the dosage, the problem setup shown illustrates the problem after appropriate conversions have been made.

1. $0.025 \text{ mg} = 25 \text{ mcg} (1,000 \text{ mcg} = 1 \text{ mg})$

   $50 \text{ mcg} : 1 \text{ tab} = 25 \text{ mcg} : x \text{ tab}$

   *or*

   $\dfrac{25 \text{ mcg}}{50 \text{ mcg}} \times 1 \text{ tab} = x \text{ tab}$

   Answer: $\dfrac{1}{2}$ tab. This is an acceptable answer, because the tabs are scored. (For administration purposes, state as $\dfrac{1}{2}$ tab.) Note that the problem could have been done without converting by using the dosage indicated on the label in mg. This would net the same answer.

   *or*

   $0.05 \text{ mg} : 1 \text{ tab} = 0.025 \text{ mg} : x \text{ tab}$

   $\dfrac{0.025 \text{ mg}}{0.05 \text{ mg}} \times 1 \text{ tab} = x \text{ tab}$

2. $5 \text{ mg} : 1 \text{ tab} = 10 \text{ mg} : x \text{ tab}$

   *or*

   $\dfrac{10 \text{ mg}}{5 \text{ mg}} \times 1 \text{ tab} = x \text{ tab}$

   Answer: 2 tabs. The dosage ordered is greater than what is available; therefore you will need more than 1 tab to administer the dosage.

3. Conversion is required. Equivalent: $1,000 \text{ mg} = 1 \text{ g}$. Therefore $1 \text{ g} = 1,000 \text{ mg}$.

   $1,000 \text{ mg} : 1 \text{ tab} = 1,000 \text{ mg} : x \text{ tab}$

   *or*

   $\dfrac{1,000 \text{ mg}}{1,000 \text{ mg}} \times 1 \text{ tab} = x \text{ tab}$

   Answer: 1 tab (DS). The dosage ordered is equivalent to the dosage available. 1 tab is equal to 1,000 mg,

which is equivalent to 1 g; therefore only 1 tab is needed to administer the dosage.

4. a. 125-mcg tablet is the appropriate strength to use ($0.125 \text{ mg} = 125 \text{ mcg}$).

   b. 1 125-mcg tab. Even though the tablets are scored, when possible, administer whole tablets.

   $125 \text{ mcg} : 1 \text{ tab} = 125 \text{ mcg} : x \text{ tab}$

   *or*

   $\dfrac{125 \text{ mcg}}{125 \text{ mcg}} \times 1 \text{ tab} = x \text{ tab}$

   Answer: 1 tab

5. a. 500-mg caps would be appropriate to use.

   b. 2 caps (500 mg each). $1,000 \text{ mg} = 1 \text{ g}$; therefore 2 caps of 500 mg each would be the least number of capsules. Using the 250-mg strength capsules would require 4 caps.

   c. 2 caps q6h = 8 caps. Multiplying the number of caps needed by the number of days gives you the number of capsules required.

   8 (number of caps per day) × 7 (number of days) = 56 (total caps needed)

   $500 \text{ mg} : 1 \text{ cap} = 1,000 \text{ mg} : x \text{ cap}$

   *or*

   $\dfrac{1,000 \text{ mg}}{500 \text{ mg}} \times 1 \text{ cap} = x \text{ cap}$

   $x = 2 \text{ caps}$

6. It would be best to administer one of the 100-mg tablets and one of the 50-mg tablets. This would allow the client to take 2 tablets to achieve the dosage ordered. Although giving the client three 50-mg tablets would be acceptable, it is not the best choice. The client always should be given the least number of tablets to achieve the desired dosage (100 mg + 50 mg = 150 mg).

7. $0.4 \text{ g} = 400 \text{ mg} (1 \text{ g} = 1,000 \text{ mg})$

   $400 \text{ mg} : 1 \text{ tab} = 400 \text{ mg} : x \text{ tab}$

   *or*

   $\dfrac{400 \text{ mg}}{400 \text{ mg}} \times 1 \text{ tab} = x \text{ tab}$

   Answer: 1 tab. 1 tab, 400 mg, is equal to 0.4 g; therefore only 1 tab is needed to administer the dosage.

8. $90 \text{ mg} : 1 \text{ tab} = 180 \text{ mg} : x \text{ tab}$

   *or*

   $\dfrac{180 \text{ mg}}{90 \text{ mg}} \times 1 \text{ tab} = x \text{ tab}$

Answer: 2 tabs. The dosage ordered is greater than what is available; therefore you will need more than 1 tab to administer the dosage.

9.  1.5 mg : 1 cap = 3 mg : $x$ cap

    *or*

    $$\frac{3\ \text{mg}}{1.5\ \text{mg}} \times 1\ \text{cap} = x\ \text{cap}$$

    Answer: 2 caps. The dosage ordered is greater than what is available; therefore you will need more than 1 cap to administer the dosage.

10. 1 mg : 1 tab = 2 mg : $x$ tab

    *or*

    $$\frac{2\ \text{mg}}{1\ \text{mg}} \times 1\ \text{tab} = x\ \text{tab}$$

    Answer: 2 tabs. The dosage ordered is more than what is available; therefore you will need more than 1 tab to administer the dosage.

11. a. 30-mg tablets

    b. Three 30-mg tablets. This strength will allow the client to take three tabs to achieve the desired dosage, as opposed to six 15-mg tabs. This dosage is logical because the maximum number of tablets administered is generally three.

    30 mg : 1 tab = 90 mg : $x$ tab

    *or*

    $$\frac{90\ \text{mg}}{30\ \text{mg}} \times 1\ \text{tab} = x\ \text{tab}$$

    Answer: three 30-mg tabs

12. 0.6 g = 600 mg (1 g = 1,000 mg)

    300 mg : 1 tab = 600 mg : $x$ tab

    *or*

    $$\frac{600\ \text{mg}}{300\ \text{mg}} \times 1\ \text{tab} = x\ \text{tab}$$

    Answer: 2 tabs. The dosage ordered is greater than what is available; therefore you will need more than 1 tab to administer the dosage.

13. 50 mg : 1 tab = 100 mg : $x$ tab

    *or*

    $$\frac{100\ \text{mg}}{50\ \text{mg}} \times 1\ \text{tab} = x\ \text{tab}$$

    Answer: You need 2 tabs to administer 100 mg. 2 tabs t.i.d. (3 times a day) = 6 tabs × 3 days = 18 tabs.

14. It would be best to administer one 80-mg tablet and one 40-mg tablet (80 + 40 = 120 mg). This would be the least number of tablets.

15. 10 mg : 1 tab = 20 mg : $x$ tab

    *or*

    $$\frac{20\ \text{mg}}{10\ \text{mg}} \times 1\ \text{tab} = x\ \text{tab}$$

    Answer: 2 tabs (extended release). The dosage ordered is larger than the available dosage; therefore more than 1 tab will be required.

16. Conversion is required. Equivalent: 1,000 mg = 1 g.

    500 mg : 1 tab = 1,000 mg : $x$ tab

    *or*

    $$\frac{1,000\ \text{mg}}{500\ \text{mg}} \times 1\ \text{tab} = x\ \text{tab}$$

    Answer: 2 tabs (extended release). The dosage ordered is greater than what is available; therefore you will need more than 1 tab to administer the dosage.

17. Conversion is required. Equivalent: 1,000 mg = 1 g. Therefore 0.2 g = 200 mg.

    100 mg : 1 tab = 200 mg : $x$ tab

    *or*

    $$\frac{200\ \text{mg}}{100\ \text{mg}} \times 1\ \text{tab} = x\ \text{tab}$$

    Answer: 2 tabs. The dosage ordered is larger than what is available; therefore you will need more than 1 tab to administer the dosage.

18. 120 mg : 1 cap = 240 mg : $x$ cap

    *or*

    $$\frac{240\ \text{mg}}{120\ \text{mg}} \times 1\ \text{cap} = x\ \text{cap}$$

    Answer: 2 delayed-release capsules. The dosage ordered is greater than what is available. You will need more than 1 cap to administer the dosage.

19. 200 mg : 1 tab = 400 mg : $x$ tab

    *or*

    $$\frac{400\ \text{mg}}{200\ \text{mg}} \times 1\ \text{tab} = x\ \text{tab}$$

    Answer: 2 tabs. The dosage ordered is more than what is available. You will need more than 1 tab to administer the dosage.

20. a. 1 tablet. The dosage ordered is contained in the one tablet.

b. two (2)

c. 49 mg of sacubitril and 51 mg of valsartan.

21. 30 mg : 1 cap = 60 mg : $x$ cap

*or*

$$\frac{60\ mg}{30\ mg} \times 1\ cap = x\ cap$$

Answer: 2 caps (delayed release). The dosage ordered is more than what is available. You will need more than 1 cap to administer the dosage.

22. It would be best to administer 3 25 mcg tablets. Although the tabs are scored, it is best to administer tabs whole rather than breaking them. Variation in dosage can occur if tablets are broken.

23. 12.5 mg : 1 tab = 25 mg : $x$ tab

*or*

$$\frac{25\ mg}{12.5\ mg} \times 1\ tab = x\ tab$$

Answer: 2 tabs. The dosage ordered is more than what is available. You will need more than 1 tab to administer the dosage.

24. 0.5 mg : 1 tab = 1 mg : $x$ tab

*or*

$$\frac{1\ mg}{0.5\ mg} \times 1\ tab = x\ tab$$

Answer: 2 tabs. The dosage ordered is more than what is available; therefore you will need more than 1 tab to administer the dosage.

25. 250 mg : 1 tab = 500 mg : $x$ tab

*or*

$$\frac{500\ mg}{250\ mg} \times 1\ tab = x\ tab$$

Answer: 2 tabs. The dosage ordered is greater than what is available. You will need more than 1 tab to administer the dosage.

26. 30 mg : 1 tab = 60 mg : $x$ tab

*or*

$$\frac{60\ mg}{30\ mg} \times 1\ tab = x\ tab$$

Answer: 2 tabs XL (extended-release). The dosage ordered is greater than what is available. You will need more than 1 tab to administer the dosage.

27. 0.25 mcg : 1 cap = 0.5 mcg : $x$ cap

*or*

$$\frac{0.5\ mcg}{0.25\ mcg} \times 1\ cap = x\ cap$$

Answer: 2 caps. The dosage ordered is greater than what is available. You will need more than 1 cap to administer the dosage.

28. 3.125 mg : 1 tab = 6.25 mg : $x$ tab

*or*

$$\frac{6.25\ mg}{3.125\ mg} \times 1\ tab = x\ tab$$

Answer: 2 tabs. The dosage ordered is greater than what is available. You will need more than 1 tab to administer the dosage.

---

**NOTE**

The setup shown for problems that required conversions reflects conversion of what the prescriber ordered to what is available. Unless stated in problems 29-35, no conversion is required to calculate the dosage.

29. 20 mg : 1 mL = 75 mg : $x$ mL

*or*

$$\frac{75\ mg}{20\ mg} \times 1\ mL = x\ mL$$

Answer: 3.75 mL = 3.8 mL. The dosage ordered is more than the available strength. You will need more than 1 mL to administer the dosage.

30. 25 mg : 5 mL = 40 mg : $x$ mL

*or*

$$\frac{40\ mg}{25\ mg} \times 5\ mL = x\ mL$$

Answer: 8 mL. The dosage ordered is more than the available strength; therefore you will need more than 5 mL to administer the required dosage.

31. 20 mEq : 15 mL = 20 mEq : $x$ mL

*or*

$$\frac{20\ mEq}{20\ mEq} \times 15\ mL = x\ mL$$

Answer: 15 mL. The dosage ordered is contained in 15 mL of the medication.

32. 1 mcg : 1 mL = 2 mcg : $x$ mL

*or*

$$\frac{2\ mcg}{1\ mcg} \times 1\ mL = x\ mL$$

Answer: 2 mL. The dosage ordered is more than the available strength; therefore you will need more than 1 mL to administer the dosage.

33. $0.5 \text{ mg} : 5 \text{ mL} = 2 \text{ mg} : x \text{ mL}$

    *or*

    $$\frac{2 \text{ mg}}{0.5 \text{ mg}} \times 5 \text{ mL} = x \text{ mL}$$

    Answer: 20 mL. The dosage ordered is greater than the available strength; therefore more than 5 mL will be needed to administer the required dosage.

34. $125 \text{ mg} : 5 \text{ mL} = 100 \text{ mg} : x \text{ mL}$

    *or*

    $$\frac{100 \text{ mg}}{125 \text{ mg}} \times 5 \text{ mL} = x \text{ mL}$$

    Answer: 4 mL. The amount ordered is less than the available strength; therefore less than 5 mL will be needed to administer the required dosage.

35. Use the microgram equivalent to calculate the dosage.

    $50 \text{ mcg} : 1 \text{ mL} = 125 \text{ mcg} : x \text{ mL}$

    *or*

    $$\frac{125 \text{ mcg}}{50 \text{ mcg}} \times 1 \text{ mL} = x \text{ mL}$$

    Answer: 2.5 mL. (2.5 mL is metric and stated with decimal.) The dosage ordered is larger than the available strength; therefore you will need more than 1 mL to administer the dosage.

36. Conversion is required. Equivalent: 1,000 mg = 1 g. Therefore 0.5 g = 500 mg.

    $125 \text{ mg} : 5 \text{ mL} = 500 \text{ mg} : x \text{ mL}$

    *or*

    $$\frac{500 \text{ mg}}{125 \text{ mg}} \times 5 \text{ mL} = x \text{ mL}$$

    Answer: 20 mL. The dosage ordered is four times larger than the available strength; therefore more than 5 mL will be needed to administer the dosage.

37. $20 \text{ mg} : 5 \text{ mL} = 60 \text{ mg} : x \text{ mL}$

    *or*

    $$\frac{60 \text{ mg}}{20 \text{ mg}} \times 5 \text{ mL} = x \text{ mL}$$

    Answer: 15 mL. The dosage ordered is more than the available strength. You will need more than 5 mL to administer the dosage.

38. The label indicates that 5 mL = 300 mg of the medication.

    $300 \text{ mg} : 5 \text{ mL} = 600 \text{ mg} : x \text{ mL}$

    *or*

    $$\frac{600 \text{ mg}}{300 \text{ mg}} \times 5 \text{ mL} = x \text{ mL}$$

    Answer: 10 mL. The dosage ordered is two times more than the available strength. You will need more than 5 mL to administer the required dosage.

39. Conversion is required. Equivalent: 1,000 mg = 1 g. Therefore 0.5 g = 500 mg.

    $400 \text{ mg} : 5 \text{ mL} = 500 \text{ mg} : x \text{ mL}$

    *or*

    $$\frac{500 \text{ mg}}{400 \text{ mg}} \times 5 \text{ mL} = x \text{ mL}$$

    Answer: 6.25 = 6.3 mL. The dosage ordered is larger than the available strength. You will need more than 5 mL to administer the dosage.

40. $40 \text{ mg} : 5 \text{ mL} = 160 \text{ mg} : x \text{ mL}$

    *or*

    $$\frac{160 \text{ mg}}{40 \text{ mg}} \times 5 \text{ mL} = x \text{ mL}$$

    Answer: 20 mL. The dosage ordered is more than the available strength; therefore you will need more than 5 mL to administer the dosage.

41. $6 \text{ mg} : 1 \text{ mL} = 75 \text{ mg} : x \text{ mL}$

    *or*

    $$\frac{75 \text{ mg}}{6 \text{ mg}} \times 1 \text{ mL} = x \text{ mL}$$

    Answer: 12.5 mL. The dosage ordered is greater than the available strength. You will need more than 1 mL to administer the dosage.

42. Conversion is necessary. Equivalent: 1,000 mg = 1 g. Therefore 0.3 g = 300 mg.

    $250 \text{ mg} : 5 \text{ mL} = 300 \text{ mg} : x \text{ mL}$

    *or*

    $$\frac{300 \text{ mg}}{250 \text{ mg}} \times 5 \text{ mL} = x \text{ mL}$$

    Answer: 6 mL. The dosage ordered is greater than the available strength; therefore you will need more than 5 mL to administer the required dosage.

43. $4 \text{ mg} : 5 \text{ mL} = 8 \text{ mg} : x \text{ mL}$

    *or*

    $$\frac{8 \text{ mg}}{4 \text{ mg}} \times 5 \text{ mL} = x \text{ mL}$$

    Answer: 10 mL. The dosage ordered is greater than the available strength; therefore you will need more than 5 mL to administer the required dosage.

44. Conversion is necessary. 1,000 mg = 1 g; therefore 0.25 g = 250 mg.

    $200 \text{ mg} : 5 \text{ mL} = 250 \text{ mg} : x \text{ mL}$

    *or*

    $$\frac{250 \text{ mg}}{200 \text{ mg}} \times 5 \text{ mL} = x \text{ mL}$$

    Answer: 6.25 = 6.3 mL. The dosage ordered is greater than the available strength. You will need more than 5 mL to administer the dosage.

45. $200 \text{ mg} : 5 \text{ mL} = 200 \text{ mg} : x \text{ mL}$

    *or*

    $$\frac{200 \text{ mg}}{200 \text{ mg}} \times 5 \text{ mL} = x \text{ mL}$$

    Answer: 5 mL. The dosage ordered is equivalent to the available strength. Label indicates 200 mg = 5 mL.

46. $20 \text{ mg} : 5 \text{ mL} = 30 \text{ mg} : x \text{ mL}$

    *or*

    $$\frac{30 \text{ mg}}{20 \text{ mg}} \times 5 \text{ mL} = x \text{ mL}$$

    Answer: 7.5 mL. The dosage ordered is greater than the available strength; therefore you will need more than 5 mL to administer the required dosage.

47. $6.25 \text{ mg} : 5 \text{ mL} = 12.5 \text{ mg} : x \text{ mL}$

    *or*

    $$\frac{12.5 \text{ mg}}{6.25 \text{ mg}} \times 5 \text{ mL} = x \text{ mL}$$

    Answer: 10 mL. The dosage ordered is greater than the available strength; therefore you will need more than 5 mL to administer the required dosage.

48. $20 \text{ mg} : 1 \text{ mL} = 30 \text{ mg} : x \text{ mL}$

    *or*

    $$\frac{30 \text{ mg}}{20 \text{ mg}} \times 1 \text{ mL} = x \text{ mL}$$

    Answer: 1.5 mL. The dosage ordered is greater than the available strength; therefore you will need more than 1 mL to administer the required dosage.

    *or*

    $100 \text{ mg} : 5 \text{ mL} = 30 \text{ mg} : x \text{ mL}$

    $$\frac{30 \text{ mg}}{100 \text{ mg}} \times 5 \text{ mL} = x \text{ mL}$$

    This would net the same answer of 1.5 mL. Note when using the dosage strength of 100 mg per 5 mL, the dosage ordered is less than the available strength; therefore you will need less than 5 mL to administer the dosage.

## Answers to Clinical Reasoning Questions

1. a. 6 tablets

   b. Question the order before administering. Double-check your calculation with another nurse. If order is correct, check with the pharmacy regarding available dosage strengths for the medication. Check a reliable and reputable medication reference for the usual dosage and action of this medication.

   c. Any calculation that requires you to administer more than the maximum number of tablets or capsules, which is usually three (3), to achieve a single dose should be questioned and calculation rechecked. An unusual number of tablets or capsules should alert the nurse to a possible error in prescribing, transcribing, or calculation.

2. a. After checking a reliable and reputable drug resource for the usual dosage, contact the pharmacy regarding the available dosage strengths for the medication.

   b. The dosage ordered would require that the tablets be broken to administer the dosage. The tablets are unscored and should not be broken. Unscored tablets will not break evenly, and there is no way to determine the dosage being administered. Breaking an unscored tablet could lead to the administration of an unintended dosage.

3. a. The right medication

   b. In preparing the medication, the nurse did not read the label carefully and administered Percodan, the wrong medication, which has a similar spelling to Percocet. By not reading the label carefully, the nurse did not notice that combination medications contain more than one medication; in this case, Percodan contained aspirin. Percocet contained Tylenol (acetaminophen).

   c. A medication error occurred because the wrong medication was administered. The client was allergic to aspirin and could have had a reaction from mild to a severe anaphylactic reaction (dyspnea, airway obstruction, shock, and in some cases, death).

   d. The error could have been prevented by carefully reading the medication label three times while preparing the medication. The nurse must use caution when administering medications that look alike or that have similar spellings. Tablets or capsules that contain more than one medication must be read carefully. (Percocet contains acetaminophen [Tylenol] and Percodan contains aspirin.)

---

**NOTE**

Refer to problems 1-48 for setup of problems if needed.

---

## Answers to Chapter Review

1. 1 tab

2. One 1.5-mg cap and one 3-mg cap

3. 1 tab

4. 2 tabs

5. 10 mL

6. 7.5 mL

7. 2 tabs

8. 2 tabs

9. a. 100 mg of glecaprevir and 40 mg of pibrentasvir

   b. 3 tabs

10. 2 tabs

11. 2 mL

12. 15 mL

13. 1 extended-release tab

14. One 0.25-mg tab and one 0.5-mg tab

15. 2 delayed-release tabs

16. 1 cap

17. 1 extended-release tab

18. a. 2 tabs

    b. 14 tabs

19. One 10-mg tab and one 20-mg tab

20. a. 2 tabs

    b. 28 tabs

21. 8.3 mL

22. 30 mL

23. One 40-mg tab and one 20-mg tab

24. 2 tabs

25. 1 cap

26. 1 long-acting cap

27. 2 sublingual films

28. 6.3 mL

29. 2 tabs

30. 1 tab

31. a. 4 oz (½ cup) of water, ginger ale, lemon-lime soda, lemonade, or orange juice only

    b. Immediately

    c. 8.8 mL

32. 2 tabs

33. 10 mL

34. 2 tabs

35. 1 tab

36. a. Find out about medications that should not be taken with Biktarvy.

    b. 3 (three) medications: bictegravir, emtricitabine, and tenofovir alafenamide

    c. bictegravir 50 mg equivalent to 52.5 mg of bictegravir, emtricitabine 200 mg, and tenofovir alafenamide 25 mg equivalent to 28 mg of tenofovir alafenamide

# CHAPTER **17**
# Parenteral Medications

## Objectives

*After reviewing this chapter, you should be able to:*

1. Identify the various types of syringes used for parenteral administration
2. Read parenteral solution labels and identify dosage strengths
3. Read and measure dosages on a syringe
4. Calculate dosages of parenteral medications already in solution
5. Identify the appropriate syringe to administer the dosage based on the dosage calculation

The term *parenteral* is used to indicate medications by any route other than through the gastrointestinal (GI) system. Parenteral is commonly used to refer to medications administered by injection with the use of a needle and syringe. Common parenteral routes include intramuscular (IM), subcutaneous (subcut), and intravenous (IV). Of the three routes, the IV route produces the desired effect more rapidly, as the medication is injected directly into the bloodstream. Intradermal (ID) is a less common injection route and is mainly used for skin testing, such as for allergy test or tuberculin skin test.

Medications administered by the parenteral route generally act more quickly than oral medications because they are absorbed more rapidly into the bloodstream. This chapter will focus on calculation of medications administered IM, subcut, and IV.

- **IM**—Indicates an injection given into a muscle, such as Demerol for pain.
- **Subcut**—Injection into the subcutaneous tissue, below the skin, such as insulin used in the management of diabetes.
- **IV**—Injection given directly into the vein. This can be direct (IV push), or the medication can be diluted in a larger volume of intravenous fluid and infused over a period of time (IV infusion). Antibiotics and other medications may be administered IV.
- **ID**—Injection administered just under the skin, or into the dermis. ID is mainly used for diagnostic purposes. Example: used to administer purified protein derivative (PPD) skin test to test for exposure to tuberculosis.

When the rapid action of a medication is necessary or a client cannot take the medication orally, the parenteral route may be preferred. For example, a client is unable to take a medication orally because of emesis (vomiting) or a nonfunctioning gastrointestinal (GI) tract, or the client is unconscious.

Medications for parenteral use are available as a sterile solution or liquid that can be absorbed and distributed without causing irritation to the tissues. Parenteral medications are also available in powder form that must be diluted with a liquid or solvent (reconstituted) before they can be used. Reconstitution of medications in powder form will be covered in Chapter 18.

## Parenteral Medication Packaging

Medications for parenteral use come packaged in a variety of devices, including ampules, vials, mix-o-vials, premeasured (prefilled) syringes, and cartridges.

1. **Ampule:** Sealed glass container that contains a typical single dose of medication. It has a constricted neck that is designed to be snapped off to allow for the withdrawal of medication. The neck is snapped off by using a plastic protective sleeve, an alcohol wipe or sterile gauze. Medication is withdrawn from an ampule using a filter needle (a needle with a filter inside) to prevent the withdrawal of glass fragments (Potter et al., 2017). If the entire amount of medication is not administered, the medication remaining must be discarded (Figure 17.1).

2. **Vial:** A vial is a plastic or glass container that has a rubber stopper (diaphragm) on the top that is punctured for the withdrawal of medication and can be for single-dose use or multi-dose use. The medication in a vial may be in liquid (solution) form (Figure 17.2) or may contain a powder that must be reconstituted before administration (discussed in Chapter 18) (Figure 17.3). Multi-dose vials contain more than one dose of the medication and contain an antimicrobial preservative to help prevent the growth of bacteria. Single-dose vials contain the amount of medication for a typical single dose and lack the antimicrobial preservative. Even though medication is in a single-dose vial, it should be measured and not just drawn up. The Centers for Disease Control and Prevention (CDC) issued recommendations for safe injection practices, which included that vials labeled "single-dose" or "single use" should be used once and are meant for one patient use (https://www.cdc.gov/injectionsafety/providers/provider_faqs_singlevials.html). When possible, the CDC also recommends multi-dose vials be for single client use and not opened or punctured in the immediate client area (e.g., client room). This practice will prevent contamination of the vial (direct or indirect), which can lead to infections in subsequent clients (https://www.cdc.gov/injectionsafety/providers/provider_faqs_multivials.html).

> **ⓘ TIPS FOR CLINICAL PRACTICE**
>
> It is important to note that for both single-dose vials and ampules, there is a little extra medication present; it is important to carefully measure the amount of medication to be withdrawn.

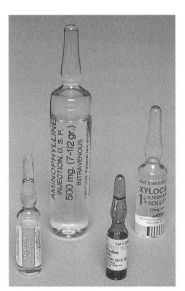

**Figure 17.1** Medication in ampules. (From Potter PA, Perry AG, Stockert PA, Hall AM: *Fundamentals of nursing*, ed 9, St Louis, 2017, Elsevier.)

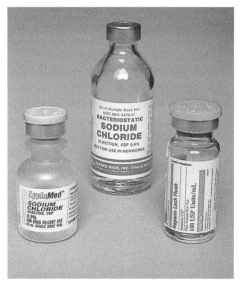

**Figure 17.2** Medication in vials. (From Potter PA, Perry AG, Stockert PA, Hall AM. *Fundamentals of nursing*, ed 9, St Louis, 2017, Elsevier.)

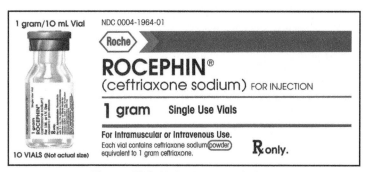

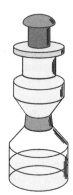

**Figure 17.3** Medication in powder form.

**Figure 17.4** Mix-o-vial. (From Willihnganz H, Gurevitz S, Clayton BD: *Clayton's Basic pharmacology for nurses*, ed 18, St Louis, 2020, Elsevier.)

3. **Mix-o-vial:** Some medications come in mix-o-vials (Figure 17.4). The vial usually contains a single dosage of medication. The mix-o-vial has two compartments separated by a rubber stopper. The top compartment contains the sterile liquid (diluent), and the bottom compartment contains the powdered medication. When pressure is applied to the top of the vial, the rubber stopper that separates the medication and liquid is released. This allows the liquid and medication to be mixed, thereby dissolving the medication.

4. **Cartridge:** A cartridge is a glass or plastic container prefilled with a single dosage of medication. Cartridges require a special holder called a *Tubex* or *Carpuject* to release the medication from the cartridge for administration. The amount of medication is calculated, and if the dosage to be administered is less than the amount contained in the unit, the unneeded portion is discarded (in the presence of another nurse when medication is a controlled substance) and then the dose of medication is administered to the client (Figure 17.5A).

5. **Prefilled syringe (premeasured):** The syringe comes from the manufacturer prefilled with medication, single-dose, and designed to be used once. The medication comes prepared for administration with a needle attached or without a needle attached, packaged with a plunger, and does not require a special holder for administration. The amount desired is calculated, the excess disposed of (in the presence of another nurse when medication is a controlled substance), and the calculated dosage is administered. Examples of medications available in prefilled syringes include vaccines, emergency medications such as sodium bicarbonate and atropine, EpiPen, insulin pens, and Amivog (used for migraine headaches) (Figure 17.5B).

In addition to the packaging discussed for parenteral medications, there are some parenteral medications that come in **auto-injectors.** An auto-injector is a medical device designed to deliver a premeasured dose of medication. Auto-injectors allow for self-injection with a single, preloaded dose of a medication that consists of a spring-loaded syringe

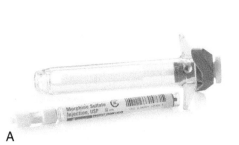

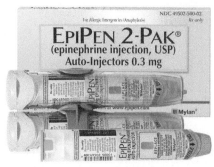

**A**

**Figure 17.5** (A) Carpuject syringe holder and needleless, prefilled sterile cartridge. (B) EpiPen 2-Pak. (A, From Hospira, Inc., Lake Forest, IL. B, From Mylan Specialty L.P., Basking Ridge, NJ.)

activated when the device is pushed firmly against the body. Examples of medications that come in auto-injectors include Epinephrine and Amivog.

> **! SAFETY ALERT!**
>
> To safely administer the ordered amount of medication from a cartridge and prefilled syringe, the amount of medication in excess of what is needed to administer the dosage should be discarded before administration.

## Syringes

Parenteral medications are administered with a syringe. The nurse has the responsibility for choosing the proper equipment required to safely administer the medication. Syringes as well as needles vary in size. The choice of needle size as well as syringe is determined by the nurse, depending on several factors, which include the route of administration, the volume of medication, the viscosity of the medication to be injected, the type of tissue being injected into, and the client's size. Nurses must be able to choose the appropriate syringe, accurately read the calibrations on the syringe, and draw up the correct volume of medication. Syringes are available in various sizes for use, have different capacities, and specific calibrations. They are made of plastic and glass, but plastic syringes are more commonly used. Syringes are disposable and designed for one-time use only. Before discussing the various types of syringes let's begin with the **parts of a syringe** (Figure 17.6).

1. **The barrel:** The outer (body) portion of the syringe that holds the medication. The barrel of the syringe is marked with lines that are referred to as calibrations (markings) that measure medication doses in milliliters (mL).
2. **The plunger:** The inner device that is moved backward to withdraw and measure the medication and is pushed to eject the medication from the syringe. The plunger fits into the barrel.
3. **The tip:** The end of the syringe that holds the needle. The needle can be twisted and locked in place (Luer-Lok) (Figure 17.7A). This design prevents the inadvertent removal of the needle (Potter, Perry, Stockert, Hall, 2017). Or the needle slips on to the tip (non–Luer-Lok) (Figure 17.7B). Some syringes also come with a needle attached that cannot be detached from the syringe.

Needles come in various lengths and diameters. The nurse chooses the needle according to the client's size, the type of tissue being injected into, and the viscosity of the medication

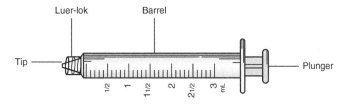

**Figure 17.6** Parts of a syringe.

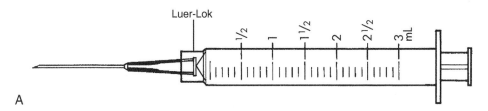

A

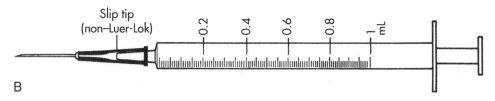

B

**Figure 17.7** (A) Luer-Lok. (B) Slip tip (non–Luer-Lok).

to be injected. Some syringes also come with a needle attached that cannot be detached from the syringe.

## Types of Syringes

Syringes are available in a variety of sizes. The nurse chooses the syringe to use based on the volume to be administered. The syringes commonly used in the clinical setting include the **3-mL** (small hypodermic) **syringe, 1-mL (tuberculin) syringe**, and the **insulin syringes**. There are larger syringes that include the 5, 6, 10, 12, up to 60 mL and larger. Syringes are calibrated in milliliters (mL) and hold varying capacities, and the calibrations vary with the size of the syringe.

- **3-mL syringe.** The 3-mL syringe is the most commonly used hypodermic syringe for the administration of medication that is more than 1 mL (Figure 17.8). Notice the calibration lines on the barrel of the 3-mL syringe. The beginning of the barrel (or first line on the syringe) is referred to as the zero line. The first calibration on all syringes is zero. Each calibration (short line) after the zero line is 0.1 mL. The longer lines indicate half (0.5 mL), and full milliliter measures up to 3 mL. Note mL is indicated on the syringe and not cubic centimeter (cc). **Milliliter (mL)** is the correct term for volume. The cubic centimeter is a three-dimensional measure of space and represents the space that a milliliter occupies. Notice also that the small hypodermic syringes up to size 3 mL also have fractions on them. There are, however, some syringes that indicate 0.5 mL, 1.5 mL, etc., instead of fractions. The use of decimals on the syringes correlates with the use of decimals in the metric system; therefore a dosage should be stated in milliliters as a decimal (e.g., 1.2 mL, 0.3 mL).

## Measuring the Amount of Medication in a Syringe

Refer to the syringe shown in Figure 17.9; notice the rubber ring. When measuring medication and reading the medication withdrawn, the forward edge of the plunger head indicates the amount of medication withdrawn. Do not become confused by the second, bottom ring or by the raised section (middle) of the suction tip. The point where the rubber plunger edge makes contact with the barrel is the spot that should be lined up with the amount desired.

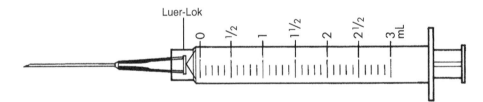

**Figure 17.8** 3-mL syringe.

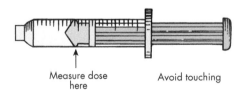

**Figure 17.9** Reading measured amount of a medication in a syringe. (From Potter PA, Perry AG, Stockert P, Hall A: *Fundamentals of nursing,* ed 9, St Louis, 2017, Elsevier.)

> **⚠ SAFETY ALERT!**
>
> Understanding the calibrations on a syringe and reading them carefully are critical to accurately measuring a medication dosage. Misreading the calibrations could lead to a medication error. The volume of medication represented by the calibrations is different depending on the size of the syringe being used. Never assume what the calibrations on a syringe mean. Check the calibrations carefully. If the medication is not accurately measured, an incorrect dosage can be administered, resulting in serious consequences to the client.

Let's examine the syringes below to illustrate specific amounts in a syringe. (Syringe **A** shows a volume of 0.7 mL filled in, and syringe **B**, 1.7 mL.)

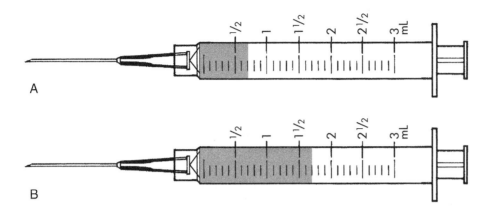

A

B

Because the small-capacity syringes are used most often to administer medications, it is very important to know how to read them to withdraw amounts accurately.

**POINTS TO REMEMBER**

- Small-capacity hypodermics are calibrated in milliliters; the 3-mL size syringe is used most often to administer dosages greater than 1 mL. Dosages administered with them must correlate to the calibration.
- Syringes are labeled with the abbreviation mL. More and more syringes are being manufactured using just mL.
- The milliliter (mL) is the correct measure for volume.
- The first calibration (line) on all syringes is zero.
- 3-mL syringe is calibrated in tenths (0.1) of a mL.

## PRACTICE **PROBLEMS**

Shade in the indicated amounts on the syringes in milliliters.

1. 0.8 mL

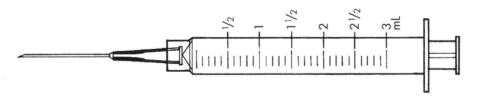

2. 1.2 mL

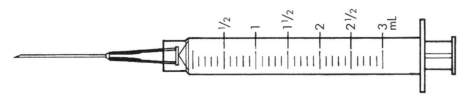

3. 1.5 mL

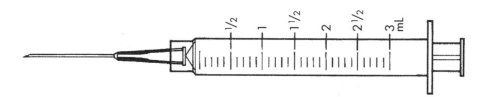

4. 2.4 mL

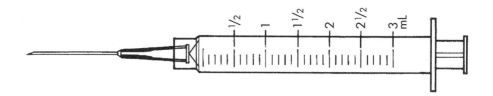

Indicate the number of milliliters shaded in on the following syringes.

5.

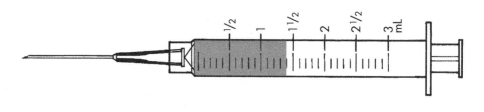

_____

6.

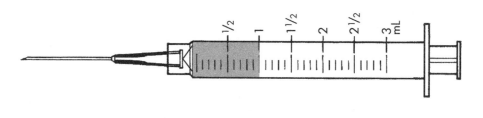

_____

7.

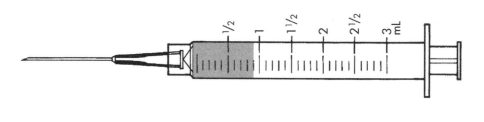

_____

8.

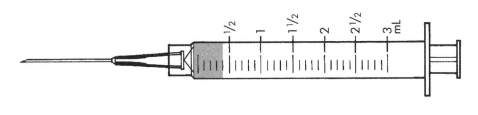

**Answers on p. 377**

**Large-Capacity Syringes.** The larger hypodermics (5, 6, 10, and 12 mL) are used when volumes larger than 3 mL are desired.

- **5-, 6-, 10-, and 12-mL syringes:** These syringes are used when volumes larger than 3 mL are desired. Of these syringes the 5 mL and 10 mL are seen most often to prepare and administer medications for intravenous (IV) administration. These syringes are sometimes referred to as *intravenous syringes*. With these syringes (5-mL, 6-mL, 10-mL, and 12-mL) each small calibration line is 0.2 mL, with the whole numbers indicated by the long calibration line and is numbered. Figure 17.10A shows 0.8 mL of medication measured in a 5-mL syringe, and Figure 17.10B shows 7.8 mL measured in a 10-mL syringe.
- **20-, 30-, and up to 60-mL syringes:** These syringes are used to administer large volumes of IV medication and other clinical uses which includes feeding clients. These syringes have small calibration lines that measure 1 mL, and every fifth mL has a longer calibration line and is numbered. These syringes also measure ounces on the syringe.

> **TIPS FOR CLINICAL PRACTICE**
>
> The larger the syringe, the larger the calibration. Example: In 5-mL and 10-mL syringes, each shorter calibration line measures two-tenths of a milliliter (0.2 mL). To be safe, always examine the calibration of the syringes and use the one best suited for the volume to be administered.

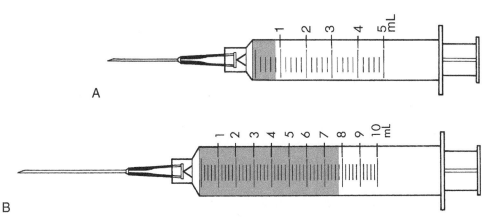

**Figure 17.10** Large hypodermics. (A) 5-mL syringe filled with 0.8 mL. (B) 10-mL syringe filled with 7.8 mL.

## ▣ PRACTICE **PROBLEMS**

Indicate the number of milliliters shaded in on the following syringes.

9.

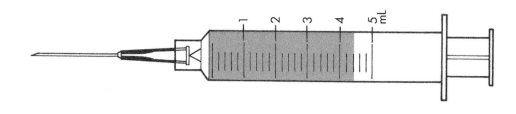

_____

10.

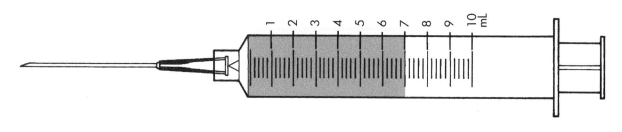

_____

11.

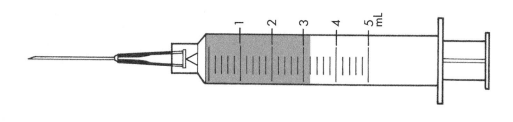

_____

**Answers on p. 377**

- **Tuberculin syringe (1 mL):** The tuberculin (TB) syringe is a narrow syringe that has a capacity of 0.5 mL or 1 mL. The 1-mL size is used most often. The syringe gets its name from its original use, which was the administration of tuberculin skin tests. Tuberculin syringes are used to accurately measure medications given in very small volumes and for medication doses contained in hundredths of a milliliter (mL) (e.g., heparin). Other medications administered with a tuberculin syringe include vaccines and small doses of medications given to children. It is also recommended that dosages less than 0.5 mL be measured and administered with a tuberculin syringe. The calibrations on a 1-mL syringe are small and close together. Dosages such as 0.42 mL and 0.37 mL can be accurately measured using a tuberculin syringe. On the tuberculin syringe each of the shorter calibration lines represent one-hundredth of a milliliter (0.01 mL); the longer calibration lines measure one-tenth of a milliliter (0.1) and are numbered. The numbers on the tuberculin syringe are decimal fractions (Figures 17.11 and 17.12).

> **① SAFETY ALERT!**
> Reading the calibration lines and measuring the correct dose with a tuberculin syringe requires extreme care. Read the calibrations carefully to avoid error.

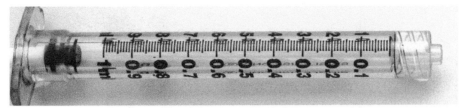

**Figure 17.11** Tuberculin syringe.

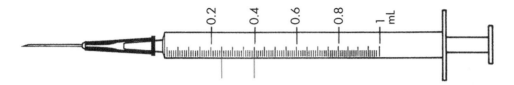

**Figure 17.12** Tuberculin syringe. The 0.4 mL calibration *(orange line)* is one of 0.1-increments; the 0.25 mL calibration *(green line)* is one of the 0.01-mL increments on the tuberculin syringe.

> **! SAFETY ALERT!**
> The calibrations on hypodermic syringes differ. Be careful when measuring medications in a syringe. Being off by even a small amount on the syringe scale can be critical. The syringe you use to administer medication must provide the calibration you need to accurately measure the dose.

**Insulin syringes:** Insulin syringes are used to administer insulin **only**. Insulin syringes are calibrated in **units**, and not mL. Insulin is ordered by the number of units to administer and not volume. Insulin syringes do not have detachable needles. The needle, hub, and barrel are inseparable. The administration of insulin, insulin orders, and insulin syringes are further discussed in the insulin chapter, Chapter 19. Insulin syringes are available in three sizes: 100 unit (1 mL), 50 unit (0.5 mL), and 30 unit (0.3 mL). The 50-unit and 30-unit insulin syringes are called Lo-Dose insulin syringes; they are designed to precisely deliver low doses (50 units or less) of insulin (Figure 17.13).

- **100-unit insulin syringe** (referred to as the standard insulin syringe): A long calibration line identifies every 10 units (i.e., 10, 20, up to 100 units). Each short line calibration is in 2-unit increments (Figure 17.13A).
- **50-unit insulin syringe:** A long calibration line identifies every 5 units (i.e., 5, 10, up to 50 units). Each short calibration line is in 1-unit increments (Figure 17.13B).
- **30-unit insulin syringe:** A long calibration line identifies every 5 units (i.e., 5, 10, up to 30 units). Each short line calibration is in 1-unit increments. Note: the calibration lines on the 30-unit insulin syringe has more spacing between the calibrations and is easy to read (Figure 17.13C).
- **\*U-500 insulin syringe:** This syringe has "U-500" indicated on the barrel of the syringe. Each calibration (short line) on the syringe is 5 units. The syringe is designed to administer U-500 insulin (discussed further in Chapter 19) and has a capacity of 250 units (Figure 17.13D).
- **Dual-scale insulin syringe:** The second type of 100-unit insulin syringe is the dual-scale version, which is calibrated in 2-unit increments. It has a scale with even numbered 2-unit increments on one side (2, 4, etc.) The opposite side is in odd-numbered 2-unit increments (1, 3 etc.). The best method for using this syringe is to measure the odd dosages on the left and even dosages using the scale on the right (Figure 17.14). Care must be taken to use the correct scale for the number of units of insulin ordered.

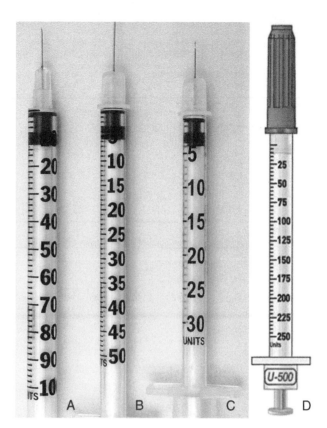

**Figure 17.13** Insulin syringes. (A) 1-mL size (100 units). (B) Lo-Dose (50 units). (C) Lo-Dose (30 units). (D) U-500. (From Macklin D, Chernecky L, Infortuna H: *Math for clinical practice*, ed 2, St Louis, 2010, Mosby.)

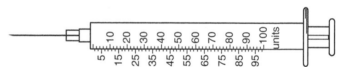

**Figure 17.14** 1-mL capacity insulin syringe (100 units) with the dual-scale odd and even calibrations.

> ⓘ **SAFETY ALERT!**
>
> Insulin is a high-alert medication. All insulin dosages should be checked by another nurse before administration to a client. Insulin is measured in units not mL.
>
> Insulin syringes are used to measure insulin **only**. Measurement of dosages that are approximate (in between lines) should be avoided. Never measure other medications measured in units in an insulin syringe (e.g., heparin).

- **Safety syringes:** Needlestick prevention is the only way to prevent transmission of blood-borne pathogens from contaminated needles. Consequently, this has resulted in special prevention techniques (e.g., no recapping of a needle after use) and development of special equipment, which includes needless syringe systems, and safety syringes with a sheath or guard that covers the needle after it is withdrawn from the skin, thereby decreasing the chance of needlestick injury. Safety syringes are available in multiple sizes and styles. An example of the safety needle technology is the safety glide syringe, which contains a protective needle guard that can be activated by a single finger to cover and seal the needle after injection (Figure 17.15). Following the administration of an injection, the nurse should **always** activate the safety device.

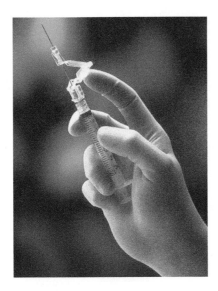

**Figure 17.15** BD Safety Glide needle. (Courtesy and copyright Becton, Dickinson and Company, Franklin Lakes, NJ.)

> ## POINTS TO REMEMBER
>
> - When parenteral medications are prepared for administration, it is important to use the correct syringe for accurate administration of the dosage.
> - Dosages must be measurable and appropriate for the syringe used.
> - Milliliters (mL) is the correct term for volume. Cubic centimeters (cc) is the amount of space that a milliliter occupies. Milliliter and cubic centimeter are not equivalent.
> - The 3-mL size syringe is the most common used for medication administration. On the 3-mL size syringe, each calibration is 0.1 mL.
> - The first line on all syringes is "zero" and referred to as the *zero line*.
> - On syringes that are 5, 6, 10, and 12 mL, each small calibration line is 0.2 mL.
> - Syringes that are 20, 30, up to 60 mL are calibrated in mL and have ounce measurements on the syringe.
> - Tuberculin syringe (1-mL) measures 0.01 mL and 0.1 mL; the calibrations are small and close together. Decimal fractions are indicated on the syringe. (Recommended for dosages less than 0.5 mL.)
> - Insulin is a high-alert medication; dosages should be checked by another nurse before administration. The insulin syringe is only used to administer insulin.
> - Insulin is administered in units, not mL.
> - Insulin syringe and tuberculin syringe are different. Confusion of the two can cause a medication error.
> - Dosages involving mL should be expressed as a decimal fraction even if the syringe has fractional markings. Milliliters is a metric measure.
> - If the dosage cannot be accurately measured, do not administer.

Before proceeding to discuss calculation of parenteral dosages, we will review some specifics in terms of reading labels. Reading the label and understanding what information is essential are important in determining the correct dosage to administer.

## Reading Parenteral Labels

The information contained on the parenteral label is similar to the information on an oral liquid label. It contains the total volume of the container and the dosage strength (amount of medication in solution) expressed in milliliters (Table 17.1). It is important to read the label carefully to determine the dosage strength and volume. Let's examine some labels.

| TABLE 17.1 | Sample Dosage Strengths |
|---|---|
| **Label** | **Interpretation** |
| Emgality 120 mg/mL | 1 mL contains 120 mg of Emgality |
| Ondansetron HCl 4 mg/2 mL | 2 mL contains 4 mg of Ondansetron HCl |
| Digoxin 500 mcg/2 mL | 2 mL contains 500 mcg of Digoxin |

The slash (/) mark used here to illustrate expression of the dosage strength as written on label. When expressing dosage strengths, do not use the slash mark. Use "per." For example, per mL is recommended by ISMP and is on the list of Error-Prone Abbreviations, Symbols, and Dose Designations. The slash mark has been mistaken for the number (1).

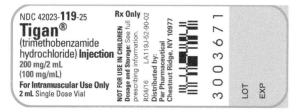

**Figure 17.16** Tigan label.

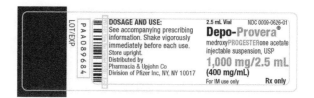

**Figure 17.17** Depo-Provera label.

The Tigan label in Figure 17.16 tells us the total size of the vial is 2 mL. The dosage strength is stated for the entire vial (200 mg per 2 mL) and per mL (100 mg per mL). The Depo-Provera label shown in Figure 17.17 indicates the total vial size is 2.5 mL. The dosage strength for the entire vial is (1,000 mg per 2.5 mL) and per mL (400 mg per mL).

Dosage strengths for parenteral medications are commonly seen expressed as the amount of medication contained in a volume of solution and expressed in milliliters. Parenteral labels can also express the dosage strength for medications in percentage strengths, ratios, units, or milliequivalents. Read labels carefully to identify the unit of measure as well as the dosage strength.

## PRACTICE **PROBLEMS**

Use the labels provided to answer the questions.

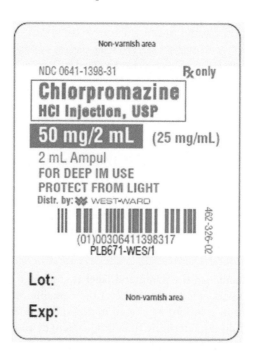

Using the chlorpromazine label above, answer the following questions:

12. a. What is the total volume of the ampul
   (ampule)?  _____

   b. What is the dosage strength?  _____

   c. If 50 mg were ordered, how many
   milliliters would this be?  _____

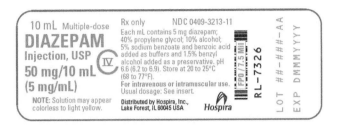

Using the Diazepam label above, answer the following questions:

13. a. What is the total volume of the vial?  _____

   b. What is the dosage strength?  _____

   c. What is the controlled substance schedule?  _____

   d. If 2.5 mL were ordered, how many
   milligrams would this be?  _____

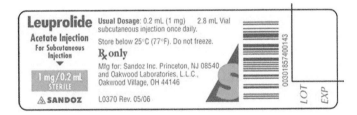

Using the Leuprolide acetate label above, answer the following questions:

14. a. What is the total volume of the vial?  _____

   b. What is the dosage strength?  _____

   c. What is the route of administration?  _____

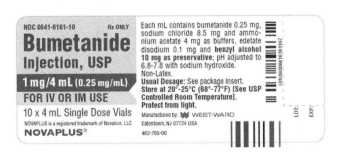

Using the Bumetanide label above, answer the following questions:

15. a. What is the total volume of the vial? _____

    b. What is the dosage strength? _____

    c. What are the directions for use? _____

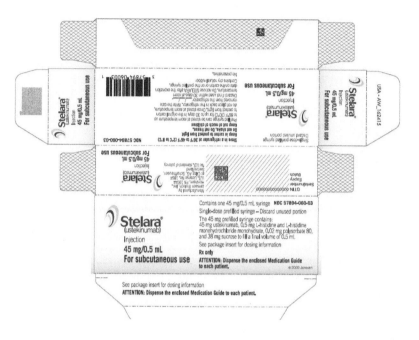

Using the Stelara label above, answer the following questions:

16. a. What is the route of administration? _____

    b. What is the dosage strength? _____

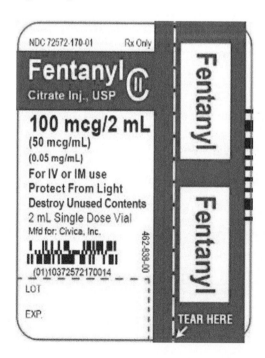

Using the Fentanyl label on the previous page, answer the following questions:

17. a. What is the dosage strength?

    b. What is the route of administration?

    c. What is the controlled substance schedule?

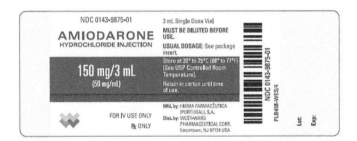

Using the furosemide label above, answer the following questions:

18. a. What is the total volume of the vial?

    b. What is the dosage strength?

    c. What are the directions for use?

    d. What type of vial is the medication packaged in?

Using the Amiodarone label above, answer the following questions:

19. a. What is the total volume of the vial?

    b. What is the dosage strength?

    c. What is the route of administration?

**Answers on p. 377**

## Medications Labeled in Percentage Strengths

Medications that are labeled as percentage solutions give information such as the percentage of the solution and the total volume of the vial or ampule. Although percentage is used, metric measures are used as well. Example: Notice the label below of lidocaine 1%, notice there are 500 mg per 50 mL (10 mg per mL). As discussed in Chapter 4, percentage solutions express the number of grams of medication per 100 mL of solution. In the lidocaine label shown, lidocaine 1% contains 1 g of medication per 100 mL of solution, 1 g per 100 mL = 1,000 mg per 100 mL = 500 mg per 50 mL (10 mg per mL).

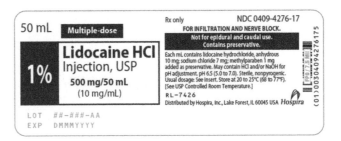

## Solutions Expressed in Ratio Strength

A medication that may be seen expressed in ratio strength is Adrenalin (epinephrine). Medications expressed this way include metric measures and are often ordered by the number of milliliters. Example: Adrenalin (epinephrine) may state 1:1,000 and indicate 1 mg per mL. Ratio solutions, as discussed in Chapter 3 on ratio and proportion, express the number of grams of the medication per total milliliters of solution. Adrenalin (epinephrine) 1:1,000 contains 1 g medication per 1,000 mL solution; 1 g: 1,000 mL = 1,000 mg : 1,000 mL = 1 mg : 1 mL. (See the label below.)

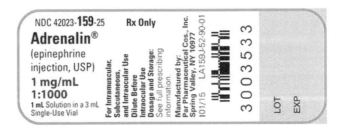

## Medications Measured in Units

Some medications measured in units for parenteral administration are heparin, Pitocin (oxytocin), insulin, and penicillin. Units measure a medication in terms of its action. Units are specific to the medication for which they are used. For example, a unit of insulin is not the same as a unit of heparin. When dosages with units are calculated, there is no conversion of units, and drugs measured in units are ordered by the number of units to be administered. See labels below, heparin 5,000 units per mL and Pitocin (oxytocin) 10 units per mL.

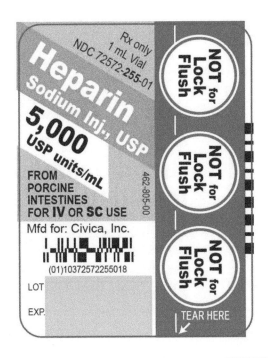

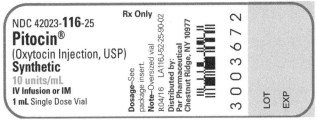

## Medications in Milliequivalents

Potassium and sodium bicarbonate are examples of medications that are expressed in milliequivalents. Like units, milliequivalents are specific measurements that have no conversion to another system and are specific to the medication used. Milliequivalents (mEq) are used to measure electrolytes (e.g., potassium) and the ionic activity of a medication. Milliequivalents are also defined as an expression of the number of grams of a medication contained in 1 mL of a normal solution. This definition is often used by a chemist or pharmacist. Refer to the potassium label below. Notice the dosage strength for the total vial is 20 mEq per 10 mL and (2 mEq per mL).

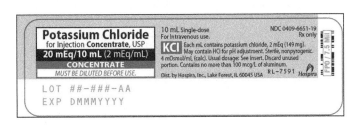

## ▦ PRACTICE **PROBLEMS**

Use the labels provided to answer the questions.

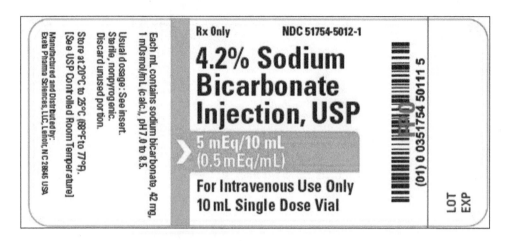

Use the sodium bicarbonate label above to answer the following questions:

20. a. What is the total volume of the vial? _____

    b. What is the dosage strength in
       milliequivalents per milliliter? _____

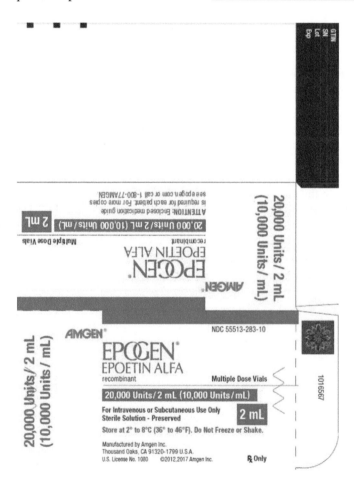

Use the Epogen label on the previous page to answer the following questions:

21. a. What is the total volume of the vial? _____

    b. What is the dosage strength? _____

    c. Directions for use _____

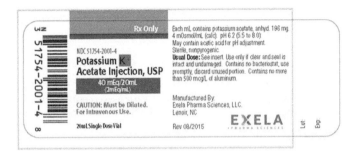

Use the potassium acetate label above to answer the following questions:

22. a. What is the total volume of the vial? _____

    b. What is the dosage strength? _____

**Answers on p. 377**

---

> **TIPS FOR CLINICAL PRACTICE**
>
> It is important to read the labels on parenteral medications carefully. Labels on parenteral medications include a variety of units to express dosage strengths. To calculate dosages to administer, it is important to know the dosage strength (the amount of medication contained in a specific volume of solution). Confusing dosage strength with total volume can lead to a medication error.

## Guidelines for Calculating and Rounding Parenteral Medications

- To calculate parenteral dosages, convert if necessary, **THINK,** and calculate using one of the methods presented (ratio and proportion, the formula method, or dimensional analysis).
- The syringe used should accurately measure the calculated dosage to administer.
- Dosage calculations sometimes result in an even answer, and you will not need to round the answer for administration. Choose the syringe in this case that allows for the accurate measurement of the calculated dose. Example: 0.35 mL can be accurately measured in a 1-mL (tuberculin) syringe, 2.2 mL can be accurately measured in a 3-mL syringe.
- When calculating parenteral dosages and the calculation does not net an answer that comes out evenly, use the following guidelines for rounding:
  a. **The 3-mL syringe** is calibrated in 0.1-increments. Round milliliters to the nearest tenth to measure in a 3-mL syringe; **never round to a whole unit.** If math calculation does not terminate evenly in the tenths place, then carry division to the hundredths place (two decimal places) and round to the nearest tenth. **Example:** 1.75 mL = 1.8 mL
  b. **The 1-mL (tuberculin) syringe** is recommended for administration of dosages less than 0.5 mL. The syringe is calibrated in 0.01-mL increments. If the math calculation does not work out evenly to the hundredths place, then the division is carried to the

thousandths (three decimal places) and rounded to the hundredths place. **Example:** 0.433 mL = 0.43 mL

   c. **Large syringes (5-, 6-, 10-, and 12-mL)** are calibrated in 0.2-mL increments. Dosages are also expressed to the nearest tenth.

- Dosages administered should be measured in milliliters and the answer labeled accordingly. The exception is insulin, which is measured in units and administered in units and administered with insulin syringes calibrated in units. (Insulin is discussed in Chapter 19.)

**TIPS FOR CLINICAL PRACTICE**

It is critical to choose the correct size syringe to ensure accurate measurement.

## Guidelines for Volume to Administer in Sites/Routes

For injectable medications, there are guidelines as to the amount of medication that can be administered in a single site/route. (See Table 17.2.) It is recommended that when the amount exceeds the amount that can be administered in a single site, divide the amount into two injections. When administering medications by injection, consider the condition of the client, site selected, and absorption and consistency of the medication. Depending on his or her condition, a client may not be able to tolerate the maximum dosage volumes.

**SAFETY ALERT!**

When the dosage for parenteral administration exceeds the guidelines of volume that can be administered in a single injection site/route, the dosage should be questioned and calculation double-checked. Dosages larger than the maximum volume are rare and can cause harm to a client.

| TABLE 17.2 | Maximum Volume for Sites/Routes |
|---|---|
| **Route/Site** | **Maximum Volume** |
| Intramuscular: | |
|    Adult | 3 mL |
|    Deltoid muscle | 1 mL |
|    Children 6 -12 years | 2 mL |
|    Children 0 -5 years | 1 mL |
| Adult: Subcutaneous (subcut) | 1 mL |
| Adult: Intravenous (IV) added to solution | May have a volume greater than 5 mL |

## Calculating Injectable Medications

Now that you have an understanding of syringes and guidelines, let's begin calculating dosages. Regardless of the method used to calculate, the following steps are used:

1. Check to make sure everything is in the same system and unit of measure.
2. Think critically and estimate what the logical volume to administer should be.
3. Calculate: use ratio and proportion, the formula method, or dimensional analysis to calculate the dosage.
4. Consider the type of syringe being used. **The cardinal rule should always be that any dosage given must be able to be measured accurately in the syringe you are using.** Let's look at some sample problems.

**Example 1:**  Order: Gentamicin 75 mg IM q8h.

          Available: Gentamicin labeled 40 mg per mL.

*Note:* No conversion is necessary here. Think—The dosage ordered is going to be more than 1 mL but less than 2 mL. Set up and solve.

### ✓ Solution Using Ratio and Proportion

Linear Format: 40 mg : 1 mL = 75 mg : $x$ mL

$$\frac{40x}{40} = \frac{75}{40}$$

$$x = \frac{75}{40}$$

$$x = 1.87 = 1.9 \text{ mL}$$

Fraction Format:

$$\frac{40 \text{ mg}}{1 \text{ mL}} = \frac{75 \text{ mg}}{x \text{ mL}}$$

$$\frac{40x}{40} = \frac{75}{40}$$

$$x = \frac{75}{40}$$

$$x = 1.87 = 1.9 \text{ mL}$$

Answer:    1.9 mL

The answer here is rounded to the nearest tenth of a milliliter. Remember that you are using a small hypodermic syringe marked in tenths of a milliliter.

### ✓ Solution Using the Formula Method

$$\frac{\text{(D) 75 mg}}{\text{(H) 40 mg}} \times \text{(Q) 1 mL} = x \text{ mL}$$

$$x = \frac{75}{40}$$

$$x = 1.87 = 1.9 \text{ mL}$$

Answer:    1.9 mL

### ✓ Solution Using Dimensional Analysis

$$x \text{ mL} = \frac{1 \text{ mL}}{40 \text{ mg}} \times \frac{75 \text{ mg}}{1}$$

$$x = \frac{75}{40}$$

$$x = 1.87 = 1.9 \text{ mL}$$

Answer:    1.9 mL

Refer to the syringe below illustrating 1.9 mL shaded in on the syringe.

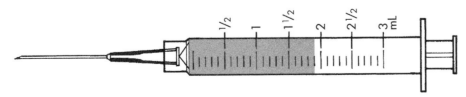

**Example 2:**   Order: Ceftriaxone 0.25 g IM stat q12h for 5 days.

Available: Ceftriaxone labeled 350 mg per 1 mL.

In this problem, a conversion is necessary. Equivalent: 1,000 mg = 1 g. Convert what is ordered to what is available: 0.25 g = 250 mg.

Think—The dosage you will need to give is less than 1 mL, and it is being given intramuscularly. The dosage therefore should fall within the range that is safe for IM administration. The solution, after making conversion, is as follows:

---

### ✓ Solution Using Ratio and Proportion

Linear Format: 350 mg : 1 mL = 250 mg : $x$ mL

$$\frac{350x}{350} = \frac{250}{350}$$

$$x = \frac{250}{350}$$

$$x = 0.71 = 0.7 \text{ mL}$$

Fraction Format: $\dfrac{350 \text{ mg}}{1 \text{ mL}} = \dfrac{250 \text{ mg}}{x \text{ mL}}$

$$\frac{350x}{350} = \frac{250}{350}$$

$$x = \frac{250}{350}$$

$$x = 0.71 = 0.7 \text{ mL}$$

**Answer:**      0.7 mL

---

### ✓ Solution Using the Formula Method

$$\frac{\text{(D) } 250 \text{ mg}}{\text{(H) } 350 \text{ mg}} \times \text{(Q) } 1 \text{ mL} = x \text{ mL}$$

$$x = \frac{250}{350}$$

$$x = 0.71 = 0.7 \text{ mL}$$

---

### ✓ Solution Using Dimensional Analysis

$$x \text{ mL} = \frac{1 \text{ mL}}{350 \text{ mg}} \times \frac{1,000 \text{ mg}}{1 \text{ g}} \times \frac{0.25 \text{ g}}{1}$$

$$x = \frac{1,000 \times 0.25}{350}$$

$$x = \frac{250}{350}$$

$$x = 0.71 = 0.7 \text{ mL}$$

**Answer:**      0.7 mL

Refer to the syringe below illustrating 0.7 mL drawn up.

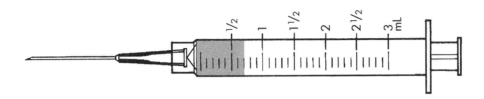

**Example 3:**  Order: Atropine sulfate 0.6 mg subcut stat.

Available: Atropine sulfate labeled 1 mg per mL.

---

## ✔ PROBLEM SETUP

1. No conversion is necessary.
2. Think—You will need less than 1 mL to administer the required dosage.
3. Set up the problem, and calculate the dosage to be administered.

---

### ✔ Solution Using Ratio and Proportion

Linear Format: 1 mg : 1 mL = 0.6 mg : $x$ mL

$$\frac{1x}{1} = \frac{0.6}{1}$$

$$x = \frac{0.6}{1}$$

$$x = 0.6 \text{ mL}$$

Fraction Format: $\dfrac{1 \text{ mg}}{1 \text{ mL}} = \dfrac{0.6 \text{ mg}}{x \text{ mL}}$

$$\frac{1}{1}\frac{x}{} = \frac{0.6}{1}$$

$$x = \frac{0.6}{1}$$

$$x = 0.6 \text{ mL}$$

**Answer:**     0.6 mL

---

### ✔ Solution Using the Formula Method

$$\frac{\text{(D) } 0.6 \text{ mg}}{\text{(H) } 1 \text{ mg}} \times \text{(Q) } 1 \text{ mL} = x \text{ mL}$$

$$x = \frac{0.6}{1}$$

$$x = 0.6 \text{ mL}$$

**Answer:**     0.6 mL

### ✓ Solution Using Dimensional Analysis

$$x\,\text{mL} = \frac{1\text{ mL}}{1\text{ mg}} \times \frac{0.6\text{ mg}}{1}$$

$$x = \frac{0.6}{1}$$

$$x = 0.6\text{ mL}$$

**Answer:**     0.6 mL

Refer to the illustration below showing 0.6 mL shaded in on the syringe.

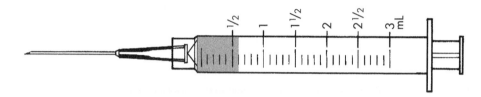

## Calculating Dosages for Medications in Units

As previously mentioned, certain medications are measured in units. Some medications measured in units include vitamins, antibiotics, insulin, and heparin. In determining the dosage to administer when medications are measured in units, use the same steps as with other parenteral medications. Dosages of certain medications such as heparin are administered with a tuberculin syringe. Heparin will also be discussed in more detail in Chapter 22. Let's look at sample problems with units.

**Example 1:**   Order: Heparin 750 units subcut daily.

Available: Heparin 1,000 units per mL

Using a 1-mL (tuberculin) syringe, calculate the dosage to be administered.

### ✓ PROBLEM SETUP

1. No conversion is required. No conversion exists for units.
2. Think—The dosage to be given is less than 1 mL. This dosage can be accurately measured in a 1-mL tuberculin syringe. Heparin is administered in exact dosages.
3. Set up the problem, and calculate the dosage to be given.

> **⊘ SAFETY ALERT!**
> Because of the action of heparin, an exact dosage is crucial; the dosage should not be rounded off.

### ✓ Solution Using Ratio and Proportion

Linear Format: 1,000 units : 1 mL = 750 units : $x$ mL

$$\frac{1,000x}{1,000} = \frac{750}{1,000}$$

$$x = \frac{75}{1,000}$$

$$x = 0.75\text{ mL}$$

$$\text{Fraction Format:} \frac{1{,}000 \text{ units}}{1 \text{ mL}} = \frac{750 \text{ units}}{x \text{ mL}}$$

$$\frac{1{,}000x}{1{,}000} = \frac{750}{1{,}000}$$

$$x = \frac{750}{1{,}000}$$

$$x = 0.75 \text{ mL}$$

**Answer:**      0.75 mL

---

### ✓ Solution Using the Formula Method

$$\frac{\text{(D) } 750 \text{ units}}{\text{(H) } 1{,}000 \text{ units}} \times \text{(Q) } 1 \text{ mL} = x \text{ mL}$$

$$x = \frac{750}{1{,}000}$$

$$x = 0.75 \text{ mL}$$

**Answer:**      0.75 mL

---

### ✓ Solution Using Dimensional Analysis

$$x \text{ mL} = \frac{1 \text{ mL}}{1{,}00\cancel{0} \text{ units}} \times \frac{75\cancel{0} \text{ units}}{1} \qquad \text{(Note cancellation of zeros to make numbers smaller.)}$$

$$x = \frac{75}{100}$$

$$x = 0.75 \text{ mL}$$

**Answer:**      0.75 mL

Refer to the syringe illustrating 0.75 mL shaded in.

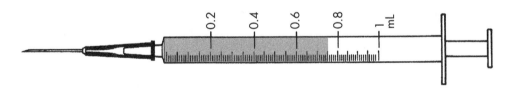

**Example 2:**  Order: Penicillin G procaine, 500,000 units IM b.i.d.

Available: Penicillin G procaine labeled 300,000 units per mL

✅ **PROBLEM SETUP**

1. No conversion is required.
2. Think—The dosage ordered is more than the available strength. Therefore more than 1 mL would be required to administer the dosage.
3. Set up the problem using ratio and proportion, the formula method, or dimensional analysis to calculate the dosage.

---

✔ **Solution Using Ratio and Proportion**

Linear Format: 300,000 units : 1 mL = 500,000 units : $x$ mL

$$\frac{300,000x}{300,000} = \frac{500,000}{300,000}$$

$$x = \frac{500,000}{300,000}$$

$$x = \frac{5}{3}$$

$$x = 1.66 = 1.7 \text{ mL}$$

Fraction Format:

$$\frac{300,000 \text{ units}}{1 \text{ mL}} = \frac{500,000 \text{ units}}{x \text{ mL}}$$

$$\frac{300,000x}{300,000} = \frac{500,000}{300,000}$$

$$x = \frac{500,000}{300,000}$$

$$x = \frac{5}{3}$$

$$x = 1.66 = 1.7 \text{ mL}$$

Answer:    1.7 mL

*Note:* Math was carried two decimal places to round to 1.7 mL. Small hypodermic was marked in tenths of a mL.

---

✔ **Solution Using the Formula Method**

$$\frac{\text{(D) } 500,000 \text{ units}}{\text{(H) } 300,000 \text{ units}} \times \text{(Q) } 1 \text{ mL} = x \text{ mL}$$

$$x = \frac{500,000}{300,000}$$

$$x = 1.66 = 1.7 \text{ mL}$$

Answer:    1.7 mL

### ✓ Solution Using Dimensional Analysis

$$x \, mL = \frac{1 \, mL}{300{,}000 \, \cancel{units}} \times \frac{500{,}000 \, \cancel{units}}{1}$$

$$x = \frac{500{,}000}{300{,}000}$$

$$x = 1.66 = 1.7 \, mL$$

Answer:     1.7 mL

Refer to the syringe illustrating 1.7 mL shaded in.

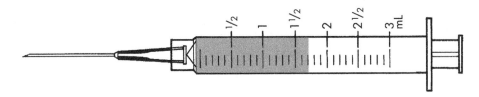

> **SAFETY ALERT!**
>
> Read orders carefully when they are expressed in units. Units should **NOT** be abbreviated in orders. To avoid confusion, The Joint Commission (TJC) has placed the abbreviations for units (U) on the "Do Not Use" list. This abbreviation is also on ISMP's (Institute for Safe Medication Practices) Error Prone Abbreviations, Symbols, and Dose Designations. Prescribers are required to write out the word units to help prevent mis- interpretation of an order—for example, "50 Ʊ" as "500 units." (Notice that the U is almost closed; it could be mistaken for a zero and misinterpreted as 500 units.) This error could be fatal.

## Mixing Medications in the Same Syringe

Two medications may be mixed in one syringe if they are compatible with each other and the total amount does not exceed the amount that can be safely administered in a site. Always consult a reliable reference in regard to compatibility of medications before mixing medications.

When mixing two medications for administration in one syringe, calculate the dosage to be administered in milliliters to the nearest tenth for each of the medications ordered. Then add the results to find the total volume to be combined and administered.

Example:     Order: Demerol 65 mg IM and Vistaril 25 mg IM q4h p.r.n. for pain.

Available: Demerol 75 mg per mL and Vistaril 50 mg per mL.

Solution: Demerol dosage 0.86 = 0.9 mL

Visatril dosage 0.5 mL

0.9 mL Demerol + 0.5 mL Vistaril = 1.4 mL (total volume)

Dosage shaded in one syringe:

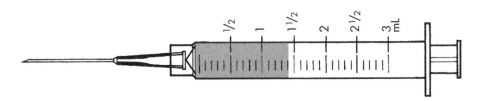

**POINTS TO REMEMBER**

- Read labels carefully. Do not confuse dosage strength with total volume.
- There is no conversion of units and milliequivalents.
- Do not exceed the dosage administration guidelines for parenteral administration. (IM—maximum 3 mL for an average-size adult, 1 mL for deltoid, 2 mL for children ages 6–12, 0–5 years 1 mL).
- Subcut maximum 1 mL for an adult.
- Calculate parenteral dosage problems using any of the methods presented (ratio and proportion, formula method, or dimensional analysis).
- 3-mL syringe calibrated in 0.1 mL. Round mL to the nearest tenth.
- 1-mL syringe calibrated in 0.01-mL and 0.1 increments. Math that does not terminate evenly in hundredths is carried to thousandths and rounded to hundredths.
- 5-, 6-, and 12-mL syringes are calibrated in 0.2 mL. Dosages are expressed to the nearest tenth.
- Two medications can be administered in the same syringe if compatible. Calculate the dosage to be administered in mL to the nearest tenth for each of the medications. Add the result to get the total volume to administer.
- Choose the correct size syringe to accurately administer the dosage. Read the calibrations carefully.

## PRACTICE **PROBLEMS**

Calculate the dosages for the problems below, and indicate the number of milliliters you will administer. Shade in the dosage on the syringe provided. Use medication labels or information provided to calculate the volume necessary to administer the dosage ordered. Express your answers in milliliters to the nearest tenth except where indicated.

23. Order: Haloperidol 5 mg IM stat.

Available:

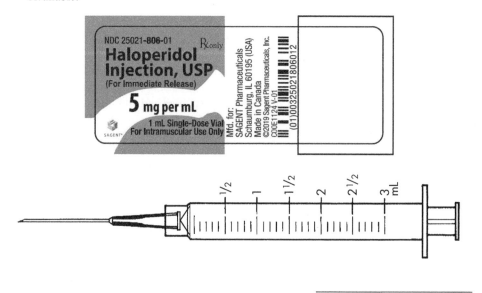

24. Order: Methylprednisolone 60 mg IM stat.

    Available:

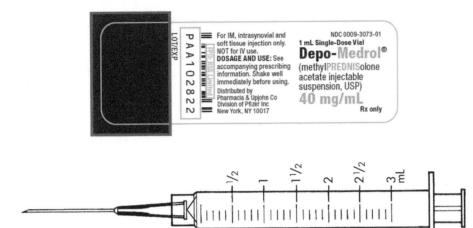

25. Order: Meperidine 50 mg IM and Hydroxine 25 mg IM q4h p.r.n. for pain.

    Available:

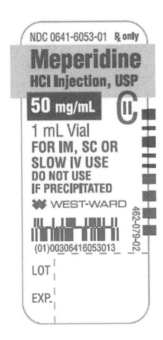

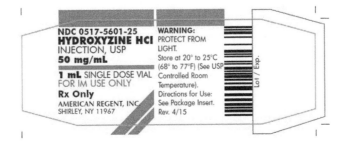

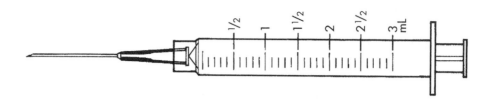

26. Order: Heparin 5,000 units subcut daily.

    Available:

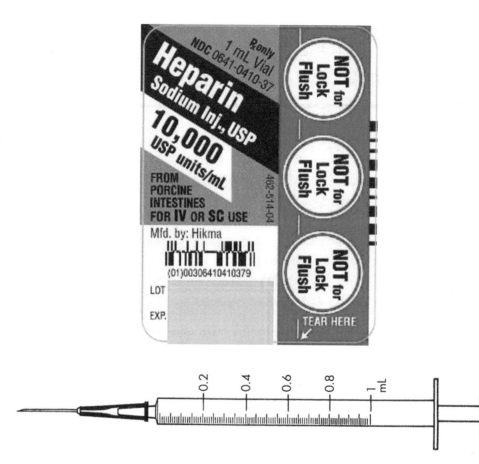

27. Order: Morphine sulfate 10 mg IM q4h p.r.n. for pain.

    Available:

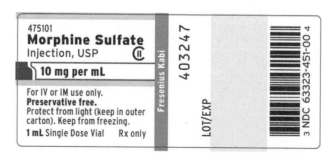

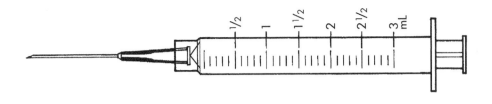

_____

**Answers on p. 378**

## 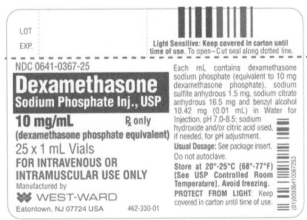 CLINICAL **REASONING**

**Scenario:** Prescriber ordered the following:

Hydroxyzine 50 mg IM q4h p.r.n. for anxiety.

The nurse, in error, administered hydralazine 50 mg IM from a vial labeled 20 mg per mL and administered 2.5 mL.

a. What client right was violated? _____

b. What contributed to the error made? _____

c. What is the potential outcome from the error? _____

d. What measures could have been taken to prevent the error? _____

**Answers on p. 378**

## NGN Case Study

**Case Scenario:** A client arrives to the postanesthesia care unit after having an appendectomy. The client has a history of postoperative nausea and vomiting. The nurse has an order to give dexamethasone 4 mg IV stat. **Using the label below, complete the following sentences by choosing from the list of options.**

LOT

EXP.

**Light Sensitive: Keep covered in carton until time of use. To open–Cut seal along dotted line.**

NDC 0641-0367-25

**Dexamethasone**
Sodium Phosphate Inj., USP

**10 mg/mL**    ℞ only
(dexamethasone phosphate equivalent)

25 x 1 mL Vials
FOR INTRAVENOUS OR
INTRAMUSCULAR USE ONLY
Manufactured by
WEST-WARD
Eatontown, NJ 07724 USA    462-330-01

Each mL contains dexamethasone sodium phosphate (equivalent to 10 mg dexamethasone phosphate), sodium sulfite anhydrous 1.5 mg, sodium citrate anhydrous 16.5 mg and benzyl alcohol 10.42 mg (0.01 mL) in Water for Injection. pH 7.0-8.5; sodium hydroxide and/or citric acid used, if needed, for pH adjustment.
Usual Dosage: See package insert.
Do not autoclave.
Store at 20°-25°C (68°-77°F) [See USP Controlled Room Temperature]. Avoid freezing.
PROTECT FROM LIGHT: Keep covered in carton until time of use.

The nurse would first determine the dosage strength of dexamethasone to be _____1_____. The nurse would calculate the correct volume to administer as _____2_____. The appropriate size syringe to use would be _____3_____.

| 1 | 2 | 3 |
|---|---|---|
| 16.5 mg per mL | 0.4 mL | 5 mL |
| 10 mg per mL | 0.25 mL | 3 mL |
| 1.5 mg per mL | 2.67 mL | 1 mL |

**Reference:** Morris D: _Calculate with confidence_, ed 8, St Louis, Elsevier, copyright 2022. _Case Study answers and rationales can be found on Evolve._

## ◉ CHAPTER **REVIEW**

Calculate the dosages for the problems that follow, and indicate the number of milliliters you will administer. Shade in the dosage on the syringe provided. Use medication labels or information provided to calculate the volume necessary to administer the dosage ordered. Express your answers to the nearest tenth except where indicated.

1. Order: Sandostatin 175 mcg subcut q12h. (Express your answer in hundredths.)

    Available:

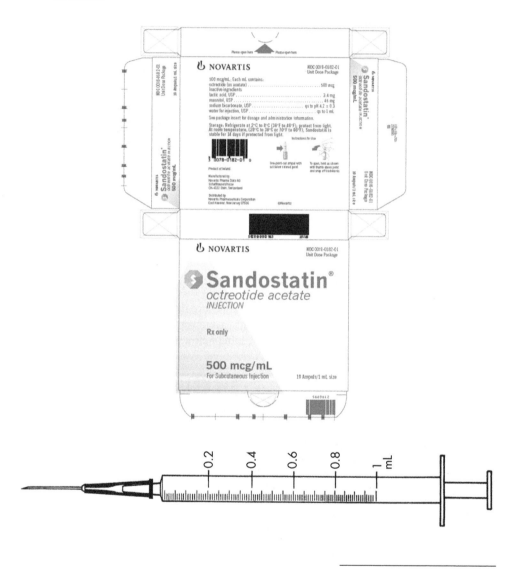

———————————————

2. Order: Ketorolac 25 mg IM q6h p.r.n. for pain.

   Available:

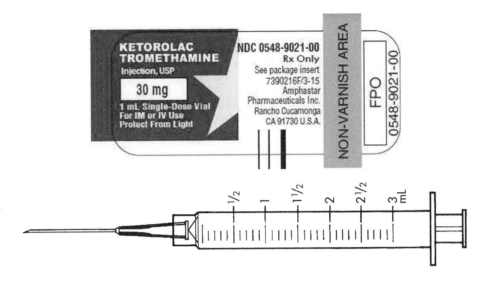

3. Order: Digoxin 125 mcg IM daily.

   Available:

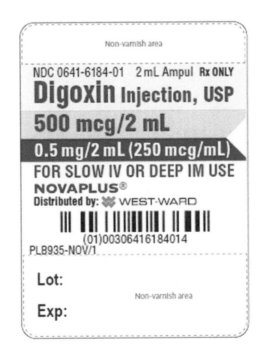

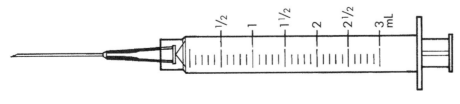

4.  Order: Bicillin C-R (900/300) 1,200,000 units IM stat.

Available:

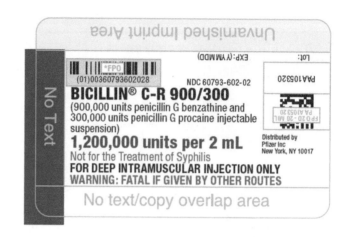

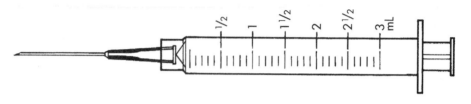

5.  Order: Methylprednisolone 100 mg IV q8h for 2 doses.

Available: *Reconstituted medication

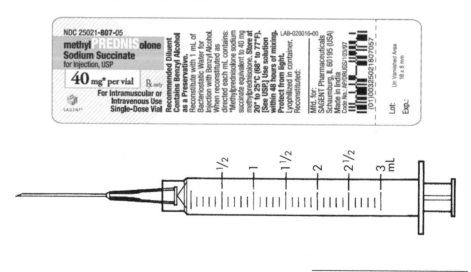

6. Order: Ondansetron 4 mg IV q4h.

    Available:

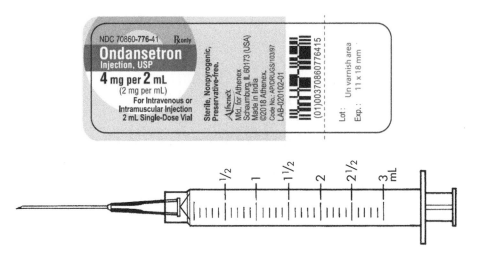

_____

7. Order: Phenytoin Sodium 200 mg IV stat.

    Available:

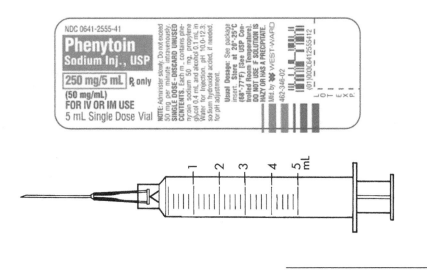

_____

8. Order: Famotidine 40 mg IV at bedtime.

Available:

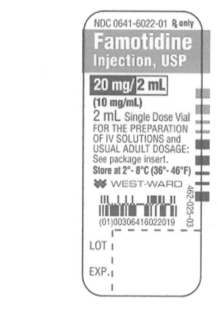

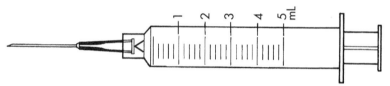

_____

9. Order: Tobramycin 50 mg IM q8h.

Available:

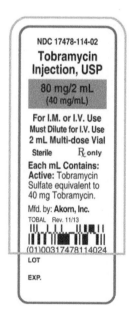

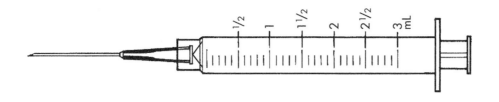

10. Order: Solu-Cortef 400 mg IV every day for a severe inflammation for 5 days.

    Available:

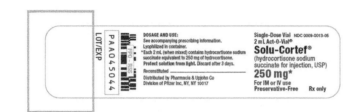

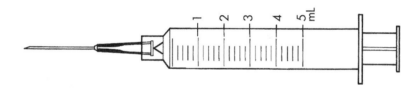

11. Order: Naloxone 0.2 mg IM stat.

    Available:

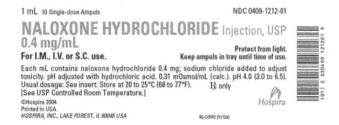

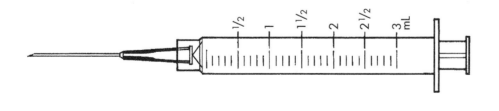

12. Order: Robinul (glycopyrrolate) 200 mcg IM on call to the O.R.

Available:

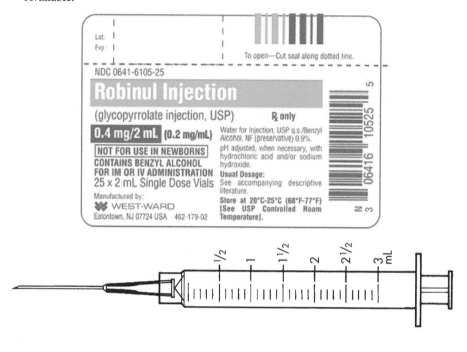

13. Order: Aranesp 30 mcg subcut stat. (Express your answer in hundredths.)

Available:

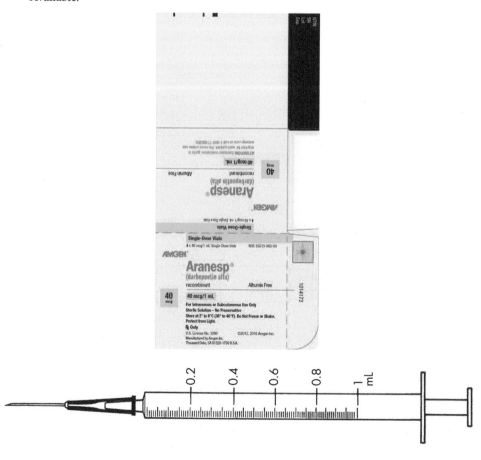

14. Order: Propranolol 250 mcg IV stat.

    Available:

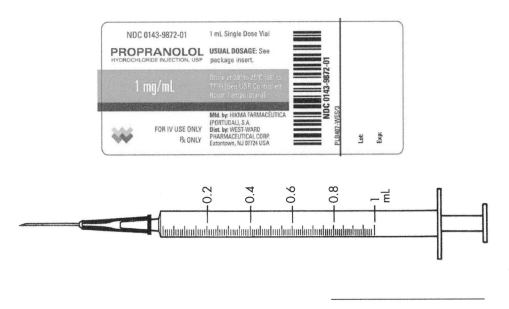

15. Order: Ativan 1.5 mg IM b.i.d. p.r.n. for agitation.

    Available:

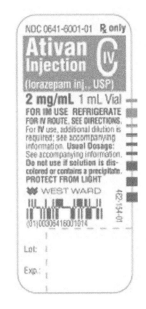

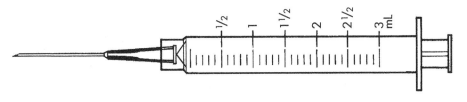

16. Order: Metoclopramide (Reglan) 15 mg IV stat.

    Available:

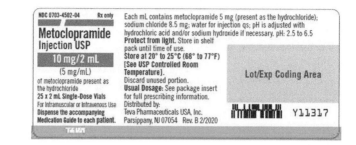

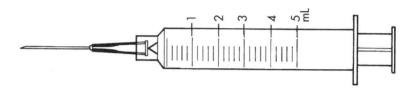

_____

17. Order: Valium (diazepam) 7.5 mg IM stat.

    Available:

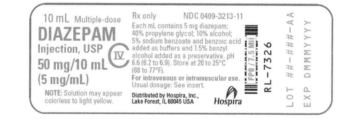

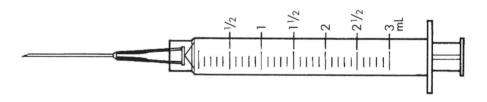

_____

18. Order: Bumetanide 1 mg IV daily.

    Available:

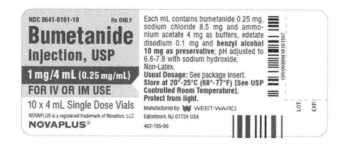

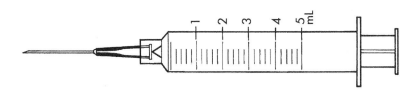

_____

19. Order: Gentamicin 55 mg IV q8h.

    Available:

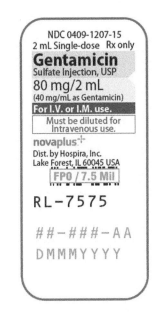

NDC 0409-1207-15
2 mL Single-dose   Rx only
**Gentamicin**
Sulfate Injection, USP
**80 mg/2 mL**
(40 mg/mL as Gentamicin)
**For I.V. or I.M. use.**
Must be diluted for
Intravenous use.
novaplus⁺
Dist. by Hospira, Inc.
Lake Forest, IL 60045 USA
FPO / 7.5 Mil

RL-7575

##-###-AA
DMMMYYYY

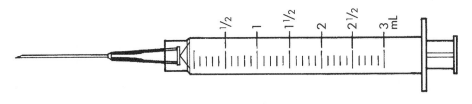

_____

20. Order: Granisetron HCl 125 mcg IV 20 minutes before start of chemotherapy.

    Available:

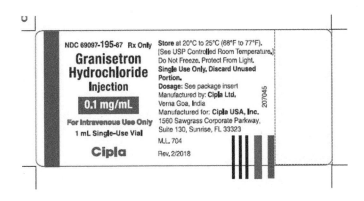

NDC 69097-**195**-67   Rx Only
**Granisetron Hydrochloride**
Injection
**0.1 mg/mL**
For Intravenous Use Only
1 mL Single-Use Vial
**Cipla**

Store at 20°C to 25°C (68°F to 77°F).
[See USP Controlled Room Temperature.]
Do Not Freeze. Protect From Light.
Single Use Only. Discard Unused Portion.
**Dosage:** See package insert
Manufactured by: Cipla Ltd.
Verna Goa, India
Manufactured for: Cipla USA, Inc.
1560 Sawgrass Corporate Parkway,
Suite 130, Sunrise, FL 33323
M.L. 704
Rev. 2/2018

207045

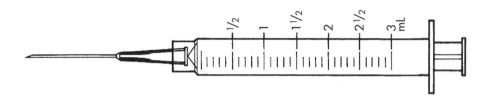

---

21. Order: Demerol (meperidine) 65 mg IM and Hydroxyzine HCl 25 mg IM q4h p.r.n. for pain.

Available:

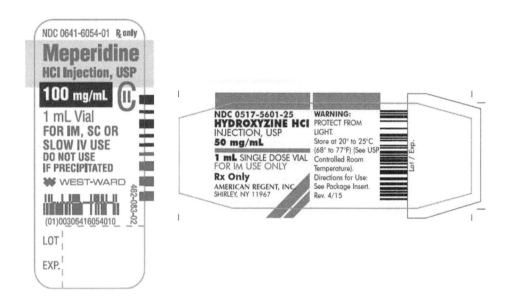

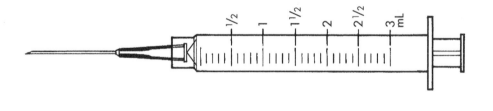

---

22. Order: Decadron (dexamethasone) 9 mg IV daily for 4 days.

    Available:

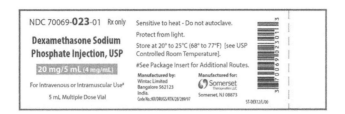

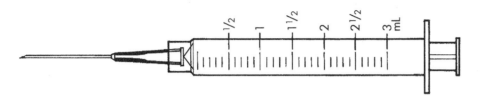

23. Order: Sublimaze (fentanyl) 60 mcg IM 30 minutes before surgery.

    Available:

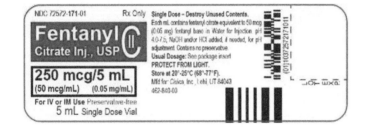

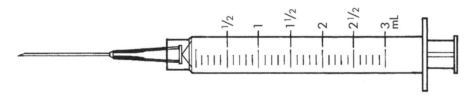

24. Order: Neupogen 300 mcg subcut every day for 2 weeks.

    Available: Prefilled syringe of Neupogen

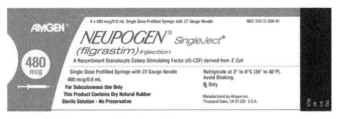

a. How many mL will the nurse administer? _____
b. How many mL will the nurse discard from the prefilled syringe? _____

25. Order: Stelara 45 mg subcut as an initial dose.

   Available: Prefilled syringe of Stelara

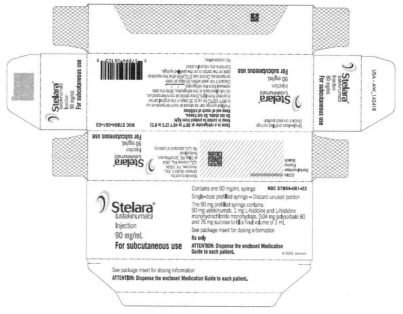

   a.  How many mL will the nurse administer? _____
   b.  How many mL will the nurse discard from the prefilled syringe? _____

26. Order: Ilumya 100 mg subcut at Week 4 for a client being treated for plaque psoriasis.

   Available: A prefilled syringe of Ilumya

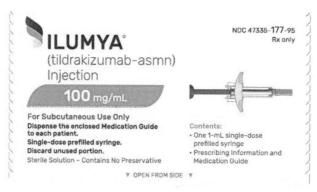

   a.  How many mL will the nurse administer? _____
   b.  How many mL will the nurse discard from the prefilled syringe? _____

**Answers on pp. 379-383**

For additional practice problems, refer to the Parenteral Dosages section of the Elsevier's Interactive Drug Calculation Application, Version 1, on Evolve.

# ⭐ ANSWERS

## Chapter 17
### Answers to Practice Problems

> **NOTE**
> Problems requiring conversion reflect conversion of what the prescriber ordered to what is available.

1.

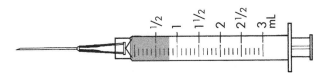

2.

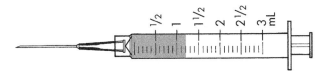

3.

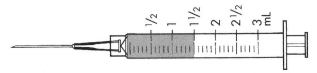

4.

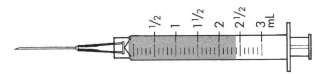

5. 1.4 mL
6. 1 mL
7. 0.9 mL
8. 0.4 mL
9. 4.4 mL
10. 7 mL
11. 3.2 mL
12. a. 2 mL
    b. 50 mg per 2 mL, 25 mg per mL
    c. 2 mL

13. a. 10 mL
    b. 50 mg per 10 mL, 5 mg per mL
    c. IV, 4
    d. 12.5 mg
14. a. 2.8 mL
    b. 1 mg per 0.2 mL
    c. subcut
15. a. 4 mL
    b. 1 mg per 4 mL, 0.25 mg per mL
    c. For IV or IM use
16. a. subcut
    b. 45 mg per 0.5 mL
17. a. 100 mcg per 2 mL, 50 mcg per mL
    b. IV or IM
    c. 11, 2
18. a. 10 mL
    b. 100 mg per 10 mL, 10 mg per mL
    c. For IV or IM use
    d. Single-dose vial
19. a. 3 mL
    b. 150 mg per 3 mL,
       50 mg per mL
    c. IV use only
20. a. 10 mL
    b. 0.5 mEq per mL
21. a. 2 mL
    b. 20,000 units per 2 mL, 10,000 units per mL
    c. For IV or subcut use only
22. a. 20 mL
    b. 40 mEq per 20 mL, 2 mEq per mL

23. 5 mg : 1 mL = 5 mg : $x$ mL

    *or*

    $$\frac{5\ mg}{20\ mg} \times 5\ mL = x\ mL$$

    Answer: 1 mL. The dosage ordered is contained in the available strength; therefore you will need 1 mL to administer the dosage.

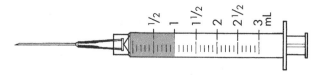

24. 40 mg : 1 mL = 60 mg : $x$ mL

    *or*

    $$\frac{60\ mg}{40\ mg} \times 1\ mL = x\ mL$$

    Answer: 1.5 mL. The dosage ordered is more than the available strength; therefore you will need more than 1 mL to administer the dosage.

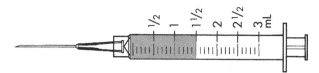

25. Meperidine : 50 mg : 1 mL = 50 mg : $x$ mL

    *or*

    $$\frac{50\ mg}{50\ mg} \times 1\ mL = x\ mL$$

    Answer: 1 mL. The dosage ordered is contained in the available strength; therefore you will need 1 mL to administer the dosage.

    Hydroxyzine: 50 mg : 1 mL = 25 mg : $x$ mL

    *or*

    $$\frac{25\ mg}{50\ mg} \times 1\ mL = x\ mL$$

Answer: 0.5 mL. The dosage ordered is less than the available strength; therefore you will need less than 1 mL to administer the dosage. The total number of milliliters you will prepare to administer is 1.5 mL (1 mL Meperidine + 0.5 mL Hydroxyzine = 1.5 mL). Medications may be administered in the same syringe as long as they are compatible.

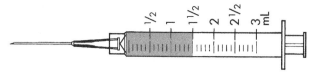

26. 10,000 units : 1 mL = 5,000 units : $x$ mL

    *or*

    $$\frac{5{,}000\ units}{10{,}000\ units} \times 1\ mL = x\ mL$$

    Answer: 0.5 mL. The dosage ordered is less than the available strength; therefore you will need less than 1 mL to administer the dosage.

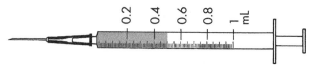

27. 10 mg : 1 mL = 10 mg : $x$ mL

    *or*

    $$\frac{10\ mg}{10\ mg} \times 1\ mL = x\ mL$$

    Answer: 1 mL. The label indicates that the dosage ordered is contained in 1 mL.

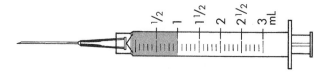

## Answers to Clinical Reasoning Questions

a. The right medication. Hydroxyzine and hydralazine have similar names but are two different medications.

b. Not reading the medication labels carefully and comparing them with the order, or medication administration record (MAR).

c. Hydralazine is an antihypertensive and could cause a fatal drop in the client's blood pressure.

d. Carefully comparing the medication label and dosage with the order or MAR three times while preparing the medication. Perhaps if the nurse had consulted a reliable drug reference, it may have alerted the nurse to the fact that hydralazine is used to treat hypertension and hydroxyzine is used for anxiety, which is what the medication was prescribed for.

## Answers to Chapter Review

1. 500 mcg : 1 mL = 175 mcg : $x$ mL

*or*

$$\frac{175 \text{ mcg}}{500 \text{ mcg}} \times 1 \text{ mL} = x \text{ mL}$$

Answer: 0.35 mL. The dosage ordered is less than the available strength. Therefore you will need less than 1 mL to administer the dosage.

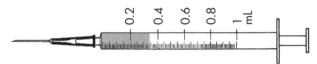

2. 30 mg : 1 mL = 25 mg : $x$ mL

*or*

$$\frac{25 \text{ mg}}{30 \text{ mg}} \times 1 \text{ mL} = x \text{ mL}$$

Answer: 0.83 mL = 0.8 mL. The dosage ordered is less than what is available. Therefore you will need less than 1 mL to administer the dosage.

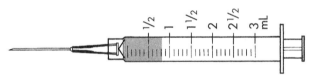

3. No conversion is required. Label indicates dosage in micrograms.

500 mcg : 2 mL = 125 mcg : $x$ mL

*or*

$$\frac{125 \text{ mcg}}{500 \text{ mcg}} \times 2 \text{ mL} = x \text{ mL}$$

Answer: 0.5 mL. The dosage ordered is less than the available strength. The dosage required would be less than 2 mL.

Alternate solution:

250 mcg : 1 mL = 125 mcg : $x$ mL

*or*

$$\frac{125 \text{ mcg}}{250 \text{ mcg}} \times 1 \text{ mL} = x \text{ mL}$$

This would net the same answer, 0.5 mL.

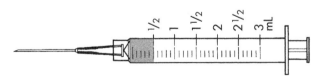

4. 1,200,000 units : 2 mL = 1,200,000 units : $x$ mL

*or*

$$\frac{1,200,000 \text{ units}}{1,200,000 \text{ units}} \times 2 \text{ mL} = x \text{ mL}$$

Answer: 2 mL. The dosage ordered is contained in 2 mL; therefore you will need 2 mL to administer the dosage.

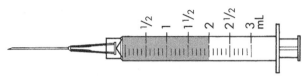

5. 40 mg : 1 mL = 100 mg : $x$ mL

*or*

$$\frac{100 \text{ mg}}{40 \text{ mg}} \times 1 \text{ mL} = x \text{ mL}$$

Answer: 2.5 mL. The amount ordered is more than the available strength; therefore you will need more than 1 mL to administer the required dosage.

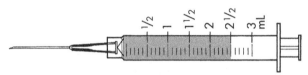

**NOTE**

You would need three (3) vials of the medication to obtain the indicated dose. The total volume available in the vial is 1 mL, which contains 40 mg.

6. 2 mg : 1 mL = 4 mg : $x$ mL

*or*

$$\frac{4 \text{ mg}}{2 \text{ mg}} \times 1 \text{ mL} = x \text{ mL}$$

Answer: 2 mL. The dosage ordered is more than the available strength; therefore you will need more than 1 mL to administer the dosage.

Alternate solution:

4 mg : 2 mL = 4 mg : $x$ mL

*or*

$$\frac{4 \text{ mg}}{4 \text{ mg}} \times 2 \text{ mL} = x \text{ mL}$$

This setup will give an answer of 2 mL.

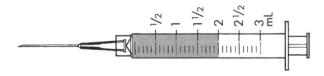

7. 250 mg : 5 mL = 200 mg : $x$ mL

*or*

$$\frac{200 \text{ mg}}{250 \text{ mg}} \times 5 \text{ mL} = x \text{ mL}$$

Answer: 4 mL. The dosage ordered is less than the available strength; therefore you will need less than 5 mL to administer the dosage.

Alternate solution:

50 mg : 1 mL = 200 mg : $x$ mL

*or*

$$\frac{200 \text{ mg}}{250 \text{ mg}} \times 1 \text{ mL} = x \text{ mL}$$

This setup will yield an answer of 4 mL.

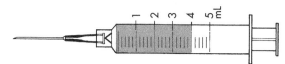

8. 20 mg : 2 mL = 40 mg : $x$ mL

*or*

$$\frac{40 \text{ mg}}{20 \text{ mg}} \times 2 \text{ mL} = x \text{ mL}$$

Answer: 4 mL. The dosage ordered is more than the available strength. Therefore you will need more than 2 mL to administer the dosage.

Alternate solution:

10 mg : 1 mL = 40 mg : $x$ mL

*or*

$$\frac{40 \text{ mg}}{10 \text{ mg}} \times 1 \text{ mL} = x \text{ mL}$$

This setup will yield an answer of 4 mL.

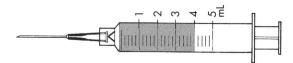

> **NOTE**
> You would need two (2) vials of the medication to administer the ordered dose. The total volume available in the vial is 2 mL, which is equal to 20 mg.

9. 40 mg : 1 mL = 50 mg : $x$ mL

*or*

$$\frac{50 \text{ mg}}{40 \text{ mg}} \times 1 \text{ mL} = x \text{ mL}$$

Answer: 1.3 mL. 1.25 mL is rounded to nearest tenth. The dosage ordered is more than the available strength per mL if you use 40 mg per mL. You will need more than 1 mL to administer the dosage.

Alternate solution:

80 mg : 2 mL = 50 mg : $x$ mL

*or*

$$\frac{50 \text{ mg}}{80 \text{ mg}} \times 2 \text{ mL} = x \text{ mL}$$

This setup still gives an answer of 1.3 mL.

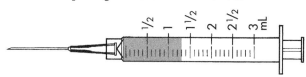

10. 250 mg : 2 mL = 400 mg : $x$ mL

*or*

$$\frac{400 \text{ mg}}{250 \text{ mg}} \times 2 \text{ mL} = x \text{ mL}$$

Answer: 3.2 mL. The dosage ordered is more than the available strength. You will need more than 2 mL to administer the dosage.

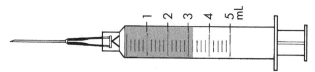

11. 0.4 mg : 1 mL = 0.2 mg : $x$ mL

*or*

$$\frac{0.2 \text{ mg}}{0.4 \text{ mg}} \times 1 \text{ mL} = x \text{ mL}$$

Answer: 0.5 mL. The dosage ordered is less than the available strength. You will need less than 1 mL to administer the dosage.

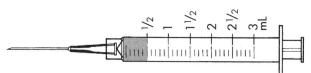

12. Conversion is required. Equivalent: 1,000 mcg = 1 mg. Therefore 200 mcg = 0.2 mg.

0.2 mg : 1 mL = 0.2 mg : $x$ mL

*or*

$$\frac{0.2 \text{ mg}}{0.2 \text{ mg}} \times 1 \text{ mL} = x \text{ mL}$$

Answer: 1 mL. Because 200 mcg = 0.2 mg, you will need 1 mL to administer the required dosage.

Alternate solution:

1 mg : 5 mL = 0.2 mg : $x$ mL

*or*

$$\frac{0.2 \text{ mg}}{1 \text{ mg}} \times 5 \text{ mL} = x \text{ mL}$$

This setup will give an answer of 1 mL.

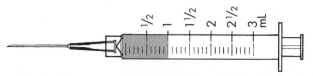

13. 40 mcg : 1 mL = 30 mcg : $x$ mL

*or*

$$\frac{30 \text{ mcg}}{40 \text{ mcg}} \times 1 \text{ mL} = x \text{ mL}$$

Answer: 0.75 mL. The dosage ordered is less than the available strength. You will need less than 1 mL to administer the dosage.

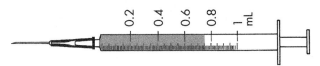

14. Conversion is required. Equivalent: 1,000 mcg = 1 mg.

Therefore 250 mcg = 0.25 mg

1 mg : 1 mL = 0.25 mg : $x$ mL

*or*

$$\frac{0.25 \text{ mg}}{1 \text{ mg}} \times 1 \text{ mL} = x \text{ mL}$$

Answer: 0.25 mL. The dosage ordered is less than the available strength; therefore you will need less than 1 mL to administer the dosage.

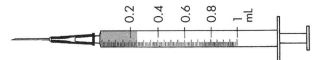

15. 2 mg : 1 mL = 1.5 mg : $x$ mL

*or*

$$\frac{1.5 \text{ mg}}{2 \text{ mg}} \times 1 \text{ mL} = x \text{ mL}$$

Answer: 0.75 mL = 0.8 mL. The dosage ordered is less than the available strength; therefore you will need less than 1 mL to administer the dosage.

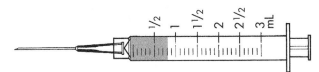

16. 10 mg : 2 mL = 15 mg : $x$ mL

*or*

$$\frac{15 \text{ mg}}{10 \text{ mg}} \times 2 \text{ mL} = x \text{ mL}$$

Answer: 3 mL. The dosage ordered is greater than the available strength. Therefore you will need more than 2 mL to administer the dosage.

Alternate solution:

5 mg : 1 mL = 15 mg : $x$ mL

*or*

$$\frac{15 \text{ mg}}{5 \text{ mg}} \times 1 \text{ mL} = x \text{ mL}$$

This setup will yield an answer of 3 mL.

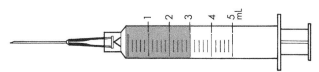

17. 5 mg : 1 mL = 7.5 mg : $x$ mL

*or*

$$\frac{7.5 \text{ mg}}{5 \text{ mg}} \times 1 \text{ mL} = x \text{ mL}$$

Answer: 1.5 mL. (State the answer as a decimal; mL is a metric measure.) The dosage ordered is greater than the available strength. Therefore you will need more than 1 mL to administer the dosage.

Alternate solution:

50 mg : 10 mL = 7.5 mg : $x$ mL

*or*

$$\frac{7.5 \text{ mg}}{50 \text{ mg}} \times 10 \text{ mL} = x \text{ mL}$$

This setup will yield an answer of 1.5 mL.

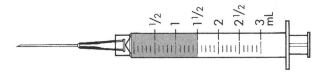

18. 0.25 mg : 1 mL = 1 mg : $x$ mL

*or*

$$\frac{1 \text{ mg}}{0.25 \text{ mg}} \times 1 \text{ mL} = x \text{ mL}$$

Answer: 4 mL. The dosage ordered is more than the available strength. Therefore you will need more than 1 mL to administer the dosage.

Alternate solution:

1 mg : 4 mL = $x$ mL

*or*

$$\frac{1 \text{ mg}}{1 \text{ mg}} \times 4 \text{ mL} = x \text{ mL}$$

This setup will yield an answer of 4 mL.

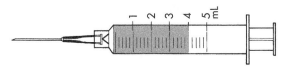

19. 40 mg : 1 mL = 55 mg : $x$ mL

*or*

$$\frac{55 \text{ mg}}{40 \text{ mg}} \times 1 \text{ mL} = x \text{ mL}$$

Alternate solution:

80 mg : 2 mL = 55 mg : $x$ mL

*or*

$$\frac{55 \text{ mg}}{80 \text{ mg}} \times 2 \text{ mL} = x \text{ mL}$$

Answer: 1.4 mL, or 1.37 rounded to the nearest tenth.

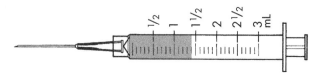

20. Conversion is required. Equivalent: 1,000 mcg = 1 mg. Therefore this should be 125 mcg not 1.25 = 0.125 mg.

0.1 mg : 1 mL = 0.125 mg : $x$ mL

*or*

$$\frac{0.125 \text{ mg}}{0.1 \text{ mg}} \times 1 \text{ mL} = x \text{ mL}$$

Answer: 1.3 mL, or 1.25 mL rounded to the nearest tenth. The dosage ordered is more than the available strength. Therefore you will need more than 1 mL to administer the dosage.

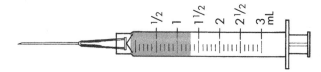

21. Demerol (meperedine):

100 mg : 1 mL = 65 mg : $x$ mL

*or*

$$\frac{65 \text{ mg}}{100 \text{ mg}} \times 1 \text{ mL} = x \text{ mL}$$

Answer: 0.7 mL, or 0.65 mL rounded to the nearest tenth. The dosage ordered is less than the available strength. Therefore less than 1 mL would be required to administer the dosage.

Hydroxyzine HCl:

50 mg : 1 mL = 25 mg : $x$ mL

*or*

$$\frac{25 \text{ mg}}{50 \text{ mg}} \times 1 \text{ mL} = x \text{ mL}$$

Answer: 0.5 mL. The dosage ordered is less than the available strength. Therefore you need less than 1 mL to administer the dosage. These two medications are often administered in the same syringe (0.7 mL of Demerol + 0.5 mL of Hydroxyzine HCl = 1.2 mL).

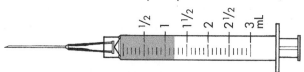

22. 4 mg : 1 mL = 9 mg : $x$ mL

*or*

$$\frac{9 \text{ mg}}{4 \text{ mg}} \times 1 \text{ mL} = x \text{ mL}$$

Answer: 2.3 mL, or 2.25 mL rounded to the nearest tenth. The dosage ordered is greater than the available strength. You would need more than 1 mL to administer the dosage.

Alternate solution:

20 mg : 5 mL = 9 mg : $x$ mL

*or*

$$\frac{9 \text{ mg}}{20 \text{ mg}} \times 5 \text{ mL} = x \text{ mL}$$

This setup would yield the same answer, 2.3 mL, or 2.25 mL rounded to the nearest tenth.

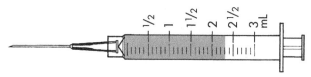

23. 50 mcg : 1 mL = 60 mcg : $x$ mL

*or*

$$\frac{60 \text{ mcg}}{50 \text{ mcg}} \times 1 \text{ mL} = x \text{ mL}$$

Answer: 1.2 mL. The dosage ordered is greater than the available strength when using 50 mcg per mL. You will need more than 1 mL to administer the dosage.

Alternate solution:

250 mcg : 5 mL = 60 mcg : $x$ mL

*or*

$$\frac{60 \text{ mcg}}{250 \text{ mcg}} \times 5 \text{ mL} = x \text{ mL}$$

This setup will still yield an answer of 1.2 mL.

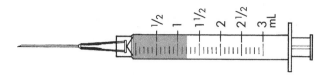

24. 480 mcg : 0.8 mL = 300 mcg : $x$ mL

    *or*

    $$\frac{300 \text{ mcg}}{480 \text{ mcg}} \times 0.8 \text{ mL} = x \text{ mL}$$

    Answers: a. 0.5 mL. The dosage ordered is less than the available strength; therefore you will need less than 0.8 mL to administer the dosage.

    b. Discard 0.3 mL

25. 90 mg : 1 mL = 45 mg : $x$ mL

    *or*

    $$\frac{45 \text{ mg}}{90 \text{ mg}} \times 1 \text{ mL} = x \text{ mL}$$

    Answers: a. 0.5 mL. The dosage ordered is less than the available strength; therefore you will need less than 1 mL to administer the dosage.

    b. Discard 0.5 mL.

26. 100 mg : 1 mL = 100 mg : $x$ mL

    *or*

    $$\frac{100 \text{ mg}}{100 \text{ mg}} \times 1 \text{ mL} = x \text{ mL}$$

    Answer: a. 1 mL. The label indicates that the dosage ordered is contained in 1 mL.

    b. Zero (0) mL will be discarded.

# CHAPTER **18**
# Reconstitution of Solutions

## Objectives

*After reviewing this chapter, you should be able to:*

1. Interpret the directions for reconstituting powdered medications from a vial, package insert, and other resources
2. Identify the dosage strength obtained after reconstituting powdered medications
3. Identify the varying directions for reconstitution and select the best directions for mixing to prepare the dosage ordered
4. Calculate dosages for reconstituted medications (single-strength and multiple-strength)
5. Determine the rate in milliliters per hour for enteral feedings
6. Calculate the amount of solute and solvent needed to prepare a desired strength for enteral feedings, irrigations, and soaks

Some medications come in a powdered form rather than in liquid form. As opposed to medications in powdered form, medications in liquid form retain their potency for a shorter time. When medications come in powdered form, *reconstitution* is necessary before they can be measured and administered to a client. The process of *reconstitution* involves adding a liquid (referred to as a diluent or solvent) to a medication in powdered form to dissolve it and form a solution. Once a medication is reconstituted, some solutions may have to be used within an hour, 1 to 14 days, or longer, depending on the medication. For example, ampicillin must be used within an hour after reconstitution, whereas EryPed, an oral suspension, is good for 35 days after reconstitution.

As a safety precaution in some institutions, the pharmacist reconstitutes most medications; however, the nurse may occasionally need to reconstitute a powdered medication. The nursing responsibility in reconstitution includes accurate interpretation of the directions for reconstitution, choosing the type and amount of diluent, and identifying the dosage strength after reconstitution to use in calculation of the ordered dosage. Medications requiring reconstitution can be for oral or parenteral use; these are not always injectable medications.

The safe preparation and administration of powdered medications require that the nurse have an understanding of the reconstitution process and terminology used:

- **Solute**—A powdered medication or liquid concentrate to be dissolved or diluted.
  **Solvent (diluent)**—A liquid that is added to the powder or liquid concentrate. The nurse **must** identify the diluent (solvent) to use. The type of diluent (solvent) varies according to the medication. The package insert or the medication label will indicate the diluent (solvent) to be used and the amount. If the information is not indicated on the label, or the package insert is unavailable, consult appropriate resources, which include the pharmacist and a medication reference (drug manual or computer website for medication, if listed). Sterile solutions (diluent/solvent) are always used to reconstitute medications for injectable use. Special diluents (solvents), when required for reconstitution, are usually packaged with the powdered medication, but medications for oral use can often be, but are not always, reconstituted with tap water.

**Solution**—The liquid that results when the diluent (solvent) dissolves the solute (powdered medication or liquid concentrate).

## Basic Principles for Reconstitution

The first step in reconstitution is to find the directions and carefully read the information on the vial or the package insert. Medications labeled and packaged with reconstitution directions may indicate "oral, IM, or IV use only." Always verify the route of administration ordered **before** reconstituting a medication. This is **critical** for parenteral routes and requires the nurse to read the directions carefully. Directions may be different based on the parenteral route of administration (i.e., IM versus IV). Follow reconstitution directions **exactly** for the route of administration to obtain the correct dosage strength.

> **⚠ SAFETY ALERT!**
> Before reconstituting a medication, read and follow the directions on the label or package insert. This includes checking the expiration date on the medication and diluent. Never assume the type or amount of diluent to be used. If the information is not available, consult appropriate resources, such as a reliable medication text, the *Physician's Desk Reference (PDR)*, a pharmacist, or the manufacturer's website, before reconstituting the medication.

1. The drug manufacturer provides directions for reconstitution, including information regarding the number of milliliters of diluent or solvent that should be added, as well as the type of solution that should be used to reconstitute the medication. The concentration (or strength) of the medication after it has been reconstituted according to the directions is also indicated on some medications. The directions for reconstitution must be followed exactly.
2. Commonly used diluents for parenteral medications include sterile water for injection and sterile sodium chloride (normal saline) for injection. Sterile water and normal saline for injection are available in preservative-free diluent used for single-use reconstitution and in bacteriostatic form with preservatives that prevent the growth of microorganisms for multiple-dose vials. Use only the diluent recommended. Using the wrong diluent can result in an incompatibility that can cause crystallization and/or clumping of the medication in solution. Some medications that require reconstitution may indicate they can be mixed with lidocaine, a local anesthetic, to reduce pain. Some medications may cause pain when injected (e.g., antibiotics). The label or package insert indicates when lidocaine can be used and the percentage. Always check with the prescriber before reconstituting a medication with lidocaine. Because lidocaine is a medication, it necessitates an order from the prescriber. If lidocaine is used, make certain to use only lidocaine. Lidocaine can come combined with epinephrine. Epinephrine causes vasoconstriction (tightening of blood vessels), which delays the absorption of the medication.

> **⚠ SAFETY ALERT!**
> Always use a sterile solution for injection and for mixing to administer a medication by the parenteral route.

3. Once you have located the reconstitution directions on the label or package insert, you need to identify the following information:
   a. The type of diluent to use for reconstitution.
   b. The amount of diluent to add. This is essential because directions relating to the amount of diluent can vary according to the parenteral route of administration. (Refer to Figure 18.1, the label for Ceftriaxone; note the amount of diluent to add for IM is 2.1 mL and for IV is 9.6 mL.)

> **⚠ SAFETY ALERT!**
> Always determine both the type and amount of diluent to be used for reconstituting medications. Read and follow the label or package insert directions carefully to ensure that your client receives the intended dosage. Consult a pharmacist or other appropriate resources if there are any questions. Never assume!

c. The length of time the medication is good for once it is reconstituted. The length of time a medication can be stored once reconstituted can vary depending on how it is stored. When medications are reconstituted, the solution must be used in a timely fashion. The potency (stability) of the medication may be several hours to several days or even a week or longer. Check the medication label, package insert, or appropriate resources for how long a medication may be used after reconstitution.

d. Directions for storing the medication after mixing. Medications must be stored appropriately once reconstituted per manufacturer's instructions to ensure optimal potency of the medication. Medications can become unstable when stored incorrectly and for long periods. Example: A label may state a medication maintains its potency 96 hours at room temperature or 7 days when refrigerated.

e. It is essential for the nurse to locate the dosage strength or concentration of the medication after it has been reconstituted as indicated by the drug manufacturer. The dosage strength after the medication is reconstituted is used in the dosage calculation.

Refer to Figure 18.1 showing the label for Ceftriaxone 1 gram. The 1 gram on the Ceftriaxone label represents the total amount of medication in the vial. As you will see, the total amount, once diluted, (reconstituted) provides a specific concentration or dosage strength. Refer to the directions for reconstitution of the Ceftriaxone for IM administration. *Note* the directions on the label say to add 2.1 mL of 1% lidocaine hydrochloride

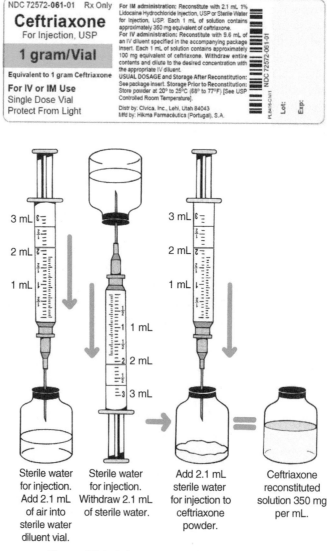

Figure 18.1 Ceftriaxone 1-g vial reconstitution.

injection or sterile water for injection and that each 1 mL contains 350 mg. The **available dosage strength (concentration)** after reconstitution is 350 mg of Ceftriaxone per 1 mL of solution. **(Remember to check with the prescriber before reconstituting a medication with lidocaine.)** Note if you were reconstituting this medication for IV administration, the amount of diluent to add and the dosage strength after reconstitution is different from the IM route.

4. If there are no directions for reconstitution on the label or on a package insert, or if any of the information (listed in number 3) is missing, consult appropriate resources such as the *PDR,* a pharmacology text, the hospital drug formulary, the pharmacy, or the manufacturer's website.

5. Injectable medications for reconstitution can come in a single-dose vial or a multiple-dose vial. When medications are in single-dose vials, there is only enough medication for **one** dose, and the contents are administered after reconstitution. In the case where the nurse reconstitutes a multiple-dose vial, there is enough medication for more than one dose. Therefore, when a multiple-dose vial is reconstituted, it is important to clearly label the vial after reconstitution with the following information:

   a. The date and time prepared, dosage strength prepared, the expiration date for the medication once reconstituted, and the time. *Note:* If all of the solution that is mixed is used, this information is not necessary. Information regarding the date and time of preparation and date and time of expiration is crucial when all of the medication is not used.

   b. Storage directions such as "Refrigerate."

   c. Your initials.

   If the medication label does not have room to clearly write the required information, add a label to the vial and indicate important information. Make certain the label is applied so that it does not obscure the medication name and dosage.

---

**TIPS FOR CLINICAL PRACTICE**

When reconstituting a multiple-dose medication vial, label it with the required information and store it appropriately. If the vial is not labeled with a date and time the medication was reconstituted and the dosage strength after reconstitution and expiration date, the medication must be discarded. The nurse should never use an unlabeled reconstituted vial.

---

6. When some powdered medications are reconstituted, the powdered medication takes up space as it dissolves and results in an increase in the amount of total (fluid) volume once it has dissolved. This is sometimes referred to as just *displacement* or as the *displacement factor.* For example, directions for 1 g of powdered medication may state to add 2.5 mL of sterile water for injection to provide an approximate volume of 3 mL (330 mg per mL). The displacement volume is 0.5 mL. The available dosage strength after reconstitution, however, is 330 mg per mL of solution. The displacement volume may not be indicated on all medication labels.

## Types of Reconstituted Medications

There are two types of powdered medications for parenteral use that require reconstitution. They are single-strength reconstitution and multiple-strength reconstitution.

*Single-strength reconstitution* medications usually have one amount of diluent to add and provide only one dosage strength. See the 1-g Ceftriaxone label shown in Figure 18.1. Notice there is only one amount of diluent to add for IM use and one dosage strength indicated after the diluent is added. For IV there is only one amount of diluent indicated and one dosage strength after the diluent is added.

*Multiple-strength reconstitution* medications have several directions for reconstitution to different dosage strengths. In other words, different amounts of diluent are indicated, allowing for the mixing of different concentrations of a medication. A multiple-strength reconstitution requires the nurse be even more attentive to the directions to select the best concentration to administer the required dosage.

## Powdered Medications for Oral Administration

Like parenteral medications, medications for oral use that come in a powder form must be reconstituted (mixed with a liquid) before administration. The diluent used to reconstitute powdered medications for oral use include tap water, distilled water, and purified water. The directions for mixing, which include the amount and type of diluent, are found on the medication label. The amount of diluent added to powdered medications for oral use provides one dosage strength. The label indicates the dosage strength after reconstitution as well as the volume of medication after reconstitution. The nurse must follow the reconstitution directions as indicated on the medication label to obtain the correct dosage strength of the medication. Reconstitution directions vary according to the medication. Other pertinent information the nurse needs to identify in addition to the dosage strength after reconstitution includes storage information for the medication once it is reconstituted, and the expiration date of the reconstituted medication (identified by the time period when the reconstituted medication will need to be discarded). The reconstitution of powdered medications for oral use usually results in multiple doses; therefore the nurse who initially mixes the medication must include the following information on the medication bottle without obscuring the label: the date and time the medication was reconstituted and the initials of the preparer. In some institutions the nurse may be required to indicate the date and time of expiration. Always follow the policy of the institution regarding the required information on reconstituted oral medications. Refer to Figure 18.2 (label for Cefaclor Oral Suspension 125 mg per 5 mL).

Let's begin with practice problems answering questions relating to single-strength reconstitution.

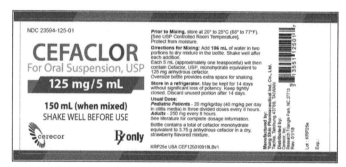

**Figure 18.2**  Directions for mixing Cefaclor Oral Suspension 125 mg per 5 mL. Notice the **directions for mixing** indicate to add 106 mL of water in two portions to the dry mixture and shake well after each addition. **The reconstituted solution** will provide a dosage strength of 125 mg per 5 mL. **The total volume** when mixed is 150 mL. **Storage directions:** Store in refrigerator. **Expiration:** Discard unused portion after 14 days.

## ⊞ PRACTICE **PROBLEMS**

Using the label for Gemcitabine, answer the following questions.

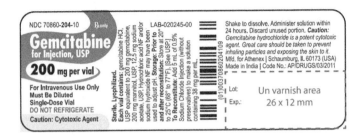

1. What is the total dosage strength of
   Gemcitabine in this vial?

   _____

2. How much diluent is added to the vial
   to prepare the medication for IV use?

   _____

3. What diluent is recommended for
   reconstitution?

   _____

4. What is the final dosage strength
   (concentration) of the prepared solution
   for IV administration?

   _____

5. How long will the reconstituted material
   retain its potency?

   _____

6. 100 mg IV is ordered for day one of
   treatment. How many milliliters will you
   give? Shade the dosage in on the syringe
   provided.

   _____

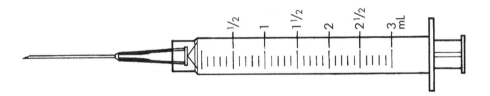

Using the label for Leucovorin calcium, answer the following questions.

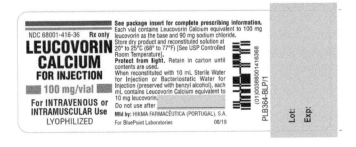

7. What is the total dosage strength of
   Leucovorin calcium in the vial?

   _____

8. How much diluent is added to the vial to reconstitute the medication?   _____

9. What diluent is recommended for reconstitution?   _____

10. What is the dosage strength (concentration) of the reconstituted solution?   _____

11. Routes of administration   _____

12. Where can you find directions for complete prescribing information?   _____

13. 15 mg IM q6h is ordered. How many milliliters will you give? Shade the dosage on the syringe provided.   _____

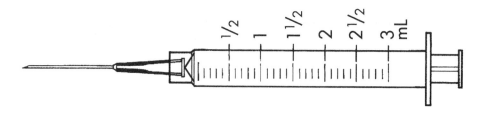

Using the label for Methylprednisolone sodium succinate, answer the following questions.

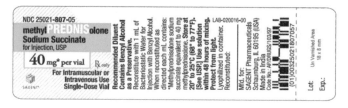

14. What is the total dosage strength of Methylprednisolone sodium succinate in the vial?   _____

15. What diluent is recommended to prepare an IV dosage?   _____

16. How many milliliters of diluent are needed to prepare an IV dosage?   _____

17. What is the dosage strength (concentration) of the solution prepared for IV administration?   _____

18. Methylprednisolone sodium succinate 35 mg IV daily is ordered. How many milliliters will you give? Shade the dosage on the syringe provided.   _____

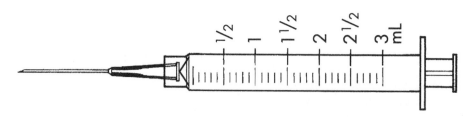

Using the label for Cefaclor, answer the following questions.

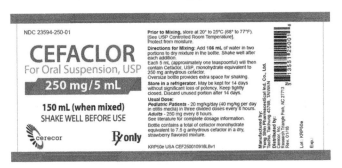

19. How much diluent must be added to
    prepare the solution?                    _____

20. What type of solution is used for the
    diluent?                                 _____

21. What is the final dosage strength
    (concentration) of the prepared solution? _____

22. How should the medication be stored
    after it is reconstituted?               _____

Using the label for Erythromycin ethylsuccinate, answer the following questions.

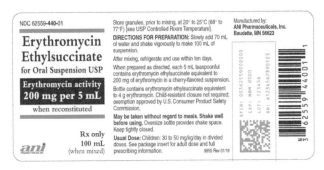

23. How much diluent must be added to
    prepare the solution?                    _____

24. What is the volume of the solution after it
    is mixed?                                _____

25. What is the final dosage strength (concentration)
    of the prepared solution?                _____

26. For how long is the reconstituted solution
    good?                                    _____

Using the label for Ceftriaxone, answer the following questions.

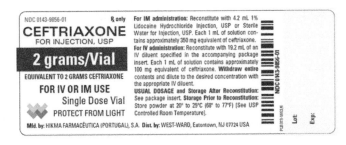

27. What is the total dosage strength of Ceftriaxone in this vial? _____

28. How much diluent must be added to the vial to prepare the medication for IM use? _____

29. How much diluent must be added to the vial to prepare the medication for IV use? _____

30. What diluent is recommended for IV reconstitution? _____

31. What is the final dosage strength (concentration) of the prepared solution for IV use? _____

Using the label for Zithromax, answer the following questions.

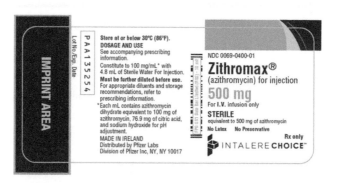

32. What is the total dosage strength of Zithromax in this vial? _____

33. How many milliliters of diluent are needed to prepare an IV dosage? _____

34. What diluent is recommended for reconstitution? _____

35. What is the final dosage strength (concentration) of the prepared solution? _____

36. Directions for use? _____

**Answers on pp. 421-422**

## Calculation of Medications When the Final Concentration (Dosage Strength) Is Not Stated

Sometimes a medication comes with directions for only one way to reconstitute it, and the label does not indicate the final dosage strength (concentration) with the reconstitution information provided on the label. The dosage strength is determined by the total amount of medication in the vial and the amount of diluent added. Refer to Figure 18.3 label for Acyclovir 500 mg.

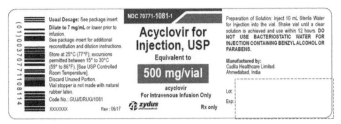

**Figure 18.3** Acyclovir 500 mg per vial. Notice there is no dosage strength stated with the reconstitution information. The dosage strength is 500 mg per 10 mL. This was determined by using the total amount of medication in the vial (500 mg) and the amount of diluent added (10 mL).

## Reconstituting Medications With More Than One Direction for Mixing (Multiple Strength Reconstitution)

Some powdered medications may come with directions for reconstitution to different solution strengths. Different volumes of diluent may be added, as specified by the drug manufacturer. The amount of diluent added determines the final dosage strength (concentration). In this case the nurse must choose the concentration or dosage strength appropriate for the dosage ordered and the individual client. The dosage strength chosen should result in a reasonable amount of solution administered to the client by the route ordered. A common medication that has directions for reconstitution to different dosage strengths is penicillin. To determine which dosage strength to use, the following guidelines may be used.

### Guidelines for Choosing Appropriate Concentrations

1. Route of administration. It is essential to verify the route of administration before reconstituting.
   a. IM—You are concerned that the amount does not exceed the maximum injection amount allowed for IM administration. However, you do not want to choose a concentration that will result in irritation when injected into a muscle. When a choice of strengths can be made, do not choose an amount that would exceed the amount allowed for IM administration or one that is very concentrated. Consider the muscle site being used and the age of the client.
   b. IV—Keep in mind that this medication is usually further diluted because, once reconstituted, the medication is then placed in additional fluid of 50 to 100 mL or more, depending on the medication being administered.
2. Choose the concentration or dosage strength that comes closest to what the prescriber has ordered. The dosage strengths are given for the amount of diluent used. Example: If the prescriber orders 300,000 units of a particular medication IM, and the choices of strength are 200,000 units per mL, 250,000 units per mL, and 500,000 units per mL, the strength closest to 300,000 units per mL is 250,000 units per mL. It allows you to administer a dosage within the range allowed for IM administration, and it is not the most concentrated.

> **! SAFETY ALERT!**
> When multiple directions are given for reconstituting medications, the smaller the amount of diluent used to reconstitute the medication, the more concentrated the resulting solution will be. Consider the route of administration when reconstituting medications. Always check the route and the directions related to reconstitution.

3. The word *respectively* may sometimes be used on a medication label for directions on reconstitution. For example, reconstitute with 23 mL, 18 mL, 8 mL of diluent to provide concentrations of 200,000 units per mL, 250,000 units per mL, 500,000 units per mL, respectively. The word *respectively* means in the order given. In terms of the directions for reconstitution, this means that if you add 23 mL diluent, it will provide 200,000 units per mL, 18 mL diluent will provide 250,000 units per mL, etc. In other words, the amounts of diluent correspond to the order in which the concentrations are written.

Remember: **When you are mixing a medication that is a multiple-strength solution, the dosage strength that you prepare must be written on the vial.**

Let's look at a sample label showing multiple reconstitution options. Refer to the label for Pfizerpen (penicillin G potassium) See Figure 18.4.

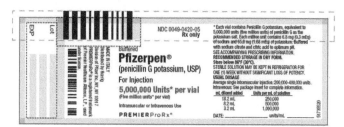

**Figure 18.4** Pfizerpen (penicillin G potassium).

Notice the label indicates the total amount of medication in the vial is 5,000,000 units. The Pfizerpen label has three choices of diluent amounts (18.2 mL, 8.2 mL, and 3.2 mL). The dosage strength (concentration) of the reconstituted medication depends on the amount of diluent used. If the nurse adds 18.2 mL of diluent, the dosage strength is 250,000 units per mL; if the nurse adds 8.2 mL of diluent, the dosage strength is 500,000 units per mL; and if the nurse adds 3.2 mL of diluent, the dosage strength is 1,000,000 units per mL. Once the nurse has chosen the amount of diluent to use and the corresponding dosage strength, the dosage strength is used to calculate the problem.

Let's assume the order is for 400,000 units IM for an adult. The best concentration in this case would be 500,000 units per mL. Refer to the label and notice to make this concentration (dosage strength), you will need to add 8.2 mL of diluent. When calculated, the client would receive 0.8 mL (3 mL is the maximum for a large adult muscle). Remember the condition of the intramuscular site and the client (age and muscle mass) **must** be considered. Depending on the status of the client, a different dosage strength may be a better choice. Notice also when you reconstitute the medication using 8.2 mL, the total volume will be 8.2 mL, which means you have enough left over for at least 9+ doses. Because this is a multiple-strength solution, the dosage strength must be indicated on the vial after you reconstitute it. Other information would include date and time prepared, expiration date and time, and initials of the preparer. This will help to ensure that the nurse using the medication after you knows the essential information (dosage strength, when the medication was reconstituted and by whom, and the expiration date).

> **(!) SAFETY ALERT!**
>
> Proper labeling is a crucial detail on a multiple-strength solution that has been reconstituted. For safe practice, never administer a reconstituted medication that lacks the appropriate information on the medication label. Instead, discard the medication. You have no way of knowing how and when the medication was mixed!

## 🔲 PRACTICE **PROBLEMS**

Using the label for Penicillin G potassium, answer the following questions.

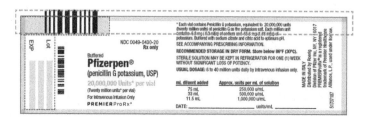

37. What are the directions for use? _____

38. If you add 33 mL of diluent to the vial, what dosage strength (concentration) will you print on the label?

    _____

39. If 2,000,000 units IV is ordered, which dosage strength (concentration) would be appropriate to use?

    _____

40. How many milliliters will you administer if 2,000,000 units are ordered?

    _____

41. How long will the medication maintain its potency if refrigerated?

    _____

Using the label for Penicillin G potassium, answer the following questions.

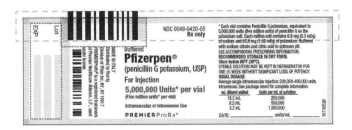

42. What are the directions for use?

    _____

43. Where would the usual dosage for IV administration be found?

    _____

44. Where will you store any unused medication?

    _____

45. How long will the medication maintain its potency?

    _____

46. What concentration strength would be obtained if you added 18.2 mL of diluent? (Write out in numbers.)

    _____

**Answers on p. 422**

## Reconstitution From Package Insert Directions and Medications With Different Reconstitution Directions Depending on Route of Administration

If the label does not contain reconstitution directions, you must obtain directions from the information insert or package insert that accompanies the vial. Sometimes the drug manufacturer may print reconstitution directions for the size of the vial as well as the route of administration. The nurse must pay attention to the amount in the vial and the route; there may be different directions based on the route of administration. Reading the directions carefully is **critical** to identification of the correct directions for reconstitution. Refer to the Ceftazidime (Tazicef) label (Figure 18.5) and insert. For example, note that the directions for mixing the Ceftazidime 1-gram vial for IM injection are different from mixing the 1-gram vial for IV infusion. Note that although the same amount of diluent is indicated for a 1-gram vial and a 2-gram vial for IV infusion, the final dosage strengths (concentrations) are different.

> **(!) SAFETY ALERT!**
> Carefully check the route ordered before reconstituting a medication and follow the directions corresponding to that route. Do not interchange the dilution instructions for IM or IV because you can harm a client.

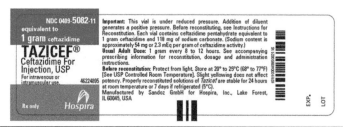

| Preparation of Solutions of Tazicef—Reconstitute with Sterile Water for Injection for IM Injection, IV Direct (Bolus) Injection, or IV Infusion | | | |
|---|---|---|---|
| **Size** | **Amount of Diluent to be Added (mL)** | **Approximate Available Volume (mL)** | **Approximate Ceftazidime Concentration (mg/mL)** |
| Intramuscular | | | |
| 1-gram vial | 3 | 3.6 | 280 |
| Intravenous | | | |
| 1-gram vial | 10 | 10.6 | 95 |
| 2-gram vial | 10 | 11.2 | 180 |

**Figure 18.5** (A) Tazicef 1 gram. (B) Portion of Tazicef package insert.

## Medications With Instructions to "See Accompanying Literature" (Package Insert) for Reconstitution and Administration

Some medications that require reconstitution may indicate the dosage strength contained in the vial and do not provide the information necessary to reconstitute the medication or information relating to administration. To prepare the powdered medication, you must see the package insert or accompanying literature. Refer to the Olanzapine (Zyprexa) label (Figure 18.6A) and the accompanying package insert information (Figure 18.6B). The label instructs you to see "accompanying literature for dosage, reconstitution instructions; method of administration, and storage conditions."

To reconstitute the medication and calculate a dosage you will need to refer to the package insert. The directions instruct you to add 2.1 mL of sterile water for injection to provide a

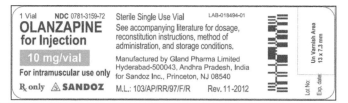

**Directions for Preparation of Olanzapine for Injection with Sterile Water for Injection:** Dissolve the contents of the vial using 2.1 mL of Sterile Water for Injection to provide a solution containing approximately 5 mg/mL of olanzapine. The resulting solution should appear clear and yellow. Olanzapine for injection reconstituted with Sterile Water for Injection should be used immediately (within 1 hour) after reconstitution. *Discard any unused portion.* The following table provides injection volumes for delivering various doses of intramuscular olanzapine for injection reconstituted with Sterile Water for Injection.

| Dose (mg) | Volume of Injection (mL) |
|---|---|
| 10 | Withdraw total contents of vial |
| 7.5 | 1.5 |
| 5 | 1 |
| 2.5 | 0.5 |

**Figure 18.6** (A) Olanzapine 10-mg label. (B) Olanzapine package insert.

solution containing approximately 5 mg per mL of Olanzapine and indicate the number of mL to withdraw to administer specific dosages of the medication IM. Notice, for example, that if you had to administer 5 mg of Olanzapine IM, when the medication has been reconstituted, you would withdraw 1 mL of the medication to administer the ordered dosage of 5 mg.

## PRACTICE **PROBLEMS**

Use the Olanzapine label and package insert in Figure 18.6A and B to answer problems 47-52.

47. What is the dosage strength of the total vial? _____

48. How much diluent must be added to this vial to prepare the medication for IM use? _____

49. What diluent is recommended for reconstitution? _____

50. For how long will the reconstituted solution be good? _____

51. How much would you withdraw for a 7.5-mg dose? _____

52. How much would you withdraw for a 2.5-mg dose? _____

**Answers on p. 422**

## Powdered Medication Delivery Systems

There has been an increase in the use of more manufacturer-prepared IV medication systems. One such system is the ADD-Vantage system. This system has two components: (1) an ADD-Vantage diluent container (e.g., an IV bag) and (2) an ADD-Vantage medication vial that contains the medication. The medication, which is in a vial, is attached to the IV bag. When this system is used, the IV solution becomes the diluent. The stopper in the vial is pulled, which allows the medication to mix with the IV fluid prior to administration (Figure 18.7).

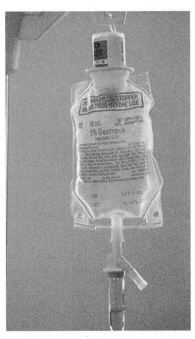

**Figure 18.7** The ADD-Vantage drug delivery system. (Courtesy Bruce Clayton.)

Examples of medications that come in the ADD-Vantage System include Vancomycin, Tazicef, and Ampicillin. The steps that are required in preparing the ADD-Vantage delivery system for IV administration can be found online and in a nursing skills textbook.

In addition to the ADD-Vantage system there are other systems used to mix powdered medications that include the Mix-O-Vial. This system was discussed in the previous chapter. A Mix-O-Vial allows for the mixing of a powdered medication (there are two compartments, the lower contains the medication in a powder, and the upper chamber contains the sterile diluent). Between the two compartments is a rubber stopper. When pressure is applied to the top of the vial (rubber diaphragm), this causes the diluent to mix with powder and produce a liquid for administration.

## Calculation of Dosages

If you are using ratio and proportion, the known ratio is also the dosage strength (concentration) obtained after you mix the medication.

- In $\dfrac{D}{H} \times Q = x$, Q is the volume of solution that contains the dosage strength.
- In dimensional analysis, the first fraction written is the solution (volume) that contains the dosage strength.

Before we proceed to calculate dosages, let's review the steps to use with medications that have been reconstituted.

1. Ratio and proportion, the formula method, or dimensional analysis may be used to calculate the dosage. However, the H (have or what is available) is the dosage strength you obtain after you mix the medication according to directions.
2. When the final concentration is not stated, the total weight of the medication in powdered form is used, and the number of milliliters diluent added.
3. As with all calculation problems, check to make sure that the ordered and the available medications are in the same system of measurement and the same units.
4. Do not forget to label your answer.

**Example 1:** To illustrate, let's calculate the dosage you would administer if you mixed penicillin and made a solution containing 1,000,000 units per mL. Order: 2,000,000 units IM q6h.

---

### ✓ Solution Using Ratio and Proportion

Linear Format: 1,000,000 units : 1 mL = 2,000,000 units : $x$ mL

(known)      (unknown)

$$\frac{1{,}000{,}000\,x}{1{,}000{,}000} = \frac{2{,}000{,}000}{1{,}000{,}000}$$    Note cancellation of zeros to make numbers smaller.)

$$x = \frac{2}{1}$$

$$x = 2 \text{ mL}$$

Fraction Format:

$$\frac{1{,}000{,}000 \text{ units}}{1 \text{ mL}} = \frac{2{,}000{,}000 \text{ units}}{x \text{ mL}}$$

$$\frac{1{,}000{,}000\,x}{1{,}000{,}000} = \frac{2{,}000{,}000}{1{,}000{,}000}$$

$$x = \frac{2}{1}$$

$$x = 2 \text{ mL}$$

**Answer:** 2 mL

### ✓ Solution Using the Formula Method

$$\frac{D}{H} \times Q = x$$

$$\frac{2,000,000 \text{ units}}{1,000,000 \text{ units}} \times 1 \text{ mL} = x \text{ mL}$$

$$x = \frac{2,000,000}{1,000,000}$$

$$x = 2 \text{ mL}$$

Answer:    2 mL

### ✓ Solution Using Dimensional Analysis

$$x \text{ mL} = \frac{1 \text{ mL}}{1,000,000 \text{ units}} \times \frac{2,000,000 \text{ units}}{1}$$

$$x = \frac{2,000,000}{1,000,000}$$

$$x = \frac{2}{1}$$

$$x = 2 \text{ mL}$$

Answer:    2 mL

**Example 2:**    Order: 0.2 g of a medication IV q6h

Available: 500 mg of the medication in powdered form that states, "Add 8 mL of diluent to yield a solution 500 mg per 8 mL."

### ✓ PROBLEM SETUP

1. A conversion is necessary. Equivalent: 1,000 mg = 1 g. Therefore 0.2 g = 200 mg.
2. Think: What would a logical answer be?
   You will need more than 1 mL but less than 8 mL.

### ✓ Solution Using Ratio and Proportion

Linear Format: 500 mg : 8 mL = 200 mg : $x$ mL

$$\phantom{Linear Format: 500 mg : 8 mL = }\text{(known)}\phantom{xxxxxx}\text{(unknown)}$$

$$\frac{500x}{500} = \frac{200 \times 8}{500}$$

$$x = \frac{1,600}{500}$$

$$x = 3.2 \text{ mL}$$

Fraction Format:

$$\frac{500 \text{ mg}}{8 \text{ mL}} = \frac{200 \text{ mg}}{x \text{ mL}}$$

$$\frac{500x}{500} = \frac{200 \times 8}{500}$$

$$x = \frac{1,600}{500}$$

$$x = 3.2 \text{ mL}$$

Answer:    3.2 mL

### ✓ Solution Using the Formula Method

$$\frac{D}{H} \times Q = x$$

$$\frac{200 \text{ mg}}{500 \text{ mg}} \times 8 \text{ mL} = x \text{ mL}$$

$$x = \frac{200 \times 8}{500}$$

$$x = \frac{1,600}{500}$$

$$x = 3.2 \text{ mL}$$

**Answer:** 3.2 mL

### ✓ Solution Using Dimensional Analysis

$$x \text{ mL} = \frac{8 \text{ mL}}{500 \text{ mg}} \times \frac{1,000 \text{ mg}}{1 \text{ g}} \times \frac{0.2 \text{ g}}{1}$$

$$x = \frac{8,000 \times 0.2}{500}$$

$$x = \frac{1,600}{500}$$

$$x = 3.2 \text{ mL}$$

**Answer:** 3.2 mL

---

**POINTS TO REMEMBER**

- Directions for reconstituting medications are provided by the drug manufacturer.
- The directions for reconstituting medications can be found on the vial, the medication container, or a package insert. If there are no instructions on the vial, container, or the package insert is not available, consult other reliable resources (pharmacy, medication reference book, *PDR*).
- Read directions carefully for reconstitution, and reconstitute the medication specific to the route of administration ordered (e.g., IM, IV). Interchanging dilution instructions for routes can have serious outcomes for client.
- The type and amount of diluent to be used for reconstitution must be followed exactly.
- Lidocaine should not be used to reconstitute a medication without an order from the prescriber.
- Read directions relating to storage and the time period for maintaining potency of medication once it is reconstituted.
- If a medication is not used in its entirety after it is reconstituted and medication remains for future use, clearly label medication with the following:
  1. Date and time of preparation
  2. Date and time of expiration
  3. Initials of the preparer
  4. Dosage strength or concentration of reconstituted solution

## Reconstitution of Noninjectable Solutions

The principles of reconstitution can be applied to nutritional liquids. Enteral feeding solutions are formulated to be administered in full strength; however, the nurse may, on occasion, need to dilute the enteral solution before administering it. Before beginning calculations, let's discuss enteral feedings.

### Enteral Feeding

Enteral nutrition involves the provision of nutrients to the gastrointestinal tract. This nutrition is provided to clients who are unable to ingest food safely or have eating difficulties. Enteral nutrition may be provided with a nasogastric, jejunal, or gastric tube. It may consist of blended foods or tube feeding formulas. Tube feedings can be administered in several ways. Depending on the client's needs, they may be given as a bolus (administration of a single large dose) by means of gravity several times per day by using a large-volume syringe, as a continuous gravity drip over a period of $\frac{1}{2}$ to 1 hour several times per day by using a pouch to hang the feeding, or as a continuous drip by infusion pump. When clients are receiving a continuous feeding, the feeding is placed in a special pouch or container and attached to a feeding pump. A common feeding pump is the Kangaroo pump (Figure 18.8). When the feeding pump is used, the feeding is delivered at a rate expressed in milliliters per hour. For the purpose of this chapter, we will focus on administering a feeding by the continuous drip method with an enteral infusion pump.

When an order is written for feedings by continuous infusion, the nurse attaches the feeding to a special pump and administers it at the prescribed rate in milliliters per hour. A sample order is Jevity at 65 mL per hour by PEG (percutaneous endoscopic gastrostomy) or by NG (nasogastric) tube. The feeding order also includes a certain volume of water with feeding (100 to 250 mL). The amount of water given with a tube feeding and how it is administered vary from one institution to the next. Check the institution's policy relating to administering enteral feedings. Some orders may be written as follows: Pulmo Care 400 mL over 8 hours followed by 100 mL of water after each feed. When the prescriber does not indicate milliliters per hour, the nurse divides the number of milliliters ordered by the number of hours and rounds answer to the nearest whole number, to determine the

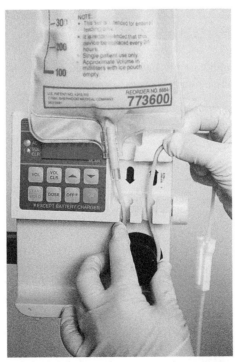

**Figure 18.8** Kangaroo pump. (From Potter PA, Perry AG, Stockert P, Hall A: *Fundamentals of nursing,* ed 9, St Louis, 2017, Elsevier.)

milliliters per hour to set the pump. In pediatrics, the order often specifies the formula and the rate. Example: Similac 24 at 20 mL per hr continuously by NG tube.

**Example 1:**   Order: Pulmocare 400 mL over 8 hours followed by 100 mL of water after each feed. Determine the rate in milliliters per hour.

$$\frac{400 \text{ mL}}{8 \text{ hr}} = 50 \text{ mL/hr}$$

The pump would be set at 50 mL/hr.

**Example 2:**   Order: Nepro 1,200 mL over 16 hours. Determine the rate in milliliters per hour.

$$\frac{1,200 \text{ mL}}{16 \text{ hr}} = 75 \text{ mL/hr}$$

The pump would be set to deliver 75 mL/hr.

In addition to nutrients, medications may be given through a tube. Liquid medications are preferred; however, some tablets may be crushed, dissolved in water, and administered.

Never assume. Not all medications are designed for administration through a tube, so check with the pharmacist or other appropriate resources. A medication's effectiveness could depend on the location of the tube (e.g., stomach, jejunum).

> **SAFETY ALERT!**
> Always verify that the medications to be administered are not sublingual, enteric-coated, or timed-release medications because such medications are absorbed differently and the effects of the medication may be altered. Consult the pharmacist or medication guide before tablets are crushed and before capsules are opened and dissolved for tube feeding administration.

## PRACTICE **PROBLEMS**

Determine the rate in milliliters per hour for the following continuous feedings. Round answers to the nearest whole number.

53.   Ensure 480 mL by NG tube over 8 hr. Follow
    with 100 mL of water after each feeding.          _____

54.   Perative 1,600 mL over 24 hr by gastrostomy.
    Follow with 250 mL of water.          _____

**Answers on p. 422**

## Determining the Strength of a Solution

Nurses or other health care professionals may be required to dilute a concentrated liquid or powder (solute) with a solution such as water or saline (solvent) so as to make a less concentrated solution. Water is a common solvent used to dilute solutions and has been referred to as the **universal solvent.** This may include preparation of irrigating solutions, soaks, and nutritional liquids. When reconstituting solutions that are noninjectable, nurses must understand that the amount of liquid (solvent) that is used to make a substance less concentrated is determined by the desired strength of the solution.

Therefore, if you add more solvent, the final solution strength will be less concentrated; the less solvent that is added, the more concentrated the final solution strength will be. An example to illustrate this concept is the directions for making one quart of ice tea from a powder. Directions call for 4 cups of water to 1 packet of powdered ice tea. If you prefer a stronger tea taste, you might add 2 cups of water (solvent) to the powder (solute), making it more concentrated. However, if you add 4 cups of water (solvent) to the powder (solute), the final solution will be more diluted and less concentrated because you added more water (solvent).

The strength of a solution can be expressed using ratios, fractions, or percents. The fraction format is usually preferred to explain the ratio of solute to the total solution. For example, a $\frac{1}{3}$ strength solution indicates 1 part solute for 3 parts of the total solution. This could be expressed as $1:3$ solution or $33\frac{1}{3}\%$ solution.

## Calculation of Solutions

Because of special circumstances in both adults and children, nutritional liquids may require dilution before they are used. These nutritional liquids may be administered orally or through feeding tubes. Nutritional solutions can be supplied in ready-to-use form, powder for reconstitution, or liquid concentrate. Nutritional formulas may be diluted with sterile or tap water. **Always consult a reference or institutional policy regarding what should be used to reconstitute a nutritional formula.**

To prepare a prescribed solution of a certain strength from a solute, first let's review some basic terms.

**Solute**—A concentrated liquid or solid substance to be dissolved or diluted
**Solvent**—A liquid substance that dissolves another substance. Commonly used solvents are sterile water and normal saline.
**Solution**—A solute plus a solvent
To prepare a solution of a specific strength, use the following steps:

1. Desired solution strength $\times$ Amount of desired solution = Solute (substance/concentrated liquid to be dissolved)

**Note:** The strength of the desired solution is written as a fraction; the amount of desired solution is expressed in milliliters or ounces, depending on the problem. This will give you the amount of solute you will need to add to the solvent to prepare the desired solution.

2. Amount of desired solution − Solute = Amount of liquid needed to dissolve substance (solvent)

**Example 1:** Order: $\frac{1}{3}$-strength Ensure 900 mL by NG tube over 8 hr

Solution:
$$\underset{\substack{\text{(desired} \\ \text{strength)}}}{\frac{1}{3}} \times \underset{\substack{\text{(amount of} \\ \text{solution)}}}{900 \text{ mL}} = \underset{\text{(solute)}}{x}$$

Step 1:
$$x = \frac{900}{3}$$
$$x = 300 \text{ mL}$$

You need 300 mL of the formula (solute).

Step 2:
$$\underset{\substack{\text{(amount of} \\ \text{solution)}}}{900 \text{ mL}} - \underset{\text{(solute)}}{300 \text{ mL}} = \underset{\substack{\text{(amount needed to dissolve} \\ \text{solvent)}}}{600 \text{ mL}}$$

Therefore you would add 600 mL water to 300 mL of Ensure to make 900 mL of $\frac{1}{3}$-strength Ensure.

**Example 2:** $3/4$-strength Isomil 4 oz p.o. q4h for 24 hr

*Note:* 4 oz q4h = 6 feedings; 4 oz × 6 = 24 oz

1 oz = 30 mL; therefore 24 oz = 720 mL

$$\frac{3}{4} \times 720 \text{ mL} = x \text{ mL}$$

$$x = \frac{2,160}{4}$$

$$x = 540 \text{ mL of the formula (solute)}$$

720 mL     − 540 mL = 180 mL
(amount of    (solute)    (amount needed
solution)                to dissolve solvent)

Therefore you would add 180 mL water to 540 mL of Isomil to make 720 mL of $3/4$-strength Isomil for a 24-hour period.

## Irrigating Solutions and Soaks

Nurses or other health care professionals may need to dilute solutions for use as a topical solution, or for irrigating body cavities or wounds. Normal saline is the preferred solution for cleaning wounds, for the application of moist dressings and packing of wounds. The use of cytotoxic solutions is discouraged. Current practice for wound irrigation recommends the use of non-cytotoxic wound cleaners such as normal saline, potable (tap) water, and sterile water. Normal saline solution is the preferred and frequently used solution for wound irrigation. Normal saline is the common term for 0.9% NaCl (full-strength) and is an isotonic solution (the same tonicity or osmolarity as blood and other body serums) and does not harm tissues. According to *Fundamentals of Nursing,* 9th edition (Potter et al., 2017), agents such as Dakin's Solution (sodium hypochlorite solution), acetic acid, povidone-iodine, and hydrogen peroxide are cytotoxic solutions. Cytotoxic solutions are toxic to cells and may interfere with healing. However, the health care provider providing wound care must always take into account the solution ordered and the nature of the wound.

**Example 1:** Using full-strength normal saline (0.9%), prepare 180 mL of $1/4$-strength normal saline solution diluted with sterile water for wound care.

**Solution:** The fraction represents the desired solution strength: $1/4$-strength means 1-part solute (normal saline) to 4 total parts solution.

1. No conversion required.

$1/4$          180 mL          $x$ mL
2. (desired   × (amount of = (solute)
   strength)     solution)

$$x = \frac{180}{4}$$

$$x = 45 \text{ mL}$$

You need 45 mL of solute (normal saline) to prepare the desired solution (180 mL of ¼ strength). The total you want to make is 180 mL. The amount of solvent you need is therefore:

180 mL − 45 mL = 135 mL (solvent/sterile water)

To make 180 mL of $1/4$-strength normal saline, mix 45 mL of full-strength normal saline and 135 mL of sterile water.

**Think:** 45 mL is $\frac{1}{4}$ of the total volume (180 mL) and 135 mL + 45 mL = 180 mL.

**Example 2:** The prescriber orders a sacral wound irrigated with $\frac{1}{3}$-strength normal saline and sterile water tid. 75 mL is needed for each irrigation (tid means three times a day). You will need to prepare 75 mL × 3 irrigations = 225 mL total solution.

How much normal saline (full-strength) and sterile water will you need?

**Solution:** The fraction represents the desired solution strength: $\frac{1}{3}$ means 1-part solute (normal saline) to 3 total parts solution.

1. No conversion required.

2. $\frac{1}{3}$      225 mL      $x$ mL
(desired × (amount of = (solute)
strength)   solution)

$$x = \frac{225}{3}$$

$$x = 75 \text{ mL}$$

You need 75 mL of solute (normal saline) to prepare the desired solution (225 mL of $\frac{1}{3}$ strength). The total you want to make is 225 mL. The amount of solvent you need is therefore:

225 mL − 75 mL = 150 mL (solvent/sterile water)

To make 225 mL of $\frac{1}{3}$-strength normal saline, mix 75 mL of full-strength normal saline and 150 mL of sterile water.

**Think:** 75 mL is $\frac{1}{3}$ of the total volume (225 mL) and 150 mL + 75 mL = 225 mL.

**SAFETY ALERT!**
Think and calculate with accuracy. Errors can be made in determining the dilution for a solution if you incorrectly calculate the amount of solute and solvent for a required solution strength.

## PRACTICE **PROBLEMS**

Prepare the following strength solutions. (Express answers in mL.)

55. $\frac{2}{3}$-strength Sustacal 300 mL p.o. q.i.d. _____

56. $\frac{3}{4}$-strength Ensure 16 oz by nasogastric (NG) tube over 8 hr _____

57. $\frac{1}{2}$-strength Ensure 20 oz by gastrostomy tube (GT) over 5 hr _____

For each of the following, indicate how you would prepare the following solutions using full-strength normal saline as the solute and sterile water as the solvent.

58. 8 oz of $\frac{1}{4}$ strength for wound cleansing _____

59. 480 mL of $\frac{1}{3}$ strength for wound irrigation _____

60. 120 mL of $\frac{3}{4}$ strength for skeletal pain care _____

61. 160 mL of $\frac{5}{8}$-strength solution _____

**Answers on p. 422**

**POINTS TO REMEMBER**

- Enteral feedings (continuous) are placed on an infusion pump and administered at a rate expressed in milliliters per hour. The prescriber usually orders the feeding rate in milliliters per hour. If not, the nurse must calculate the rate at which to deliver the feeding.
- To prepare a solution of a specific strength, write the desired solution strength as a fraction and multiply it by the amount of desired solution. This will give you the amount of solute needed.
- The amount of desired solution − solute = amount of liquid needed to dissolve the substance (solvent).
- Think and calculate with accuracy to avoid making errors in determining the dilution for a required solution strength.

## ☐ CLINICAL **REASONING**

1. **Scenario:** Order: Ceftazidime 250 mg IM q8h.

   The nurse had the package insert below and a 1-g vial.

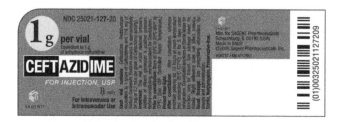

| Preparation of Solutions of Ceftazidime for Injection | | | |
|---|---|---|---|
| **Size** | **Amount of Diluent to be Added (mL)** | **Approximate Available Volume (mL)** | **Approximate Ceftazidime Concentration (mg/mL)** |
| Intramuscular | | | |
| 1-gram vial | 3 | 3.6 | 280 |
| Intravenous | | | |
| 1-gram vial | 10 | 10.8* | 100 |
| 2-gram vial | 10 | 11.5** | 170 |

The nurse reconstituted the medication (Ceftazidime) with 10.8 mL of diluent and administered 2.5 mL to the client.

a. What error occurred here? _____

b. What concentration should have been made? _____

c. What concentration did the nurse make and for which route? _____

d. What is the potential outcome of the error? _____

e. What measures could have been taken to prevent the error? _____

**Answers on p. 423**

## ⊙ CHAPTER **REVIEW**

Use the labels where provided to obtain the necessary information. Shade the dosage on syringes where provided. Round the answers to the nearest tenth where indicated.

1. Order: methylprednisolone sodium succinate 170 mg for 5 days.

Available:

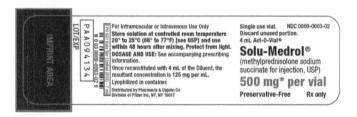

a. How many milliliters will you administer? _____

b. Shade the dosage calculated on the syringe provided.

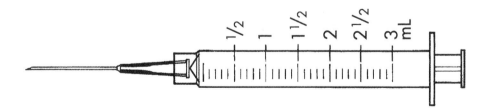

2. Order: Ampicillin 375 mg IM q6h

Available:

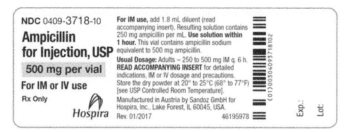

a. How much diluent must be added to
   the vial for IM administration?                    _____

b. What is the final concentration of the
   solution prepared for IM administration?          _____

c. How many milliliters will you administer?         _____

d. Shade the dosage calculated on the syringe provided.

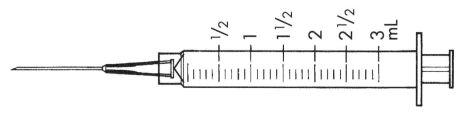

3. Order: Cefdinir 0.3 g p.o. q12h for 10 days.

Available:

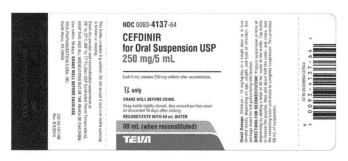

a. How much diluent must be added to prepare the solution? _____

b. What diluent is recommended for reconstitution? _____

c. What is the dosage strength of the reconstituted solution? _____

d. How many milliliters will you administer? _____

e. How long will the medication maintain its potency? _____

4. Order: penicillin G potassium 275,000 units IM q6h.

   Available:

   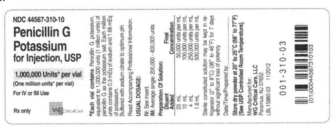

   a. Which dosage strength would be best to choose? _____

   b. How many milliliters of diluent would be
      needed to make the dosage strength? _____

   c. How many milliliters will you administer? _____

   d. Shade the dosage calculated on the syringe provided.

   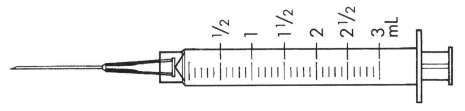

5. Order: Vivitrol 380 mg IM every 4 weeks for a client who is alcohol dependent.

   Available: Vivitrol and enclosed diluent to use for reconstitution of medication

   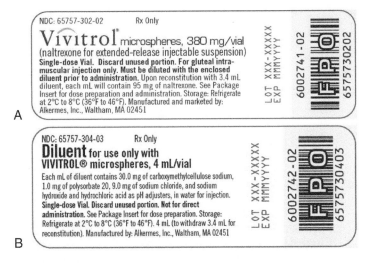

   a. How much diluent must be added to
      the vial for gluteal IM administration?          _____

   b. How many milliliters of diluent will
      be discarded?                                    _____

   c. What is the final dosage strength (concentration)
      of the reconstituted solution?                   _____

   d. How many milliliters will you need
      to administer?                                   _____

   e. After verifying that the dosage ordered is
      the recommended dosage, how will you
      administer the dosage? Provide a rationale.      _____

   f. What syringe will you use?                       _____

6. Order: Cefazolin 0.5 g IM q6h.

   Available:

   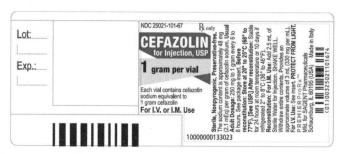

   a. What is the total dosage strength of
      Cefazolin in this vial?

   _____

   b. How many milliliters of diluent must
      be added for IM use?

   _____

   c. What diluent is recommended for
      reconstitution?

   _____

   d. What is the final dosage strength of the
      reconstituted solution?

   _____

   e. What is the displacement volume?

   _____

   f. How many milliliters will you administer?

   _____

   g. Shade the dosage calculated on the syringe provided.

   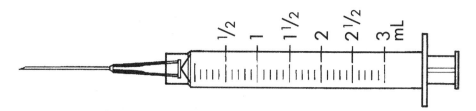

7. Order: Amoxicillin/clavulanate 0.5 g p.o. q12h (calculation based on Amoxicillin).

   Available:

   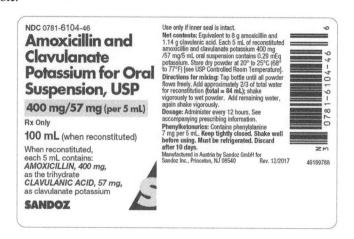

   a. How many milliliters of diluent must
      be added?

   _____

b. What is the dosage strength after reconstitution?  _____

c. How many milliliters are needed to administer the required dosage?  _____

8. Order: Cefepime 1.5 g IV q12h.

   Available: Refer to medication label and portion of the package insert.

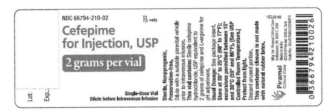

| Preparation of Solutions of Ceftazidime for Injection | | | |
|---|---|---|---|
| **Single-Dose Vials for Intravenous (IV)/ Intramuscular (IM) Administration** | **Amount of Diluent to be Added (mL)** | **Approximate Cefepime Concentration (mg/mL)** | **Amount of Reconstituted Volume to be Withdrawn (mL)** |
| Cefepime vial content | | | |
| 1 g (IV) | 10 | 100 | 10.5 |
| 1 g (IM) | 2.4 | 280 | 3.6 |
| 2 g (IV) | 10 | 160 | 12.5 |

a. How many milliliters will you administer?  _____

b. Shade the dosage calculated on the syringe provided.

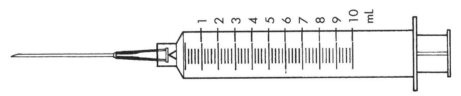

9. Order: Penicillin G potassium 1.8 million units IV q6h.

   Available:

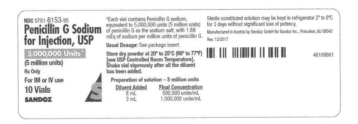

a. Which dosage strength would be best to choose? _____

b. How many milliliters of diluent would be
   needed to make the dosage strength?            _____

c. How many milliliters will you add to the IV?   _____

d. Shade the dosage calculated on the syringe provided

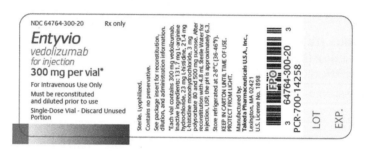

10. Order: Entyvio 300 mg IV Week 1 for a client with Crohn's disease.

    Available: Refer to label and an excerpt from the reconstitution directions.

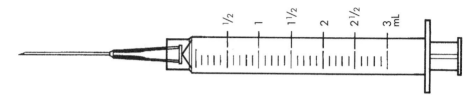

   Directions for reconstitution: Reconstitute with 4.8 mL of sterile water for injection.
   Allow solution to sit for up to 20 minutes at room temperature. Once it is dissolved, withdraw 5 mL (300 mg) of reconstituted Entyvio. Discard any remaining
   portion of the reconstituted solution in vial.

   a. What is the total dosage strength of this vial?    _____

   b. What are the directions for use?                   _____

   c. What is the dosage strength of the prepared
      solution?                                          _____

   d. How many mL will you prepare for
      administration?                                    _____

11. Order: Vancomycin 0.45 g IV q6h.

Available:

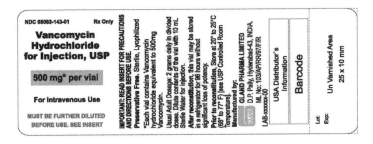

a. How many milliliters of diluent
   must be added to the vial?          _____

b. What diluent is recommended for
   reconstitution?                     _____

c. What is the final concentration of
   the prepared solution?              _____

d. How many milliliters will you
   add to the IV?                      _____

e. Shade the dosage calculated on the syringe provided.

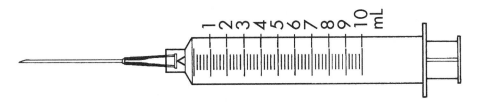

12. Order: Levothyroxine sodium 0.05 mg IV daily.

Available:

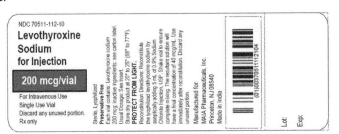

a. How many milliliters will you add to the IV? _____

b. Shade the dosage calculated on the syringe provided.

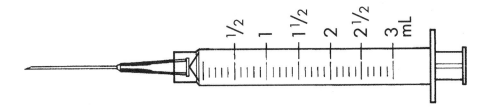

13. Order: Acyclovir 0.25 g IV q8h for 5 days.

    Use the directions from the insert provided.

    Available:

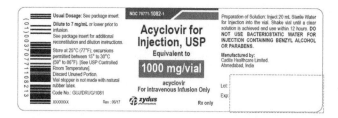

**Method of Preparation:** Each 10 mL vial contains acyclovir sodium equivalent to 500 mg of acyclovir. Each 20 mL vial contains acyclovir sodium equivalent to 1000 mg of acyclovir. The contents of the vial should be dissolved in Sterile Water for Injection as follows:

| Contents of Vial | Amount of Diluent |
| --- | --- |
| 500 mg | 10 mL |
| 1000 mg | 20 mL |

The resulting solution in each case contains 50 mg acyclovir per mL (pH approximately 11). Shake the vial well to assure complete dissolution before measuring and transferring each individual dose. DO NOT USE BACTE-RIOSTATIC WATER FOR INJECTION CONTAINING BENZYL ALCOHOL OR PARABENS.

a. How many milliliters will you add to the IV? _____

b. Shade the dosage calculated on the syringe provided.

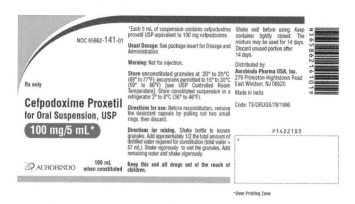

14. Vantin (cefpodoxime proxetil) 200 mg by nasogastric tube q12h.

    Available:

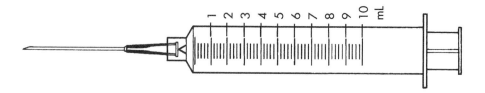

How many milliliters will you
administer? _____

15. Order: Nafcillin 1 g IV q4h.

Available: Refer to label and portion of the package insert for Nafcillin.

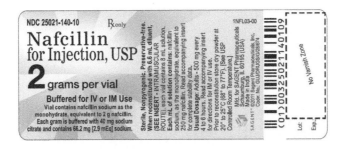

**DIRECTIONS FOR USE**

**For Intramuscular Use**

Reconstitute with Sterile Water for Injection, USP, 0.9% Sodium Chloride Injection, USP, or Bacteriostatic Water for Injection, USP (with benzyl alcohol or parabens); add 3.4 mL to the 1-g vial for 4 mL resulting solution and 6.6 mL to the 2-g vial for 8 mL resulting solution. All reconstituted vials have a concentration of 250 mg per mL.

**For Direct Intravenous Use**

The required amount of drug should be diluted in 15 to 30 mL of Sterile Water for Injection, USP or Sodium Chloride Injection, USP and injected over a 5- to 10-minute period. This may be accomplished through the tubing of an intravenous infusion if desirable.

**For Administration by Intravenous Drip**

Reconstitute as directed above (For Intravenous Use) prior to diluting with intravenous solutions.

a. What is the total dosage strength of this vial?        _____

b. How many milliliters of diluent must be added to the vial?        _____

c. What diluent is recommended for reconstitution?        _____

d. What is the dosage strength after reconstitution?        _____

e. What is the displacement volume?        _____

f. How many milliliters will you add to the IV?        _____

g. Shade the dosage calculated on the syringe provided.

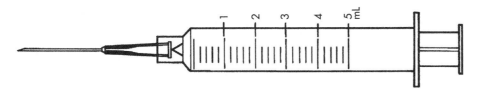

16. Order: Vfend 200 mg IV q12h.

Available:

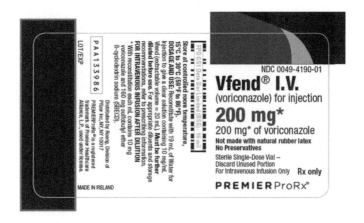

a. How many milliliters of diluent
   must be added to the vial?                    _____

b. How many milliliters will you
   add to the IV?                                 _____

17. Order: Zosyn 3.375 g IV q6h.

Available:

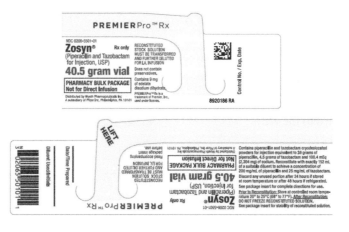

a. How many milliliters of diluent are
   recommended for reconstitution?               _____

b. What is the dosage strength of the vial?      _____

c. How many milliliters will you add
   to the IV? (The dosage is based on
   the two medications together.)                 _____

18.  Order: Zithromax (azithromycin) 500 mg p.o. stat for 1 dose.

Available:

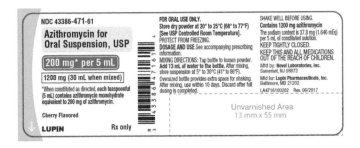

How many milliliters will you administer?     _____

19.  Order: Unasyn 1.5 g IV q6h.

Available:

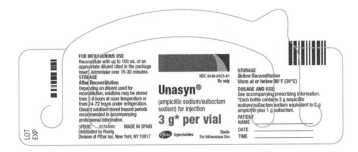

Refer to excerpt from package insert of Unasyn.

| Unasyn Vial Size | Volume of Diluent to Be Added | Withdrawal Volume |
| --- | --- | --- |
| 1.5 g | 3.2 mL | 4 mL |
| 3 g | 6.4 mL | 8 mL |

How many milliliters will you
add to the IV?     _____

20.  Order: Ceftriaxone 1 g IV 30 minutes before surgery.

Available:

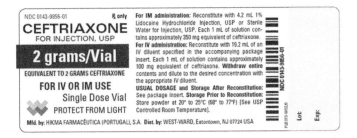

How many milliliters will you
administer?     _____

21. Order: Amphotericin B 45.5 mg IV every day.

Available:

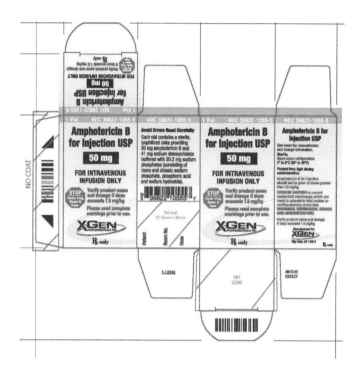

**Preparation of Solutions**

Reconstitute as follows: An initial concentrate of 5 mg amphotericin B per mL is first prepared by rapidly expressing 10 mL Sterile Water for Injection USP *without a bacteriostatic agent* directly into the lyophilized cake, using a sterile needle (minimum diameter: 20 gauge) and syringe. Shake the vial immediately until the colloidal solution is clear. The infusion solution, providing 0.1 mg amphotericin B per mL, is then obtained by further dilution (1:50) with 5% Dextrose Injection USP *of pH above 4.2.* The pH of each container of Dextrose Injection should be ascertained before use. Commercial Dextrose Injection usually has a pH above 4.2; however, if it is below 4.2, then 1 or 2 mL of buffer should be added to the Dextrose Injection before it is used to dilute the concentrated solution of amphotericin B. The recommended buffer has the following composition:

| | |
|---|---|
| Dibasic sodium phosphate (anhydrous) | 1.59 g |
| Monobasic sodium phosphate (anhydrous) | 0.96 g |
| Water for Injection USP | qs 100.0 mL |

Use the excerpt from the package insert to answer the questions and calculate the number of milliliters you will administer.

a. How many milliliters of diluent must be added for the initial concentration?

_____

b. What is the recommended diluent?

_____

c. What is the final concentration of the prepared solution per milliliter?

_____

d. How many milliliters will you administer (initial dose)?

_____

22. Order: Oxacillin 0.35 g IM q6h.

    Available:

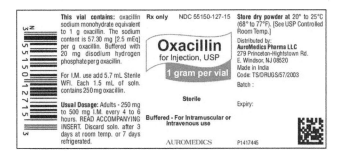

    a. How many milliliters will you administer IM? _____

    b. Shade the dosage calculated on the syringe provided.

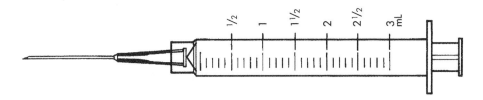

23. Order: Streptomycin 0.75 g IM daily for 1 week.

    Available:

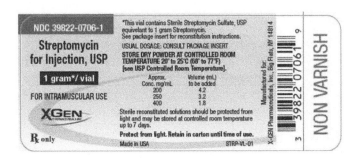

    Directions: Dilute with 1.8 mL of sterile water for injection.

    a. How many milliliters will you administer IM? _____

    b. Shade the dosage calculated on the syringe provided.

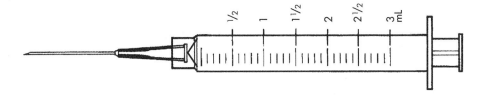

24. Order: Visudyne 10 mg IV × 1 dose.

Available:

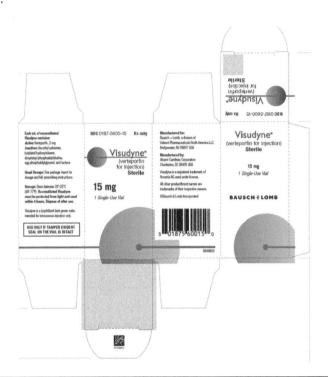

> Reconstitute each vial of Visudyne with 7 mL of sterile water for Injection
> to provide 7.5 mL containing 2 mg/mL. Reconstituted Visudyne must be
> protected from light and used within 4 hours. It is recommended that
> reconstituted Visudyne be inspected visually for particulate matter and
> discoloration prior to administration. Reconstituted Visudyne is an opaque
> dark green solution. Visudyne may precipitate in saline solutions. Do not
> use normal saline or other parenteral solutions, except 5% Dextrose for
> Injection, for dilution of the reconstituted Visudyne. Do not mix Visudyne
> in the same solution with other drugs.

a. How many milliliters will you administer IV? _____

b. Shade the dosage calculated on the syringe provided.

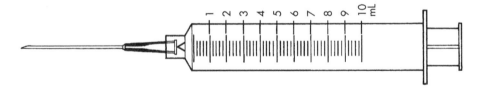

Prepare the following solutions from the nutritional formulas. (Express answers in mL.)

25. Order: $\frac{1}{4}$-strength Ensure 12 oz by nasogastric tube over 6 hr. _____

26. Order: $\frac{2}{3}$-strength Isomil 6 oz p.o. q4h for 24 hr.
    (State answer for single feeding.) _____

27. A client has an order for Jevity 1,000 mL by continuous feeding through a gastros-
    tomy tube over 16 hours, followed by 250 mL of free water. The feeding is placed on

an infusion pump. Calculate the mL per hr to set the pump at. (Round answer to nearest whole number.) _____

28. Order: ⅛-strength Ensure 4 oz by nasogastric tube q4h for 24h. (State answer for single feeding.) _____

Indicate how you would prepare each of the following using full-strength normal saline (0.9%) (solute) and sterile water (solvent).

29. Clean sacral wound with 4 oz of ½-strength normal saline q6h. You make enough solution for 24 hours. _____

30. Irrigate foot wound with 0.24 L of ¼-strength daily. _____

31. 18 oz of ⅔-strength solution for wound irrigation _____

32. 0.5 L of ¼-strength solution for wound irrigation _____

**Answers on pp. 423-428**

---

## ⭐ ANSWERS

## Chapter 18
### Answers to Practice Problems

1. 200 mg per vial
2. 5 mL
3. 0.9% sodium chloride injection without preservatives
4. 38 mg per mL
5. 24 hours
6. 2.6 mL

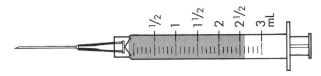

7. 100 mg per vial
8. 10 mL
9. Sterile water for injection or Bacteriostatic water for injection preserved with benzyl alcohol
10. 10 mg per mL
11. IV or IM use
12. See package insert.

13. 1.5 mL

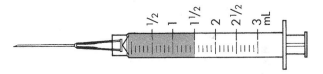

14. 40 mg per vial
15. Bacteriostatic water for injection with benzyl alcohol
16. 1 mL
17. 40 mg per mL
18. 0.9 mL

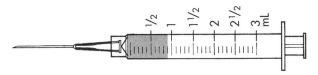

19. 106 mL

20. water

21. 250 mg per 5 mL (1 tsp)

22. Refrigerate and keep tightly closed.

23. 70 mL

24. 100 mL

25. 200 mg per 5 mL (1 tsp)

26. 10 days (refrigerated)

27. 2 g per vial

28. 4.2 mL

29. 19.2 mL

30. IV diluents specified in the accompanying package insert

31. 100 mg per mL

32. 500 mg per vial

33. 4.8 mL

34. sterile water for injection

35. 100 mg per mL

36. IV infusion only

37. For Intravenous Infusion Only

38. 500,000 units per mL

39. 1,000,000 units per mL; this strength is closest to what is ordered.

40. 2 mL

41. 7 days (1 week)

42. Intramuscular or Intravenous use

43. See package insert for complete information.

44. refrigerator

45. 7 days (1 week)

46. 250,000 units per mL

47. 10 mg per vial

48. 2.1 mL

49. sterile water for injection

50. 1 hour

51. 1.5 mL

52. 0.5 mL

53. $\dfrac{480 \text{ mL}}{8 \text{ hr}} = 60 \text{ mL/hr}$

54. $\dfrac{1,600 \text{ mL}}{24 \text{ hr}} = 66.6 = 67 \text{ mL/hr}$

55. 300 mL qid = 300 mL × 4 = 1,200 mL

$$\tfrac{2}{3} \times 1,200 \text{ mL} = x \text{ mL}$$

$$x = \frac{2,400}{3}$$

$x = 800$ mL of formula needed

1,200 mL − 800 mL = 400 mL (water)

Therefore you will add 400 mL of water to 800 mL of Sustacal to make 1,200 mL of $\tfrac{2}{3}$-strength Sustacal.

56. 1 oz = 30 mL; therefore 16 oz = 480 mL

$$\tfrac{3}{4} \times 480 \text{ mL} = x \text{ mL}$$

$$x = \frac{1,440}{4}$$

$$x = 360 \text{ mL}$$

$x = 360$ mL of formula needed.

480 mL − 360 mL = 120 mL. You would need 360 mL of formula and 120 mL of water to make 480 mL of $\tfrac{3}{4}$-strength Ensure.

57. 1 oz = 30 mL; therefore 20 oz = 600 mL

$$\tfrac{1}{2} \times 600 \text{ mL} = x \text{ mL}$$

$$x = \frac{600}{2}$$

$$x = 300 \text{ mL}$$

$x = 300$ mL

600 mL − 300 mL = 300 mL (10 oz of water)

Answer: You would need 300 mL of Ensure and 300 mL of water to make 600 mL of $\tfrac{1}{2}$-strength Ensure.

58. 1 oz = 30 mL; therefore 8 oz = 240 mL

$$\tfrac{1}{4} \times 240 \text{ mL} = x \text{ mL}$$

$$x = \frac{240}{4}$$

$x = 60$ mL

60 mL normal saline (solute) + 180 mL sterile water (solvent) = 240 mL $\tfrac{1}{4}$-strength solution.

59. $\tfrac{1}{3} \times 480 \text{ mL} = x \text{ mL}$

$$x = \frac{480}{3}$$

$x = 160$ mL

160 mL normal saline (solute) + 320 mL sterile water (solvent) = 480 mL $\tfrac{1}{3}$-strength solution.

60. $\tfrac{3}{4} \times 120 \text{ mL} = x \text{ mL}$

$$x = \frac{360}{4}$$

$x = 90$ mL

90 mL normal saline (solute) + 30 mL sterile water (solvent) = 120 mL $\tfrac{3}{4}$-strength solution.

61. $\tfrac{5}{8} \times 160 \text{ mL} = x \text{ mL}$

$$x = \frac{800}{8}$$

$x = 100$ mL

100 mL normal saline (solute) + 60 mL sterile water (solvent) = 160 mL $\tfrac{5}{8}$-strength solution.

## Answers to Clinical Reasoning Questions

1. a. The wrong dosage was administered because the nurse chose the incorrect dilution instructions. The dilution instructions used were for IV instead of IM.

   b. The concentration for IM should have been made (add 3 mL of diluents to give a concentration of 280 mg per mL).

   c. The nurse added 10.8 mL of a diluent and made the concentration for IV administration 100 mg per mL.

   d. The client received almost three times the mL of medication IM (2.5 mL instead of 0.9 mL).

   Interchanging dilution instructions for IV and IM administration can have serious outcomes ranging from irritation of muscles to formation of a sterile abscess.

   e. This type of error could have been prevented by the nurse by reading the label carefully for the correct amount of diluents for the route ordered. Nurses must always check the route ordered and follow the directions that correspond to that route. The dilution instructions for IV and IM should never be interchanged.

> **NOTE**
> For problems in which conversion is indicated, answers are shown with order converted to what is available. Calculations could also be performed using dimensional analysis.

## Answers to Chapter Review

1. 125 mg : 1 mL = 170 mg : $x$ mL

$$\frac{125x}{125} = \frac{170}{125}$$

$$x = 1.36 = 1.4 \text{ mL}$$

*or*

$$\frac{170 \text{ mg}}{125 \text{ mg}} \times 1 \text{ mL} = x \text{ mL}$$

   a. Answer: 1.4 mL. The dosage ordered is greater than the available strength; therefore you will need more than 1 mL to administer the dosage ordered.

   b.

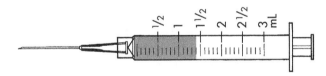

2. a. 1.8 mL

   b. 250 mg per 1 mL

   c. 250 mg : 1 mL = 375 mg : $x$ mL

$$\frac{250x}{250} = \frac{375}{250}$$

$$x = 1.5 \text{ mL}$$

*or*

$$\frac{375 \text{ mg}}{250 \text{ mg}} \times 1 \text{ mL} = x \text{ mL}$$

   d. Answer: 1.5 mL. The dosage ordered is greater than the available strength; you will need more than 1 mL to administer the dosage.

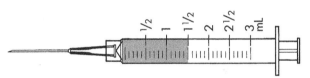

3. Conversion is required 1 g = 1,000 mg; therefore 0.3 g = 300 mg

   a. 49 mL

   b. water

   c. 250 mg per 5 mL

$$250 \text{ mg} : 5 \text{ mL} = 300 \text{ mg} : x \text{ mL}$$

$$\frac{250x}{250} = \frac{1,500}{250}$$

$$x = 6 \text{ mL}$$

*or*

$$\frac{300 \text{ mg}}{250 \text{ mg}} \times 5 \text{ mL} = x \text{ mL}$$

   d. Answer: 6 mL. The dosage ordered is greater than the available strength. You will need more than 5 mL to give the dosage ordered.

   e. 10 days

4.  a. 250,000 units per mL

    b. 4 mL

    c.    250,000 units : 1 mL = 275,000 units : $x$ mL

$$\frac{250{,}000x}{250{,}000} = \frac{275{,}000}{250{,}000}$$

$$x = \frac{275}{250}$$

$$x = 1.1 \text{ mL}$$

*or*

$$\frac{275{,}000 \text{ units}}{250{,}000 \text{ units}} \times 1 \text{ mL} = x \text{ mL}$$

    d. Answer: 1.1 mL. The dosage ordered is greater than what is available; therefore you will need more than 1 mL to administer the dosage.

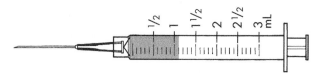

5.  a. 3.4 mL

    b. 0.6 mL

    c. 95 mg per mL

$$95 \text{ mg} : 1 \text{ mL} = 380 \text{ mg} : x \text{ mL}$$

$$\frac{95x}{95} = \frac{380}{95}$$

$$x = 4 \text{ mL}$$

or

$$\frac{380 \text{ mg}}{95 \text{ mg}} \times 1 \text{ mL} = x \text{ mL}$$

    d. Answer: 4 mL. The dosage ordered is greater than the available strength; therefore you will need more than 1 mL to administer the dosage ordered.

    e. 4 mL exceeds the maximum amount of 3 mL allowed for administration to an adult IM in one site. If more than 3 mL is needed to deliver the ordered dose IM, then the amount to administer is divided equally between two (2) syringes and administered into separate IM sites. In this case, 2 mL would be drawn up in each syringe, and 2 mL would be administered in the right gluteal and 2 mL in the left gluteal.

    f. 3-mL syringe (You will need two syringes and will draw up 2 mL in each syringe.)

6.  a. 1 g per vial

    b. 2.5 mL

    c. Sterile water for injection

    d. 330 mg per mL

    e. 0.5 mL

    Conversion is required. Equivalent 1 g = 1,000 mg, therefore 0.5 g = 500 mg

$$330 \text{ mg} : 1 \text{ mL} = 500 \text{ mg} : x \text{ mL}$$

$$\frac{330x}{330} = \frac{500}{330}$$

$$x = 1.51 = 1.5 \text{ mL}$$

*or*

$$\frac{500 \text{ mg}}{330 \text{ mg}} \times 1 \text{ mL} = x \text{ mL}$$

    f. Answer: 1.5 mL. The dosage ordered is greater than the available strength; therefore you will need more than 1 mL to administer the dosage ordered.

    g.

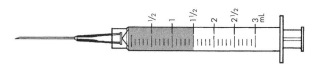

7.  Conversion is required. Equivalent: 1,000 mg = 1 g; therefore 0.5 g = 500 mg

    a. 84 mL

    b. 400 mg per 5 mL

    c. 6.3 mL

$$400 \text{ mg} : 5 \text{ mL} = 500 \text{ mg} : x \text{ mL}$$

$$\frac{400x}{400} = \frac{2{,}500}{400}$$

$$x = 6.25 = 6.3 \text{ mL}$$

*or*

$$\frac{500 \text{ mg}}{400 \text{ mg}} \times 5 \text{ mL} = x \text{ mL}$$

    Answer: 6.3 mL. The dosage ordered is greater than the available strength. You will need more than 5 mL to give the dosage.

8.  Conversion is required. Equivalent: 1,000 mg = 1 g; therefore 1.5 g = 1,500 mg

    a.    160 mg : 1 mL = 1,500 mg : $x$ mL

$$\frac{160\, x}{160} = \frac{1{,}500}{160}$$

$$x = 9.37 = 9.4 \text{ mL}$$

*or*

$$\frac{1{,}500 \text{ mg}}{160 \text{ mg}} \times 1 \text{ mL} = x \text{ mL}$$

    Answer: 9.4 mL. The dosage ordered is greater than the available strength; therefore you will need more than 1 mL to administer the dosage ordered.

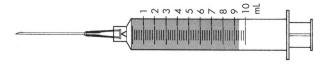

9. a. 1,000,000 units per mL. It is closest to what the prescriber ordered. The route ordered is IV; you would not choose a weak solution. The medication when administered IV is further diluted when added to the IV solution for administration (50–100 mL). Usually the maximum concentration is used for IV. You will have medication left over; therefore the dosage strength you mixed must be indicated on the medication label.

b. 3 mL

1,000,000 units : 1 mL = 1,800,000 units : $x$ mL

$$\frac{1,000,000x}{1,000,000} = \frac{1,800,000}{1,000,000}$$

$$x = \frac{18}{10}$$

$$x = 1.8 \text{ mL}$$

*or*

$$\frac{1,800,000 \text{ units}}{1,000,000 \text{ units}} \times 1 \text{ mL} = x \text{ mL}$$

c. Answer 1.8 mL. The dosage ordered is greater than the available strength; therefore you will need more than 1 mL to administer the dosage ordered.

d.

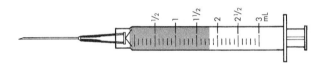

10. a. 300 mg per vial

b. For intravenous use only

c. 300 mg per 5 mL

d. No calculation required. The dosage ordered is contained the 5 mL of solution withdrawn from the vial after the medication is reconstituted.

11. a. 10 mL

b. Sterile water for injection

c. 500 mg per 10 mL

d. Conversion is required. Equivalent: 1,000 mg = 1 g; therefore 0.45 g = 450 mg

500 mg : 10 mL = 450 mg : $x$ mL

$$\frac{500\,x}{500} = \frac{4,500}{500}$$

$$x = 9 \text{ mL}$$

*or*

$$\frac{450 \text{ mg}}{500 \text{ mg}} \times 10 \text{ mL} = x \text{ mL}$$

Answer: 9 mL. The dosage ordered is less than the available strength; therefore you need less than 10 mL to administer the dosage ordered.

e.

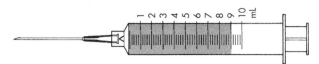

12. Conversion is required. Equivalent: 1,000 mcg = 1 mg; therefore 0.05 mg = 50 mcg.

a. 40 mcg : 1 mL = 50 mcg : $x$ mL

$$\frac{40x}{40} = \frac{50}{40}$$

$$x = 1.25 = 1.3 \text{ mL}$$

*or*

$$\frac{50 \text{ mcg}}{40 \text{ mcg}} \times 1 \text{ mL} = x \text{ mL}$$

Answer: 1.3 mL; 1.25 mL rounded to the nearest tenth. The dosage ordered is more than the available strength; therefore you will need more than 1 mL to administer the dosage ordered.

b.

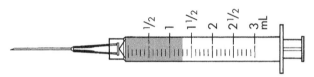

13. Conversion is required. Equivalent: 1,000 mg = 1 g; therefore 0.25 g = 250 mg.

a. 50 mg : 1 mL = 250 mg : $x$ mL

$$\frac{50x}{50} = \frac{250}{50}$$

$$x = 5 \text{ mL}$$

*or*

$$\frac{250 \text{ mg}}{50 \text{ mg}} \times 1 \text{ mL} = x \text{ mL}$$

Answer: 5 mL. The dosage ordered is greater than the available strength; therefore you will need more than 1 mL to administer the dosage ordered.

b.

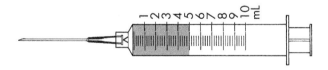

14.    $100 \text{ mg} : 5 \text{ mL} = 200 \text{ mg} : x \text{ mL}$

$$\frac{100x}{100} = \frac{1,000}{100}$$

$$x = 10 \text{ mL}$$

*or*

$$\frac{200 \text{ mg}}{100 \text{ mg}} \times 5 \text{ mL} = x \text{ mL}$$

Answer: 10 mL. The dosage ordered is greater than the available strength; therefore you will need more than 5 mL to administer the dosage ordered.

15. a. 2 g per vial

b. 6.6 mL

c. Sterile Water for Injection, 0.9% Sodium Chloride Injection, or Bacteriostatic Water for Injection (with benzyl alcohol or parabens)

d. 250 mg per mL

e. 1.4 mL

f. Conversion is required. Equivalent: 1 g = 1,000 mg; therefore 1 g ordered = 1,000 mg

$250 \text{ mg} : 1 \text{ mL} = 1,000 \text{ mg} : x \text{ mL}$

$$\frac{250x}{250} = \frac{1,000}{250}$$

$$x = 4 \text{ mL}$$

*or*

$$\frac{1,000 \text{ mg}}{250 \text{ mg}} \times 1 \text{ mL} = x \text{ mL}$$

Answer: 4 mL. The dosage ordered is more than the available strength; therefore you will need more than 1 mL to administer the dosage ordered.

g.

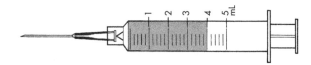

16. a. 19 mL

b.    $10 \text{ mg} : 1 \text{ mL} = 200 \text{ mg} : x \text{ mL}$

$$\frac{10x}{10} = \frac{200}{10}$$

$$x = 20 \text{ mL}$$

*or*

$$\frac{200 \text{ mg}}{10 \text{ mg}} \times 1 \text{ mL} = x \text{ mL}$$

Answer: 20 mL. The dosage ordered is greater than the available strength; therefore you will need more than 1 mL to administer the dosage ordered.

17. a. 152 mL

b. 40.5 g per vial

c. Conversion is required. 1,000 mg = 1 g; 3.375 g = 3,375 mg

The piperacillin and tazobactam are added together for calculation. When reconstituted, the result is 200 mg per mL of piperacillin and 25 mg per mL of tazobactam.

200 mg per mL + 25 mg per mL = 225 mg per mL.

$225 \text{ mg} : 1 \text{ mL} = 3,375 \text{ mg} : x \text{ mL}$

$$\frac{225x}{225} = \frac{3,375}{225}$$

$$x = 15 \text{ mL}$$

*or*

$$\frac{3,375 \text{ mg}}{225 \text{ mg}} \times 1 \text{ mL} = x \text{ mL}$$

Answer: 15 mL. The dosage ordered is greater than the available strength; therefore more than 1 mL is needed to administer the dosage ordered.

18.    $200 \text{ mg} : 5 \text{ mL} = 500 \text{ mg} : x \text{ mL}$

$$\frac{200x}{200} = \frac{2,500}{200}$$

$$x = 12.5 \text{ mL}$$

*or*

$$\frac{500 \text{ mg}}{200 \text{ mg}} \times 5 \text{ mL} = x \text{ mL}$$

Answer: 12.5 mL. The dosage ordered is greater than what is available; therefore you will need more than 5 mL to administer the dosage ordered.

19.    $3 \text{ g} : 8 \text{ mL} = 1.5 \text{ g} : x \text{ mL}$

$$\frac{3x}{3} = \frac{12}{3}$$

$$x = 4 \text{ mL}$$

*or*

$$\frac{1.5 \text{ g}}{3 \text{ g}} \times 8 \text{ mL} = x \text{ mL}$$

Answer: 4 mL. The dosage ordered is less than the available strength; therefore you will need less than 8 mL to administer the dosage ordered. (Ordered dosage is half of the available strength.)

20. Conversion is required. Equivalent: 1 g = 1,000 mg; therefore the 1 g ordered = 1,000 mg

$100 \text{ mg} : 1 \text{ mL} = 1,000 \text{ mg} : x \text{ mL}$

$$\frac{100x}{100} = \frac{1,000}{100}$$

$$x = 10 \text{ mL}$$

*or*

$$\frac{1,000 \text{ mg}}{100 \text{ mg}} \times 1 \text{ mL} = x \text{ mL}$$

Answer: 10 mL. The dosage ordered is greater than the available strength; therefore you will need more than 1 mL to administer the ordered dosage.

21. a. 10 mL

   b. Sterile Water for Injection without a bacteriostatic agent

   c. 5 mg per mL

   d.   5 mg : 1 mL = 45.5 mg : $x$ mL
   $$\frac{5x}{5} = \frac{45.5}{5}$$
   $$x = 9.1 \text{ mL}$$
   *or*
   $$\frac{45.5 \text{ mg}}{5 \text{ mg}} \times 1 \text{ mL} = x \text{ mL}$$

   Alternate solution

   50 mg : 10 mL = 45.5 mg : $x$ mL
   $$\frac{50x}{50} = \frac{455}{50}$$
   $$x = 9.1 \text{ mL}$$
   *or*
   $$\frac{45.5 \text{ mg}}{50 \text{ mg}} \times 10 \text{ mL} = x \text{ mL}$$

   This setup would net the same answer of 9.1 mL.

   Answer: 9.1 mL is the dose for the initial concentration (before further dilution). The dosage ordered is greater than the available strength; therefore you need more than 1 mL to administer the dosage ordered. This medication would have to be further diluted according to the instructions as follows: The infusion solution, providing 0.1 mg amphotericin B per mL, is then obtained by further dilution (1 : 50) with 5% dextrose injection. This may be accomplished by adding 49 mL dextrose and water injection to each 1 mL (5 mg) of amphotericin B solution. The concentrated amphotericin solution to dilute is the 9.1 mL. Therefore we need to add it. 9.1 × 49 mL = 445.9 = 446 mL of IV solution before administering the medication IV.

22. Conversion is required. Equivalent: 1,000 mg = 1 g; therefore 0.35 g = 350 mg

   a.   250 mg : 1.5 mL = 350 mg : $x$ mL
   $$\frac{250x}{250} = \frac{525}{250}$$
   $$x = 2.1 \text{ mL}$$
   *or*
   $$\frac{350 \text{ mg}}{250 \text{ mg}} \times 1.5 \text{ mL} = x \text{ mL}$$

   Answer: 2.1 mL. The dosage ordered is greater than the available strength; therefore you will need more than 1.5 mL to administer the dosage ordered.

   b.

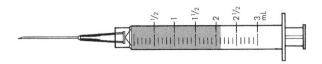

23. Conversion is required. Equivalent: 1 g = 1,000 mg; therefore 0.75 g = 750 mg

   a.   400 mg : 1 mL = 750 mg : $x$ mL
   $$\frac{400x}{400} = \frac{750}{400}$$
   $$x = 1.87 = 1.9 \text{ mL}$$
   *or*
   $$\frac{750 \text{ mg}}{400 \text{ mg}} \times 1 \text{ mL} = x \text{ mL}$$

   Answer: 1.9 mL; 1.87 rounded to the nearest tenth. The dosage ordered is greater than the available strength. Therefore you will need more than 1 mL to administer the dosage ordered.

   b.

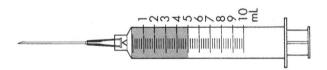

24. a.   2 mg : 1 mL = 10 mg : $x$ mL
   $$\frac{2x}{2} = \frac{10}{2}$$
   $$x = 5 \text{ mL}$$
   *or*
   $$\frac{10 \text{ mg}}{2 \text{ mg}} \times 1 \text{ mL} = x \text{ mL}$$

   Answer: 5 mL. The dosage ordered is greater than the available strength. Therefore you will need more than 1 mL to administer the dosage ordered.

   b.

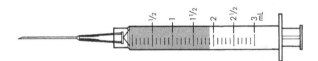

25. 1 oz = 30 mL; therefore 12 oz = 360 mL
   $$\frac{1}{4} \times 360 \text{ mL} = x \text{ mL}$$
   $$\frac{360}{4} = x$$
   $$x = 90 \text{ mL}$$

   $x$ = 90 mL; you need 90 mL of Ensure.

   360 mL − 90 mL Ensure = 270 mL of water.

   Answer: 90 mL Ensure + 270 mL water = 360 mL ¼-strength Ensure.

26. 1 oz = 30 mL; therefore 6 oz = 180 mL

$$\frac{2}{3} \times \frac{180}{1} = \frac{360}{3} = 120 \text{ mL Isomil}$$

180 mL − 120 mL = 60 mL water

You would add 60 mL of water to 120 mL Isomil to make 180 mL of $\frac{2}{3}$-strength Isomil for each feeding po q4h.

27. $\dfrac{1{,}000 \text{ mL}}{16 \text{ hr}} = 62.5 \text{ mL/hr}$

Answer: 63 mL/hr (62.5 rounded to nearest whole number)

28. 1 oz = 30 mL; therefore 4oz = 120 mL

$$\frac{1}{8} \times \frac{120}{1} = \frac{120}{8} = 15 \text{ mL Ensure}$$

120 mL − 15 mL = 105 mL water

You would add 105 mL of water to 15 mL Ensure to make 120 mL of $\frac{1}{8}$-strength Ensure for each feeding by nasogastric tube q4h.

29. q6h = 4 times in 24 hours; therefore 4 oz × 4 = 16 oz.

1 oz = 30 mL; therefore 16 oz = 480 mL

480 mL × $\frac{1}{2}$ = $x$ mL

$$x = \frac{480}{2}$$

$x = 240$ mL

240 mL normal saline (solute) + 240 mL sterile water (solvent) = 480 mL $\frac{1}{2}$-strength solution

30. Conversion is required. Equivalent: 1 L = 1,000 mL; therefore 0.24 L = 240 mL

240 mL × $\frac{1}{4}$ = $x$ mL

$$x = \frac{240}{4}$$

$x = 60$ mL

60 mL normal saline (solute) + 180 mL sterile water (solvent) = 240 mL $\frac{1}{4}$-strength solution.

31. 1 oz = 30 mL; therefore 18 oz = 540 mL

540 mL × $\frac{2}{3}$ = $x$ mL

$$x = 540 \times \frac{2}{3}$$

$$x = \frac{1{,}080}{3}$$

$x = 360$ mL

360 mL normal saline (solute) + 180 mL sterile water (solvent) = 540 mL $\frac{2}{3}$-strength solution.

32. Conversion is required. Equivalent: 1 L = 1,000 mL.

Therefore 0.5 L = 500 mL

500 mL × $\frac{1}{4}$ = $x$ mL

$$x = \frac{500}{4}$$

$x = 125$ mL

125 mL normal saline (solute) + 375 mL sterile water (solvent) = 500 mL $\frac{1}{4}$-strength solution.

# CHAPTER **19**
# Insulin

## Objectives

*After reviewing this chapter, you should be able to:*

1. Identify important information on insulin labels
2. Identify various methods for insulin administration
3. Read calibrations on 30-, 50-, and 100-unit syringes
4. Read calibrations on a U-500 insulin syringe
5. Measure doses using a 30-, 50-, and 100-unit insulin syringe
6. Measure doses using a U-500 insulin syringe
7. Measure insulin in single doses
8. Measure combined insulin dosages

## Introduction

Insulin, which is used in the treatment of diabetes mellitus (DM), is a hormone secreted by the islets of Langerhans in the pancreas. It is a necessary hormone for glucose use by the body. Individuals who do not produce adequate insulin experience an increase in their blood sugar (glucose) level. These individuals may require the administration of insulin. According to the Centers for Disease Control and Prevention (CDC), it is estimated that 26 million Americans have type 2 diabetes (insufficient production of insulin, causing high blood sugar). In addition, according to the American Diabetes Association (ADA), 1.5 million Americans are diagnosed with diabetes every year. With the increase in the incidence of diabetes, one can also expect that there will be an increase in the use of insulin. Insulin is considered to be a vital and life-saving medication for persons with diabetes. Therefore accuracy in administration of insulin is **critical** because inaccurate dosage administration can lead to serious life-threatening effects or death. Any error that occurs in medication administration, regardless of the reason for it, may result in harm to a client; however, there are some medications that have been designated "high-alert medications." Insulin is considered a "high-alert medication" by the Institute for Safe Medication Practices (ISMP). Medications that are considered high-alert medications have a high risk of causing injury or death to a client and are also identified as those with which health care providers often make errors. ISMP defines high-alert medications as "drugs that bear a heightened risk of causing significant patient harm when they are used in error." The consequences associated with errors with these medications are usually more devastating than those that occur with other medications. High-alert medications require that safeguards be in place to ensure that when they are used, there is a focus on safely using them and preventing harm to the clients who receive them. Nurses as well as other health care providers **must** be highly attentive when calculating dosages and administering high-alert medications. Always follow the policy of the institution for administering high-alert medications to decrease the chance of error and harm to the client. This chapter will focus on basic concepts related to the safe administration of insulin.

Despite the focus of health care institutions on initiatives aimed at improving safety in the administration of insulin and preventing errors, it has been noted that the occurrence of errors with insulin persists. In addition to insulin being considered a high-alert medication, insulin has also been known to be associated with more medication errors than most other medications. The U.S. Pharmacopeia Medication Errors Reporting Program states that approximately 50% of all medication errors involve insulin. The ISMP developed *Guidelines for Optimizing Safe Subcutaneous Insulin Use in Adults* (June 5, 2017), aimed at assisting health care facilities in the prevention of insulin errors and improving patient outcomes, which also included recommendations for the safe use of subcutaneous insulin in the hospital and during transition of care. Causes for insulin errors were also identified, which included administration of the wrong insulin product, improper dosing (underdosing and overdosing), dose omissions, and wrong route (intramuscular versus subcutaneous). These guidelines can be viewed on the ISMP website: https://www.ismp.org/guidelines/subcutaneous-insulin.

*Diabetes in Control* (News and Information for Medical Professionals), in October 2019 in an article titled "A Review of Insulin Errors," identified errors with insulin from information provided by Novo Nordisk, an insulin manufacturer, which included clinician errors, bad drawing-up procedure, improper monitoring (not checking blood glucose 2 hours after injection), and using the wrong insulin (http://www.diabetesincontrol.com/a-review-of-insulin-errors/). The current literature identifies a variety of errors that continue to occur with insulin therapy. The errors presented are just a sample of the causes of errors with insulin. Even currently there are still reports to ISMP on the misadministration of insulin. This has serious implications for nurses as well as other health care providers. Some practices to promote safety include reading insulin labels carefully (some brand names may sound and look alike), client monitoring, and administration of U-500 insulin with a U-500 syringe.

## Types of Insulin

Insulins distributed in the United States are synthetic "human insulins" or their analogs, which are chemically altered DNA. Insulin from a human source is designated on the label as recombinant DNA (rDNA origin).

- Humalog insulin (lispro) is a fast-acting insulin analog. Lispro acts within 5 to 15 minutes. Lispro can be administered 5 minutes before meals, whereas regular insulin can be administered 30 to 60 minutes before meals. Like regular human insulin, Lispro is clear and can be administered intravenously as well as subcutaneously. Other rapid-acting insulin analogs include aspart (NovoLog) and glulisine (Apidra). Like lispro and regular insulin, these analogs are clear and can also be administered intravenously as well as subcutaneously.
- Lantus (insulin glargine) is an analog of human insulin, classified as long-acting, and permits once-daily dosing. It can be administered at any time during the day for 24-hour coverage without a peak; however, it must be administered at the same time every day. In addition, it is clear in appearance, intended for subcutaneous use **only**, and cannot be mixed with other insulins. The packaging is distinct; the vial is tall, narrow, and the name Lantus is printed in purple letters. Levemir (detemir), which is also long-acting, is also generally given once daily. However, it does not last as long as Lantus, so clients may require a nighttime dose. Like Lantus, Levemir cannot be mixed with other insulins.
- Tresiba (insulin degludec injection), a long-acting insulin analog, was approved in 2015 by the US Food and Drug Administration (FDA). Tresiba is administered subcutaneously once daily at any time of day. It should not be diluted or mixed with other insulins and is available in the FlexTouch pen in two concentrations: 100 units per mL and 200 units per mL. Also available in vial U-100 (multiple-dose 10-mL vial).

## Labels

It is essential that the nurse know the essential information on an insulin label and where to locate it. Information such as the origin of insulin, type, brand and generic names, the dosage strength or concentration, and storage information is indicated on the label.

Figure 19.1 shows information that can be found on an insulin label. Notice the following:

- The trade name is followed by a large capital letter. In Figure 19.1, Humulin N is the trade name. The larger capital letter N following the trade name identifies the type of insulin by action and time. The large capital letter N indicates NPH (intermediate-acting). These letters are important identifiers for insulin.

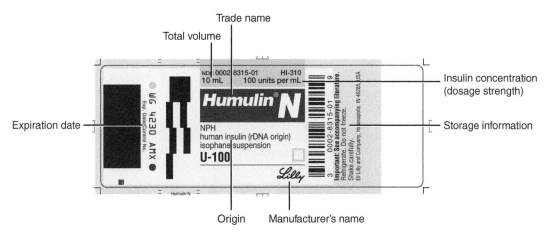

**Figure 19.1** Label for U-100 insulin. (NPH)

- Notice the use of uppercase letters for the letter N for NPH. You will see the large capital letter R to indicate Regular insulin.
- Concentration (dosage strength) of the insulin is also indicated; notice U-100 (which means 100 units per mL). 100 units per mL is also indicated on the label. Every type of insulin is measured in units.
- The expiration date is also indicated on insulin labels and is important to check. Review the important information identified on the label in Figure 19.1.

## U-500 Insulin

U-500 insulin is a short-acting regular insulin that is concentrated and not for ordinary use. It is indicated to improve glycemic control in clients with diabetes mellitus requiring more than 200 units of insulin per day. U-500 insulin is **five (5) times more potent** than U-100 insulin. Accidental substitution of U-500 for U-100 could result in a fatal overdose. According to The Institute for Safe Medication Practices (ISMP), as the obesity epidemic continues and insulin resistance problems worsen, larger doses of insulin are more frequently required to meet glycemic goals and this has led to an increased use of U-500 insulin. U-500 insulin means 500 units per mL. U-500 insulin should only be administered using the U-500 syringe. The U-500 syringe has a green needle shield cover (cap) and U-500 indicated on the barrel of the syringe in green. Refer to Figure 19.2 for a U-500 insulin label.

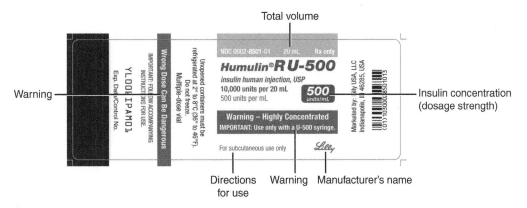

**Figure 19.2** Label for U-500 insulin.

Notice the following on the U-500 insulin label:

- Notice the U-500 is indicated in green.
- Concentration (dosage strength) U-500 (500 units per mL). The 500 units per mL is also indicated in green. This insulin is **5 times more potent than the U-100.** The dosage strength is also indicated for the total vial (10,000 units per 20 mL). The total volume of the vial is 20 mL.
- Warnings are indicated in red: "Highly concentrated, use only with a U-500 syringe, wrong dose can be dangerous, and follow accompanying instructions for use."
- The directions for use are also indicated on the label, for subcutaneous use only.
  U-500 insulin comes in a 20-mL multiple-dose vial containing 10,000 units of insulin and a 3-mL U-500 Kwikpen containing 1,500 units of insulin.

> **! SAFETY ALERT!**
>
> It is critical that the nurse use **extreme caution** when administering U-500 insulin to prevent unintentional overdose, which can result in irreversible insulin shock and death of a client.
>
> U-500 insulin, 500 units per mL, is five (5) times more potent than U-100 insulin, which is 100 units per mL. **U-500 insulin is administered with a U-500 syringe only.** Read the calibrations on the syringe carefully.

> **! SAFETY ALERT!**
>
> Careful reading of insulin labels is essential to avoid a medication error that could be life-threatening. Always read the label carefully and compare it with the medication order to ensure selection of the right type of insulin, correct action time, and concentration (strength).

## Insulin Action Times

Insulins are classified by their actions as rapid-acting, short-acting, intermediate-acting, and long-acting insulin. Rapid-acting insulin and short-acting insulin are referred to as **bolus** types of insulin. These types of insulin are administered just a few minutes before a meal.

Intermediate- and long-acting insulins are considered **basal** types of insulin. Basal type insulins last longer in the body and provide a steady level of insulin throughout the day. Intermediate- and long-acting insulin can only be administered subcutaneously. Nurses must be familiar with the action times of insulins. Figure 19.3 shows samples of labels for insulin grouped by action times. As stated, note the use of N for NPH Insulin and R for Regular, indicated in bold uppercase letters. Regular and NPH insulin are the two types that have traditionally been used most frequently, and they are often mixed.

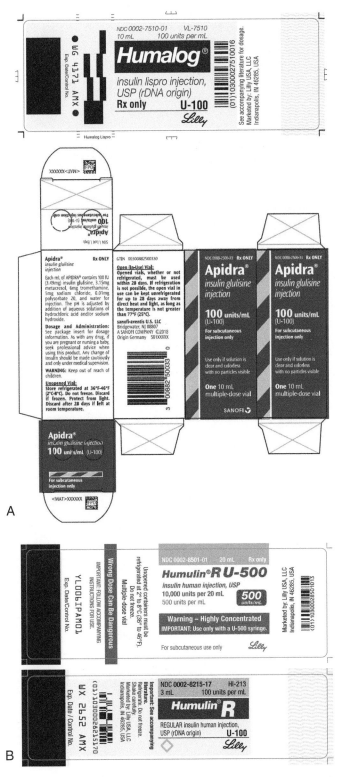

**Figure 19.3** (A) Rapid-acting (fast-acting). (B) Short-acting. *Continued*

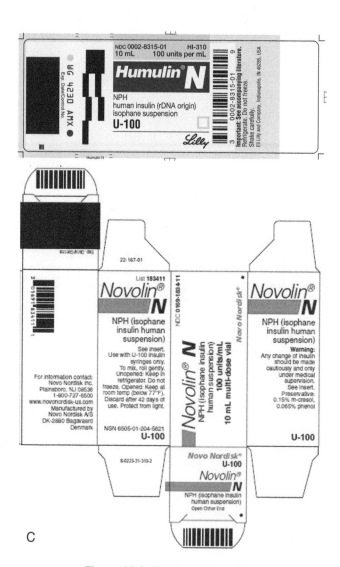

**Figure 19.3** (C) Intermediate-acting.

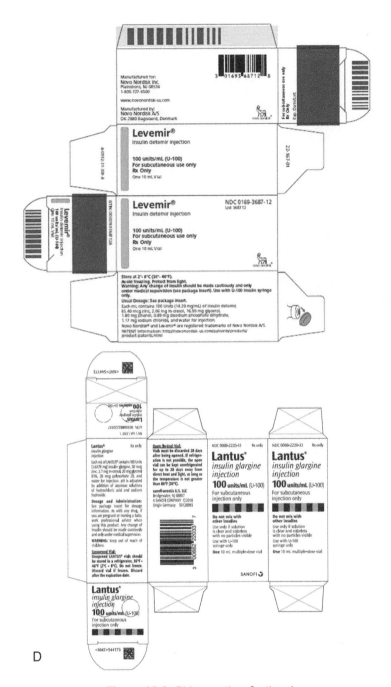

**Figure 19.3** (D) Long-acting. *Continued*

---

# PRACTICE **PROBLEMS**

Using the labels provided, identify the insulin trade name and action time (short acting, rapid acting, intermediate acting, or long acting).

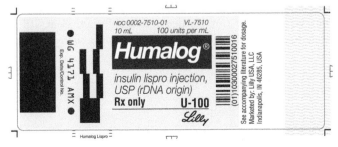

1. Trade name _____     Action time _____

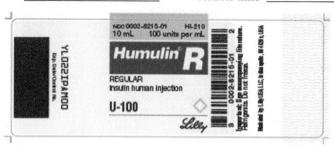

2. Trade name _____     Action time _____

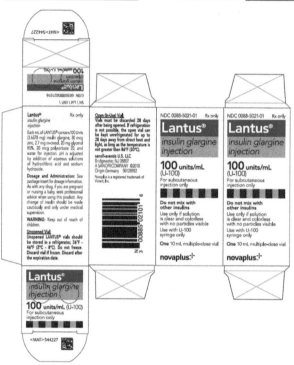

3. Trade name _____     Action time _____

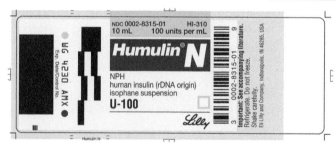

4. Trade name _____     Action time _____

**Answers on p. 461**

## Appearance of Insulin

Regular insulin, Humalog (lispro), Lantus (insulin glargine), Apidra (insulin glulisine), aspart (Novolog), and Levemir (insulin detemir) insulin are clear. All other insulin is cloudy. They include NPH and fixed-combination insulins such as Humulin 70/30 and Humalog 75/25.

## Premixed, Fixed, and Combination Insulins

Fixed-combination insulins are shown in Figure 19.4. These insulins have become popular for clients who must mix fast-acting and intermediate-acting insulins. The purpose of the fixed-combination insulins is to simulate the varying levels of insulin within the bodies of diabetic persons. The availability of the premixed-combination insulins has also decreased the need for clients to mix insulins, as well as decreased the number of required injections. Premixed combination insulins are available in vials and pens for administration and contain both mealtime and basal insulin. This combination can only be administered subcutaneously or by insulin pen. Read labels carefully on combination insulins to identify differences. Selecting the incorrect combination could result in a serious or life-threatening error. Always read an insulin label carefully and compare it to the medication order to avoid errors in administration.

> **SAFETY ALERT!**
>
> Carefully read all insulin labels to ensure selection of the correct type of insulin. The action of insulin varies according to the type of insulin and combination.

To understand fixed-combination insulin orders, it is important for the nurse to read the labels to understand what types of insulin are included in the combination and that they have different action times. For example, Humalog 50/50 concentration in Figure 19.4A means there is a mixture of 50% insulin lispro protamine, an intermediate-acting human insulin analog, and 50% insulin lispro, a rapid-acting human insulin analog. Humulin 70/30 concentration (Figure 19.4B) is a mixture of 70% human insulin isophane, an intermediate-acting human insulin, and 30% regular human insulin, a short-acting human insulin.

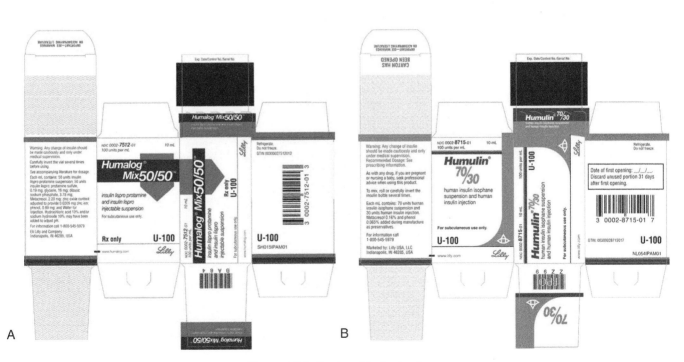

A    B

**Figure 19.4** Fixed-combination insulins.

## Insulin Administration

The major route of administration of insulin is by subcutaneous injection; it is never administered intramuscularly. Regular U-100 insulin, aspart, and glulisine can be administered intravenously.

### Insulin Pumps

Insulin can also be administered by a pump. A CSII pump (continuous subcutaneous insulin infusion) is an insulin pump. An insulin pump is not an IV pump. Figure 19.5A, shows an insulin pump and a blood glucose monitor. Insulin pumps deliver rapid- or short-acting insulin continuously for 24 hours a day through a catheter placed under the skin. This eliminates the need for multiple daily injections of insulin. Pumps can be programmed to deliver a basal rate and/or a bolus dose. Basal insulin is delivered continuously over 24 hours to keep blood glucose levels in range between meals and overnight. The basal rate can be programmed to deliver different rates at different times. Bolus doses can be delivered at mealtime to provide control for additional food intake. The two types of pumps are implantable and external (portable). There are varied insulin pumps that have become available on the market. An example of a pump currently available is the Omnipod system. This system is a tubeless, waterproof insulin pump that can be worn under the clothing. The insulin pump has a reservoir, referred to as a pod, that supplies up to 72 hours of insulin to the body continuously. A handheld device referred to as the Personal Diabetes Manager (PDM) is used to program the Omnipod with customized insulin delivery instructions and monitor the operation of the system. More information about this system can be found at https://www.myomnipod.com/home. According to ISMP, more patients are using ambulatory insulin infusion pumps; however, many inpatient practitioners are unfamiliar with their functionality and the safest way to care for such patients in an inpatient setting. Errors that have been reported with insulin pumps have included patients self-administering insulin by pump without telling the nurse; the nurse administering the same insulin dose by a subcutaneous injection; and changes in the patient's condition that require

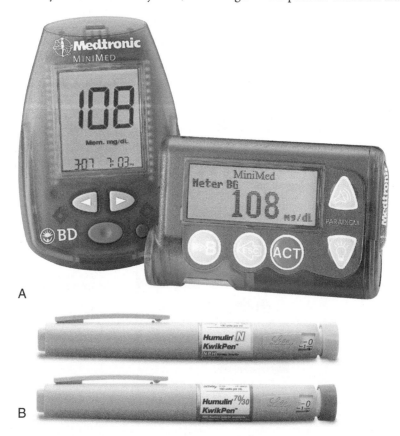

**Figure 19-5** (A) Paradigm® 515 insulin pump and Paradigm Link™ blood glucose monitor. (B) Prefilled Kwik Pens, Humulin N and Humulin 70/30. (Copyright Eli Lilly and Company. All rights reserved. Used with permission. Humulin is a registered trademark of Eli Lilly and Company.)

reassessment of the use of the device. In the 2017 publication by ISMP, *Guidelines for Optimizing Safe Subcutaneous Insulin Use in Adults*, it was recommended that organizational policies are in place to guide the care of patients with personal subcutaneous insulin pumps. ISMP also developed additional guidelines on the safe use of an insulin pump in 2016, which were vetted. These recommendations can be viewed on the ISMP website: https://www.ismp.org/resources/safe-management-patients-external-subcutaneous-insulin-pump-during-hospitalization.

## Insulin Pen

Insulin can also be delivered by an insulin pen. When capped, the insulin pen looks very much like an ink pen. Use of the insulin pens affords clients an easy and accurate method for self-administration of insulin. Insulin pens come in two forms, disposable and reusable. Disposable pens contain a prefilled cartridge and are thrown out after they are emptied. Reusable pens require replacement of the insulin cartridge each time it is emptied. The needles in insulin pens are extremely short and thin. Figure 19.5B shows examples of prefilled insulin pens. The insulin pen has a dose selector knob that is used to "dial" the desired dose of units. The dose dial is turned until the correct number of units is displayed in the dose window. Some of the newer pens have a digital dose display that can be easily misinterpreted if the pen is held upside down. For example, a dose of 27 units looks like 72 units on the digital display if the pen is held incorrectly and read upside down. Client education on the use of the insulin pen (correct way to hold the pen and read the display) is a **must.** This will help in the prevention of dosing errors. Once the pen has been cleared of any air in the cartridge (primed) and the dose set, the insulin is injected by pressing on the injection button. When the injection is completed, the needle is removed and cap replaced. Insulin pens are available in many styles and colors. All insulin pens are designed for single client use and cannot be shared with other clients, even if a new needle is attached.

Although insulin pens were designed for client self-administration of insulin, in an effort to decrease errors with insulin and improve medication safety, many hospitals are also switching from the administration of insulin from vials to pens. Many hospital pharmacies are also supplying insulin pens for nurses to administer insulin.

According to the ISMP's 2017 publication *Guidelines for Optimizing Safe Subcutaneous Insulin Use in Adults,* in institutions that use insulin pens for administration of insulin, there was a need for processes to be in place to reduce the risk of an insulin pen being used on more than one patient, and avoidance of pen mix-ups between patients. Recommendations by ISMP include insulin pens being dispensed to the clinical units with a patient-specific, barcode label (that has been applied in the pharmacy, using a barcode verification process that confirms the correct pen type has been selected based on the patient's order) and steps have been taken to ensure that only the correct specific label can be scanned at the bedside. Patient-specific insulin pens are stored on clinical units in a manner that prevents their inadvertent use on more than one patient. With the use of insulin pens increasing and being used in some institutions, it is important that nurses embrace practices to ensure their safe use on clients.

## Glucose Monitoring Systems

In addition, there are also glucose monitoring systems available on the market that have decreased the need for pricking of the finger to check blood glucose levels. They include the FreeStyle 14-day glucose monitoring system and the Dexcom G6 continuous glucose monitoring system, which can be worn up to 10 days. Both of these systems use a sensor that is worn under the skin and provides continual monitoring of blood glucose levels. Further information on these glucose monitoring systems can be found on their websites: https://www.freestylelibre.us and https://www.dexcom.com/g6-cgm.

## Measuring Insulin in a U-100 Syringe

The insulin syringes and their calibration was introduced in Chapter 17. Recall from Chapter 17 that insulin syringes are available in three sizes (100 unit, 1 mL; 50 unit, 0.5 mL; and 30 unit, 0.3 mL). These syringes are calibrated exclusively for U-100 insulin (100 units per mL) and marked U-100. Typically, these syringes also have orange caps. U-100 insulin should be measured in U-100 syringes and **not** in syringes calibrated in milliliters, such as a 1-mL or 3-mL syringe. U-500 insulin was previously administered using a tuberculin (1-mL) syringe. In 2016 the US Food and Drug Administration approved a dedicated syringe for the administration of Humulin R U-500 insulin. The U-500 insulin syringe is **only** used for the administration of U-500 insulin.

Measuring U-100 insulin with the insulin syringe makes it easy to obtain a correct dosage without mathematical calculation. To prepare the U-100 insulin when only one dosage is required, the U-100 insulin syringe is used to draw up the ordered U-100 insulin to the unit calibration that corresponds to the ordered dose. The nurse **must** carefully select the correct insulin and withdraw the correct amount. It is not necessary to use dosage calculation formulas or ratio and proportion to calculate the volume for administering U-100 insulin. The insulin syringe is designed to measure insulin in units, and insulin is ordered in units. After drawing up insulin, the nurse should provide the order, vial, and syringe to another nurse to verify the insulin dosage before administering to client to avoid errors. In other words, the dosage should always be double-checked by another nurse.

Let's look at the U-100 insulin syringes. An essential skill is correctly reading the syringe calibrations on U-100 syringes.

1. **Lo-Dose syringe**—It has a capacity of 50 units (0.5 mL). Each calibration on the syringe measures 1 unit. There is also a 30-unit (0.3 mL) syringe, which is used to accurately measure very small amounts of insulin. It is marked in units up to 30 units. Each calibration is 1 unit.
2. **1-mL (100-unit) capacity syringe**—The 100-unit syringe comes with even and odd numbers on it. There are two types of 1-mL syringes in current use.
   a. The single-scale syringe is calibrated in 2-unit increments. Any dosage measured in an odd number of units is measured between the even calibrations. This would not be the desired syringe for clients with vision problems.
   b. The double-scale syringe (dual syringe) has odd-numbered units on the left in 2-unit increments (1, 3, etc.) and even-numbered units on the right in 2-unit increments (2, 4, etc.). To avoid confusion, the scale on the left should be used for odd numbers of units (e.g., 13 units) and the scale on the right for even numbers of units (e.g., 26 units). When even numbers of units are measured, each calibration is then measured as 2 units.
3. **U-500 insulin syringe**—This has a capacity of 250 units. The U-500 insulin syringes have a green cap, and U-500 is marked on the barrel of the syringe. Each calibration on the syringe measures 5 units (0.01 mL) of U-500 insulin. You can administer 5 to 250 units in one injection. If more than 250 units is required, the client will need more than one injection. This syringe is used for the administration of U-500 insulin **only**.

> ## ! SAFETY ALERT!
> Administer insulin in an insulin syringe used only for the administration of U-100 insulin. Do not use an insulin syringe to measure other medications that are measured in units. Syringes of 30 and 50 units measure a smaller volume of insulin but are intended for the measurement of U-100 insulin only. Use the smallest capacity insulin syringe available to ensure the accuracy of dosage preparation.

To review what the four types of U-100 insulin syringes look like and the U-500 syringe, see Figure 19.6.

### Lo-Dose Syringe

Let's look at some insulin dosages measured in the syringes to help you visualize the amounts in a syringe. Syringe *A* shows 30 units and syringe *B* shows 37 units in a Lo-Dose syringe.

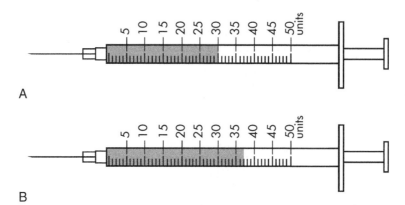

A

B

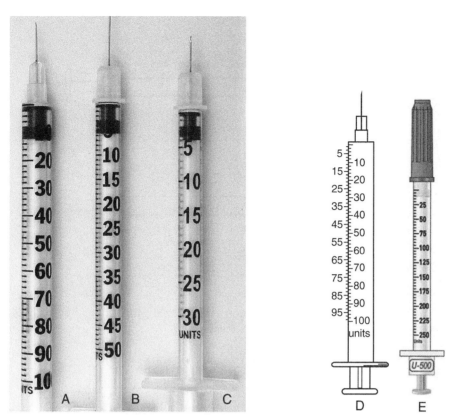

**Figure 19.6** Types of insulin syringes. (A) Single-scale (100 units). (B) Lo-Dose insulin syringe (50 units). (C) Lo-Dose insulin syringe (30 units). (D) Double-scale syringe (100 units). (E) U-500 insulin syringe (250 units).

## 🖩 PRACTICE **PROBLEMS**

Using the syringes below, indicate the dosages shown by the arrows.

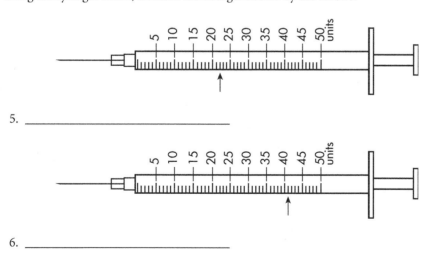

5. _____

6. _____

Using the syringes below, shade in the dosages indicated.

7. 17 units

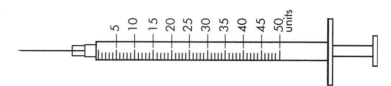

8. 47 units

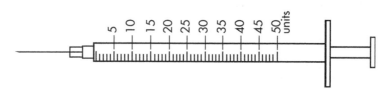

**Answers on p. 461**

## Single-Scale 1-mL Syringe

Now let's look at what dosages would look like on a single-scale 1-mL syringe. The syringes below show 32 units in syringe *A* and 56 units in syringe *B*.

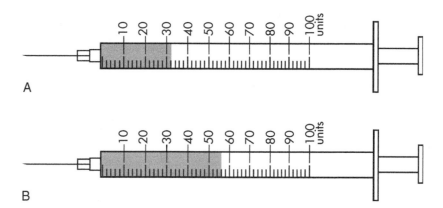

## Double-Scale 1-mL Syringe

Now let's look at the dosage indicated on a double-scale (100-unit) 1-mL syringe. Syringe *C* shows 37 units; notice that the scale on the left is used. Syringe *D* shows 54 units; notice that the scale on the right is used.

> **! SAFETY ALERT!**
> Look carefully at the increments when using a dual syringe.

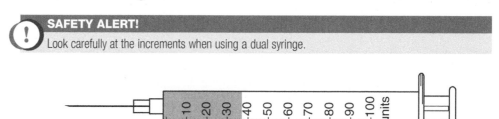

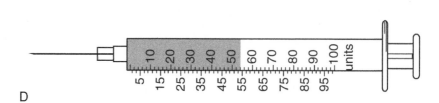

## ⊞ PRACTICE **PROBLEMS**

Indicate the following dosages shaded on the 100-unit (1-mL) syringes.

9. _____

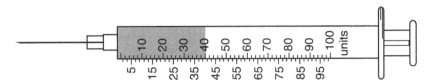

10. _____

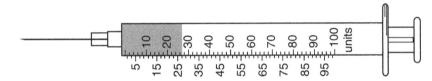

11. _____

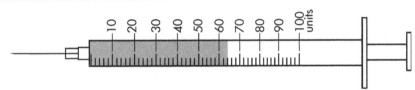

12. _____

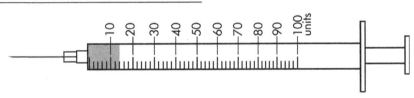

Shade the specified dosages on each of the U-100 syringes below.

13. 88 units

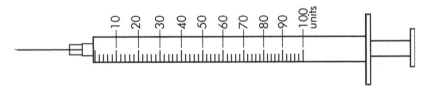

14. 44 units

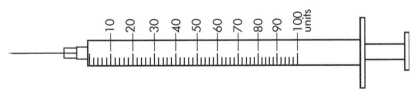

15. 30 units

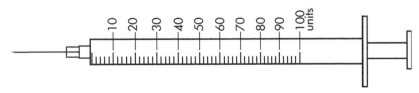

**Answers on p. 461**

### U-500 Syringe

Let's look at insulin dosages measured in the U-500 syringe. Syringe *A* shows 55 units, and syringe *B* shows 125 units in a U-500 syringe.

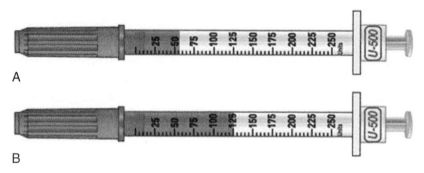

A

B

## PRACTICE PROBLEMS

Using the syringes below, indicate the dosages shown by the arrows.

16.

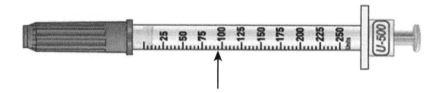

17.

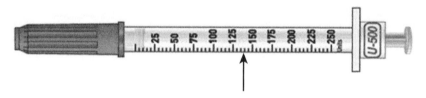

Using the syringes below, shade in the dosages indicated.

18. 15 units

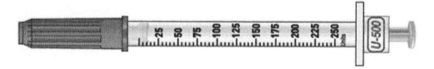

19. 155 units

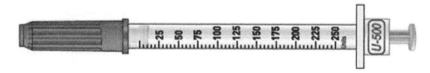

**Answers on p. 461**

## Insulin Orders

Like any written medication order, an insulin order must be written clearly and contain certain information to prevent errors in administration. An error in administration can cause harmful effects to a client. Insulin orders should contain the following information:

    a. The name of the insulin. Example: Humulin R (indicating human origin, with the R indicating regular). Some orders may be written simply as Humulin Regular.

    b. The number of units to be administered. Example: Humulin Regular 20 units.

c. **The route of administration (subcut).** Insulin is usually administered subcutaneously; however, regular insulin, aspart, and glulisine can be administered intravenously, as well.

d. **The frequency or time of administration.** Example: q AM ½ hour before breakfast.

e. The **insulin concentration** is written following the name of the insulin with regular insulin U-500. According to ISMP, the insulin concentration (example: Humulin R U-100) does not follow the name of the insulin on the medication administration record (MAR) or other medication lists on which insulin doses are recorded, with the exception of regular insulin U-500. ISMP reported having errors in which the concentration (strength) of the insulin had been mistaken for the dose when written following the name of the insulin. In addition, the most common concentration available and used is U-100.

**Example of Insulin Orders:** Humulin R 20 units subcut q AM ½ hour before breakfast. Humulin R U-500 215 units subcut daily ½ hour before breakfast.

- When the prescriber orders premixed (combination insulins), the name of the insulin identifying the fixed combination, the number of units to administer, the route of administration, and the frequency of administration should be specified in the order. **Example:** Humalog Mix 50/50 20 units subcut q AM 30 minutes before breakfast.

There are times when the prescriber will order two insulins, such as a rapid-acting or short-acting insulin combined with an intermediate-acting insulin. These insulins are administered in the same syringe. The prescriber specifies the name of each insulin, the number of units to be administered, the route of administration, and the frequency of administration. **Example:** Humulin R 18 units and Humulin N 40 units subcut daily at 7:30 AM.

To ensure the safe administration of insulin, the nurse must correctly interpret the insulin order and recognize any use of error-prone abbreviations (which include use of "u" for units and "sc" for subcutaneous) that might cause an error in administration of insulin because of misinterpretation.

> **SAFETY ALERT!**
>
> To avoid misinterpretation, the abbreviation "U," which stands for units, should not be used when insulin orders are written. The word *units* should be written out. Errors have occurred as a result of the "U" being mistaken for a "0" in a handwritten order. Example: 6U subcut stat of Humulin Regular. The U is almost completely closed and could be misread as 60 units. The recommendation to write out the word *units* has also been issued by the Institute for Safe Medication Practices (ISMP) and should be included on each accredited organization's "do not use" list approved by The Joint Commission (TJC).

## Insulin Coverage Practices

Sometimes, in addition to standing insulin orders, clients may require additional insulin "to cover" their increased blood glucose (sugar) level.

The terms Correction Insulin and Sliding Scale Practices are different approaches used for the same purpose, which is to correct high blood glucose. According to the literature, there are differences between the two practices. Correction insulin is an extra dose of insulin given based on the preprandial (preceding a meal) glucose value, and it is often given in addition to the usual dose that a client takes to cover their meal. A dose of quick-acting insulin such as Novolog, Humalog, or Apidra is administered to lower blood sugar. Correction insulin is said to resemble a sliding scale and has been referred to as a sliding scale.

Traditionally, the use of the sliding scale has been for glycemic control. Sliding scale insulin is generally defined as a set of orders that indicate a certain dosage of insulin is administered based on the client's blood glucose level (the amount of glucose in a given amount of blood, recorded in mg in a deciliter or mg/dL). Orders for the sliding scale may also indicate capillary blood glucose (CBG) to indicate the checking of blood glucose for the sliding scale. Most sliding scales use regular (short-acting) insulin or lispro (rapid-acting) insulin. The prescriber specifies the dosage of insulin, which can increase or decrease based on a specific blood glucose level range. Sliding scales are individualized to the client. When orders for sliding scale are written, the order must include the type of insulin to be administered, the amount of insulin (in units), and the specific blood glucose range. In addition, the order should include the frequency for blood glucose checks. A sample sliding scale is shown below. Using the sliding scale, if the blood glucose level for the client is 135 mg/dL, you would not administer any insulin because 135 mg/dL is less than 180 mg/dL. However, if the client's blood glucose level is 200 mg/dL, you would administer 2 units of regular insulin immediately because 200 mg/dL is between 181 and 240 mg/dL.

**Sample Insulin Sliding Scale**

**Humulin Regular U-100 according to finger stick q8h**

| | |
|---|---|
| 0-180 mg/dL | No coverage |
| 181-240 mg/dL | 2 units subcut |
| 241-300 mg/dL | 4 units subcut |
| 301-400 mg/dL | 6 units subcut |
| Greater than 400 mg/dL | 8 units subcut stat and notify doctor |
| | Repeat finger stick in 2 hr |

> **(i) TIPS FOR CLINICAL PRACTICE**
>
> When orders are written for sliding scale, the abbreviation "SS" should not be used to mean sliding scale. In the apothecary system, ss means 1/2, and ss could also be mistaken for the number 55. Write out sliding scale.

Note that the process for documenting the insulin administered varies among institutions. Know the institution's policies and protocols regarding the use of the sliding scale.

Despite current evidence cited in the literature indicating the sliding scale as not being effective in achieving glycemic control, and discouragement regarding its use by the American Diabetes Association (ADA), the sliding scale continues to be a common practice in some health care institutions to correct hyperglycemia (high blood glucose) in hospitalized clients.

## Current Recommendations Regarding Use of the Sliding Scale

ISMP's 2017 *Guidelines for Optimizing Safe Subcutaneous Insulin use in Adults* recommends eliminating the use of sliding scale insulin doses based on blood glucose values as the only strategy for managing hyperglycemia. This concurs with the American Association of Clinical Endocrinologists (AACE), the American Diabetes Association (ADA), and the Endocrine Society. "Scheduled subcutaneous administration of insulin is the preferred method for achieving and maintaining glucose control in non-critically ill patients with diabetes or stress hyperglycemia." It has been found that the use of a sliding scale insulin regimen alone results in undesirable hypoglycemia (low blood glucose) and hyperglycemia (high blood glucose) and high risk of hospital complications. Scheduled subcutaneous insulin administration with basal insulin, nutritional (meal), and correctional components has been shown to promote the best outcomes in non–critically ill clients and to be safe and effective in managing hyperglycemia in non-critical hospital patients.

The basal insulin component uses a long-acting insulin analog to control the fasting plasma glucose level, and the nutritional component uses rapid-acting insulin to cover nutritional intake and correct hyperglycemia. The basal plus rapid-acting insulin is referred to as *basal/bolus insulin therapy,* which closely approximates normal physiological insulin production and controls hyperglycemia. The correction dose is determined by the patient's insulin sensitivity and current blood glucose level. Insulin sensitivity is calculated by adding up the patient's total daily insulin requirement and dividing that amount into 1,500 (for type 2 DM) or 1,700 (for type 1 DM). The use of this management combines the basal insulin with mealtime (prandial insulin).

In summary, the basal-prandial insulin therapy is a physiological approach to insulin therapy that uses multiple daily injections to cover both basal and prandial therapy. The basal prandial insulin therapy is a regimen that has evidence to support it as being optimal to achieving glycemic control in clients with diabetes.

## Preparing a Single Dosage of Insulin in an Insulin Syringe

Measuring insulin in an insulin syringe is different from the administration of most other injectable medications. There is no calculation or conversion required because the syringe measures units of insulin, rather than volume of solution. An order must be written following the previously stated guidelines. Frequent errors have occurred with insulin dosages, and insulin is considered a high-alert medication. Because of this, special attention should be used when preparing dosages of insulin. Insulin dosage errors can be avoided by following two important rules to ensure safe administration of insulin.

> **RULE**
> **Avoiding Insulin Dosage Errors**
> - Insulin dosages **MUST** be checked by two nurses. To be considered an independent verification, the check by the second nurse must occur independently, away from the first nurse, with no prior knowledge of calculations to verify the dosage.
> - In the preparation of combination dosages (two insulins), two nurses must verify each step of the process.

**Example 1:**  Order: Humulin R 40 units subcut in AM $\frac{1}{2}$ hr before breakfast

Available: Humulin R labeled U-100

To measure 40 units, withdraw insulin to the 40-unit mark on the U-100 syringe. A Lo-Dose syringe can also be used to draw up this dose, as shown below.

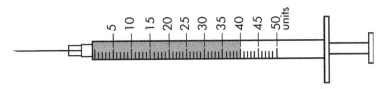

**Example 2:**  Order: Humulin N 70 units subcut daily at 7:30 AM

Available: Humulin N labeled U-100

There is no calculation or conversion required here. Draw up the required amount using a U-100 (1-mL) syringe.

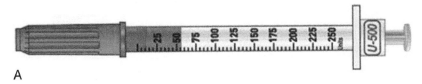

A

**Example 3:**  Order: Humulin R 5 units subcut stat

Available: Humulin R labeled U-100

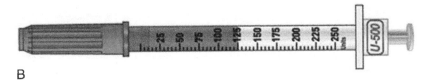

B

## Measuring Two Types of Insulin in the Same Syringe

Sometimes individuals may require two different types of insulin for control of their blood sugar levels: for example, NPH and regular. To decrease the number of injections, it is common to mix two insulins in a single syringe. To mix insulin in one syringe, remember:

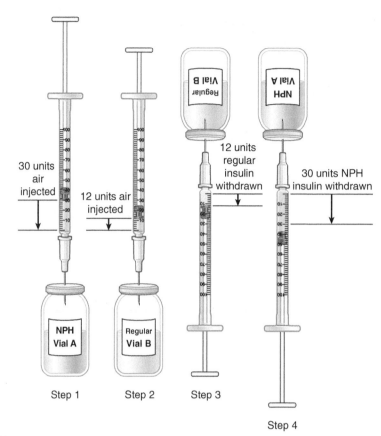

**Figure 19.7** Mixing insulins. Order: Humulin N 30 units subcut, Humulin R, 12 units subcut. **Step 1,** Inject 30 units of air into Humulin N first; do not allow needle to touch insulin. **Step 2,** Inject 12 units of air into Humulin R. **Step 3,** Withdraw 12 units; withdraw needle. **Step 4,** Insert needle into vial of Humulin N and withdraw 30 units. Total 30 units Humulin N (NPH) + 12 units Humulin R (Regular) = 42 units. (Modified from Harkreader H, Hogan MA: *Fundamentals of nursing: caring and clinical judgment,* ed 3, St. Louis, 2007, Saunders.)

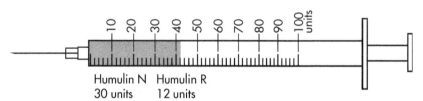

**Figure 19.8** Total of two insulins combined. Total = 42 units (30 units Humulin N + 12 units Humulin R).

> **RULE**
>
> **Safety When Combining Two Insulins in the Same Syringe**
>
> Draw up clear insulin first, and then draw up cloudy insulin. Rapid- and short-acting insulins are clear (regular, aspart, lispro). Intermediate-acting (NPH) insulin is cloudy.
> THINK: First rapid-acting or short-acting insulin, then intermediate-acting insulin.
> THINK: The insulin that acts **first** is drawn up **first.**

Drawing regular insulin up first prevents contamination of the regular insulin with other insulin. This sequence is extremely important.

To prepare insulin in one syringe (mixing insulin), complete the following steps (Figures 19.7 and 19.8):

1. Cleanse tops of both vials with an alcohol wipe.
2. Inject air equal to the amount being withdrawn into the vial of cloudy insulin first. When the air is injected, the tip of the needle should not touch the solution.

3. Remove the needle from the vial of cloudy insulin.
4. Using the same syringe, inject an amount of air into the regular insulin (clear) equal to the amount to be withdrawn, invert or turn the bottle up in the air, and draw up the desired amount.
5. Remove the syringe from the regular insulin, and check for air bubbles. If air bubbles are present, gently tap the syringe to remove them.
6. Next, withdraw the desired dosage from the vial of cloudy insulin.
7. The total number of units in the syringe will be the sum of the two insulin orders.

*Note:* Provide the order, vial of insulin, and syringe to another nurse for independent verification each time you draw up an insulin dose.

> ⚠ **SAFETY ALERT!**
>
> **DO NOT combine** long-acting insulin types or dilute them with any other insulin preparation. The effects can be life threatening.

> ⓘ **TIPS FOR CLINICAL PRACTICE**
>
> • Cloudy insulin should be rolled gently between the palms of the hands to mix it before it is drawn up. *Do not* shake insulin. Shaking creates bubbles in addition to breaking down the particles and causing clumping.
> • Insulins mix instantly; they do not remain separated. Therefore insulin that has been overdrawn cannot be returned to the vial. You must discard the entire medication and start over.

**Example 1:** The order is to administer 18 units of Humulin R subcut and 22 units subcut of Humulin N.

The total amount of insulin is 40 units (18 units [Humulin R] + 22 units Humulin N = 40 units).

To administer this dosage, a Lo-Dose syringe or a U-100 (1-mL) syringe can be used. However, because the dosage is 40 units, the Lo-Dose would be more desirable. (See the syringes that follow, illustrating this dosage.)

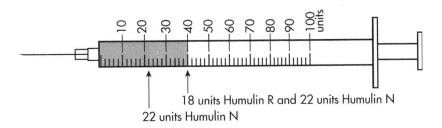

18 units Humulin R and 22 units Humulin N
22 units Humulin N

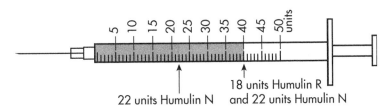

22 units Humulin N    18 units Humulin R and 22 units Humulin N

> ⓘ **TIPS FOR CLINICAL PRACTICE**
>
> When mixing insulins, follow the steps outlined. Committing one of the following phrases to memory may help you remember the steps: (1) last injected is **first** drawn up; (2) run fast first (regular), then slow down (NPH); (3) clear to cloudy; or (4) it is alphabetical: clear, cloudy. Also remember, when mixing insulins, only the same type should be mixed together – for example, Humulin and Humulin.

## Non-Insulin Medications

There are medications being used for the treatment of diabetes mellitus that are not insulin but deserve a brief mention in this chapter. These medications may be used in patients having trouble getting to their goal with insulin therapy. These medications may also be used to lower the A1C. A1C stands for glycated hemoglobin. According to the literature, "A1C measures the amount of glucose that attaches to hemoglobin, part of the red blood cells. The more glucose that attaches the higher the A1C." A1C test is used to diagnose diabetes as well as assess how well a person is managing their diet, food, activity, and blood glucose levels. The A1C can help in determining potential complications from diabetes (such as kidney, cardiovascular, and other problems). There are some medications that decrease the risks of major adverse cardiovascular (CV) events as well as decrease the risk of major CV events in clients with diabetes who have established CV disease. These medications are not insulin, and some may be given as adjunct therapy to diet and exercise to improve glycemic control while improving the A1C or with insulin therapy. Examples of these medications include oral forms that must be taken daily, such as Jardiance (empagliflozin), and Farxiga (dapagliflozin) (Figure 19.9). Injectable forms include Victoza (liraglutide), which is injected once a day subcutaneously, and Trulicity (dulaglutide) (Figure 19.10), which is administered once weekly subcutaneously. Note that only a few examples of these medications are provided here.

As nurses, we need to remember the importance of taking steps to prevent errors that can occur in dosage administration. Extra care must be taken to prevent errors with high-alert medications. The results can be fatal to a client. Reading insulin labels carefully, obtaining independent verification of dosages by another nurse before administering insulin, recognizing the use of dangerous abbreviations associated with insulin and the errors they can cause, and performing practices that support safety and prevent harm to a client are part of the QSEN competency of safety. Safety competencies have been incorporated in this chapter to ensure that you consider safety in each aspect of insulin administration.

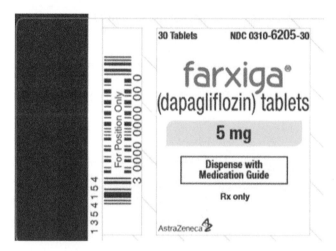

**Figure 19.9** Farxiga 5-mg tablets.

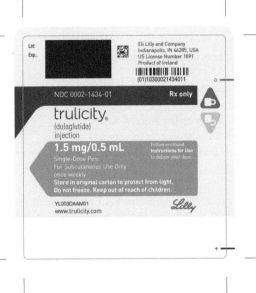

**Figure 19.10** Trulicity single-dose pen, 1.5 mg per 0.5 mL.

---

**⚙ POINTS TO REMEMBER**

- U-100 means 100 units per mL.
- Carefully read the prescriber's orders.
- To ensure accuracy, U-100 insulin should be given only with an insulin syringe. Insulin syringes should not be used to measure other medications measured in units.
- U-100 insulin is designed to be given with syringes marked U-100.
- Insulin dosages must be exact. Read the calibration on the insulin syringes carefully.
- Lo-Dose syringes are desirable for small dosages up to 50 units. The Lo-Dose 30-unit syringe may be used for dosages up to 30 units. Although Lo-Dose insulin syringes (30 units and 50 units) can hold a smaller volume, they are intended for U-100 insulin only.
- A U-100 (1-mL capacity) syringe is desirable when the dosage exceeds 50 units.
- Drawing up insulin correctly is critical to safe administration of insulin to clients.
- When insulins are mixed, regular insulin (clear) is always drawn up first, then cloudy.
- Do not shake insulin. Roll the insulin gently between the palms of the hands to mix.
- When insulins are mixed, the total volume is the sum of the two insulin amounts in units.
- Regular insulin, aspart, and glulisine are approved for IV administration.
- Read insulin labels to ensure that you have the correct type of insulin, to avoid medication errors. Only mix the same types of insulin (e.g., Humulin R and Humulin N).
- Use the smallest-capacity syringe possible to ensure accuracy.
- Insulin orders should be written with units spelled out, not abbreviated U.
- Do not mix long-acting insulin with any other insulin or dilute with any other insulin preparation.
- Avoid insulin dosage errors; always obtain an independent verification by a second nurse.
- U-500 insulin means 500 units per mL. U-500 is 5x more potent than U-100.
- Use U-500 syringe to measure and administer U-500 insulin.
- Current evidence supports basal-prandial insulin therapy, which improves client outcomes and is an optimal strategy for achieving glycemic control in diabetic clients.

## CLINICAL **REASONING**

1. **Scenario:** The prescriber wrote the following insulin order:
   Humulin 10 0 subcut ā breakfast.
   The nurse assumed the order was for regular insulin 100 units and administered the insulin to the client.
   Later, it was discovered the insulin dose desired was NPH 10 units.
   a. What error occurred here? _____
   b. What client medication rights were violated? _____
   c. What is the potential outcome of the error? _____
   d. What measures could have been taken to prevent the error that occurred? _____

2. **Scenario:** A client is to receive Humulin R 10 units subcut and Humulin N 14 units subcut before breakfast. In drawing up the insulins in the same syringe, the nurse used the following technique:
   a. Injected 10 units of air into the regular vial.
   b. Injected 14 units of air into the NPH vial.
   c. Withdrew 14 units of NPH insulin, then the 10 units of regular insulin.
      (a) What is the error in the technique of drawing up the two insulins? _____
      (b) What is the potential outcome from the technique used? _____

**Answers on pp. 461-462**

## CHAPTER **REVIEW**

Using the syringes below and the labels where provided, indicate the dosage you would prepare and shade the dosage on the syringe provided. All insulin available is U-100 unless specified otherwise.

1. Order: Humulin N 56 units subcut daily every AM ½ hour before breakfast.

   Available:

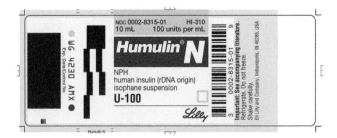

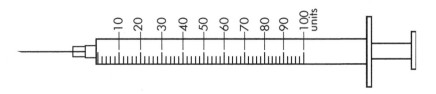

2. Order: Humulin R 18 units subcut and Humulin N 40 units subcut daily at 7:30 AM.
   (Indicate the total insulin dosage.)

   Available:

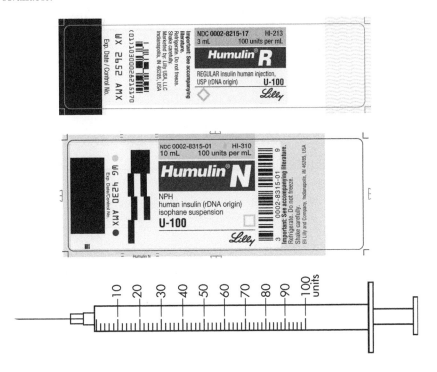

3. Order: Novolin R 9 units subcut daily.

   Available:

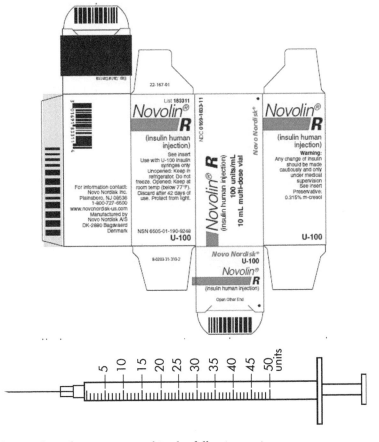

Indicate the number of units measured in the following syringes.

4. Units measured   _____

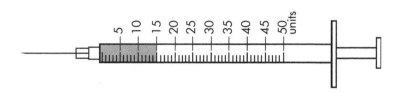

5. Units measured   _____

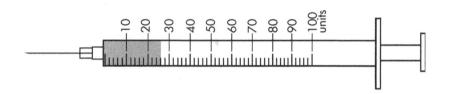

6. Units measured   _____

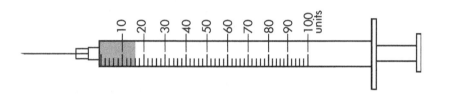

7. Units measured   _____

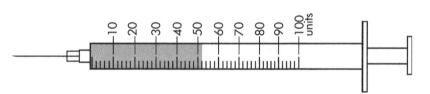

8. Units measured   _____

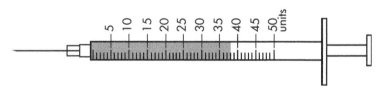

9. Units measured   _____

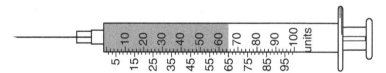

10. Units measured   _____

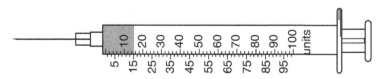

Calculate the dosage of insulin where necessary, and shade the dosage on the syringe provided. Labels have been provided for some problems.

11. Order: Humulin R 10 units subcut at 7:30 AM.

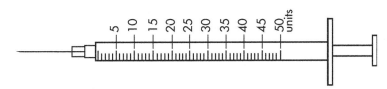

12. Order: Humulin R 16 units subcut and Humulin N 24 units subcut a.c. 7:30 AM. (Indicate the total insulin dosage.)

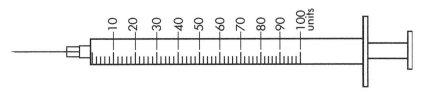

13. Order: Humulin R 10 units subcut and Humulin N 15 units subcut a.c. 7:30 AM. (Indicate the total insulin dosage.)

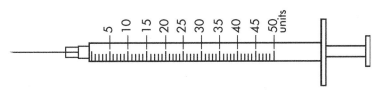

14. Order: Humulin R 5 units subcut and Humulin N 25 units subcut a.c. 7:30 AM. (Indicate the total insulin dosage.)

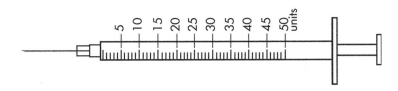

15. Order: Novolin R 40 units subcut and Novolin N 10 units subcut at 7:30 AM. (Indicate the total insulin dosage.)

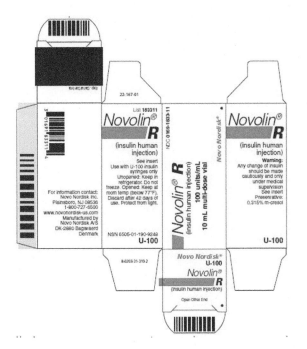
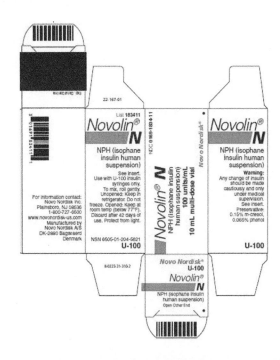

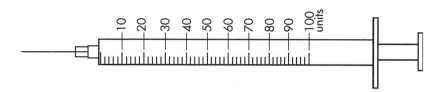

16. Order: Humulin N 48 units subcut and Humulin R 30 units subcut a.c. 7:30 AM. (Indicate the total insulin dosage.)

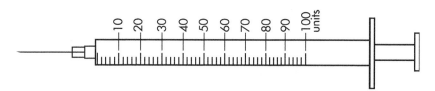

17. Order: Novolin R 16 units subcut and Novolin N 12 units subcut 7:30 AM. (Indicate the total insulin dosage.)

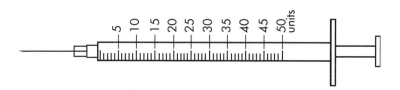

18. Order: Novolin R 17 units subcut 5 PM.

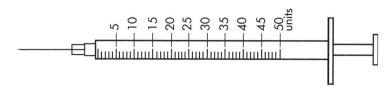

19. Order: Humalog 15 units subcut daily at 7:30 AM.

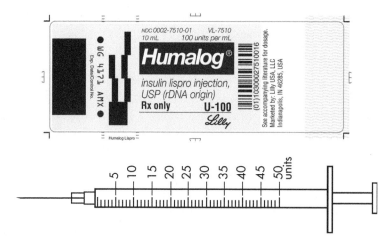

20. Order: Humulin R 26 units subcut and Humulin N 48 units subcut daily. (Indicate the total insulin dosage.)

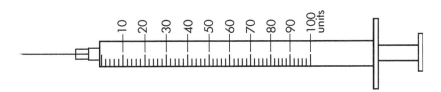

21. Order: Humulin 70/30 27 units subcut at 5 PM.

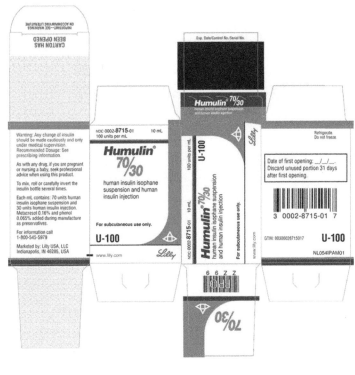

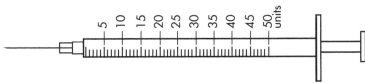

22. Order: Novolin R 21 units subcut and Novolin N 35 units subcut daily at 7:30 AM. (Indicate the total insulin dosage.)

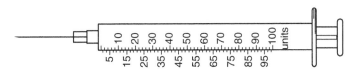

23. Order: Novolin R 5 units subcut and Novolin N 35 units subcut 7:30 AM. (Indicate the total insulin dosage.)

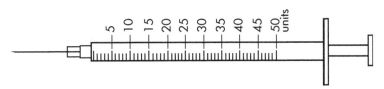

24. Order: NovoLog 36 units subcut 7:30 AM before breakfast.

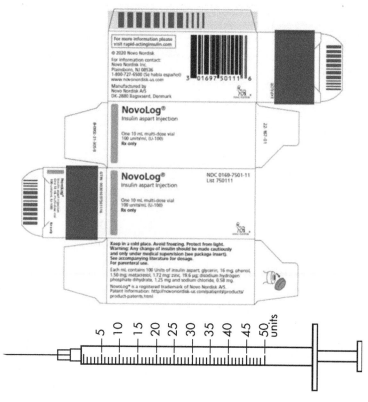

25. A client has a sliding scale for insulin dosages. The order is for Humulin Regular insulin q6h as follows:

| Finger stick | 0-180 mg/dL | no coverage |
|---|---|---|
| Blood sugar (mg/dL) | 181-240 mg/dL | 2 units subcut |
| | 241-300 mg/dL | 4 units subcut |
| | 301-400 mg/dL | 6 units subcut |
| | Greater than 400 mg/dL | 8 units subcut and repeat finger stick in 2 hr |

At 11:30 AM, the client's finger stick is 364 mg/dL. Shade the syringe to indicate the dosage that should be given.

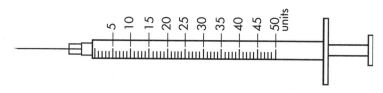

26. Order: Humulin R 32 units subcut every morning at 7:30 AM.

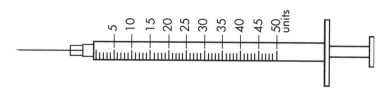

27. Order: Humulin R 9 units subcut 5 PM.

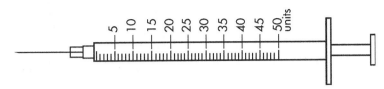

28. Order: Humulin N 11 units subcut at bedtime.

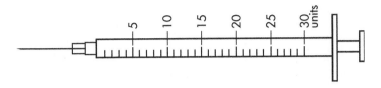

29. Order: Humulin 70/30 20 units subcut ½ hr before breakfast.

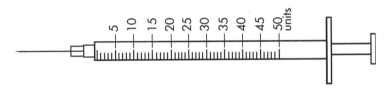

30. Order: Humulin R 10 units subcut and Humulin N 42 units subcut at 4:30 PM. (Indicate the total insulin dosage.)

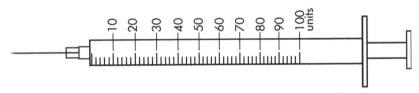

31. Order: Novolin R 8 units subcut and Novolin N 15 units subcut at 7:30 AM. (Indicate the total insulin dosage.)

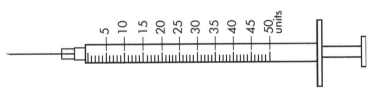

32. Order: Humulin R 30 units subcut and Humulin N 40 units subcut every day at 8:00 AM. (Indicate the total insulin dosage.)

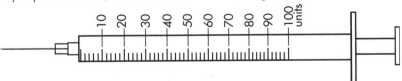

33. A client has a sliding scale for insulin dosages. The order is for Humulin R q6h as follows:

| Finger stick Blood sugar (mg/dL) | | |
|---|---|---|
| | 201-250 mg/dL | 4 units subcut |
| | 251-300 mg/dL | 6 units subcut |
| | 301-350 mg/dL | 8 units subcut |
| | 351-400 mg/dL | 10 units subcut |
| | Greater than 400 mg/dL | call MD |

At 6:00 PM, the client's blood sugar is 354 mg/dL. Shade the syringe to indicate the dosage that should be administered.

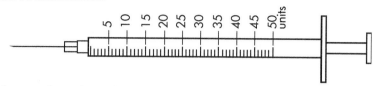

For problems 34 through 38, shade the dosage in on the syringe; available is:

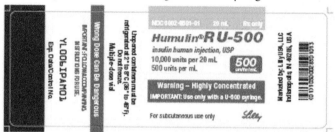

34. Order: Humulin R U-500 200 units subcut stat.

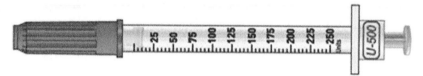

35. Order: Humulin R U-500 225 units subcut stat.

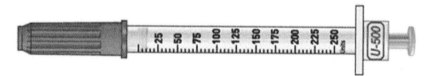

36. Order: Humulin R U-500 235 units subcut stat.

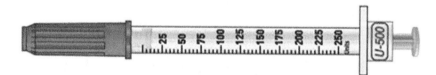

37. Order: Humulin R U-500 175 units subcut qAM before breakfast.

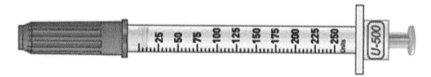

38. Order: Humulin R U-500 165 units subcut stat.

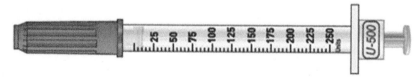

**Answers on pp. 462-463**

ⓔvolve

For additional practice problems, refer to the the Dosages Measured in Units section of the Elsevier's Interactive Drug Calculation Application, Version 1, on Evolve.

---

## ⭐ ANSWERS

## Chapter 19
### Answers to Practice Problems

1. Humalog, rapid-acting (fast-acting)

2. Humulin R Regular, short-acting

3. Lantus, long-acting

4. Humulin N, NPH, intermediate-acting

5. 22 units

6. 41 units

7.

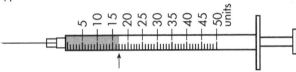

8.

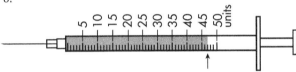

9. 40 units

10. 27 units

11. 64 units

12. 14 units

13.

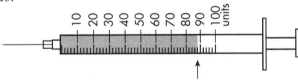

14.

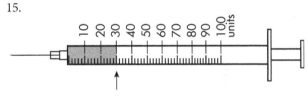

15.

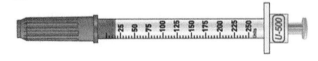

16. 95 units

17. 140 units

18.

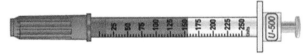

19.

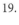

### Answers to Clinical Reasoning Questions

1. a. The wrong insulin was administered. Failure to clarify an insulin order when the type of insulin was not specified, and the dosage was not clear because the U for units was used. U almost closed and caused the "U" to be mistaken for "0."

   b. The right medication, the right dosage.

   c. The client received 10 times the dose of an insulin (regular) that was not ordered. Regular insulin is short acting, and NPH is intermediate acting and was desired. Administering the insulin would likely cause a dangerously low glucose level (hypoglycemia). Results could be tremors, confusion, sweating, and death. This incident constitutes malpractice.

   d. The error could have been prevented by remembering that all the essential components of an insulin order should have been in the order (name of insulin, number of units to be administered, route of administration, and frequency or time. When one element is missing, never assume. The order should have been clarified with the prescriber. Further, the dosage should have been double-checked with another nurse. In addition, units should have been written out in the order to avoid misinterpretation of "U" as a zero (0). Many insulin errors occur when the nurse fails to clarify an incomplete order or misinterprets the dosage when units is abbreviated.

2. a. The nurse should have injected the 14 units of air into the NPH vial and then injected 10 units of air into the regular vial and drawn up the 10 units of regular insulin first. First regular, then NPH.

Another nurse should have been present during the mixing and to verify the dosage drawn.

b. Contamination of insulins. Regular (rapid acting) is drawn up first to prevent it from becoming contaminated with the intermediate-acting insulin. This can also result in reversing the doses of the two insulins being drawn up and result in incorrect insulin dosages.

## Answers to Chapter Review

1.

2.

3.

4. 15 units

5. 26 units

6. 16 units

7. 52 units

8. 38 units

9. 65 units

10. 15 units

11.

12. 40 units

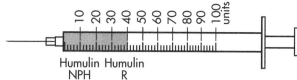

13. 25 units

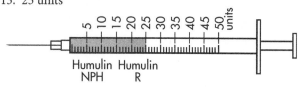

14. 30 units

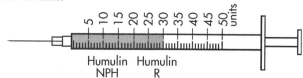

15. 50 units

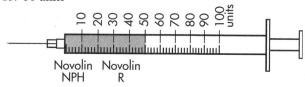

16. 78 units

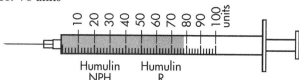

17. 28 units

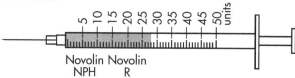

18.

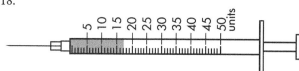

19.

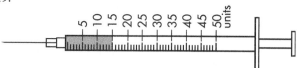

20. 74 units

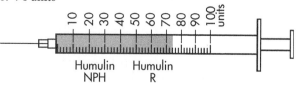

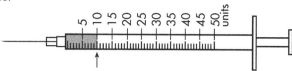

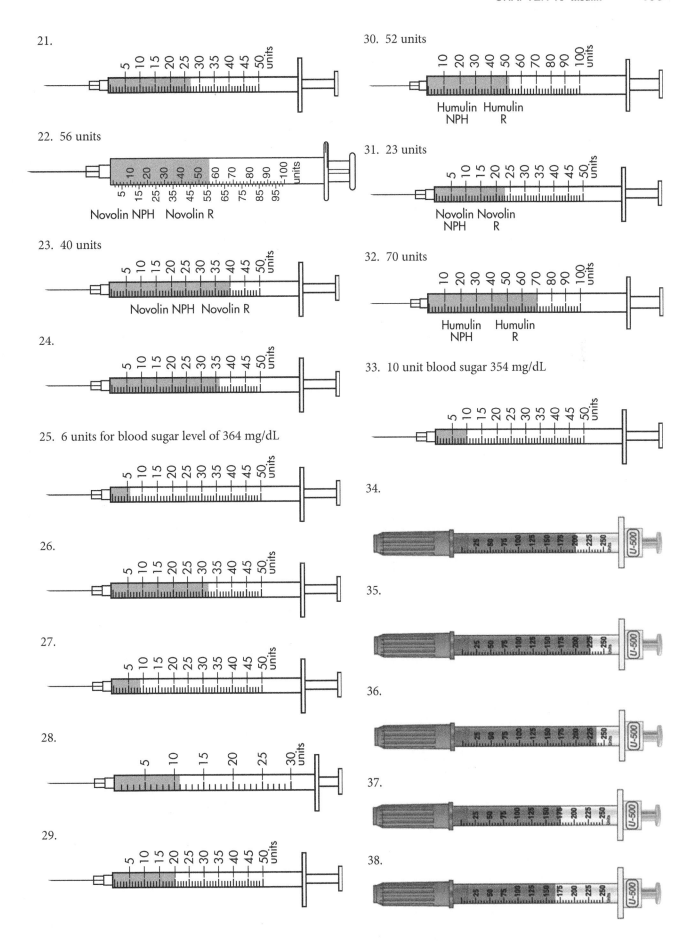

21.

22. 56 units

Novolin NPH   Novolin R

23. 40 units

Novolin NPH  Novolin R

24.

25. 6 units for blood sugar level of 364 mg/dL

26.

27.

28.

29.

30. 52 units

Humulin   Humulin
NPH       R

31. 23 units

Novolin  Novolin
NPH        R

32. 70 units

Humulin    Humulin
NPH        R

33. 10 unit blood sugar 354 mg/dL

34.

35.

36.

37.

38.

# Intravenous, Heparin, and Critical Care Calculations and Pediatric and Adult Calculations Based on Weight

The ability to accurately calculate flow rates for intravenous medications is essential to both heparin administration and critical care calculations.

# CHAPTER **20**

# Intravenous Solutions and Equipment

## Objectives

*After reviewing this chapter, you should be able to:*

1. Identify common intravenous (IV) solutions and abbreviations
2. Calculate the amount of specific components in IV solutions
3. Define the following terms associated with IV therapy: peripheral line, central line, primary line, secondary line, saline/heparin locks, IV piggyback (IVPB), and IV push
4. Differentiate among various devices used to administer IV solutions (e.g., patient-controlled analgesia [PCA] pumps, syringe pumps, volumetric pumps)
5. Identify best practices that prevent IV administration errors and ensure client safety

A general discussion of intravenous therapy will make it easier to understand the calculations associated with IV therapy, which will be discussed in Chapter 21. Intravenous (IV) therapy is the infusion of fluids (solutions), nutrients (i.e., *vitamins, electrolytes, carbohydrates, fatty acids*), blood or blood products, or medications through a vein. IV fluids can be ordered to infuse continuously or intermittently. The reasons for the ordering and administration of IV fluids are varied and include:

- To maintain fluid and electrolyte balance. Fluids that are given to help sustain normal levels of fluids and electrolytes are called *maintenance fluids.*
- To replace lost fluids—when a client has lost fluids as a result of vomiting, diarrhea, or hemorrhage, IV fluids are administered to replenish fluid volume, and referred to as *replacement fluids.*
- To prevent depletion in clients who have the potential to become depleted, such as a client who is allowed nothing by mouth (NPO) for surgery or prior to the administration of chemotherapy.
- Act as a medium for administering medications directly into the bloodstream.

Fluids administered directly into the bloodstream have a rapid effect that is necessary during emergencies or other critical care situations when medications are needed. The advantage of administering medications by this route is the immediate availability of the medication to the body and the rapidity of action. However, IV administration of medications can be rapidly fatal to the client if the incorrect medication or dosage is administered. There are numerous medications available for IV use. Each medication has guidelines relating to its use. Health care providers are responsible to know about the medications they administer and the protocol relating to IV administration of medications.

IV medication protocols are valuable references, often posted in the medication room of an institution, found in a medication reference book, and online. They provide nurses with specifics about usual medication dosage, dilution for IV administration, compatibility, and specific observations of a client that need to be made during medication administration. **Always adhere to the protocol for administering IV medications.**

## IV Delivery Methods

IV fluids and medications can be administered by continuous and intermittent infusion.

- *Continuous IV infusions* replace or maintain fluids and electrolytes. As the name implies, a continuous infusion is an IV solution that flows continuously until it is changed.
- *Intermittent IV infusions* (e.g., IV piggyback [IVPB], IV push) are used to administer medications and supplemental fluids. Intermittent peripheral infusion devices, known as saline or heparin locks, are used to maintain venous access without the need for continuous infusion.
- Hypodermoclysis (HDC), or clysis, is the subcutaneous infusion of fluids. It is considered to be an easy hydration technique suitable for mildly to moderately dehydrated adult clients, especially the elderly; for clients who are unable to take adequate fluids orally; and for clients for whom it is difficult or impractical to insert an intravenous line. The advantages of hypodermocylsis include: it can be administered at home by family members or a nurse; it is simple to insert; and it lessens the need for hospitalization of a client for hydration.

## IV Solutions

There are several types of IV fluids. The type of fluid used is individualized according to the client and the reasons for its use. IV solutions are available in glass bottles and plastic bags. IV plastic bags are more commonly used. IV solutions come prepared in plastic bags and are in various sizes, including 1,000 mL, 500 mL, 250 mL, 100 mL, 50 mL, and 25 mL. The larger-volume IV bags (500 and 1,000 mL) are usually used for continuous IV infusion in adults. The smaller-volume IV bags (usually 50 or 100 mL) are used for IV piggyback (IVPB), also referred to as a secondary IV line, and used to dilute medications for intermittent IV administration. Most IV solution bags are clearly labeled with the exact components of the IV solution, the amount of solution in the bag, storage and handling information, and the expiration date. The large-volume IV bags also have numbered markings on the side of the bag. The smaller IV bags have the same information as the large-volume IV bags, with the exception that they do not have the numbered line markings on the side of the bag. *Note:* The amount of IV solution, as well as the type of solution a medication is diluted in, depends on the medication being administered and is determined by the drug manufacturer. When IV solutions are written in orders and medical records (electronic or handwritten), abbreviations are used. You may encounter various abbreviations; however, the percentage and initials, regardless of how they are written, have the same meaning: "D" is for dextrose, "W" is for water, "S" is for saline, and "NS" is for normal saline. Ringer's lactate (lactated Ringer's), a commonly used electrolyte solution, is abbreviated "RL" or "LR" and occasionally "RLS." Refer to Box 20.1, and learn the common abbreviations for IV solutions. Figures 20.1 to 20.6 show various IV solutions. Abbreviations are often used when health care providers discuss IV solutions. It is important for nurses to know the common IV solution components and the solution concentration strengths represented by such abbreviations. Refer to Box 20.1 and learn the common abbreviations for IV solutions. Since the name for IV solutions is usually discussed and ordered using abbreviations, it is imperative that the nurse carefully read the label on IV solutions to ensure that the correct solution is administered and that the correct solution is infusing on clients who have IV therapy in progress.

> **(!) SAFETY ALERT!**
>
> Administration of the **right IV fluids** to the **right client at the right rate** and **monitoring** the client during the therapy is a safety priority and are essential nursing responsibilities. If a client receives the incorrect IV fluid, an IV infusion too rapidly, and is not monitored closely, reactions can vary from mild to severe (death). Follow the same six rights of medication administration when administering IV therapy to clients. IV fluids are considered to be medications.

| BOX 20.1 | **Abbreviations for Common IV Solutions** |
|---|---|
| NaCl | Sodium chloride |
| NS | Normal saline (0.9% NaCl) |
| $\frac{1}{2}$ NS | $\frac{1}{2}$ Normal saline (0.45% NaCl) |
| $D_5W$ or 5% D/W | Dextrose 5% in water |
| $D_5RL$ or D5RL | Dextrose 5% and lactated Ringer's (Ringer's lactate) |
| RL or RLS | Lactated Ringer's solution (electrolytes) |
| $D_5NS$ | Dextrose 5% in normal saline (0.9% NaCl) |
| $D_5$ and $\frac{1}{2}$ NS (0.45%) | Dextrose 5% in $\frac{1}{2}$ normal saline (0.45% NaCl) |

***Note:*** IV bags are labeled as sodium chloride (NaCl) but frequently referred to as normal saline (NS).

## IV Solution Components

Intravenous fluids generally contain glucose (dextrose), sodium chloride (NaCl), water, and/or electrolytes. The components of IV fluids are indicated on the label of the IV fluid. IV fluids vary in terms of their components and the concentration of the components.

## IV Solution Strength

The abbreviation letters indicate the components in the IV solution, and the numbers indicate the solution strength or concentration of the components in the IV fluid. The numbers may be written as subscripts; for example, $D_5W$ (dextrose 5% in water).

Normal saline solutions are written with 0.9 and the percent sign included (e.g., 0.9% NS). NS is the abbreviation used for normal saline. Normal saline is also referred to as sodium chloride (NaCl). Saline is available in different percentages. Normal saline is the common term used for 0.9% sodium chloride.

Another common saline IV concentration is 0.45% NaCl, often written as 1/2 NS (0.45% is half of 0.9%). Other saline solution strengths include 0.33% NaCl, also abbreviated as 1/3 NS, and 0.225% NaCl, also abbreviated as 1/4 NS. Some IV orders, therefore, may be written as 1/2 NS, 1/4 NS, or 1/3 NS. IV solutions can contain saline only (see Figure 20.5) or saline mixed with dextrose, which would be indicated with percentage of dextrose (e.g., $D_5$ 0.9% sodium chloride) (see Figures 20.3 and 20.4).

> ⓘ **SAFETY ALERT!**
> Pay close attention to IV abbreviations. The letters indicate the solution components, whereas the numbers indicate the solution strength.

Let's examine some IV labels (see Figures 20.1 to 20.7). Recall from Chapter 4 that solution strength expressed as percent (%) indicates the number of grams (g) per 100 milliliters (mL).
- $D_5W$. This abbreviation means dextrose 5% in water, which means each 100 mL of solution contains 5 g dextrose (Figure 20.1).
- $D_5RL$. This abbreviation means 5% dextrose in lactated Ringer's. Lactated Ringer's is a solution containing electrolytes, including potassium chloride and calcium chloride (Figure 20.2).
- 5% Dextrose and 0.9% sodium chloride. This solution contains 5 g of dextrose and 0.9 g (or 900 mg) of sodium chloride per 100 mL solution (Figure 20.3).
- 5% Dextrose and 0.45% sodium chloride. This solution contains 5 g of dextrose and 0.45 g (or 450 mg) of sodium chloride per 100 mL solution (Figure 20.4).
- NS or 0.9% NaCl. This solution contains 0.9 g (or 900 mg) of sodium chloride per 100 mL (Figure 20.5).

## IV Solution Additives

Some IV solutions are available, premixed by the manufacturer, with additives such as medications or electrolytes. Figure 20.6 shows an IV solution premixed with potassium chloride (KCl), a commonly prescribed additive to IV fluids. In many institutions, IV solutions are available premixed with potassium. Premixed additives are clearly marked on IV solutions as shown in Figure 20.6 and Figure 20.7. Potassium chloride is a *high-alert medication*. Notice the label on the IV has the "20 mEq potassium" indicated in red. Notice the solution with the

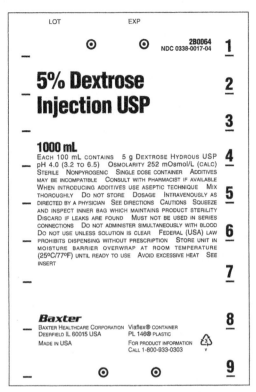

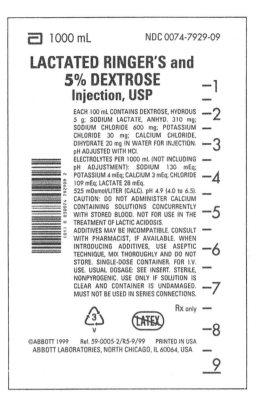

**Figure 20.1** 5% Dextrose (D$_5$W).

**Figure 20.2** Lacated Ringer's and 5% dextrose (D$_5$LR).

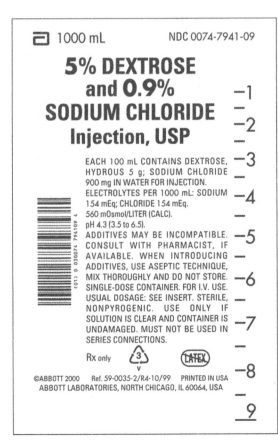

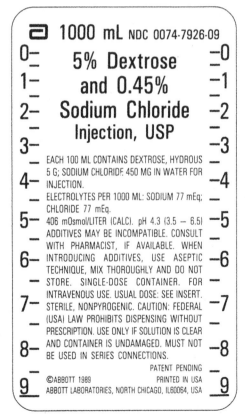

**Figure 20.3** 5% Dextrose in 0.9% sodium chloride (D$_5$NS).

**Figure 20.4** 5% Dextrose in 0.45% sodium chloride (D$_5$ 1/2 NS).

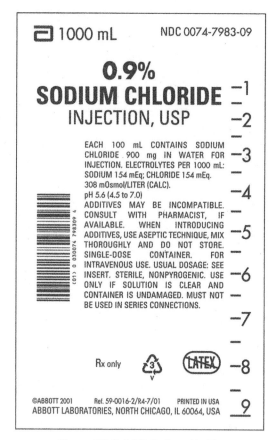

**Figure 20.5** 0.9% Sodium chloride.

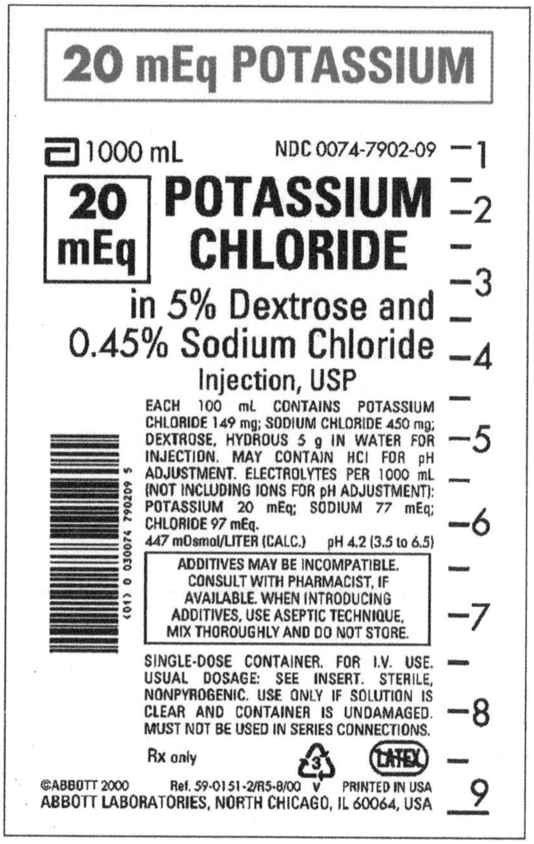

**Figure 20.6** 20 mEq Potassium chloride in 5% dextrose and 0.45% sodium chloride.

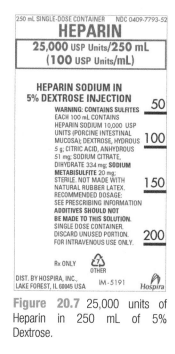

**Figure 20.7** 25,000 units of Heparin in 250 mL of 5% Dextrose.

additive potassium (Figure 20.6) is the same as the IV solution shown in Figure 20.4, 5% dextrose and 0.45% sodium chloride without potassium. **Do not confuse these two solutions. Always read the labels carefully.** Figure 20.7 shows an IV solution premixed with heparin (heparin 25,000 units in 250 mL of 5% dextrose). Heparin is also a *high-alert medication* that is an anticoagulant (blood thinner) that prevents the formation of blood clots. Notice the amount of heparin added to the IV solution is also indicated in red. Notice the dosage strength is indicated per total amount of the bag (25,000 units per 250 mL) and per mL (100 units per mL). Also notice it also indicates on the IV solution, *"Additives should not be made to this solution."* Heparin will be further discussed in Chapter 22. Additives can also be inserted in the IV bag through an injection port by the nurse or a pharmacist. If this is done, a label clearly indicating the name and amount of additive, date, time, and signature of the person who added the additive must be applied to the solution container.

> **SAFETY ALERT!**
>
> Before placing any additives in an IV solution (vitamins, medications, electrolytes), be sure the additives are compatible with the solution. Some incompatible additives may cause the solution to become cloudy or crystallize. Always verify the compatibility of the additive and solution.

## IV Orders

The prescriber is responsible for writing the order. However, administering and monitoring an IV is a nursing responsibility. An IV order (Figure 20.8, shows sample IV orders) **must** specify the following:

- Name of the IV solution
- Name of medication to be added, if any
- Amount (volume) to be administered
- Time period during which the IV is to infuse

> **SAFETY ALERT!**
>
> Remember the following when adding potassium to an IV:
> - It should be compatible with the solution and well diluted.
> - Monitor client during infusion; rapid infusion of potassium can cause death due to cardiac depression, arrhythmias, and arrest.
> - Check IV site frequently; medication is extremely irritating.
> - Administer IV using an infusion control device.
> - Never administer potassium concentrate IV push.
> - **DO NOT** add potassium to an IV bag that is already infusing. Injecting potassium into an upright infusing IV solution causes the medication to concentrate in the lower portion of the IV bag, resulting in the client receiving a concentrated medication solution, which can be harmful.

## Charting of IV Solution

IV fluids are charted on the intake and output (I&O) sheet; in some institutions, they are also charted on the medication administration record (MAR). Figure 20.9 is a sample I&O charting record. In institutions where there is computer charting, this information is entered into the electronic record.

## Calculating Percentage of Solute in IV Fluids

The amount of each ingredient in an IV fluid can be calculated; however, it is not necessary because the label on the IV solution indicates the amount of each ingredient. Calculation of the percentage of solutions was presented in Chapter 4, which deals with percentages.

As you may recall, it is possible to determine the percentage of substances such as dextrose in IV solutions. It is important to remember that **solution strength expressed as a percentage means grams of solute per 100 mL of fluid.** Therefore 5% dextrose solution will have 5 g of dextrose in each 100 mL. In addition to the amount of dextrose in the

| Order | Interpretation |
|---|---|
| D$_5$W 1,000 mL IV q8h | Infuse 1,000 mL 5% dextrose in water intravenously every 8 hours. |
| 0.9% NS 1,000 mL IV with 20 mEq KCl per L q8h | Infuse 1,000 mL 0.9% normal saline IV solution with 20 milliequivalents of potassium chloride added per liter every 8 hours. |

**Figure 20.8** Sample IV orders.

solution, amounts of other components, such as sodium chloride, can be determined. To calculate the amount of a specific component in an IV solution, a ratio and proportion or dimensional analysis can be used.

**Example 1:** Calculate the amount of dextrose in 500 mL $D_5W$. Remember % = g per 100 mL; therefore 5% dextrose = 5 g dextrose per 100 mL.

### ✓ Solution Using Ratio and Proportion

Linear Format: 5 g:100 mL = $x$ g:500 mL   *or*   Fraction Format: $\dfrac{5\,g}{100\,mL} = \dfrac{x\,g}{500\,mL}$

$$\frac{100x}{100} = \frac{2{,}500}{100}$$

$$x = 25\,g$$

500 mL $D_5W$ contains 25 g of dextrose

Remember that ratios and proportions can be stated in linear or fraction format.

### ✓ Solution Using Dimensional Analysis

5% dextrose = 5 g dextrose per 100 mL. Enter it as the starting fraction, and determine the number of grams in the solution.

$$x\,g = \frac{5\,g}{\cancel{100\,mL}} \times \frac{\overset{5}{\cancel{500\,mL}}}{1}$$

$$x = 25\,g\ dextrose$$

500 mL $D_5W$ contains 25 g dextrose

**Example 2:** Calculate the amount of sodium chloride (NaCl) in 1,000 mL NS.

$$0.9\% = 0.9\,g\ NaCl\ per\ 100\,mL$$

Juice glass – 180 mL   Small water cup – 120 mL
Water glass – 210 mL   Jello cup – 150 mL
Coffee cup – 240 mL   Ice cream – 120 mL
Soup bowl – 180 mL   Creamer – 30 mL

**Date:** 8/17/20 _____

Client information

| INTAKE | | | | | OUTPUT | | | | |
|---|---|---|---|---|---|---|---|---|---|
| Time | Type | Amt | Time | IV/ Blood type | Amount absorbed | Time | Urine | Stool | Other |
| | | | 7A | 1,000 mL D5W | 800 mL | 9A | 400 mL | | |
| | | | 12P | IVPB | 100 mL | 1P | 500 mL | | |
| | | | | | | | | | |
| | | | | | | | | | |
| | | | | | | | | | |
| | | | | | | | | | |
| | | | | | | | | | |
| 8 hr total | | | | | 900 mL | | 900 mL | | |

**Figure 20.9** Sample of charting IV fluids on an I&O record.

### ✔ Solution Using Ratio and Proportion

Linear Format: 0.9 g : 100 mL = $x$ g : 1,000 mL   *or*   Fraction Format: $\dfrac{0.9\ g}{100\ mL} = \dfrac{x\ g}{1,000\ mL}$

$$\frac{100x}{100} = \frac{900}{100}$$

$$x = 9\ g\ NaCl$$

1,000 mL of NS contains 9 g of sodium chloride

### ✔ Solution Using Dimensional Analysis

0.9% = 0.9 g NaCl per 100 mL. Use the grams of solute per 100 mL of fluid as the starting fraction.

$$x\ g = \frac{0.9\ g}{\overset{}{\underset{1}{\cancel{100\ mL}}}} \times \frac{\overset{10}{\cancel{1,000\ mL}}}{1}$$

$$x = 9\ g\ NaCl$$

1,000 mL of NS contains 9 g of NaCl

**Example 3:** Calculate the amount of dextrose and sodium chloride in 1,000 mL of 5% dextrose and 0.45% normal saline (D5 and $\frac{1}{2}$ NS or $D_5$ 1/2 NS).

### ✔ Solution Using Ratio and Proportion

$$D_5 = dextrose\ 5\% = 5\ g\ dextrose\ per\ 100\ mL$$

$$0.45\%\ NS = 0.45\ g\ NaCl\ per\ 100\ mL$$

Linear Format: Dextrose: 5 g : 100 mL = $x$ g : 1,000 mL   *or*   Fraction Format: $\dfrac{5\ g}{100\ mL} = \dfrac{x\ g}{1,000\ mL}$

$$\frac{100x}{100} = \frac{5,000}{100}$$

$$x = 50\ g\ dextrose$$

Linear Format: NaCl: 0.45 g : 100 mL = $x$ g : 1,000 mL   *or*   Fraction Format: $\dfrac{0.45\ g}{100\ mL} = \dfrac{x\ g}{1,000\ mL}$

$$\frac{100x}{100} = \frac{450}{100}$$

$$x = 4.5\ g\ NaCl$$

1,000 mL $D_5$ 0.45% NS contains 50 g of dextrose and 4.5 g of NaCl

### ✔ Solution Using Dimensional Analysis

$$5\%\ dextrose = 5\ g\ dextrose\ per\ 100\ mL$$

$$0.45\%\ NS = 0.45\ g\ NaCl\ per\ 100\ mL$$

$$Dextrose: x\ g = \frac{5\ g}{\overset{}{\underset{1}{\cancel{100\ mL}}}} \times \frac{\overset{10}{\cancel{1,000\ mL}}}{1}$$

$$x = 50\ g\ dextrose$$

$$NaCl: x\ g = \frac{0.45\ g}{\overset{}{\underset{1}{\cancel{100\ mL}}}} \times \frac{\overset{10}{\cancel{1,000\ mL}}}{1}$$

$$x = 4.5\ g\ NaCl$$

1,000 mL $D_5$ 0.45% NS contains 50 g of dextrose and 4.5 g of NaCl

## Vascular Access Devices

IV fluids may be infused through a peripheral vein or central vein using a vascular access device (VAD), also known as a venous access device.

**Peripheral line**—Generally used for short-term therapy. The infusion site of a peripheral line is a vein in the arm, hand, or scalp in an infant; or if other sites are not accessible, and on rare occasions, a vein in the leg.

**Central line**—Provides direct access to large major veins. Used for long-term therapy. For a central line, a special catheter is used to access a large vein near the heart, such as the subclavian or jugular vein. A central line is used for infusion of large amounts of fluids and for infusion of highly concentrated electrolyte replacements, chemotherapy (infusion of medications for cancer), and total parenteral nutrition (TPN). TPN is an IV solution that provides nutrients. Parenteral nutrition solutions consist of glucose, amino acids, minerals, vitamins, and/or fat emulsions. Examples of central catheters include single-lumen, triple-lumen, Hickman, Broviac, and Groshong catheters.

- **Peripherally inserted central catheter (PICC line)**—When a peripheral vein is used to access a central vein. A PICC line is inserted into the antecubital vein in the arm and is advanced into the superior vena cava.
- **Port-A-Cath**—Used to deliver medication to a central vein. The device is surgically placed under the skin, usually on the upper chest. When the device is in place, there is no part of the central venous catheter that is outside the body. The device is accessed using a special needle (to administer medications or draw blood) that goes through the skin and into the port.

**Saline lock**—Intermittent venous access device (Figure 20.10) used for the purpose of administering IV medication intermittently or for access to a vein in an emergency situation and can be used to administer medications IV push (IV bolus). A saline lock is a short IV line that is attached to an IV catheter that is capped off on the end and can be accessed by a needle or needleless system to administer medications intermittently. Various institutions use a needleless system for administration of medications through the access devices such as the saline lock as well as the primary line. Intermittent venous access devices are referred to as *med locks, saline locks, heparin locks, IV lock,* and *intermittent peripheral infusion devices* (IPIDs). Venous access devices are referred to as saline locks because they are periodically flushed with sterile normal saline solution for injection, or with heparin (heparin lock) to keep the line patent. Due to bolusing of clients when heparin is used, heparin (a potent anticoagulant despite its use in dilute form) is now used at most institutions on the initial insertion of the catheter. For subsequent flushing of the port, normal saline solution is used (1 to 3 mL, depending on institution policy).

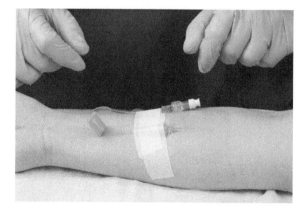

**Figure 20.10** Intermittent lock covered with a rubber diaphragm. (From Potter PA, Perry AG, Stockert P, Hall A: *Fundamentals of nursing,* ed 9, St. Louis, 2017, Elsevier.)

When medications are administered through an intermittent access device, the device must be flushed before and after medication is given. **Always refer to the policy at your institution or health care agency regarding the frequency, volume, and concentration of saline or heparin to be used to maintain the IV lock.**

Medications can be administered through a port used for direct injection of medication by syringe or directly into the vein by venipuncture. This is referred to as IV **push** or **bolus.** IV push indicates that a syringe is attached to the lock and pushed in over a certain period of time. IV bolus indicates that a large volume of IV fluid or medication is infused over a specific time through an IV administration set attached to the lock. There are guidelines, however, relating to the acceptable rate for IV push administration. **Check appropriate references for the rate for IV push medication administration.** Also check the institution's policy and a pharmacology reference regarding administration by IV push or bolus.

### Monitoring IVs

The nurse is responsible for monitoring the client during an IV infusion. IV site and the infusion should be checked according to hospital policy for the volume of remaining fluid, the correct infusion rate, and for signs of complications. It is the nurse's responsibility to maintain and regulate IV infusions.

## Administration of IV Fluids

IV fluids are administered by an IV infusion set, which includes the sealed IV bag containing the fluids (Figure 20.11A). The **IV infusion set (IV tubing)** (Figure 20.11B) allows the IV fluid to flow from the IV bag to the IV catheter placed in the client's vein. The IV tubing is attached to the bottom of the IV bag. A **spike** at the top of the IV tubing is used to insert the tubing into the fluid container. At the top of the tubing is a **drip chamber** that allows the nurse to observe the drops of fluid and count the drops per minute (gtt/min) for manually regulated IVs. **The roller clamp** squeezes the tubing, to allow for the IV flow rate to be increased or decreased, and is used to regulate the gtt/min that fall into the drip chamber. Some IV tubing has a **sliding clamp** attached as well, which can be used to temporarily stop the IV infusion. **Injection ports** are located on the IV tubing and on most IV solution bags. Injection ports allow for injection of medications directly into the bag of solution or line. The injection ports also allow for the attachment of secondary IV lines that contain fluids or medications to the primary line. The tubing used for the primary line is long tubing, whereas the secondary tubing used for intravenous piggyback (IVPB) is short IV tubing with a drip chamber, and a clamp.

IV fluids infuse by gravity flow. This means that for the IV solution to infuse, it must be hung above the level of the client's heart, which will allow for adequate pressure to be exerted for the IV to infuse. The height of the IV bag therefore has a relationship to the rate of flow. The higher the IV bag is hung, the greater the pressure; therefore the IV will infuse at a more rapid rate. The lower the IV bag is hung, the less the pressure, and the IV will infuse at a slower rate.

### Primary and Secondary Lines

**Primary lines**—As previously stated, the primary line is usually the IV solution, which is continually infusing. The primary line is usually a large volume of fluid. Frequently used primary IV bags are 500 or 1,000 mL (see Figure 20.11A). Examples of medications added include multivitamins (MVI) and electrolytes, such as potassium chloride. These medications

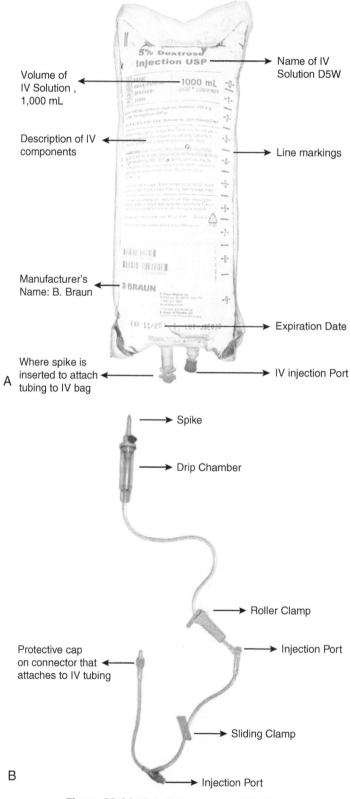

Name of IV Solution D5W

Volume of IV Solution , 1,000 mL

Description of IV components

Line markings

Manufacturer's Name: B. Braun

Expiration Date

Where spike is inserted to attach tubing to IV bag

A

IV injection Port

Spike

Drip Chamber

Roller Clamp

Protective cap on connector that attaches to IV tubing

Injection Port

Sliding Clamp

B

Injection Port

**Figure 20.11** (A) D$_5$W IV solution. (B) IV tubing.

are usually diluted in a large volume of fluid (1,000 mL), particularly potassium chloride, because of the side effects and untoward reactions that can occur. In many institutions, IV solutions containing potassium chloride are stocked by the pharmacy and obtained on request by the unit, eliminating the need for potassium chloride to be added to an IV bag. The IV tubing used for the primary line is long tubing. Injection ports on the tubing allow for the attachment of a secondary line or for the administration of medications with the use of a syringe, or needleless entry.

**Secondary lines**—These attach to the primary line at an injection port. They are also known as IV piggyback (IVPB). The main purpose of secondary lines is to infuse medications on an intermittent basis (e.g., antibiotics every 6 hr). Secondary IVs usually contain a smaller volume of IV fluid (50–250 mL) than the primary. Amounts of 50 to 100 mL are seen most often. The amount of solution used for the IVPB is determined by the medication being added. The IVPB is hung higher than the primary line so that it is given a greater pressure than the primary, thereby allowing it to infuse first. To do this, an extender is attached to the primary bag to lower it below the secondary (Figure 20.12). Secondary lines can also be used to infuse other IV fluids, as long as they are compatible with the fluid on the primary line. The tubing used for secondary IVs is shorter than for primary IVs.

**Premixed IVPBs**—Many IVPBs come premixed by the manufacturer or the pharmacist depending on the institution, or the nurse may have to prepare them.

Whether an IVPB is premixed or prepared by the nurse, the IV bag must be labeled with appropriate information which includes the name of the medication, the dosage strength of the medication, and the solution the medication is diluted in. Premixed IVPBs often come labeled with this information. The rate for an IVPB to infuse should be checked using appropriate resources. The manufacture's insert provides recommended times for infusion if not stated in the prescriber's order. This information can also be found online.

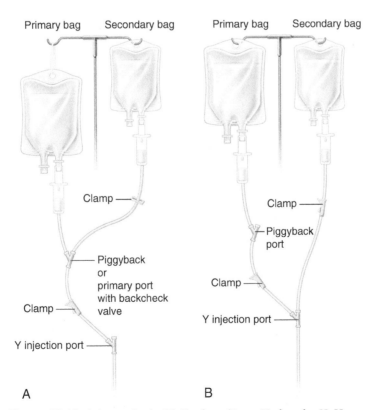

**Figure 20.12** (A) Piggyback. (B) Tandem. (From Harkreader H, Hogan MA: *Fundamentals of nursing: Caring and clinical judgment*, ed 3, St. Louis, 2007, Saunders.)

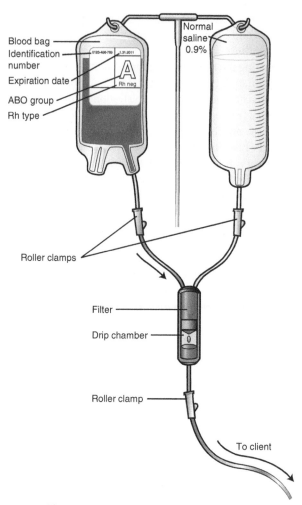

**Figure 20.13**  Setup for blood administration.

### Blood Administration Tubing

The administration of blood and blood products is commonly done with a special tubing called Y-tubing. The "Y" refers to two spikes above the drip chamber of the IV tubing. One spike is attached to the blood container, and the other is attached to a container of normal saline (NaCl) solution. Normal saline is used to flush the IV tubing before and after the transfusion. Tubing for blood administration has an in-line filter (to remove small clots [microemboli] and particles from the blood before it's infused into the client). Blood may be administered by gravity or electronic pump (Figure 20.13). Blood transfusions and blood products are regulated in the same manner as any other intravenous infusion and also involve calculation of flow rates and infusion times.

### Systems for Administering Medications by Intravenous Piggyback

Other types of secondary medication setups used in some institutions include:

- **ADD-Vantage system.** This system requires a special type of IV bag that has a port for inserting the medication (usually in powder form and mixed with the IV solution as a diluent). The contents of the vial are therefore mixed into the total solution and then infused (Figure 20.14).

  The Baxter Mini-Bag Plus is also used to administer piggyback medication. The mini-bag, which is dispensed by the pharmacy, has a vial of unreconstituted medication attached to a special port. You break an internal seal and mix the medication and diluent just before administration. The medication vial remains attached to the mini-bag (Figure 20.15).

- **Volume-control devices** are referred to by their trade names (Buretrol, Burette, or Volutrol), depending on the institution. These volume-control devices usually have a maximum capacity of 150 mL and attach below the primary infusion bag. Volume-control devices have a safety factor in that the volume of fluid administered can be limited, therefore decreasing the chance of infusing a large volume of fluid accidentally to a client. The volume-control fluid chamber is filled with small volumes of fluid for administration. They can also be used intermittently for medication purposes. There is a port on the fluid chamber that allows medication to be injected and a certain amount of IV fluid to be added (Figure 20.16). They are used often in the pediatric and critical care settings. These devices allow for precise control of the infusion and medication.

The rate for an IVPB to infuse should **always** be verified if not stated in the prescriber's orders. The nurse has the responsibility for calculating the **right** infusion rate for the IVPB.

> **! SAFETY ALERT!**
>
> When an infusion rate is not stated for IVPB, check appropriate resources, which include: the manufacturer's insert, a pharmacology book, online resources, or the hospital pharmacy. The nurse is responsible for any error that occurs in reference to IV administration including incorrect rate of infusion.

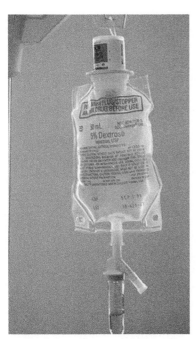

**Figure 20.14** The ADD-Vantage drug delivery system. (Courtesy Bruce Clayton.)

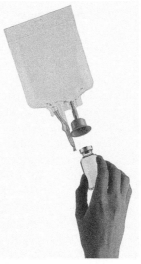

**Figure 20.15** Mini-Bag Plus. (From Baxter Healthcare Corporation, Deerfield, IL.)

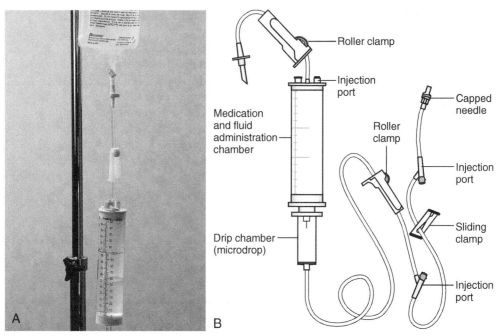

**Figure 20.16** **(A)** Volume-controlled device. **(B)** Parts of a volume-control set. (**A**, From Potter PA, Perry AG, Stockert P, Hall A: *Fundamentals of nursing*, ed 9, St. Louis, 2017, Elsevier.)

## Methods Used for the Administration of Intravenous Fluids

There are two methods used for the infusion of IV fluids and IVPBs to clients. IV fluids can be administered by gravity or by the use of electronic devices such as infusion pumps.

- IV **infusion by gravity**—Requires the nurse to calculate the IV flow rate in drops per minute (gtt/min).
- IV **infusion by pump**—With infusion pumps the nurse sets the IV flow rate in milliliters per hour (mL/hr).

The calculation of the IV flow rate in gtt/min and mL/hr will be discussed in Chapter 21.

Electronic Infusion Devices. There are several electronic infusion devices on the market used to administer and regulate intravenous fluid and/or medication infusions (e.g., IV Infusion Pumps), which are used for a variety of purposes. Electronic infusion pumps are used to deliver fluids and medications into a client's body at a controlled rate. There are many types of IV pumps, which include volumetric pumps, patient-controlled analgesia (PCA) pumps, and syringe pumps. Smart infusion pumps are available on the market, which are equipped with safety features designed to reduce infusion-related medication errors. Smart pumps (Figure 20.17) have software that includes a reference library of IV medications and dosing guidelines and alerts the nurse when a pump setting is programmed outside of the pre-configured limits. According to ISMP (2020), smart infusion pumps are now used in more than 80% of US hospitals.

- **Electronic volumetric pumps**—Electronic infusion devices that infuse fluids into the vein under pressure and against resistance and do not depend on gravity. The manufacturer provides specialized tubing that must be used with this device. The rate on a volumetric pump is set in mL/hr (Figure 20.18). There is a wide range of electronic pumps. Because the pump delivers in mL/hr, milliliter calculation that results in a decimal fraction must be rounded to a whole milliliter, unless the pump has decimal capabilities. There are some IV pumps available that are capable of delivering IV fluids in tenths of a mL. These pumps may be seen in some intensive care units.
- **Syringe pumps**—Hold a prefilled syringe and apply pressure to the plunger to deliver small volumes of fluid or medication at a set rate (Figure 20.19). These pumps are often used for neonatal and pediatric clients for delivery of small volumes at low rates. These pumps are also useful in other areas, which include intensive care units, labor and delivery, and hospice. The rate on syringe pumps is set at mL/hr.

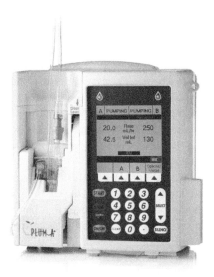

Figure 20.17  Smart pump.

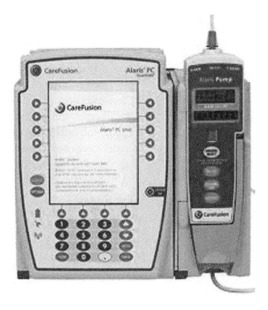

Figure 20.18  Infusion pump.

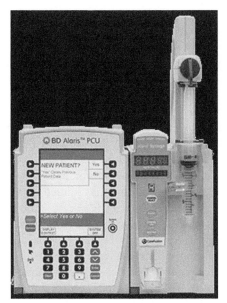

Figure 20.19  Syringe pump.

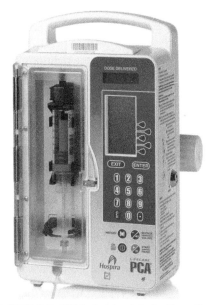

Figure 20.20  CADD Solis PCA Ambulatory Infusion Pump (from Smiths Medical, Dublin OH.)

- **Patient-controlled analgesia (PCA) pumps**—A form of pain management that allows the client to self-administer IV pain medications with the push of control button (Figure 20.20). The PCA pump is programmed to allow dosages of narcotics only within specific limits to be delivered to prevent overdosage. The dosage and frequency of administration are programmed into the pump. The pump also stores information that includes the frequency and dosage of medication delivered to the client.

Infusion Devices for the Home Care Setting.  Infusion devices used in the outpatient and home care setting include insulin pumps and elastomeric balloon pumps. With the elastomeric balloon device, fluid is held in a stretchable balloon reservoir, and pressure from the walls of the balloon causes fluid delivery. No infusion rates are set on these devices. An example of the elastomeric pump is the ON-Q Pump. The ON-Q pump is a non-narcotic elastomeric portable pump that is being used to provide postoperative pain relief. The device automatically and continuously delivers a slow rate of local anesthetic to a patient's surgical site or in close proximity to nerves providing targeted pain relief for up to 5 days depending on the size of the pump. A small catheter is placed under the skin and attached to the pump. The pump is completely portable and can be clipped to the clothing or placed in a small carrying case. Clients using infusion devices at home **must** be educated about the device to ensure safe use, and both device and client **must** be monitored to ascertain proper functioning.

While infusion pumps were designed to improve client safety, infusion pumps are not without problems and have been associated with medication errors. Despite improvements in design and the use of smart pumps, performance problems still occur that have resulted in both over- and underinfusion. Pump efficacy is a primary and continual concern of the US Food and Drug Administration (FDA) and the Institute for Safe Medication Practices (ISMP). Problems include programming errors, calculation errors resulting from unit of measure inconsistency between the drug library and the EHR (i.e., a bolus dose ordered in mg, but the smart pump requires mg/kg), and selection errors when choosing among multiple listed concentrations in the drug library for the same medication are some of the errors identified by ISMP (2020) with the smart pump. In response to the numerous and varied errors associated with the smart pump, the ISMP revised and expanded the *Guidelines for Optimizing Safe Implementation and Use of Smart Infusion Pumps* in February 2020. The complete guidelines can be viewed on the ISMP at https://www.ismp.org/node/972.

As stated both the FDA and ISMP have published recommendations for best practices relating to infusion pumps, which include verifying that the infusion pump is programmed for the right dosage, at the right rate and volume to be infused, obtaining an independent double-check of infusion pump settings by a second clinician when infusing high-risk medications, and client monitoring as well as the infusion. Infusion Pump recommendations related to safety when using infusion pumps can be found at https://www.fda.gov/medical-devices/infusion-pumps/infusion-pump-risk-reduction-strategies-clinicians.

Other strategies that have been identified to increase safety during the use of infusion pumps include, when using multiple-channel pumps, labeling each infusion line, and prominently displaying IV fluid and medication labels on the infusion pump and the tubing at the port of entry. Hospital or clinical in-service education is required for the use of all infusion devices.

As nurses we must use best practices for client safety with the use of infusion pumps. Nurses need to apply the six "rights" of safe medication administration when using infusion pumps. The **right client** should always receive the **right fluid** and/or medication by the appropriate IV pump programmed to deliver the **right dosage and volume** with the **right documentation** and continual monitoring. **Do not** rely solely on the pump.

> **!** **SAFETY ALERT!**
>
> An institution may use many different infusion pumps. The nurse **must** know how to use them correctly to prevent client harm and a fatal outcome.

---

**POINTS TO REMEMBER**

- IV orders are written by the doctor or other prescriber certified to do so (e.g., nurse practitioner, physician's assistant).
- IV orders must specify the name of the solution, medications (if any are to be added), the amount to be administered, and the infusion time.
- Several electronic devices are on the market for infusing IV solutions. Always familiarize yourself with the equipment before use.
- Follow the institution's protocol for IV administration.
- Nurses have the primary responsibility for monitoring the client during IV therapy.
- Nurses are responsible for any errors that occur in administration of IV fluids (e.g., inadequate dilution, too rapid infusion).
- Pay close attention to IV abbreviations. The letters indicate the solution components, and the numbers indicate the solution strength.
- Solution strength expressed as a percentage (%) indicates grams of solute per 100 mL of fluid.
- Principles relating to flow rate and infusion times are also applicable to parenteral nutrition solutions and blood and blood products.
- Apply the six rights of medication administration to IV infusion pumps. The nurse is responsible to ensure client safety when a client is receiving fluids and/or medications by an infusion pump.

---

# PRACTICE **PROBLEMS**

Answer the following questions as briefly as possible.

1. What does PCA stand for? _____

2. An IV initiated in a client's lower arm is called what type of line?

   _____

3. IVPB is an abbreviation for _____ .

4. A client has an IV of 1,000 mL 0.9% NS. The initials identify what type of solution?

   _____

5. A secondary line is hung _____ than the primary line.

6. Volumetric pumps infuse fluids into the vein by _____ .

Identify the components and percentage strength of the following IV solutions:

7. $D_{20}W$ _____

8. $D_5W$ 10 mEq KCl _____

9. How many grams of dextrose does 500 mL $D_{10}W$ contain? _____

Calculate the amount of dextrose and/or sodium chloride in the following IV solutions:

10. 750 mL $D_5$ NS

    dextrose _____

    NaCl _____

11. 250 mL D$_{10}$W

dextrose _____

12. 1,000 mL D$_5$ 0.33% NS

dextrose _____

NaCl _____

13. 500 mL D$_5$ ½ NS

dextrose _____

NaCl _____

**Answers on p. 487**

---

## ⚕ CLINICAL **REASONING**

**Scenario:** A client returned to the unit after surgery connected to a patient-controlled analgesia (PCA) pump. An order was written to attach a solution of 100 mL 0.9% normal saline (NS) with morphine 100 mg to the pump and infuse at a rate of 1 mg per 6 min. The ordered solution was inserted into the device and the rate set. The client had been instructed on the use of the PCA pump. The client continued to complain of severe pain on each shift despite the pump indicating that medication was being received at the set rate. The client received intermittent boluses of morphine to relieve pain.

Twenty-four hours later, a nurse opened the PCA pump, found the full bag of IV solution in place, and noticed that the tubing had not been primed.

What should have been done in this situation?

_____

_____

_____

**Answer on p. 487**

---

## ◎ CHAPTER **REVIEW**

For questions 1 through 4, specify the letter of the solution (*A* through *D*) corresponding to the fluid abbreviation.

1. D$_5$ ½ NS _____

2. D$_5$W _____

3. RL _____

4. D$_5$ NS _____

**A**

LOT    EXP

2B2324
NDC 0338-0117-04
DIN 00061085

**1**

# Lactated Ringer's Injection USP

**2**

**3**

**1000 mL**

EACH 100 mL CONTAINS   600 mg SODIUM CHLORIDE USP   310 mg SODIUM LACTATE   30 mg POTASSIUM CHLORIDE USP   20 mg CALCIUM CHLORIDE USP   pH 6.5 (6.0 TO 7.5)   mEq/L   SODIUM 130   POTASSIUM 4   CALCIUM 2.7   CHLORIDE 109   LACTATE 28   OSMOLARITY 273 mOsmol/L (CALC)   STERILE   NONPYROGENIC   SINGLE DOSE CONTAINER   **NOT FOR USE IN THE TREATMENT OF LACTIC ACIDOSIS**   ADDITIVES MAY BE INCOMPATIBLE   CONSULT WITH PHARMACIST IF AVAILABLE   WHEN INTRODUCING ADDITIVES USE ASEPTIC TECHNIQUE   MIX THOROUGHLY   DO NOT STORE   DOSAGE   INTRAVENOUSLY AS DIRECTED BY A PHYSICIAN   SEE DIRECTIONS   CAUTIONS   SQUEEZE AND INSPECT INNER BAG WHICH MAINTAINS PRODUCT STERILITY   DISCARD IF LEAKS ARE FOUND   MUST NOT BE USED IN SERIES CONNECTIONS   DO NOT ADMINISTER SIMULTANEOUSLY WITH BLOOD   DO NOT USE UNLESS SOLUTION IS CLEAR   FEDERAL (USA) LAW PROHIBITS DISPENSING WITHOUT PRESCRIPTION   STORE UNIT IN MOISTURE BARRIER OVERWRAP AT ROOM TEMPERATURE (25°C/77°F) UNTIL READY TO USE   AVOID EXCESSIVE HEAT   SEE INSERT

**4**

**5**

**6**

**7**

***Baxter***
BAXTER HEALTHCARE CORPORATION
DEERFIELD IL 60015 USA
MADE IN USA
DISTRIBUTED IN CANADA BY
BAXTER CORPORATION
TORONTO ONTARIO CANADA

Viaflex® CONTAINER
PL 146® PLASTIC
FOR PRODUCT INFORMATION
CALL 1-800-933-0303

**8**

**9**

---

**B**

LOT    EXP

2B1073
NDC 0338-0085-03

**1**

# 5% Dextrose and 0.45% Sodium Chloride Injection USP

**2**

**3**

**500 mL**

EACH 100 mL CONTAINS   5 g DEXTROSE HYDROUS USP   450 mg SODIUM CHLORIDE USP   pH 4.0 (3.2 TO 6.5)   mEq/L   SODIUM 77   CHLORIDE 77   HYPERTONIC   OSMOLARITY   406 mOsmol/L (CALC)   STERILE   NONPYROGENIC   SINGLE DOSE CONTAINER   ADDITIVES MAY BE INCOMPATIBLE   CONSULT WITH PHARMACIST IF AVAILABLE   WHEN INTRODUCING ADDITIVES USE ASEPTIC TECHNIQUE   MIX THOROUGHLY   DO NOT STORE   DOSAGE   INTRAVENOUSLY AS DIRECTED BY A PHYSICIAN   SEE DIRECTIONS   CAUTIONS   SQUEEZE AND INSPECT INNER BAG WHICH MAINTAINS PRODUCT STERILITY   DISCARD IF LEAKS ARE FOUND   MUST NOT BE USED IN SERIES CONNECTIONS   DO NOT USE UNLESS SOLUTION IS CLEAR   FEDERAL (USA) LAW PROHIBITS DISPENSING WITHOUT PRESCRIPTION   STORE UNIT IN MOISTURE BARRIER OVERWRAP AT ROOM TEMPERATURE (25°C/77°F) UNTIL READY TO USE   AVOID EXCESSIVE HEAT   SEE INSERT

**4**

***Baxter***
BAXTER HEALTHCARE CORPORATION
DEERFIELD IL 60015 USA
MADE IN USA

Viaflex® CONTAINER
PL 146® PLASTIC
FOR PRODUCT INFORMATION
CALL 1-800-933-0303

---

**C**

LOT    EXP

2B0064
NDC 0338-0017-04

**1**

# 5% Dextrose Injection USP

**2**

**3**

**1000 mL**

EACH 100 mL CONTAINS   5 g DEXTROSE HYDROUS USP   pH 4.0 (3.2 TO 6.5)   OSMOLARITY 252 mOsmol/L (CALC)   STERILE   NONPYROGENIC   SINGLE DOSE CONTAINER   ADDITIVES MAY BE INCOMPATIBLE   CONSULT WITH PHARMACIST IF AVAILABLE   WHEN INTRODUCING ADDITIVES USE ASEPTIC TECHNIQUE   MIX THOROUGHLY   DO NOT STORE   DOSAGE   INTRAVENOUSLY AS DIRECTED BY A PHYSICIAN   SEE DIRECTIONS   CAUTIONS   SQUEEZE AND INSPECT INNER BAG WHICH MAINTAINS PRODUCT STERILITY   DISCARD IF LEAKS ARE FOUND   MUST NOT BE USED IN SERIES CONNECTIONS   DO NOT ADMINISTER SIMULTANEOUSLY WITH BLOOD   DO NOT USE UNLESS SOLUTION IS CLEAR   FEDERAL (USA) LAW PROHIBITS DISPENSING WITHOUT PRESCRIPTION   STORE UNIT IN MOISTURE BARRIER OVERWRAP AT ROOM TEMPERATURE (25°C/77°F) UNTIL READY TO USE   AVOID EXCESSIVE HEAT   SEE INSERT

**4**

**5**

**6**

**7**

***Baxter***
BAXTER HEALTHCARE CORPORATION
DEERFIELD IL 60015 USA
MADE IN USA

Viaflex® CONTAINER
PL 146® PLASTIC
FOR PRODUCT INFORMATION
CALL 1-800-933-0303

**8**

**9**

---

**D**

LOT    EXP

2B1064
NDC 0338-0089-04

**1**

# 5% Dextrose and 0.9% Sodium Chloride Injection USP

**2**

**3**

**1000 mL**

EACH 100 mL CONTAINS   5 g DEXTROSE HYDROUS USP   900 mg SODIUM CHLORIDE USP   pH 4.0 (3.2 TO 6.5)   mEq/L   SODIUM 154   CHLORIDE 154   HYPERTONIC   OSMOLARITY   560 mOsmol/L (CALC)   STERILE   NONPYROGENIC   SINGLE DOSE CONTAINER   ADDITIVES MAY BE INCOMPATIBLE   CONSULT WITH PHARMACIST IF AVAILABLE   WHEN INTRODUCING ADDITIVES USE ASEPTIC TECHNIQUE   MIX THOROUGHLY   DO NOT STORE   DOSAGE   INTRAVENOUSLY AS DIRECTED BY A PHYSICIAN   SEE DIRECTIONS   CAUTIONS   SQUEEZE AND INSPECT INNER BAG WHICH MAINTAINS PRODUCT STERILITY   DISCARD IF LEAKS ARE FOUND   MUST NOT BE USED IN SERIES CONNECTIONS   DO NOT USE UNLESS SOLUTION IS CLEAR   FEDERAL (USA) LAW PROHIBITS DISPENSING WITHOUT PRESCRIPTION   STORE UNIT IN MOISTURE BARRIER OVERWRAP AT ROOM TEMPERATURE (25°C/77°F) UNTIL READY TO USE   AVOID EXCESSIVE HEAT   SEE INSERT

**4**

**5**

**6**

**7**

***Baxter***
BAXTER HEALTHCARE CORPORATION
DEERFIELD IL 60015 USA
MADE IN USA

Viaflex® CONTAINER
PL 146® PLASTIC
FOR PRODUCT INFORMATION
CALL 1-800-933-0303

**8**

**9**

5. A client has a PCA in use following surgery. What is this device used to control?

_____

6. When an IV medication is injected directly into the vein through a port, it is called an IV _____ or _____.

7. The two major intravenous access sites are _____ and _____.

8. A client is to receive an antibiotic IVPB. In order for the antibiotic to infuse first, how must it be hung in relation to the existing IV solution bag? _____

Calculate the amount of dextrose and/or sodium chloride in each of the following IV solutions:

9. 0.5 L D$_5$ 1/4 NS

   dextrose _____ g

   NaCl _____ g

10. 750 mL D$_5$ 1/2 NS

   dextrose _____ g

   NaCl _____ g

**Answers on p. 488**

⊝volve

For additional practice problems, refer to the Intravenous Flow Rates section of the Elsevier's Interactive Drug Calculation Application, Version 1, on Evolve.

## ⭐ ANSWERS

### Chapter 20
#### Answers to Practice Problems

1. patient-controlled analgesia
2. peripheral
3. intravenous piggyback
4. 0.9% normal saline, 0.9% sodium chloride (NaCl)
5. higher
6. pressure
7. 20% dextrose in water
8. 5% dextrose in water with 10 mEq potassium chloride (KCl)
9. 50 g
10. Dextrose: 5 g : 100 mL = $x$ g : 750 mL

$$\frac{100x}{100} = \frac{3,750}{100}$$

$$x = 37.5 \text{ g dextrose}$$

*or*

$$\frac{5\text{ g}}{100 \text{ mL}} = \frac{x\text{ g}}{750 \text{ mL}}$$

NaCl: 0.9 g : 100 mL = $x$ g : 750 mL

$$\frac{100x}{100} = \frac{675}{100}$$

$$x = 6.75 \text{ g NaCl}$$

*or*

$$\frac{0.9\text{ g}}{100 \text{ mL}} = \frac{x\text{ g}}{750 \text{ mL}}$$

750 mL $D_5NS$ contains 37.5 g of dextrose and 6.75 g NaCl (saline).

11. 10 g : 100 mL = $x$ g : 250 mL

$$\frac{100x}{100} = \frac{2,500}{100}$$

$$x = 25 \text{ g dextrose}$$

*or*

$$\frac{10\text{ g}}{100 \text{ mL}} = \frac{x\text{ g}}{250 \text{ mL}}$$

250 mL $D_{10}W$ contains 25 g dextrose.

12. Dextrose: 5 g : 100 mL = $x$ g : 1,000 mL

$$\frac{100x}{100} = \frac{5,000}{100}$$

$$x = 50 \text{ g dextrose}$$

*or*

$$\frac{5\text{ g}}{100 \text{ mL}} = \frac{x\text{ g}}{1,000 \text{ mL}}$$

NaCl: 0.33 g : 100 mL = $x$ g : 1,000 mL

$$\frac{100x}{100} = \frac{330}{100}$$

$$x = 3.3 \text{ g NaCl}$$

*or*

$$\frac{0.33\text{ g}}{100 \text{ mL}} = \frac{x\text{ g}}{1,000 \text{ mL}}$$

1,000 mL $D_5$ 0.33% NS contains 50 g dextrose and 3.3 g NaCl (saline).

13. Dextrose: 5 g : 100 mL = $x$ g : 500 mL

$$\frac{100x}{100} = \frac{2,500}{100}$$

$$x = 25 \text{ g dextrose}$$

*or*

$$\frac{5\text{ g}}{100 \text{ mL}} = \frac{x\text{ g}}{500 \text{ mL}}$$

NaCl: 0.45 g : 100 mL = $x$ g : 500 mL

$$\frac{100x}{100} = \frac{225}{100}$$

$$x = 2.25 \text{ g NaCl}$$

*or*

$$\frac{0.45\text{ g}}{100 \text{ mL}} = \frac{x\text{ g}}{500 \text{ mL}}$$

500 mL $D_5$ 1/2 NS contains 25 g dextrose and 2.25 g of NaCl (saline).

### Answer to Clinical Reasoning Question

Troubleshooting should have been done by the nurses caring for the client. If the client's pain was not being relieved, the device should have been checked for possible malfunctioning and to determine whether the machine had been set up properly. It is mandatory that all programming be double-checked by nurses and the pump be monitored frequently to ensure that it is functioning. The client's continual complaint of severe pain with no relief should have been a key to the nurses caring for the client.

## Answers to Chapter Review

1. B
2. C
3. A
4. D
5. pain
6. push *or* bolus
7. peripheral and central
8. higher
9. 25 g dextrose; 1.125 g NaCl

Equivalent: 1 L = 1,000 mL

Therefore 0.5 L = 500 mL

Dextrose:

5 g : 100 mL = x g : 500 mL

$$\frac{100x}{100} = \frac{2{,}500}{100}$$

$$x = 25 \text{ g dextrose}$$

*or*

$$\frac{5 \text{ g}}{100 \text{ mL}} = \frac{x \text{ g}}{500 \text{ mL}}$$

NaCl:

0.225 g : 100 mL = x g : 500 mL

$$\frac{100x}{100} = \frac{112.5}{100}$$

$$x = 1.125 \text{ g NaCl}$$

*or*

$$\frac{0.225 \text{ g}}{100 \text{ mL}} = \frac{x \text{ g}}{500 \text{ mL}}$$

500 mL D$_5$ 1/4 NS contains 25 g dextrose and 1.125 g NaCl (saline).

10. 37.5 g dextrose; 3.375 g NaCl

Dextrose:

5 g : 100 mL = x g : 750 mL

$$\frac{100x}{100} = \frac{3{,}750}{100}$$

$$x = 37.5 \text{ g of dextrose}$$

*or*

$$\frac{5 \text{ g}}{100 \text{ mL}} = \frac{x \text{ g}}{750 \text{ mL}}$$

NaCl:

0.45 g : 100 mL = x g : 750 mL

$$\frac{100x}{100} = \frac{337.5}{100}$$

$$x = 3.375 \text{ g NaCl}$$

*or*

$$\frac{0.45 \text{ g}}{100 \text{ mL}} = \frac{x \text{ g}}{750 \text{ mL}}$$

750 mL D$_5$ 1/2 NS contains 37.5 g dextrose and 3.375 g NaCl (saline).

# CHAPTER **21**
# Intravenous Calculations

## Objectives

*After reviewing this chapter, you should be able to:*

1. Calculate the intravenous (IV) flow rate by infusion pump in milliliters per hour (mL/hr)
2. Identify the two types of IV administration tubing used for infusion by gravity
3. Identify from IV tubing packages the drop factor in drops per milliliter (gtt/mL)
4. Calculate the IV flow rate for IV infusion by gravity in drops per minute (gtt/min) using a formula and shortcut method
5. Calculate the IV flow rate for medications administered IV piggyback (IVPB)
6. Calculate the infusion and completion times for an IV
7. Recalculate IV flow rates and determine the percentage (%) of increase or decrease
8. Calculate the rate for medications administered IV push

This chapter will present the calculations performed with intravenous therapy. As stated previously, nurses have the responsibility to make sure that clients are receiving the correct rate. Several methods to calculate IV rates are presented in the chapter: ratio and proportion, dimensional analysis, and the formula. Let's now begin our calculations with determining IV rates in milliliters per hour (mL/hr).

## IV Flow Rate Calculation

As previously discussed, the prescriber's order for an IV includes the following:

- The name of the IV solution
- The volume to infuse
- Medications to be added, if any
- Time for the IV to infuse

Continuous IV, which is often referred to as the primary IV, usually contains a large volume of fluid (500 mL or 1,000 mL). IV fluids are usually ordered to be administered at rates expressed in mL/hr. The time for the IV to infuse may be indicated as the total number of hours (i.e., $D_5W$ 3,000 mL in 24 hr), or mL/hr (i.e. $D_5$ ½ NS 1,000 mL at 125 mL/hr). Small volumes of fluid (usually 50 mL or 100 mL) are often used when the IV fluid contains medications such as antibiotics. Rates for IV fluids are usually expressed in drops per minute (gtt/min) when an infusion device is not used. When an infusion device such as a pump is used, the flow rate must be expressed in mL/hr.

### Calculating Flow Rates for Infusion Pumps in mL/hr

When a client is using an electronic infuser, such as a volumetric pump, the prescriber orders the volume and can include mL/hr or the total number of hours for the IV to infuse. If the order states the number of mL/hr for the infusion, such as previously stated $D_5$ ½ NS at 125 mL/hr, there is no calculation required by the nurse. The nurse programs the pump to deliver the ordered rate. However, if the order states the total number of hours for the IV to infuse ($D_5W$ 3,000 mL in 24 hr), the nurse will need to calculate the mL/hr to program the pump.

For most electronic devices that regulate the flow of IV solutions, the rate is expressed in milliliters per hour (mL/hr). For the purpose of this text, the equipment being used is programmable in whole mL/hr; therefore mL/hr should be rounded to a whole number unless indicated that the infusion pump has decimal capability. To determine mL/hr the following information is needed:

- The volume (amount) of solution in milliliters
- The time for the IV to infuse in hours

The simplest way to determine the mL/hr is by using the formula, although ratio-and-proportion and dimensional analysis can be used:

---

### Formula to Determine mL/hr

$$x \text{ mL/hr} = \frac{\text{Volume (amount) of solution (mL)}}{\text{Time in hours}}$$

Round mL/hr to the nearest **whole number.** If the answer does not result in a whole number, carry division to tenths place and round to the nearest whole number. If pump has decimal capability, round answer to the **nearest tenth.**

---

### ! SAFETY ALERT!

There are some IV pumps in use that are capable of delivering IV fluids in tenths of a milliliter. Always be familiar with the IV equipment being used at the institution before rounding milliliters per hour (mL/hr) to the nearest whole mL/hr.

---

Let's begin with the calculation of IV flow rates in mL/hr.

**Example 1:** Client with an infusion pump has an order for 3,000 mL $D_5W$ over 24 hours.

### Solution:

1. Think: Pump is regulated in mL/hr.
2. No conversion required; the volume is in milliliters, and the time is in hours.
3. To use the formula method to determine mL/hr: $x$ mL/hr = volume in mL.

$$x \text{ mL/hr} = \frac{\text{volume in mL}}{\text{time (hr)}}$$

4. To determine mL/hr using ratio and proportion, the volume ordered and hours to infuse is the known ratio; 3,000 mL : 24 hr (stated first), and the unknown is $x$ mL : 1 hr. (stated as the second ratio) or:

$$\frac{3,000 \text{ mL}}{24 \text{ hr}} = \frac{x \text{ mL}}{1 \text{ hr}}$$

5. To determine mL/hr using dimensional analysis, identify what you are looking for, and write it to the left of the equation in a fraction format. Label factor:

$$\frac{x \text{ mL}}{\text{hr}}$$

Place problem as starting fraction (if no conversion required). If conversion is required, the starting fraction is the conversion factor, and the problem is inserted as the second fraction in the equation. Refer to the setups of Example 1 using the various methods.

---

### Formula Method

$$x \text{ mL/hr} = \frac{3,000 \text{ mL}}{24 \text{ hr}}$$

$$x = \frac{3,000}{24}$$

$$x = 125 \text{ mL/hr}$$

**Ratio and Proportion (Linear Format)**

$$3{,}000 \text{ mL} : 24 \text{ hr} = x \text{ mL} : 1 \text{ hr}$$

$$\frac{24\,x}{24} = \frac{3{,}000}{24}$$

$$x = \frac{3{,}000}{24}$$

$$x = 125 \text{ mL/hr}$$

**Ratio and Proportion (Fraction Format)**

$$\frac{3{,}000 \text{ mL}}{24 \text{ hr}} = \frac{x \text{ mL}}{1 \text{ hr}}$$

$$\frac{24\,x}{24} = \frac{3{,}000}{24}$$

$$x = \frac{3{,}000}{24}$$

$$x = 125 \text{ mL/hr}$$

**Dimensional Analysis**

$$\frac{x \text{ mL}}{\text{hr}} = \frac{3{,}000 \text{ mL}}{24 \text{ hr}}$$

$$x = \frac{3{,}000}{24}$$

$$x = 125 \text{ mL/hr}$$

In this problem no conversion was required, the ordered amount is in mL/hr, which is the same as the desired; therefore the problem is solved by division, and no cancellation of units is required.

To infuse 3,000 mL of $D_5W$ in 24 hr, the pump would be set to deliver 125 mL/hr. Sometimes a conversion may be necessary before calculating mL/hr. Let's look at a problem showing the calculation of mL/hr when a conversion is required.

**Example 2:** Client with an infusion pump is to receive 0.5 L 0.9% NS over 8 hours.

**Solution:**

1. Convert 0.5 L to 500 mL using any of the methods presented in earlier chapters.
   Use the conversion factor 1 L = 1,000 mL. Convert 0.5 L to mL by moving the decimal three places to the right (metric to metric). Decimal movement can be used. Review methods of converting if necessary.
2. Set up the problem and solve using one of the calculation methods.

**Formula Method**

$$x \text{ mL/hr} = \frac{500 \text{ mL}}{8 \text{ hr}}$$

$$x = \frac{500}{8} = 62.5$$

$$x = 63 \text{ mL/hr}$$

mL/hr is rounded to the nearest whole number of mL.

**Ratio and Proportion (Linear Format)**

$$500 \text{ mL} : 8 \text{ hr} = x \text{ mL} : 1 \text{ hr}$$

$$\frac{8x}{8} = \frac{500}{8}$$

$$x = \frac{500}{8} = 62.5$$

$$x = 63 \text{ mL/hr}$$

mL/hr is rounded to the nearest whole number of mL.

**Ratio and Proportion (Fraction Format)**

$$\frac{500 \text{ mL}}{8 \text{ hr}} = \frac{x \text{ mL}}{1 \text{ hr}}$$

$$\frac{8x}{8} = \frac{500}{8}$$

$$x = \frac{500}{8} = 62.5$$

$$x = 63 \text{ mL/hr}$$

mL/hr is rounded to the nearest whole number of mL.

**Dimensional Analysis**

$$x \text{ mL/hr} = \frac{1,000 \text{ mL}}{1 \cancel{L}} \times \frac{0.5 \cancel{L}}{8 \text{ hr}}$$

$$x = \frac{1000 \times 0.5}{8}$$

$$x = \frac{500}{8} = 62.5$$

$$x = 63 \text{ mL/hr}$$

mL/hr is rounded to the nearest whole number. Notice the conversion factor is written $\frac{1,000 \text{ mL}}{1L}$ to cancel L, leaving mL/hr.

To infuse 500 mL of 0.9% NS, the pump would be set to deliver 63 mL/hr. As previously stated, pumps deliver in whole mL unless indicated the pump has decimal capability.

### Determining mL/hr When the Time Period Is Less Than 1 Hour

Often when medications are administered IV, such as IVPB (e.g., for antibiotics), the time period for the IV to infuse is less than 1 hour. When the period is less than 1 hour and an electronic infusion device is used, the IV rate must still be determined in mL/hr. **Remember that there are 60 minutes in 1 hour.** The rate can be determined using ratio and proportion. (The known ratio is the ordered rate, mL/min, and the second is the unknown ratio, x mL/60 min). Dimensional analysis can also be used to determine the rate in mL/hr. (The first factor in the equation is the ordered mL/min, and the second factor is 60 min/1 hr). The rate can also be determined using the formula:

$$x \text{ mL/hr} = \frac{\text{Total mL to infuse}}{\text{Number of min to infuse}} \times 60 \text{ min/hr}$$

Let's look at an example. The various methods for calculating the infusion rate will be shown.

**Example 3:** A client is to receive an antibiotic in 100 mL of 0.9% NS over 45 min by infusion pump. Determine the IV flow rate.

### Solution:
1. Think: The infusion pump infuses in mL/hr. Use a ratio and proportion, the formula method, or dimensional analysis to determine mL/hr.
2. Remember: 1 hr = 60 min.

**Ratio and Proportion (Linear Format)**

$$100 \text{ mL} : 45 \text{ min} = x \text{ mL} : 60 \text{ min}$$

$$45x = 100 \times 60$$

$$\frac{45x}{45} = \frac{6,000}{45} = 133.3$$

$$x = 133 \text{ mL/hr}$$

### Ratio and Proportion (Fraction Format)

$$\frac{100 \text{ mL}}{45 \text{ min}} = \frac{x \text{ mL}}{60 \text{ min}}$$

$$45x = 100 \times 60$$

$$\frac{45x}{45} = \frac{6{,}000}{45} = 133.3$$

$$x = 133 \text{ mL/hr}$$

### Formula Method

$$x \text{ mL/hr} = \frac{100 \text{ mL}}{\underset{3}{\cancel{45} \text{ min}}} \times \frac{\overset{4}{\cancel{60} \text{ min/hr}}}{1}$$

$$x = \frac{100 \times 4}{3} = \frac{400}{3} = 133.3$$

$$x = 133 \text{ mL/hr}$$

*Note:* min is cancelled, leaving mL/hr.

### Dimensional Analysis

$$\frac{x \text{ mL}}{hr} = \frac{100 \text{ mL}}{\underset{3}{\cancel{45} \text{ min}}} \times \frac{\cancel{60} \text{ min}}{1 \text{ hr}}$$

$$x = \frac{100 \times 4}{3} = \frac{400}{3} = 133.3$$

$$x = 133 \text{ mL/hr}$$

*Note:* min is cancelled, leaving mL/hr.

The infusion pump would be set at 133 mL/hr to infuse 100 mL in 45 minutes. The volume of 100 mL will be infused.

> **SAFETY ALERT!**
> The usual rate in mL/hr ranges from 50 to 200 mL/hr. If the rate exceeds this amount, double-check the order and your calculation before programming the rate into an infusion pump.

> **POINTS TO REMEMBER**
> - IV infusion pumps deliver IV flow rates in mL/hr.
> - IV orders indicate: the name of the IV solution, the volume to infuse, medications to be added, if any, and the time for the IV to infuse. The prescriber may indicate the time for an IV to infuse in mL/hr, or the total number of hours for the IV to infuse.
> - To determine flow rates for an electronic infusion device such as the infusion pump, determine mL/hr using the formula:
>
> $$x \text{ mL/hr} = \frac{\text{Total volume to infuse (mL)}}{\text{Time (hours)}}$$
>
> - If the time for the IV to infuse is less than 1 hour and the infusion pump is used, the infusion rate still must be determined in mL/hr. Ratio and proportion, the formula method, or dimensional analysis can be used to determine the infusion rate. Remember that 60 min = 1 hr.
> - Milliliters per hour (mL/hr) are rounded to the nearest whole number. If math does not result in a whole number, carry math to the tenths place and round to the nearest whole number.
> - Some infusion pumps have decimal capability and can deliver IV rates in tenths of a mL. If the answer obtained is not in the tenths place, carry math to the hundredths place and round to the tenths.
> - Always be familiar with the infusion device being used by an institution before rounding mL/hr to a whole number.

## PRACTICE **PROBLEMS**

Calculate the flow rate in mL/hr. (Equipment used is programmable in whole mL/hr.)

1. 1,800 mL of $D_5W$ in 24 hr by infusion pump _____

2. 2,000 mL $D_5W$ in 24 hr by infusion pump _____

3. 500 mL RL in 12 hr by infusion pump _____

4. 1,500 mL $D_5RL$ in 24 hr by infusion pump _____

5. 750 mL $D_5W$ in 16 hr by infusion pump _____

**Answers on p. 538**

## Manually Regulated IVs

When an electronic infusion device is not used, the nurse uses a gravity-flow system and must manually regulate the infusion rate. To do this, the nurse must calculate the ordered IV flow rate in drops per minute (gtt/min). IV flow rates in gtt/min are based on the IV tubing calibration, referred to as the *drop factor*. The **drop factor** is the number of drops per milliliter (gtt/mL) that a particular IV tubing delivers and therefore will vary depending on the type of IV tubing.

The drop size is determined by the size of the tubing or the small needle inside the drop chamber releasing the drops. See Figure 21.1. Note the large opening for drops in Figure 21.1A, the drops are large (**macrodrops**). The drops delivered through the small needle in Figure 21.1B are very small drops (**microdrops**). The drop factor of the IV tubing is stated in large numbers on the IV tubing package (Figure 21.2). The drop factor of the IV tubing is needed to calculate gtt/min.

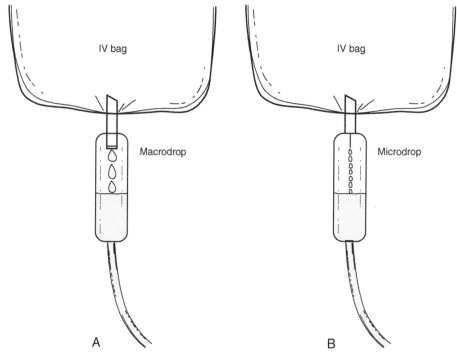

**Figure 21.1** Comparison of (A) macrodrops and (B) microdrops.

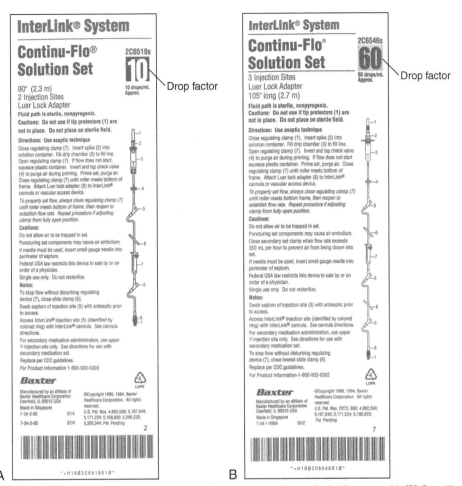

**Figure 21.2** IV administration sets (package). **(A)** Set with drop factor of 10 (10 gtt =1 mL). **(B)** Set with drop factor of 60 (60 gtt = 1 mL).

As stated previously, at the top of the IV tubing is a drip chamber (also referred to as a drop chamber), where the nurse observes and counts the number of drops falling into the drip chamber per minute or fraction of a minute placing a watch at the level of the drip chamber. The flow rate is regulated by a hand-operated slide clamp or a roller clamp, which is opened or closed so the drops fall at the desired rate.

> ⚠ **SAFETY ALERT!**
>
> IV infusions that are manually regulated must be monitored regularly. The flow rate of a manually regulated IV can be affected by the height of the IV infusion, the location of the site, and changes in the client position, which can result in impediment of the IV flow rate or excessive amounts of fluid being delivered to the client.

### IV Tubing

The two common types of tubing used to administer IV fluids (regulated manually) are:
- Macodrop tubing
- Microdrop tubing

### Macrodrop Tubing

Macrodrop is the standard tubing used for general IV administration. With macrodrop tubing the size of the drop and the number of gtt/mL varies according to the manufacturer. Macrodrops are large drops, and there are fewer drops in 1 mL (see Figure 21.1A). Macrodrop tubing have the following drop factors:

- 10 gtt/mL
- 15 gtt/mL
- 20 gtt/mL

Since the drop factor for macrodrop tubing differs according to the manufacturer, always read the IV tubing package and identify the drop factor of the tubing. Never assume to know the drop factor, because not all macrodrop tubing has the same factor.

> **! SAFETY ALERT!**
>
> To accurately administer IV fluids at the correct rate to a client, the nurse **must** know the drop factor of the IV tubing. Knowing the drop factor of the IV tubing used can prevent an error in IV rate determination and the client receiving IV fluid at the incorrect rate. **Never** assume the drop factor for macrodrop tubing.

### Microdrop Tubing

Microdrop tubing delivers tiny drops through a small needle in the drip chamber and therefore has more drops in 1 mL (see Figure 21.1B). It is used to administer either small or precise amounts of fluid. For example, it is used in critical care, for the elderly, and for pediatric infusions. Microdrop tubing, because of the size of the drops (very small/ tiny) is sometimes referred to as pedidrip tubing. Microdrop tubing, regardless of the manufacturer, is only available in one drop factor (60 gtt/mL). With microdrop tubing the number of mL/hr is the same as gtt/min (i.e., if the infusion rate is 100 mL/hr, the IV rate is 100 gtt/min).

> • 60 gtt/mL

> **⚙ POINTS TO REMEMBER**
>
> • Drop factor = gtt/mL of the IV tubing. This information is written on the package of the IV tubing.
> • Knowing the drop factor of the IV tubing is the **FIRST** step in accurate administration of IV fluids in gtt/min. IVs that infuse by gravity are manually regulated, and the IV flow rate is determined in gtt/min.
> • Macrodrops are large and have drop factors of 10, 15, and 20 gtt/mL.
> • Microdrops are tiny and have only one drop factor, 60 gtt/mL.

---

##  PRACTICE **PROBLEMS**

Refer to the drop factor provided and identify the type of tubing.

6. 15 gtt/ mL _____

7. 60 gtt/mL _____

8. 10 gtt/mL _____

**Answers on p. 538**

### Calculating Flow Rates in Drops Per Minute Using a Formula and Dimensional Analysis

To calculate the IV flow rate in gtt/min for an IV infusing by gravity, a formula method can be used or dimensional analysis. To calculate the flow rate in gtt/min for the IV infusion regardless of the method used (formula method or dimensional analysis), the nurse needs to know the following:

• Drop factor of the IV tubing
• Volume (number of mL) to infuse
• Time the IV is to infuse (minutes or hours)

The formula for calculating the IV flow rate is:

$$x \text{ gtt/min} = \frac{\text{volume of solution (mL)} \times \text{drop factor}}{\text{time (min)}}$$

Before beginning to calculate gtt/min, let's review some basic guidelines:

### Guidelines for Calculating gtt/min

- Drops per minute are **always** expressed in whole numbers. Think: You cannot regulate an IV to half a drop or count half a drop; therefore **you can only count whole drops.**
- Principles of rounding are applied if the calculation for gtt/min does not result in a whole number. Carry calculation to the tenths place, and round answer to the nearest whole number (i.e., 19.6 is rounded to 20 gtt/min).
- Answers must be labeled. The label is usually drops per minute unless otherwise specified. Example: 17 gtt/min. To reinforce the differences in drop factor, the type of tubing is sometimes included as part of the label. Examples: 17 macrogtt/min, 100 microgtt/min.
- Common conversion factors used include 1 L = 1,000 mL, and 1 hr = 60 min.

First let's look at some sample problems using the formula method and dimensional analysis.

**Example 1:** Order: $D_5W$ 1,000 mL to infuse at 100 mL/hr. Drop factor: 10 gtt/mL. At what rate in gtt/min should the IV infuse?

- Notice the numbers in the problem are placed in the formula.
- Remember the formula solves for gtt/min and the time is indicated in minutes. 60 min = 1 hr; therefore 1 hr is changed to 60 min in the formula (100 mL/60 min).
- When mL is cancelled out, the flow rate is determined in gtt/min.
- Reduction is done where possible.
- The answer is labeled.
- *Note:* The volume of 1,000 mL was not used in the calculation; the mL/hr was stated in the order.

### Setup Using Formula Method

$$x \text{ gtt/min} = \frac{100 \text{ mL} \times 10 \text{ gtt/mL}}{60 \text{ min}}$$

$$x = \frac{100 \times \overset{1}{\cancel{10}}}{\underset{6}{\cancel{60}}}$$

$$x = \frac{100 \times 1}{6}$$

$$x = \frac{100}{6} = 16.6 = 17$$

$$x = 17 \text{ gtt/min; } 17 \text{ macrogtt/min}$$

To deliver 100 mL/hr, the IV rate would be regulated at 17 gtt/min; 17 macrogtt/min.

### Dimensional Analysis

Let's look at the previous example using dimensional analysis.

**Example 1:** Order: $D_5W$ 1,000 mL to infuse at 100 mL/hr. Drop factor: 10 gtt/mL. At what rate in gtt/min should the IV infuse?

- Notice $x$ gtt is written to the left of the equation, followed by the equal sign (=) (labeled $x$ gtt/min because that is what you're looking for).
- The **first** factor starts with gtt and is the drop factor, which is written, placing gtt in the numerator. 10 gtt/1 mL.
- The next fraction is written so that the denominator matches the previous fraction (what you are looking for). The order is to infuse 100 mL in 1 hr. The 1 hr is entered as 60 min in the denominator because you are calculating gtt/min (100 mL/60 min).

- Cancel the units and you are left with the desired gtt/min.
- Reduction is done if possible.
- Label the answer.

### Dimensional Analysis

$$\frac{x \text{ gtt}}{\text{min}} = \frac{10 \text{ gtt}}{1 \text{ mL}} \times \frac{100 \text{ mL}}{60 \text{ min}}$$

$$x = \frac{100 \times \overset{1}{\cancel{10}}}{\underset{6}{\cancel{60}}}$$

$$x = \frac{100 \times 1}{6}$$

$$x = \frac{100}{6} = 16.6 = 17$$

$$x = 17 \text{ gtt/min; } 17 \text{ macrogtt/min}$$

**Note:** An alternate way of setting up the problem, without changing the hourly rate to 60 min, would be to add 1 hr = 60 min conversion factor to the equation: $\dfrac{1 \text{ hr}}{60 \text{ min}}$

### Alternate Setup Using Dimensional Analysis

$$\frac{x \text{ gtt}}{\text{min}} = \frac{10 \text{ gtt}}{1 \text{ mL}} \times \frac{100 \text{ mL}}{1 \text{ hr}} \times \frac{1 \text{ hr}}{60 \text{ min}}$$

Notice the hourly rate is entered in mL/hr in the equation; the fraction 1 hr/60 min is inserted into the equation. The units are cancelled, leaving gtt/min. The calculation would be the same as the previous setup.

**Example 2:**  Order: 1.5 L 0.9% NaCl to infuse in 10 hr. Drop factor: 15 gtt/mL. At what rate in gtt/min should the IV infuse at?

- Notice this problem contains a large volume of fluid, and the order contains the total number of hours to infuse as opposed to mL/hr as shown in Example 1.
- A conversion is also required before the problem can be solved. L must be converted to mL. Use the conversion factor 1 L = 1,000 mL; therefore 1.5 L = 1,500 mL.
- When using the **formula method**, the IV rate can be determined in two ways:
  a. First convert the flow rate to mL/hr, and then calculate the gtt/min using the formula.

  *or*

  b. Convert the number of hours to minutes using the conversion factor 60 min = 1 hr. Multiply the number of hours by 60 min/hr and then place the calculated minutes into the formula. In this problem, 10 hr is multiplied by 60 min/hr to obtain the 600 minutes used in the formula: 10 hr × 60 min/hr.
- For **dimensional analysis,** if the mL/hr is not expressed as mL/min, insert the conversion factor 1 hr/60 min.

Let's look at the above problem using the formula method and dimensional analysis.

### Formula Method Using Two Steps

**Step 1:** Calculate the mL/hr:

$$x \, \text{mL/hr} = \frac{1{,}500 \, \text{mL}}{10 \, \text{hr}}$$

$$x = 150 \, \text{mL/hr}$$

Convert mL/hr to mL/min. 1 hr = 60 min (150 mL/hr = 150 mL/60 min)

**Step 2:** Place into formula:

$$x \, \text{gtt/min} = \frac{150 \, \cancel{\text{mL}} \times 15 \, \text{gtt/}\cancel{\text{mL}}}{60 \, \text{min}}$$

$$x = \frac{150 \times \overset{1}{\cancel{15}}}{\underset{4}{\cancel{60}}}$$

$$x = \frac{150 \times 1}{4}$$

$$x = \frac{150}{4} = 37.5 = 38$$

$$x = 38 \, \text{gtt/min}; \, 38 \, \text{macrogtt/min}$$

### Formula Method Using hr Converted to min

$$x \, \text{gtt/min} = \frac{1{,}500 \, \cancel{\text{mL}} \times 15 \, \text{gtt/}\cancel{\text{mL}}}{600 \, \text{min}}$$

$$x = \frac{1{,}500 \times \overset{1}{\cancel{15}}}{\underset{40}{\cancel{600}}}$$

$$x = \frac{1{,}500 \times 1}{40}$$

$$x = \frac{1{,}500}{40} = 37.5 = 38$$

$$x = 38 \, \text{gtt/min}; \, 38 \, \text{macrogtt/min}$$

To infuse 1,500 mL in 10 hr, the IV rate would be regulated at 38 gtt/min; 38 macrogtt/min.

### Dimensional Analysis Using mL/min

Calculate mL/hr: 1,500 mL ÷ 10 hr = 150 mL/hr.
Convert mL/hr to mL/min (150 mL/hr = 150 mL/60 min).
Proceed using the steps shown in Example 1.

$$\frac{x \, \text{gtt}}{\text{min}} = \frac{15 \, \text{gtt}}{1 \, \text{mL}} \times \frac{150 \, \text{mL}}{60 \, \text{min}}$$

$$\frac{x \, \text{gtt}}{\text{min}} = \frac{\overset{1}{\cancel{15}} \, \text{gtt}}{1 \, \cancel{\text{mL}}} \times \frac{150 \, \cancel{\text{mL}}}{\underset{4}{\cancel{60}} \, \text{min}}$$

$$x = \frac{150 \times 1}{4}$$

$$x = \frac{150}{4} = 37.5 = 38$$

$$x = 38 \, \text{gtt/min}; \, 38 \, \text{macrogtt/min}$$

**Dimensional Analysis Using mL/hr**

$$\frac{x\,gtt}{min} = \frac{15\,gtt}{1\,mL} \times \frac{150\,mL}{1\,hr} \times \frac{1\,hr}{60\,min}$$

$$\frac{x\,gtt}{min} = \frac{15\,gtt}{1\,\cancel{mL}} \times \frac{150\,\cancel{mL}}{1\,\cancel{hr}} \times \frac{1\,\cancel{hr}}{60\,min}$$

$$x = \frac{\overset{1}{\cancel{15}} \times 150 \times 1}{\underset{4}{\cancel{60}}}$$

$$x = \frac{150 \times 1}{4}$$

$$x = \frac{150}{4} = 37.5 = 38$$

$$x = 38\,gtt/min;\ 38\,macrogtt/min$$

**Dimensional Analysis Using the Total Volume and Total Number of hr**

$$\frac{x\,gtt}{min} = \frac{15\,gtt}{1\,mL} \times \frac{1,500\,mL}{10\,hr} \times \frac{1\,hr}{60\,min}$$

$$\frac{x\,gtt}{min} = \frac{15\,gtt}{1\,\cancel{mL}} \times \frac{1,500\,\cancel{mL}}{10\,\cancel{hr}} \times \frac{1\,\cancel{hr}}{60\,min}$$

Proceed with calculation as shown in previous examples.

## Example 3:

Order: The following IVs for 24 hours. Drop factor: 15 gtt/mL
- 1,000 mL D$_5$W c̄ 10 mEq potassium chloride (KCl)
- 500 mL D$_5$NS c̄ 1 ampule of multivitamin (MVI)
- 500 mL D$_5$W

What rate will you regulate the IV to deliver the ordered IV fluid?

In this problem, the order is written for different amounts and types of fluid to be given in a certain time period. Notice that medications are also ordered to be added to the solutions: potassium chloride and multivitamin. When medications such as potassium chloride and vitamins are added to the IV solutions, they are generally not considered in the total volume. (Some institutions consider the medication in the volume if it is 10 mL or more. Always check the policy of the institution.)

To calculate the IV rate, add up the IV fluid to obtain the total volume (2,000 mL). The total number of hours for the IV infusion is given (24 hours). To convert 24 hr to min, multiply: 24 h̶r̶ × 60 min/h̶r̶ = 1,440 min.

## Formula Method Using Two Steps

**Step 1:** Calculate the mL/hr:

$$x \text{ mL/hr} = \frac{2,000 \text{ mL}}{24 \text{ hr}} = 83.3$$

$$x = 83 \text{ mL/hr}$$

Convert mL/hr to mL/min. 60 min = 1 hr (83 mL/hr = 83 mL/60 min).

**Step 2:** Place into formula

$$x \text{ gtt/min} = \frac{83 \text{ mL} \times 15 \text{ gtt/mL}}{60 \text{ min}}$$

$$x = \frac{83 \times \overset{1}{\cancel{15}}}{\underset{4}{\cancel{60}}}$$

$$x = \frac{83 \times 1}{4}$$

$$x = \frac{83}{4} = 20.7 = 21$$

$$x = 21 \text{ gtt/min; 21 macrogtt/min}$$

## Formula Method Using hr Converted to min

$$x \text{ gtt/min} = \frac{2,000 \text{ mL} \times 15 \text{ gtt/mL}}{1,440 \text{ min}}$$

$$x = \frac{2,000 \times \overset{1}{\cancel{15}}}{\underset{96}{\cancel{1,440}}}$$

$$x = \frac{2,000 \times 1}{96}$$

$$x = \frac{2,000}{96} = 20.8 = 21$$

$$x = 21 \text{ gtt/min; 21 macrogtt/min}$$

To infuse 2,000 mL in 24 hours, the IV would be regulated at 21 gtt/min; 21 macrogtt/min.

## Dimensional Analysis Using mL/min

$$\frac{x \text{ gtt}}{\text{min}} = \frac{15 \text{ gtt}}{1 \text{ mL}} \times \frac{83 \text{ mL}}{60 \text{ min}}$$

$$\frac{x \text{ gtt}}{\text{min}} = \frac{\overset{1}{\cancel{15}} \text{ gtt}}{1 \text{ mL}} \times \frac{83 \text{ mL}}{\underset{4}{\cancel{60}} \text{ min}}$$

$$x = \frac{83 \times 1}{4}$$

$$x = \frac{83}{4} = 20.7 = 21$$

$$x = 21 \text{ gtt/min; 21 macrogtt/min}$$

**Dimensional Analysis Using mL/hr**

$$\frac{x \text{ gtt}}{\text{min}} = \frac{15 \text{ gtt}}{1 \text{ mL}} \times \frac{83 \text{ mL}}{1 \text{ hr}} \times \frac{1 \text{ hr}}{60 \text{ min}}$$

$$\frac{x \text{ gtt}}{\text{min}} = \frac{\overset{1}{\cancel{15}} \text{ gtt}}{1 \text{ mL}} \times \frac{83 \cancel{\text{ mL}}}{1 \cancel{\text{ hr}}} \times \frac{1 \cancel{\text{ hr}}}{\underset{4}{\cancel{60}} \text{ min}}$$

$$x = \frac{83 \times 1}{4}$$

$$x = \frac{83}{4} = 20.7 = 21$$

$$x = 21 \text{ gtt/min; } 21 \text{ macrogtt/min}$$

**Dimensional Analysis Using the Total Volume and Total Number of hr**

$$\frac{x \text{ gtt}}{\text{min}} = \frac{15 \text{ gtt}}{1 \text{ mL}} \times \frac{2,000 \text{ mL}}{24 \text{ hr}} \times \frac{1 \text{ hr}}{60 \text{ min}}$$

$$\frac{x \text{ gtt}}{\text{min}} = \frac{15 \text{ gtt}}{1 \cancel{\text{ mL}}} \times \frac{2,000 \cancel{\text{ mL}}}{24 \cancel{\text{ hr}}} \times \frac{1 \cancel{\text{ hr}}}{60 \text{ min}}$$

Proceed with calculation as shown in previous examples.

## Example 4:

Order: 50 mL NS to infuse over 20 minutes.
Drop factor: 20 gtt/mL. What rate will you regulate the IV to infuse?

Notice, in this example, you have a small volume of fluid, and the time for the IV to infuse is in minutes. This problem can be solved using the same methods (formula method and dimensional analysis) shown in the previous examples.

**Formula Method**

$$x \text{ gtt/min} = \frac{50 \cancel{\text{ mL}} \times 20 \text{ gtt/}\cancel{\text{mL}}}{20 \text{ min}}$$

$$x = \frac{50 \times \overset{1}{\cancel{20}}}{\underset{1}{\cancel{20}}}$$

$$x = \frac{50 \times 1}{1}$$

$$x = \frac{50}{1} = 50$$

$$x = 50 \text{ gtt/min; } 50 \text{ macrogtt/min}$$

**Dimensional Analysis**

$$\frac{x \text{ gtt}}{\text{min}} = \frac{20 \text{ gtt}}{1 \text{ mL}} \times \frac{50 \text{ mL}}{20 \text{ min}}$$

$$\frac{x \text{ gtt}}{\text{min}} = \frac{20 \text{ gtt}}{1 \cancel{\text{ mL}}} \times \frac{\overset{5}{\cancel{50 \text{ mL}}}}{\underset{2}{\cancel{20 \text{ min}}}}$$

$$x = \frac{20 \times 5}{2}$$

$$x = \frac{100}{2} = 50$$

$$x = 50 \text{ gtt/min; } 50 \text{ macrogtt/min}$$

To infuse 50 mL NS in 20 minutes, the IV would be regulated at 50 gtt/min; 50 macrogtt/min.

## ▣ PRACTICE PROBLEMS

Calculate the flow rate in gtt/min using the formula method or dimensional analysis.

9. $D_5RL$ at 75 mL/hr. The drop factor is 10 gtt/mL.

     _____

10. $D_5$ ½ NS at 30 mL/hr. The drop factor is a microdrop.

     _____

11. 1,000 mL $D_5$ 0.33% NS in 6 hr. The drop factor is 15 gtt/mL.

     _____

12. An IV medication in 60 mL of 0.9% NS is to be administered in 45 min. The drop factor is a microdrop.

     _____

13. 1,000 mL of Ringer's lactate solution (RL) is to infuse in 16 hr. The drop factor is 15 gtt/mL.

     _____

14. 3,000 mL $D_5$ and ½ NS in 24 hr. The drop factor is 10 gtt/mL.

     _____

15. Infuse 2,000 mL $D_5W$ in 12 hr. The drop factor is 15 gtt/mL.

     _____

**Answers on pp. 538-539**

## Calculation of IV Flow Rates Using a Shortcut Method

This shortcut method can be used where the IV sets all have the same drop factor. Example: an institution where all the macrodrop sets deliver 10 gtt/mL. This method can also be used with microdrop sets (60 gtt/mL). It is important to note that this method can be used only if the rate of the IV infusion is expressed in mL/hr (mL/60 min).

To use this method, you must know the drop factor constant for the administration set you are using. The drop factor constant is sometimes referred to as the *division factor*. To obtain the drop factor constant (division factor) for the IV administration set being used, divide 60 by the drop factor calibration from the IV infusion set. Box 21.1 shows the constant calculated based on the drop factor for the IV tubing.

| BOX 21.1 Drop Factor Constants | |
| --- | --- |
| **Drop Factor of Tubing** | **Drop Factor Constant** |
| 10 gtt/mL | $\frac{60}{10} = 6$ |
| 15 gtt/mL | $\frac{60}{15} = 4$ |
| 20 gtt/mL | $\frac{60}{20} = 3$ |
| 60 gtt/mL | $\frac{60}{60} = 1$ |

**RULE**

After the drop factor constant is determined, the gtt/min can be calculated in one step:

$$x \text{ gtt/min} = \frac{\text{mL/hr}}{\text{gtt factor constant}}$$

Let's look at examples of calculating the gtt/min using the stated rule:

### Example 1:
Order: Administer $D_5W$ at 125 mL/hr. Drop factor: 15 gtt/mL
The drop factor constant: 4.
In this example, the drop factor constant is 4. The set calibration is 15 gtt/mL (60 ÷ 15 = 4).

### Solution:

$$x \text{ gtt/min} = \frac{125 \text{ mL/hr}}{4} = 31.2 = 31$$

$$x = 31 \text{ gtt/min; } 31 \text{ macrogtt/min}$$

### Solution Using Dimensional Analysis:

$$\frac{x \text{ gtt}}{\text{min}} = \frac{\overset{1}{\cancel{15}} \text{ gtt}}{1 \cancel{\text{ mL}}} \times \frac{125 \cancel{\text{ mL}}}{\underset{4}{\cancel{60}} \text{ min}} = 31.2 = 31$$

*or*

$$125 \text{ mL} \div 4 = 31.2 = 31$$

$$x = 31 \text{ gtt/min; } 31 \text{ macrogtt/min}$$

Remember that the shortcut method discussed (using the drop factor constant) can be used to calculate the gtt/min for any volume of fluid that can be stated in mL/hr or mL/60 min.

**RULE**

The shortcut method can be used if the volume of fluid is large; however, an additional step of calculating mL/hr first must be done and then calculate the gtt/min using the shortcut method.

**Example 2:**  Order: RL 1,500 mL to infuse in 12 hr. Drop factor: 20 gtt/mL. Drop factor constant: 3.

In this example, the volume of fluid is 1,500 mL and the total hours to infuse is 10 hr. Before using the shortcut method, the mL/hr must be calculated. 1,500 mL ÷ 12 = 125 mL/hr. The set calibration is 20 gtt/mL. 60 ÷ 20 = 3.

### Solution:

$$x \text{ gtt/min} = \frac{125 \text{ mL/hr}}{3} = 41.6 = 42$$

$$x = 42 \text{ gtt/min; } 42 \text{ macrogtt/min}$$

### Solution Using Dimensional Analysis:

Determine mL/hr expressed as mL/60 min.

$$\frac{x \text{ gtt}}{\text{min}} = \frac{\overset{1}{\cancel{20}} \text{ gtt}}{1 \cancel{\text{ mL}}} \times \frac{125 \cancel{\text{ mL}}}{\underset{3}{\cancel{60}} \text{ min}} = \frac{125}{3} = 31.2 = 31 \text{ gtt/min}$$

$$x = 31 \text{ gtt/min; } 31 \text{ macrogtt/min}$$

The shortcut method can also be used for small volumes of fluid and when the time period is less than 1 hour. If the volume of fluid to infuse is small and the time period is less than 1 hour (60 minutes), the volume and time must each be multiplied to get mL/hr.

**Example 3:** Order: 20 mL $D_5W$ in 30 minutes. Drop factor 60 gtt/mL. Drop factor constant: 1.

In this example the volume of fluid is small, and the time period is less than 60 min. The set calibration is 60 gtt/mL. $60 \div 60 = 1$.

**Solution:** To express 20 mL in 30 minutes in mL/hr, you multiply the volume and the time by 2.

$$20 \text{ mL}/30 \text{ min} = (20 \times 2) / (2 \times 30) = 40 \text{ mL/hr (60 min)}$$

$$x \text{ gtt/min} = \frac{40 \text{ mL/hr}}{1} = 40$$

$$x = 40 \text{ gtt/min; 40 microgtt/min}$$

**Step 1:** Change 20 mL/30 min to 40 mL/hr as shown above.

**Step 2:** Express 40 mL/hr as 40 mL/60 min.

$$\frac{x \text{ gtt}}{\text{min}} = \frac{\overset{1}{\cancel{60} \text{ gtt}}}{1 \cancel{\text{ mL}}} \times \frac{40 \cancel{\text{ mL}}}{\cancel{60} \text{ min}} = \frac{40}{1} = 40$$

$$x = 40 \text{ gtt/min; 40 microgtt/min}$$

***Note:*** In the above problem to administer 40 mL/hr, the IV would be set at 40 gtt/min. When the drop factor of the infusion set used is 60 gtt/mL, the number of gtt/min is equal (=) to the mL/hr.

---

## 🖩 PRACTICE **PROBLEMS**

Calculate the rate in gtt/min using the shortcut method.

16. Order: $D_5W$ 200 mL/hr.
    Drop factor: 10 gtt/mL        _____

17. Order: 0.9% NS 140 mL/hr.
    Drop factor: 20 gtt/mL        _____

18. Order: 1,000 mL $D_5W$ in 10 hr.
    Drop factor: 10 gtt/mL        _____

19. Order: 40 mL $D_5W$ in 20 min.
    Drop factor: 10 gtt/mL        _____

Calculate the flow rate in gtt/min.

20. Order: To infuse in 16 hr. Drop factor: 10 gtt/mL

    • $D_5W$ 500 mL c̄ 10 potassium chloride (KCl)

    • $D_5W$ 1,000 mL

    • $D_5W$ 1,000 mL c̄ 1 ampule of multivitamin (MVI)  _____

21. Order: 1,000 mL $D_5$ 0.9% NS for 3 L at
    100 mL/hr. Drop factor: microdrop        _____

**Answers on p. 539**

**POINTS TO REMEMBER**

- To calculate the IV flow rate in gtt/min, the nurse must know the drop factor of the IV tubing, the volume to infuse, and the time for the IV to infuse.
- Drop factor is expressed as gtt/mL and indicated on the package of the IV tubing.
- Calculation of gtt/min can be done using the formula method or dimensional analysis.
- Formula for calculating gtt/min is as follows:

$$x\ gtt/min = \frac{\text{volume of solution (mL)} \times \text{drop factor}}{\text{time in minutes}}$$

- With the formula method, determine the IV rate by converting the flow rate to mL/hr (60 min), and then calculate gtt/min using the formula. **OR** Convert the number of hours to minutes using the conversion factor 60 min = 1 hr, and then place the calculated minutes into the formula.
- For dimensional analysis, if the mL/hr is not expressed as mL/min, insert the conversion factor 1 hr/60 min into the equation.
- Drops per minute are always expressed as whole numbers.
- A shortcut method can be used to calculate flow rates infusing in mL/hr or mL/60 min using the drop constant.
- To determine the drop constant factor, divide 60 by the calibration of the IV set.
- To use the shortcut method for small volumes and time periods less than 1 hr, the volume and the time must each be multiplied to get mL/hr.

## Calculating IV Flow Rates Using a Dial-Flow Controller

Dial-flow controllers are also known as IV manual flow regulators or just IV flow regulators, as well as just flow controllers. There are a wide variety of dial-flow controllers available for use and are either part of the IV tubing or added on (Figure 21.3). These devices are regulated manually and are not infusion pumps. Use of the device is based on several factors, which include severity of illness, type of therapy, and the setting. Dial-flow devices are designed to regulate the flow of IV fluid instead of using the roller clamp. The flow rate can be adjusted from 5 to 250 mL/hr. To use the device, you set or dial the desired flow rate in mL/hr, which is an estimate, and then the rate must be verified by counting drops per minute. Drops per minute would be calculated using one of the methods presented in the chapter.

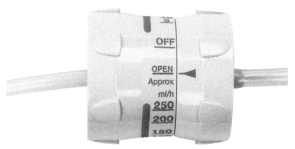

**Figure 21.3** Flow controller. (Courtesy and © Becton, Dickinson and Company, Franklin Lakes, NJ.)

If used, it is important to remember that use of the device does not relinquish the nurse from his or her responsibility, which is to monitor the IV to ensure there is accurate delivery of the ordered infusion rate.

Let's look at an example using this device.

**Example:** Order: D₅W 1,000 mL to infuse at 100 mL/hr. Drop factor: 15 gtt/mL.
1. Turn the dial of the controller to 100 mL/hr.
2. Use the formula or dimensional analysis to determine gtt/min.

3. Verify accuracy of controller by counting the drops either for a minute or a fraction, such as 20 seconds. Divide the number of drops per minute by 3 (25 gtt ÷ 3 = 8.3 = 8 gtt). You find the number of drops is 8; the controller is delivering the correct rate for 20 seconds. If the rate is not correct for 20 seconds, the controller dial can be adjusted. The rate will have to be monitored periodically during the infusion.

---
**Formula Method**
---

$$x\text{ gtt/min} = \frac{100 \text{ mL} \times 15 \text{ gtt/mL}}{60 \text{ min}}$$

$$x = \frac{100 \times \overset{1}{\cancel{15}}}{\underset{4}{\cancel{60}}}$$

$$x = \frac{100 \times 1}{4}$$

$$x = \frac{100}{4} = 25$$

$$x = 25 \text{ gtt/min; 25 macrogtt/min}$$

---
**Dimensional Analysis**
---

$$\frac{x\text{ gtt}}{\text{min}} = \frac{15 \text{ gtt}}{1 \text{ mL}} \times \frac{100 \text{ mL}}{60 \text{ min}}$$

*or*

$$\frac{x\text{ gtt}}{\text{min}} = \frac{15 \text{ gtt}}{1 \text{ mL}} \times \frac{100 \text{ mL}}{1 \text{ hr}} \times \frac{1 \text{ hr}}{60 \text{ min}}$$

Refer to examples for steps in solving.

To infuse 100 mL/hr, the IV flow rate would be set at 25 gtt/min; 25 macrogtt/min.

> **!  SAFETY ALERT!**
> The flow rate on the controller is in **mL/hr, not gtt/min**. Failure to verify the drop rate can result in client not receiving the correct rate, which can result in the client receiving insufficient or excessive IV fluid. To ensure client safety during IV administration, the controller as well as the client **must** be monitored.

## Calculating Intermittent IV Infusions Piggyback

A medication such as an antibiotic can be administered by attaching it to a port on the primary line (referred to as Intravenous Piggyback [IVPB]) and infusing it by gravity or infused using an electronic infusion device. IVPBs may come premixed from the drug manufacturer, or medications are added to a small volume bag by the nurse, or in some institutions by the pharmacist and sent to the unit.

If the prescriber does not include the type and amount of solution for the medication to be placed in or the rate for infusion, the nurse must check a medication reference or the manufacturer's guidelines. Even if medications are premixed (with medication added to the solution by the drug manufacturer or pharmacy), the nurse is responsible for ensuring that the IVPB is infusing at the correct rate. When medications are premixed, the nurse calculates the infusion rate by using the volume of solution containing the medication. Regardless of whether the IVPB is mixed by the nurse, is premixed, or the ADD-Vantage system is used, the IVPB must be in the correct amount of solution and infused at the correct rate. The volume of IV solution used for an IVPB is usually 50 to 100 mL to infuse over 20, 30, 60 minutes, or longer depending on the type and amount of medication added.

As already stated, depending on the volume of the medication being added (for an IVPB mixed by the nurse), at some institutions the medication is considered in the volume of IV fluid when determining the IV rate. *Note:* For the purpose of this text, it will be indicated when to consider the medication in the IV volume and the type and amount of solution for dilution of the piggyback, and infusion rate will be indicated in the order.

Let's look at the examples shown for determining the rate for the IVPB.

**Example 1:** Order: Keflin 2 g IVPB in 100 mL D$_5$W over 30 min. Drop factor: 15 gtt/mL. Determine the IV flow rate.

## Solution:
- In this problem, there is no conversion needed; the volume of solution is in mL.
- The amount of medication added, 2 g, is not needed to calculate the IV flow rate. The 100 mL of fluid that the Keflin is placed in is used as the volume.
- A drop factor is stated; therefore the IV rate will be calculated in gtt/min.
- The volume of IV fluid, which is stated in mL, the time (min), and the drop factor are the required information needed to calculate the IV flow rate, using the formula method or dimensional analysis.

| Formula Method |
|---|

$$x\,\text{gtt/min} = \frac{100\,\cancel{\text{mL}} \times 15\,\text{gtt/}\cancel{\text{mL}}}{30\,\text{min}}$$

$$x = \frac{100 \times \overset{1}{\cancel{15}}}{\underset{2}{\cancel{30}}}$$

$$x = \frac{100 \times 1}{2}$$

$$x = \frac{100}{2}$$

$$x = 50\,\text{gtt/min; } 50\,\text{macrogtt/min}$$

| Dimensional Analysis |
|---|

$$\frac{x\,\text{gtt}}{\text{min}} = \frac{15\,\text{gtt}}{1\,\cancel{\text{mL}}} \times \frac{100\,\cancel{\text{mL}}}{30\,\text{min}}$$

$$x = \frac{100 \times \overset{1}{\cancel{15}}}{\underset{2}{\cancel{30}}}$$

$$x = \frac{100 \times 1}{2}$$

$$x = \frac{100}{2}$$

$$x = 50\,\text{gtt/min; } 50\,\text{macrogtt/min}$$

To infuse 100 mL in 30 minutes the IV rate would be regulated at 50 gtt/min; 50 macrogtt/min. Now let's look at the same problem if an electronic infusion device was used.

**Example 2:** Order: Keflin 2 g IVPB in 100 mL D$_5$W over 30 min by infusion pump.

Determine the IV flow rate.

Solution:
- An electronic infusion device is being used; the rate will need to be determined in mL/hr.
- As with Example 1, the amount of medication, 2 g, is not needed to calculate the IV flow rate.
- Remember there are 60 minutes in 1 hr.
- The rate can be determined using ratio and proportion, the formula below, or dimensional analysis.

$$x \text{ mL/hr} = \frac{\text{Total mL to infuse}}{\text{Number of min to infuse}} \times 60 \text{ min/hr}$$

**Ratio and Proportion (Linear Format)**

$$100 \text{ mL} : 30 \text{ min} = x \text{ mL} : 60 \text{ min}$$

$$30\, x = 100 \times 60$$

$$\frac{30x}{30} = \frac{6,000}{30}$$

$$x = 200 \text{ mL/hr}$$

**Ratio and Proportion (Fraction Format)**

$$\frac{100 \text{ mL}}{30 \text{ min}} = \frac{x \text{ mL}}{60 \text{ min}}$$

$$x = 200 \text{ mL/hr}$$

**Formula Method**

$$x \text{ mL/hr} = \frac{100 \text{ mL}}{\cancel{30 \text{ min}}^{1}} \times \frac{\cancel{60 \text{ min}}^{2}\text{/hr}}{1}$$

$$x = \frac{200}{1}$$

$$x = 200 \text{ mL/hr}$$

**Notice** min is cancelled, leaving mL/hr.

**Dimensional Analysis**

$$\frac{x \text{ mL}}{\text{hr}} = \frac{100 \text{ mL}}{\cancel{30 \text{ min}}_{1}} \times \frac{\cancel{60 \text{ min}}^{2}}{1 \text{ hr}}$$

$$x = 200 \text{ mL/hr}$$

**Notice** min is cancelled, leaving mL/hr.

The pump would be set at 200 mL/hr to infuse 100 mL in 30 min. **Note:** The actual volume of 100 mL will be infused.

## ⊞ PRACTICE **PROBLEMS**

Calculate the rate in gtt/min for the following medications being administered IVPB. Use the labels where provided. (Add the volume of medication being added to IV solutions, where indicated.)

22. Order: Erythromycin 200 mg in
    250 mL D$_5$W to infuse over 1 hr.
    Drop factor: 10 gtt/mL                         _____

23. Order: Ampicillin 1 g in 50 mL D$_5$W to infuse over 45 minutes. Drop
    factor: 10 gtt/mL. For IV, reconstitute with 10 mL of diluent to get 1 g per 10 mL.
    (Consider the medication added in the volume of fluid.)

    a. How many milliliters of medication
       must be added to the solution?             _____

    b. Calculate the rate in gtt/min at which
       the IV should infuse.                      _____

24. Order: Clindamycin 900 mg in 75 mL D$_5$W over 30 minutes. Drop factor:
    10 gtt/mL

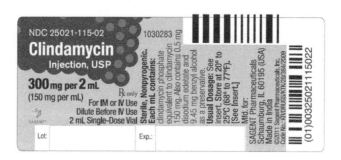

    a. How many milliliters of medication
       must be added to the solution?             _____

    b. Determine the IV rate.                     _____

25. Order: Vancomycin 500 mg IVPB q24hr. The reconstituted vancomycin provides
    50 mg per mL. The medication is placed in 100 mL of D$_5$W to infuse over 60 min-
    utes. Drop factor: 15 gtt/mL. (Consider the medication added in the volume of fluid.)

    a. How many milliliters of medication
       must be added to the solution?             _____

    b. Calculate the rate in gtt/min at which
       the IV should infuse.                      _____

26. Order: Fungizone (amphotericin B) 20 mg in 300 mL D$_5$W over 6 hr by infusion pump. The reconstituted material contains 50 mg per 10 mL.

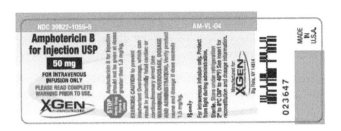

   a. How many milliliters will you add
      to the IV solution?                    _____

   b. Determine the IV rate.                 _____

27. Order: Septra (sulfamethoxazole and trimethoprim) 300 mg in 300 mL D$_5$W over 1 hr q6h. Drop factor: 10 gtt/mL. Calculate the dose using trimethoprim.

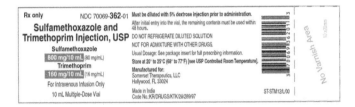

   a. How many milliliters of medication
      will be added to the IV? (Round the
      answer to the nearest tenth.)          _____

   b. Consider the medication added to the volume of IV fluid.
      Calculate the rate in gtt/min at
      which the IV should infuse.            _____

28. Order: Retrovir (zidovudine) 100 mg IV q4h over 1 hr. Available medication states each mL contains 10 mg of zidovudine.

   a. How many milliliters of medication will be added to the IV solution?
      _____

   b. The medication is placed in 100 mL
      of D$_5$W. Drop factor: 10 gtt/mL
      (Consider the medication added to
      the volume of IV fluid.)               _____

**Answers on pp. 539-540**

## Determining the Amount of Medication in a Specific Amount of Solution

Sometimes medications are added to IV solutions, and the prescriber orders a certain amount of medication to be administered in a certain time period. In order to calculate the volume of fluid needed to deliver a specific amount of medication, a ratio and proportion can be used or dimensional analysis.

**Example 1:** Order: 20 mEq of potassium chloride in 1,000 mL D$_5$W to infuse at 2 mEq/hr. Calculate the mL/hr to deliver 2 mEq of potassium chloride/hr.

Solution:

Set up a ratio and proportion using the linear or fraction format:
- With use of the ratio and proportion, the known ratio is the amount of medication in the total volume of solution, and the unknown ratio is what the prescriber ordered.
- Dimensional analysis of the first factor is the total volume of solution and the amount of medication, and the second factor is what the prescriber ordered.

**Ratio and Proportion (Linear Format)**

$$20 \text{ mEq} : 1,000 \text{ mL} = 2 \text{ mEq} : x \text{ mL}$$
$$20x = 1,000 \times 2$$
$$\frac{20x}{20} = \frac{2,000}{20}$$
$$x = \frac{2,000}{20} = 100$$
$$x = 100 \text{ mL/hr}$$

**Ratio and Proportion (Fraction Format)**

$$\frac{20 \text{ mEq}}{1,000 \text{ mL}} = \frac{2 \text{ mEq}}{x \text{ mL}}$$
$$x = 100 \text{ mL/hr}$$

**Dimensional Analysis**

$$\frac{x \text{ mL}}{\text{hr}} = \frac{1,000 \text{ mL}}{\overset{}{\underset{10}{20 \text{ mEq}}}} \times \frac{\overset{1}{2 \text{ mEq}}}{1 \text{ hr}}$$
$$x = \frac{1,000 \times 1}{10}$$
$$x = \frac{1,000}{10} = 100$$
$$x = 100 \text{ mL/hr}$$

Notice cancelling mEq leaves mL/hr.

100 mL/hr will deliver 2 mEq /hr of potassium chloride.

**Example 2:** Order: 100 units of Humulin regular insulin in 500 mL ½ NS to infuse at 10 units/hr. Calculate the mL/hr to deliver 10 units of insulin/hr.

**Ratio and Proportion (Linear Format)**

$$100 \text{ units} : 500 \text{ mL} = 10 \text{ units} : x \text{ mL}$$
$$100x = 500 \times 10$$
$$\frac{100x}{100} = \frac{5,000}{100}$$
$$x = \frac{5,000}{100} = 50$$
$$x = 50 \text{ mL/hr}$$

## Ratio and Proportion (Fraction Format)

$$\frac{100 \text{ units}}{500 \text{ mL}} = \frac{10 \text{ units}}{x \text{ mL}}$$

$$x = 50 \text{ mL/hr}$$

## Dimensional Analysis

$$\frac{x \text{ mL}}{\text{hr}} = \frac{\overset{5}{\cancel{500}} \text{ mL}}{\underset{1}{\cancel{100}} \cancel{\text{units}}} \times \frac{10 \cancel{\text{units}}}{1 \text{ hr}}$$

$$x = 50 \text{ mL/hr}$$

50 mL/hr will deliver 10 units/hr of insulin.

### POINTS TO REMEMBER

- When preparing medications for intermittent infusion:
a. Reconstitute the medication using the label or package insert if needed.
b. Calculate the amount of medication to administer.
c. Verify the recommended infusion rate with the manufacturer's recommendations or a medication reference.
d. Determine the IV rate using the IV formula or dimensional analysis.
- If the intermittent infusion is being administered by an electronic infusion device, the flow rate is determined in mL/hr using ratio and proportion, dimensional analysis, or the formula method for time periods less than 1 hour.

$$x \text{ mL/hr} = \frac{\text{Total mL to infuse}}{\text{Number of min to infuse}} \times 60 \text{ min/hr}$$

- To determine the volume (amount) of IV fluid to administer the prescribed amount of medication in mL/hr, use ratio and proportion or dimensional analysis.

## PRACTICE **PROBLEMS**

Solve the following problems using the steps indicated.

29. Order: 15 mEq of potassium chloride in 1,000 mL of D₅ ½ NS to be administered at a rate of 2 mEq/hr.

    How many mL/hr should the
    IV infuse at?                    _____

30. Order: 10 units of Humulin regular insulin per hour. 50 units of insulin is placed in 250 mL NS.

    How many mL/hr should the
    IV infuse at?                    _____

**Answers on pp. 540-541**

## Determining the Unknown for Time and Volume

You may need to calculate the following:

    a. **Time in hours**—How long it will take a certain amount of fluid to infuse or how long it may last

    b. **Volume**—The total number of milliliters a client will receive in a certain time period

    These unknown elements can be determined by the use of the formula method or dimensional analysis.

## Formula:

$$x \text{ gtt/min} = \frac{\text{Volume of solution in mL} \times \text{Drop factor}}{\text{Time (min)}}$$

## Calculating a Problem with an Unknown Using the Formula Method and Dimensional Analysis

1. Take the information given in the problem and place it in the formula.
2. Place an $x$ in the formula in the position of the unknown. If you are trying to determine time in hours, place $x$ in the position for minutes; once you find the minutes, divide the number of minutes by 60 (60 minutes = 1 hr) to get the number of hours. If you are trying to determine the volume the client would receive, place an $x$ in the position for amount of solution, and label $x$ mL.
3. Set up an algebraic equation so that you can solve for $x$.
4. Solve the equation.
5. Label the answer in hours or milliliters for volume.

  **Example 1:**  Determining hours:

An IV is regulated at 20 microgtt/min. How many hours will it take for 100 mL to infuse?

| Formula Method |
| --- |

$$20 \text{ microgtt/min} = \frac{100 \text{ mL} \times 60 \text{ gtt/mL}}{x \text{ min}}$$

$$\frac{20x}{20} = \frac{100 \times \overset{3}{\cancel{60}}}{\underset{1}{\cancel{20}}}$$

$$x = \frac{100 \times 3}{1} = \frac{300}{1}$$

$$x = 300 \text{ min}$$

Convert min to hr; 60 min = 1 hr.

$$300 \text{ min} \div 60 \text{ min/hr} = 5 \text{ hr}$$

*Note:* In the position of drop factor, 60 gtt/mL was placed, IV was infusing in microgtt, and the infusion set had to be a microdrip (60 gtt/mL).

### Dimensional Analysis

$x$ hr is what you are looking for. The **first** starting fraction is 1 hr/60 min, the **second** fraction is 1 min/20 gtt to match the denominator of the starting fraction. The **third** fraction is 60 gtt/1 mL to match the denominator in the fraction before it. The **last fraction** is 100 mL/1, to match mL in the fraction before it. Cancel the units, reduce if possible, and perform mathematical process.

$$x\ \text{hr} = \frac{1\ \text{hr}}{\underset{1}{60\ \text{min}}} \times \frac{1\ \text{min}}{\underset{1}{20\ \text{gtt}}} \times \frac{\overset{1}{60\ \text{gtt}}}{1\ \text{mL}} \times \frac{\overset{5}{100\ \text{mL}}}{1}$$

$$x = 5\ \text{hours}$$

*Note:* When calculating time and the answer results in hr and min, express entire time in hr (i.e., 1 hr and 30 min = 1.5 hr, or 1½ hr; 1½ hr is the preferred way to state answer).

**Example 2:** Determining volume:

An IV is regulated at 17 macrogtt/min. The drop factor is 15 gtt/mL. How much fluid volume in milliliters will the client receive in 8 hr?

### Formula Method

$$17\ \text{macrogtt/min} = \frac{x\ \text{mL} \ \times \ 15\ \text{gtt/mL}}{480\ \text{min}}$$

$$17 = \frac{x \times \overset{1}{15}}{\underset{32}{480}}$$

$$\frac{17}{1} = \frac{x}{32}$$

$$x = 17 \times 32 = 544$$

$$x = 544\ \text{mL}$$

*Note:* Formula uses min. 8 hr was changed to 480 min. 8 hr × 60 min/hr = 480 min

### Dimensional Analysis

$x$ mL is what you are looking for here. Enter the drop factor as the **first** starting fraction 1 mL/15 gtt. The **second** fraction is 17 gtt/1 min, so it matches the denominator of the first fraction. The **third** fraction is 480 min/1 so that it matches the denominator before it. **An alternate** to changing min to hr is to enter the conversion 60 min/1 hr, and enter 8 hr/1 to match the denominator before it. Cancel if possible, and perform the mathematical process.

$$x\ \text{mL} = \frac{1\ \text{mL}}{\underset{1}{15\ \text{gtt}}} \times \frac{17\ \text{gtt}}{1\ \text{min}} \times \frac{\overset{32}{480\ \text{min}}}{1}$$

$$x = 544\ \text{mL}$$

*Note:* Some problems for calculating an unknown may be solved without using the formula method or dimensional analysis; however, the use of one or the other is recommended.

**POINTS TO REMEMBER**

**Determining the Unknown**

- Use the IV formula and place the information given into the position of the formula.

$$x \text{ gtt/min} = \frac{\text{Volume of solution (mL)} \times \text{drop factor}}{\text{Time (min)}}$$

Use $x$ for unknown values.

1. For determining time—place an $x$ in the minutes position, and then divide the minutes by 60 to determine the time in hours.
2. For volume—place an $x$ in the position for amount of solution and label $x$ mL. Convert the hours to minutes.
- Set up an algebraic equation and solve for $x$.
- Answers for time are labeled in hours, with mL for volume, unless instructed otherwise.
- Dimensional analysis can also be used to determine the unknown.

## 🖩 PRACTICE **PROBLEMS**

Solve for the unknown in the following problems as indicated.

31. You find that there is 150 mL of $D_5W$ left in an IV. The IV is infusing at 60 microgtt/min. How many hours will the fluid last?    _____

32. 0.9% NS is infusing at 35 macrogtt/min. The drop factor is 15 gtt/mL. How many milliliters of fluid will the client receive in 5 hours?    _____

33. There is 90 mL of $D_5$ 0.33% NS left in an IV that is infusing at 60 microgtt/min. The drop factor is 60 gtt/mL. How many hours will the fluid last?    _____

**Answers on p. 541**

## Recalculating an IV Flow Rate

Flow rates on IVs change when a client stands, sits, or is repositioned in bed if IVs are infusing by gravity. Therefore, nurses must frequently check the flow rates. Sometimes IVs infuse ahead of schedule, or they may be behind schedule if they are not monitored closely. When this happens, the IV flow rate must be recalculated. To recalculate the flow rate, the nurse uses the volume remaining and the time remaining. Recalculation may be done with uncomplicated infusions. IVs that require exact infusion rates should be monitored by an electronic infusion device.

**⚠ SAFETY ALERT!**

Never arbitrarily increase or decrease an IV to get it back on schedule without assessing a client and checking with the prescriber. Increasing or decreasing the rate without thought can result in serious harm to a client, including overhydration or underhydration. Check the policy of the institution. Avoid off-schedule IV rates by regularly monitoring the IV at least every 30 to 60 minutes.

When an IV is significantly ahead of or behind schedule, you may need to notify the prescriber, depending on the client's condition and the use of appropriate nursing judgment. **Always assess the client** before making any change in an IV rate. Changes depend on the client's condition. Check the institution's policy regarding the percentage of adjustment that can be made. Each situation must be individually evaluated, and appropriate action must be taken.

**A safe rule is that the recalculated flow rate should not vary from the original rate by more than 25%. If the recalculated rate varies by more than 25% from the original rate, the prescriber should be notified. The order may require revision.** If a client is stable, recalculate the IV rate, using the remaining volume and time, and then proceed to calculate gtt/min using the formula method or dimensional analysis. Refer to content in this chapter (calculating gtt/min) if necessary. Let's go over the steps to recalculate an IV rate if allowed by your institution policy, and the client is stable.

**To recalculate an IV flow rate:**
- Use the remaining volume and remaining hours, and calculate the rate in mL/hr.

$$x\,mL/hr = \frac{\text{Remaining volume}}{\text{Remaining time (hr)}}$$

- Use the mL/hr to calculate gtt/min for the recalculated rate, using the formula or the shortcut method:

$$\text{Formula: } x\,gtt/min = \frac{\text{Volume of solution (mL)} \times \text{drop factor}}{\text{Time in minutes}}$$

- Shortcut method:

$$x\,gtt/min = \frac{mL/hr}{\text{gtt factor constant}}$$

- Determine whether the new rate calculation is greater or lesser than 25%. Use the amount of increase or decrease divided by the original rate.

$$\frac{\text{Amount of} \uparrow \text{or} \downarrow}{\text{Original rate}} = \% \text{ of change of original rate } \text{(round to nearest whole percent)}$$

Let's look at some examples. *Note:* All examples assume the institution allows a 25% IV flow variation, and the clients are stable.

**Example 1:** 1,000 mL of $D_5$ RL was to infuse in 8 hr at 31 gtt/min (31 macrogtt/min). The drop factor is 15 gtt/mL. After 4 hr, you notice 700 mL of fluid left in the IV. Recalculate the flow rate for the remaining solution. *Note:* The infusion is behind schedule. After 4 hr, half of the volume (or 500 mL) should have infused.

Solution:

| Solution to Example 1: Using the Shortcut Method |
|---|

**Determine recalculated rate:**

**Time remaining:** 8 hr − 4 hr = 4 hr

**Volume remaining:** 1,000 mL − 300 mL = 700 mL

700 mL ÷ 4 hr = 175 mL/hr

Drop factor: 15 gtt/mL; therefore the drop factor constant is 4.

$$x\,gtt/min = \frac{175\,mL/hr}{4} = 43.7 = 44$$

$x = 44$ gtt/min; 44 macrogtt/min **(recalculated rate)**

**Determine the percentage of the change:**

$$\frac{44 - 31}{31} = \frac{13}{31} = 0.419 = 42\%$$

**Dimensional Analysis**

$$\text{Time remaining: } 8 \text{ hr} - 4 \text{ hr} = 4 \text{ hr}$$

$$\text{Volume remaining: } 1{,}000 \text{ mL} - 300 \text{ mL} = 700 \text{ mL}$$

$$\frac{x \text{ gtt}}{\text{min}} = \frac{\overset{1}{\cancel{10}} \text{ gtt}}{1 \text{ mL}} \times \frac{700 \text{ mL}}{4 \text{ hr}} \times \frac{1 \text{ hr}}{\underset{4}{\cancel{60}} \text{ min}} = 43.7 = 44$$

$$x = 44 \text{ gtt/min; 44 macrogtt/min}$$

**Course of Action**

Assess the client.

Notify the prescriber.

**Do not** increase the IV rate; the increase is **greater than 25%.**

Increasing the IV could result in serious consequences for the client. Assessment of the client is always done first to determine the client's ability to tolerate an increase in fluid. In this situation the prescriber should be notified, a new order is needed, the recalculated rate is greater than 25%.

**Example 2** **(IV Ahead of Schedule):** An IV of 1,000 mL $D_5W$ is to infuse from 8 AM to 4 PM (8 hr). The drop factor is 10 gtt/mL. The rate is set at 20 gtt/min (20 macrogtt/min). In 5 hr, you notice that 700 mL has infused. Recalculate the flow rate for the remaining solution.

Solution:

**Shortcut Method**

Determine recalculated rate:

**Time remaining:** 8 hr − 5 hr = 3 hr
**Volume remaining:** 1,000 mL − 700 mL = 300 mL

$$300 \text{ mL} \div 3 = 100 \text{ mL/hr}$$

Drop factor: 10 gtt/mL; therefore the drop factor constant is 6.

$$x \text{ gtt/min} = \frac{100 \text{ mL/hr}}{6} = 16.6 = 17$$

$$x = 17 \text{ gtt/min; 17 macrogtt/min } \textbf{(recalculated rate)}$$

Determine the percentage of change:

$$\frac{17 - 20}{20} = \frac{-3}{20} = -0.15 = -15\%$$

**Dimensional Analysis**

**Time remaining:** 8 hr − 5 hr = 3 hr
**Volume remaining:** 1,000 mL − 700 mL = 300 mL

$$\frac{x \text{ gtt}}{\text{min}} = \frac{\overset{1}{\cancel{10}} \text{ gtt}}{1 \text{ mL}} \times \frac{\overset{100}{\cancel{300}} \text{ mL}}{\underset{1}{\cancel{3}} \text{ hr}} \times \frac{1 \text{ hr}}{\underset{6}{\cancel{60}} \text{ min}} = 16.6 = 17$$

$$x = 17 \text{ gtt/min; 17 macrogtt/min}$$

**Course of Action**

Assess the client.

Adjust the rate if allowed by institutional policy, and assess during the remainder of the infusion.

Notify prescriber if required.

In this situation, the flow rate must be decreased from 20 gtt/min (20 macrogtt/min) to 17 gtt/min (17 macrogtt/min), and the change is not greater than 25% of the original rate. −15% is within the acceptable 25% of change. However, the client's condition must still be assessed to determine the ability to tolerate the change, and the prescriber may still require notification.

## Alternate to Determining the Percentage of Change

As already stated, you can adjust the flow rate as much as (+) or (–)25%. Think 25% = ¼. Therefore you can verify the safety of the recalculated rate by using a method that eliminates the need to use percents. To do this, do the following:

- Divide the original rate by 4, then add, and subtract the result from the original rate. This will provide a range for the acceptable rate adjustment. Let's use the two examples we just did.

### Example 1:

The original rate was 31 gtt/min (macrogtt/min), and the recalculated rate is 44 gtt/min (macrogtt/min).

**Original rate ± (original rate ÷ 4) = Acceptable IV rate adjustment**

31 + (31 ÷ 4) = 31 + 7.75 = 38.75 = 39 gtt/min (macrogtt/min)

31 − (31 ÷ 4) = 31 − 7.75 = 23.25 = 23 gtt/min (macrogtt/min)

The safe acceptable IV rate adjustment is 23 to 39 gtt/min (macrogtt/min). 44 gtt/min is above the acceptable adjustment range, and 25%. The prescriber should be notified to provide a new order.

### Example 2:

The original rate was 20 gtt/min (macrogtt/min), and the recalculated rate is 17 gtt/min (17 macrogtt/min).

**Original rate ± (original rate ÷ 4) = Acceptable IV rate adjustment**

20 + (20 ÷ 4) = 20 + 5 = 25 gtt/min (macrogtt/min).

20 − (20 ÷ 4) = 20 − 5 = 15 gtt/min (macrogtt/min).

The safe acceptable IV rate adjustment is 15 to 25 (macrogtt/min). It is safe to slow the rate to 17 gtt/min (macrogtt/min), which is less than 25%.

---

### POINTS TO REMEMBER

- Monitor IV therapy every 30 to 60 min to maintain the ordered IV rate.
- Do not arbitrarily speed up or slow down an IV that is behind or ahead of schedule.
- Know the hospital policy regarding recalculation of IV flow rate. An IV should not vary more than 25% from its original rate.
- To recalculate an IV rate:
- Determine mL/hr:

$$x\,mL/hr = \frac{\text{Remaining volume}}{\text{Remaining time (hrs)}}$$

- Use mL/hr and recalculate the rate in gtt/min, using formula or shortcut method.

$$x\,gtt/min = \frac{\text{Volume of solution (mL)} \times \text{drop factor}}{\text{Time in minutes}}$$

$$x\,gtt/min = \frac{mL/hr}{\text{gtt factor constant}}$$

- Determine the % of change

$$\frac{\text{Amount of} \uparrow \text{or} \downarrow}{\text{Original rate}} = \% \text{ of change (rounded to the nearest whole \%)}$$

- Alternate to use of percent: Divide the original rate by 4, then add and subtract the result from the original rate to get the acceptable IV rate adjustment.
- Contact the prescriber for a new IV order, if the recalculated rate exceeds 25%.

## PRACTICE **PROBLEMS**

For each of the problems, recalculate the IV flow rates in gtt/min rates using either method presented, determine the percentage of change, and state your course of action. *Note:* The institution allows 25% variation and clients are stable.

34. 500 mL of 0.9% NS was ordered to infuse in 8 hr at the rate of 16 gtt/min (16 macrogtt/min). The drop factor is 15 gtt/mL. After 5 hr, you find 250 mL of fluid left.

a. _____ gtt/min

b. _____ % variation

c. _____ Course of action

35. 250 mL of $D_5W$ was to infuse in 3 hr at the rate of 21 gtt/min (21 macrogtt/min). Drop factor: 15 gtt/mL. With $1\frac{1}{2}$ hr remaining, you find 200 mL left.

a. _____ gtt/min

b. _____ % variation

c. _____ Course of action

36. 1,000 mL $D_5$ 0.33% NS was to infuse in 12 hr at 28 gtt/min (28 macrogtt/min). After 4 hr, 250 mL has infused. Drop factor: 20 gtt/mL

a. _____ gtt/min

b. _____ % variation

c. _____ Course of action

37. 500 mL $D_5$ 0.9% NS to infuse in 5 hr at 100 gtt/min (100 microgtt/min). After 2 hr, 250 mL has infused. Drop factor: 60 gtt/mL

a. _____ gtt/min

b. _____ % variation

c. _____ Course of action

**Answers on pp. 541-542**

## Calculating Infusion and Completion Time

IV fluids are ordered by the prescriber for administration indicating a specific rate in mL/hr, such as 1,000 mL $D_5W$ to infuse at 100 mL/hr. **The nurse needs to be able to determine the amount of time (hours and minutes) that it would take for a certain volume of IV solution to infuse, which is referred to as *infusion time*.** Knowing the infusion time is important for the nurse, which includes reasons such as allowing the preparation for hanging a new solution as one infusion is being completed and preventing things such as the line clotting off as a result of not knowing when an IV was to be completed. Infusion times can be calculated using any of the following methods:

- Ratio and proportion: The known ratio, which is written first, is the ordered rate in mL/hr, and the second ratio is the unknown, which is the total number of mL to infuse in $x$ hr, total mL/$x$ hr. The ratio and proportion can be written in linear or fraction format.

- Formula method: $\dfrac{\text{Total number of mL to infuse}}{\text{mL/hr (infusion rate)}} = \text{Infusion time}$
- Dimensional analysis: The unknown is $x$ hr; therefore the first fraction will be the ordered rate, hr/mL, the second fraction will be total mL/1.

Let's look at some examples of calculating infusion time.

**Example 1:** Calculate the infusion time for an IV of 1,000 mL $D_5W$ to infuse at a rate of 125 mL/hr.

**Ratio and Proportion (Linear Format)**

$$125 \text{ mL} : 1 \text{ hr} = 1,000 \text{ mL} : x \text{ hr}$$
$$125\,x = 1,000$$
$$\frac{125x}{125} = \frac{1,000}{125}$$
$$x = 8 \text{ hr (infusion time)}$$

**Formula Method**

1,000 mL (total mL to infuse)
125 mL/hr (mL/hr to infuse)

$$\frac{1,000 \text{ mL}}{125 \text{ mL/hr}} = 1,000 \div 125 = 8 \text{ hr}$$

Infusion time = 8 hr

**Ratio and Proportion (Fraction Format)**

$$\frac{125 \text{ mL}}{1 \text{ hr}} = \frac{1,000 \text{ mL}}{x \text{ hr}}$$

Solve by cross-multiplication.

**Dimensional Analysis**

$$x \text{ hr} = \frac{1 \text{ hr}}{\cancel{125} \text{ mL}} \times \frac{\overset{8}{\cancel{1000} \text{ mL}}}{1}$$
$$x = 8 \text{ hr}$$
mL is cancelled here, leaving hr.

When an infusion time result is not an even whole number but instead the infusion rate includes a decimal fraction; the decimal fraction represents a fraction of an hour and must be converted to minutes. This calculation of infusion time is done as follows:
- Determine the infusion time using any of the methods already presented, and carry division two decimal places.
- Calculate the minutes using, conversion factor; 60 min = 1 hr. (Multiply the fraction of an hr by 60 min/hr) or use any of the methods presented.
- Using the rules of rounding, round the minutes to the nearest whole number of minutes.

Let's look at an example.

**Example 2:**  1,000 mL $D_5$ ½ NS to infuse at 150 mL/hr. Calculate the infusion time for the IV.

### Ratio and Proportion (Linear Format)

- Determine the infusion time

  150 mL : 1 hr = 1,000 mL : $x$ hr

  150 $x$ = 1,000

  $$\frac{150x}{150} = \frac{1,000}{150}$$

  $x$ = 6.66 hr
- Calculate the minutes

  1 hr : 60 min = 0.66 hr : $x$ min

  $x$ = 0.66 × 60 = 39.6

  $x$ = 40 min (rounded to whole number)

Infusion time is 6 hr and 40 min.

### Formula Method

- Determine infusion time

  $$\frac{1,000 \text{ mL}}{150 \text{ mL/hr}} = 6.66$$

  $x$ = 6.66 hr
- Calculate the minutes

  0.66 hr × 60 min/hr = 39.6 = 40

Infusion time is 6 hr and 40 min.

### Ratio and Proportion (Fraction Format)

Solve by cross-multiplication.

- Determine infusion time

  $$\frac{150 \text{ mL}}{1 \text{ hr}} = \frac{1,000 \text{ mL}}{x \text{ hr}}$$

  $x$ = 6.66 hr
- Calculate the minutes

  $$\frac{60 \text{ min}}{1 \text{ hr}} = \frac{x \text{ min}}{0.66 \text{ hr}} = 39.6 = 40$$

  $x$ = 40 min

Infusion time is 6 hr and 40 min.

### Dimensional Analysis

- Determine infusion rate

  $$x \text{ hr} = \frac{1 \text{ hr}}{150 \text{ mL}} \times \frac{1,000 \text{ mL}}{1}$$

  $x$ = 6.66 hr
- Calculate the minutes

  $$x \text{ min} = \frac{60 \text{ min}}{1 \text{ hr}} \times \frac{0.66 \text{ hr}}{1} = 39.6 = 40$$

  $x$ = 40 min

Infusion time is 6 hr and 40 min.

## Completion Time

Once the infusion time has been calculated, the nurse can use this information to determine the completion time. Completion time is the when the infusion is completed (i.e., the client has received all of the IV fluid). This would be determined as follows: Add the calculated infusion time to the time the infusion was started. If the IV was started at 7:00 AM, add the 6 hours and 40 minutes to that time (7:00 AM). The IV would be completed at 1:40 PM. It is easier to calculate completion time using military time: 7:00 AM = 0700; now add 6 hours and 40 minutes to arrive at the answer of 1340.

> Start time          0700
> Infusion time     +0640
> **Completion time:** 1340 or 1:30 PM

> **Calculating Completion Time**
>
> To calculate the completion time, add the infusion time to the time the IV was (military time).

*Note:* Converting traditional time to military time, and a discussion of completion time, appears in Chapter 8.

Let's look at some examples.

**Example 1:** An IV of 1,000 mL of $D_5W$ is started at 1000 to infuse over 8 hr. Determine the completion time.

**Solution:**

> Start time          1000
> Infusion time +0800

**Completion time:** 1800 or 6:00 PM

**Example 2:** An IV of 1,000 mL of 0.9% NS is started at 2130 to infuse over 12 hr. Determine the completion time.

**Solution:**

> Start time          2130
> Infusion time +1200
>                      3330 (time here is greater than 2400)

As you recall, when the time period is greater than 2400, you must subtract 2400 from the total (the day ends at 2400). This will give you the completion time for the next day.

Using the answer from the problem, which is  3330

> Subtract  –2400
> **Completion time:**  0930 or 9:30 AM the next day

**Example 3:** An IV of $D_5\frac{1}{2}$ NS is started at 0430 to infuse in 6 hr and 40 min. Determine the completion time.

**Solution:**

> Start time          0430
> Infusion time +0640
>                      1070 (the minutes here are greater than 60)

As you recall, when the minutes are greater or equal to 60, subtract 60 from the number of minutes, which in this example is 70 min, and then add the 1 hour obtained when you subtracted the 60 minutes to get the completion rate, as follows:

    1070
    −0060 minutes (1 hr)
    1010
    +0100 (the 1 hr obtained when you subtracted the 60 min)

**Completion time:** 1110 or 11:10 AM

**Alternate to Example 3:**     Add start time: 0430

                               Infusion time +0640

                                           1070

Convert 70 min to 1 hr and 10 min and add to 10 hr.  1000

                                           +0110

**Completion time:** 1110 or 11:10 AM

As you will notice in the examples provided, you were given the infusion time as well as the time for the infusion to start in military time. Let's look at an example in which you will need to determine the infusion time before calculating the completion time.

### Example 4:

500 mL D$_5$W to infuse at 80 mL/hr is started at 7:30 AM. Determine the completion time. State time in military and traditional time.

### Solution:

- First determine the infusion time using any of the methods already presented (ratio and proportion, formula method, or dimensional analysis)

**Ratio and Proportion (Linear Format)**

$$80 \text{ mL} : 1 \text{ hr} = 500 \text{ mL} : x \text{ hr}$$
$$80x = 500$$
$$\frac{80x}{80} = \frac{500}{80} = 6.25$$
$$x = 6.25 \text{ hr}$$

Calculate the minutes.

$$1 \text{ hr} : 60 \text{ min} = 0.25 \text{ hr} : x \text{ min}$$
$$x = 0.25 \times 60 = 15$$
$$x = 15 \text{ min}$$

Infusion time is 6 hr and 15 min.

**Formula Method**

$$\frac{500 \text{ mL}}{80 \text{ mL/hr}} = 500 \div 8 = 6.25 \text{ hr}$$

Calculate the minutes.

$$60 \text{ min/hr} \times 0.25 \text{ hr} = 15 \text{ min}$$

Infusion time is 6 hr and 15 min.

## Ratio and Proportion (Fraction Format)

Solve by cross-multiplication.

$$\frac{80 \text{ mL}}{1 \text{ hr}} = \frac{500 \text{ mL}}{x \text{ hr}}$$

$$x = 6.25 \text{ hr}$$

Calculate the minutes.

$$\frac{60 \text{ min}}{1 \text{ hr}} = \frac{x \text{ min}}{0.25 \text{ hr}}$$

$$x = 15 \text{ min}$$

Infusion time is 6 hr and 15 min.

## Dimensional Analysis

$$x \text{ hr} = \frac{1 \text{ hr}}{80 \text{ mL}} \times \frac{500 \text{ mL}}{1}$$

$$x = 6.25 \text{ hr}$$

Calculate the minutes:

$$x \text{ min} = \frac{60 \text{ min}}{1 \text{ hr}} \times \frac{0.25 \text{ hr}}{1}$$

$$x = 15 \text{ min}$$

Infusion time is 6 hr and 15 min.

- Now determine the completion time (add the infusion time to the start time).

Start time: 0730

Infusion time: $\dfrac{+0615}{1345}$ = 1:45 PM

*Note:* The start time (7:30 AM) was changed to military time: to convert AM time omit colon and AM, add a zero to beginning to make a 4-digit number. To convert PM time to traditional time, subtract 1200 and add PM. If necessary, review the conversion of time (traditional and military) in Chapter 8.

## PRACTICE **PROBLEMS**

Determine infusion and completion time for the following IVs. State the time in traditional and military time.

38. An IV of 500 mL NS is to infuse at 60 mL/hr.

    a. Determine the infusion time.  _____

    b. The IV was started at 10:00 PM. When
       would the IV infusion be completed?  _____

39. An IV of 250 mL D$_5$W is to infuse at 80 mL/hr.

    a. Determine the infusion time.  _____

    b. The IV was started at 2:00 AM. When
       would the IV infusion be completed?  _____

40. An IV of 1,000 mL D$_5$ RL is to infuse at 60 mL/hr.

    a. Determine the infusion time.  _____

    b. The IV was started at 6:00 AM.
       At what time would this
       IV infusion be completed?  _____

41. An IV of 500 mL D$_5$W is to infuse at 75 mL/hr.

    a.  Determine the infusion time.    _____

    b.  The IV was started at 2:00 PM.
        At what time would the
        IV infusion be completed?    _____

**Answers on p. 542**

## Calculating Infusion Time When Rate in mL/hr Is Not Indicated for Large Volumes of Fluid

There are situations in which the prescriber may order the IV solution and not indicate the rate in mL/hr. The only information may be the total number of milliliters to infuse, the flow rate (gtt/min) of the IV, and the number of gtt/mL that the tubing delivers. In this situation, before the infusion time is calculated, the following must be done:

- Convert gtt/min to mL/min.
- Convert mL/min to mL/hr.
- Use the formula or other methods shown to determine the infusion time.

**Example:**    A client is receiving 1,000 mL of RL. The IV is infusing at 21 macrogtt/min (21 gtt/min). The administration set delivers 10 gtt/mL. Calculate the infusion time.

**Step 1: Change gtt/min to mL/min.**
**Ratio and Proportion (Linear Format)**
10 gtt : 1 mL = 21 gtt : $x$ mL

$$\frac{10x}{10} = \frac{21}{10}$$

$$x = 2.1 \text{ mL/min}$$

*Note:* Ratio and proportion could also be set up in fraction format.

**Step 2: Convert mL/min to mL/hr.**
2.1 mL/~~min~~ $\times$ 60 ~~min~~/hr = 126 mL/hr

**Step 3: Calculate the infusion time.**

$$\frac{1,000 \text{ ~~mL~~}}{126 \text{ ~~mL~~/hr}} = 1,000 \div 126 = 7.93 \text{ hr}$$

**Convert hr to min.**
0.93 ~~hr~~ $\times$ 60 min/~~hr~~ = 55.8 = 56 min

Infusion time is 7 hr and 56 min.

---

### Solution Using Dimensional Analysis

$x$ hr is being calculated. The **first fraction** is 1 hr/60 min; the **second fraction** is written so that min is in the numerator: 1 min/21 gtt. The **third fraction** is written so that it matches the denominator of the second fraction; the drop factor is written 10 gtt/mL. **The final fraction** is written so that the denominator matches the proceeding fraction. The mL is provided by the volume to infuse (1,000 mL), the fraction is written 1,000 mL/1.

**Calculate the infusion time.**

$$x \text{ hr} = \frac{1 \text{ hr}}{\underset{6}{60 \text{ ~~min~~}}} \times \frac{1 \text{ ~~min~~}}{21 \text{ ~~gtt~~}} \times \frac{\overset{1}{10 \text{ ~~gtt~~}}}{1 \text{ ~~mL~~}} \times \frac{1,000 \text{ ~~mL~~}}{1} = 7.93 \text{ hr}$$

**Convert hr to minutes.**

$$x \text{ min} = \frac{60 \text{ min}}{1 \text{ ~~hr~~}} \times \frac{0.93 \text{ ~~hr~~}}{1} = 55.8 = 56 \text{ min}$$

$$x = 56 \text{ min}$$

Infusion time is 7 hr and 56 min.

## PRACTICE **PROBLEMS**

Determine the infusion time for the following IVs.

42. A client is receiving 250 mL of NS at
    17 macrogtt/min. Drop factor: 15 gtt/mL _____

43. A client is receiving 1,000 mL D$_5$W at
    20 macrogtt/min. Drop factor: 10 gtt/mL _____

44. A client is receiving 100 mL D$_5$W at
    10 macrogtt/min. Drop factor: 15 gtt/mL _____

**Answers on pp. 542-543**

## Calculating Infusion Time for Small Volumes of Fluid

There may be times when it is necessary for the nurse to determine the infusion time for small volumes of fluid that will infuse in less than an hour. To do this the nurse must first do the following:
- Calculate the mL/min.
- Divide the total volume by the mL/min to obtain the infusion time. The infusion time will be in minutes.

Example: An IV antibiotic of 30 mL is infusing at 20 macrogtt/min. Drop factor is 10 gtt/mL. Determine the infusion time.

**Step 1: Calculate the mL/min.**

10 gtt :1 mL = 20 gtt : $x$ mL

$$\frac{10\ x}{10} = \frac{20}{10}$$

$x = 2$ mL/min

**Step 2: Divide the total volume by mL/min to determine the infusion time.**

30 mL ÷ 2 mL/min = 15 min

Infusion time is 15 min.

---

**Solution Using Dimensional Analysis**

Since a small volume is being infused in less than 1 hr and there is a drop factor the time will be in minutes. The conversion factor 60 min = 1 hr is not needed.

$$x\ min = \frac{1\ min}{\underset{2}{20\ gtt}} \times \frac{\overset{1}{10\ gtt}}{1\ mL} \times \frac{30\ mL}{1}$$

$$x = \frac{30}{2} = 15$$

$x = 15$ min

Infusion time is 15 min.

PRACTICE **PROBLEM**

Determine the infusion time for the following:

45. An IV medication of 20 mL is infusing at
    35 microgtt/min. Drop factor: 60 gtt/mL  _____

**Answers on p. 543**

## Monitoring the Infusion of IV Solutions

Whether a client is receiving fluids by gravity or with the use of an infusion device, the nurse has the responsibility to monitor the client to ensure the right fluid is infusing at the right rate. When the client is receiving IV fluids by infusion pump, the rate is set in mL/hr and the pump delivers the amount each hour that it is programmed to deliver. When IVs infuse by gravity, the nurse often monitors the IV therapy visually. The IV bag is marked in increments of 50 to 100 mL and provides a visual for the nurse that includes the amount of fluid that has infused and the amount remaining in the bag. Some health care institutions use a commercially prepared label on IVs, referred to as flow meter, and time tape, which is a strip of paper applied to the IV bag. The flow meter and time tape include information such as starting time for the IV and the ending time. These strips applied to the side of the IV bag allow the nurse to visually identify the hourly fluid level.

## Charting IV Therapy

The documentation of IV therapy varies from institution to institution. Some institutions chart IV therapy on a special record or flow sheet for IV therapy. Medications that are administered intermittently by IVPB may be charted on medication administration records according to the order (i.e., standing medication, prn). At institutions where a computerized system is used, IV therapy is charted directly into the computer (this includes IV solutions with or without medications). Assessments relating to IV therapy that include the status of the site and complications are also charted on either a form for IV therapy or in the computer. Regardless of what method is used for documentation, it is a nursing responsibility to accurately document all IV therapy that is administered to a client.

> **POINTS TO REMEMBER**
>
> - The infusion rate can be calculated using ratio and proportion, dimensional analysis, or the formula method:
>
> $$\frac{\text{Total number of mL to infuse}}{\text{mL/hr (infusion rate)}} = \text{Infusion time}$$
>
> - Express fractional hours for infusion rate in minutes using 60 min = 1 hr. Multiply the fractional hour by 60 min/hr, and round to the nearest whole number.
> - To calculate the completion time, add the start time and infusion time. Time can be stated as military or traditional time.
> - Calculation of completion times provides the nurse with the opportunity to plan ahead, (i.e., having the next IV solution ready to hang once solution is completed).
> - Monitoring of IV fluids is a nursing responsibility. Tape and flow meters allow for a visual of the status of IV infusions.

## IV Push Medications

When medications are administered by IV push (IVP), the medication is injected directly into a vein, the medication is rapidly absorbed in the bloodstream, and the client experiences a rapid result from the medication. Several terms are used for IVP, including IV bolus and direct IV injection. IVP administration is used to deliver diluted and undiluted medication over a brief period (seconds or minutes). Drug references provide the acceptable rate for IV push medication administration. Because of the rapidity of action, an error in calculation can result in a serious outcome for the client. Most IV push medications should be administered over a period of 1 to 5 minutes (or longer), depending on the medication. The volume of the prescribed medication should be calculated in increments of 15 to 30 seconds. This allows for the use of a watch to provide accurate administration. The prescriber orders the medication, dosage, route, frequency, and time to administer a medication for IVP. To ensure client safety, the nurse should always consult a drug reference for the following:

- The recommended rate for administering the medication
- The directions for dilution of the medication including, the amount and type of solution

> ⚠ **SAFETY ALERT!**
>
> **Never** infuse IV push medications more rapidly than recommended. Carefully read the drug reference for proper dilution, and the time for administration of medications IV push. IV medications are potent and rapid acting.

## Administration of Medications by IV Push

Injection ports on IV tubing can be used for direct injection of the medication with a syringe which is called IV push. When using the primary line, administer the medication through the port closest to the client. An IV push medication can also be administered using a saline or heparin lock, which can be attached to the IV catheter. A saline lock indicates that saline is used to flush or maintain IV catheter patency, whereas a heparin lock indicates that heparin is used to maintain the IV catheter patency. Know the policy of the institution regarding the use of saline or heparin. Medications can be administered IV push by attaching the syringe to the lock and pushing in the medication. The lock is usually flushed after administration of the medication. Medications can be administered by IV push by registered nurses who have been specially trained in this practice at some institutions. The actual administration of IV push medications is beyond the scope of this text. For a detailed description on the technique, consult a clinical skills textbook or view the skill online. This text provides a brief discussion of medications by IV push and some examples.

> ⚠ **SAFETY ALERT!**
>
> Remember heparin is a **high-alert medication**. Heparin lock flush solution is usually in dosage strengths of 10 or 100 units per mL. **Always read** the label carefully. Know the agency policy for the use of heparin to maintain an IV lock.

When administering medications by direct IV infusion, remember the following:

- **The compatibility of the IV solution and the medication must be verified.**
- The tubing will require a flush after direct administration to ensure that all the medication has been given and none remains in the tubing.
- The amount of time needed to administer a medication by direct IV infusion can be determined by using ratio and proportion or dimensional analysis. Let's look at some examples.

**Example 1:**  Order: 200 mg of a medication IV push stat.

Available: The medication available is 300 mg per 2 mL.

*The literature recommends diluting the medication to a total of 20 mL. Compatible solution recommended is sodium chloride (0.9%) injection. Inject over a period of not less than 2 minutes. An injection time of 5 minutes is ordered.*

a. How many mL of the medication will you administer?
b. How many mL of sodium chloride must you add to obtain the desired volume?
c. To administer the infusion in 5 minutes, how many mL should you infuse every minute?
d. How much should you infuse every 15 seconds?
   a. First determine the number of mL to administer the dosage.

**Ratio and Proportion (Linear Format)**

$$300 \text{ mg} : 2 \text{ mL} = 200 \text{ mg} : x \text{ mL}$$

$$300x = 200 \times 2$$

$$\frac{300x}{300} = \frac{400}{300} = 1.33$$

$$x = 1.3 \text{ mL}$$

**Formula Method**

$$\frac{200 \text{ mg}}{300 \text{ mg}} \times 2 \text{ mL} = x \text{ mL}$$

**Dimensional Analysis**

$$x \text{ mL} = \frac{2 \text{ mL}}{300 \text{ mg}} \times \frac{200 \text{ mg}}{1}$$

**Ratio and Proportion (Fraction Format)**

$$\frac{300 \text{ mg}}{2 \text{ mL}} = \frac{200 \text{ mg}}{x \text{ mL}}$$

1.3 mL would be equal to 200 mg of the medication

b. According to the literature, the total volume of the diluent and medication is 20 mL. If the literature stated to dilute in 20 mL, then the total volume would be the medication and the diluent.

$$20 \text{ mL (desired diluent)}$$
$$\underline{-1.3 \text{ mL (medication dosage)}}$$
$$\textbf{18.7 mL (amount of diluent to add)}$$

18.7 mL of sodium chloride is needed to obtain the desired volume.

c. Determine the number of mL to administer the infusion in 1 minute.

**Ratio and Proportion (Linear Format)**

$$20 \text{ mL} : 5 \text{ min} = x \text{ mL} : 1 \text{ min}$$

$$5x = 20$$

$$\frac{5x}{5} = \frac{20}{5} = 4$$

$$x = 4 \text{ mL per min}$$

**Ratio and Proportion (Fraction Format)**

$$\frac{20 \text{ mL}}{5 \text{ min}} = \frac{x \text{ mL}}{1 \text{ min}}$$

**Dimensional Analysis**

$$x\,\text{mL} = \frac{\overset{4}{\cancel{20}}\,\text{mL}}{\underset{1}{\cancel{5}\,\cancel{\text{min}}}} \times \frac{1\,\cancel{\text{min}}}{1} = 4$$

$$x = 4\,\text{mL per min}$$

Place the desired unit mL to the left of the equal sign. Place the mL ordered as the first fraction (20 mL in 5 min); place mL in the numerator, place 1 min in the numerator of the next unit.

4 mL per min to administer the infusion in 5 min.

d. Determine the volume to infuse every 15 sec.

**Ratio and Proportion (Linear Format)**

$$4\,\text{mL} : 60\,\text{sec} = x\,\text{mL} : 15\,\text{sec}$$

$$60x = 4 \times 15$$

$$\frac{60x}{60} = \frac{60}{60} = 1$$

$$x = 1\,\text{mL every 15 sec}$$

**Ratio and Proportion (Fraction Format)**

$$\frac{4\,\text{mL}}{60\,\text{sec}} = \frac{x\,\text{mL}}{15\,\text{sec}}$$

**Dimensional Analysis**

**Note:** In this question you are asked to determine sec. (Express 4 mL per min as 4 mL per 60 sec. 60 sec = 1 min. The starting fraction would be 4 mL/60 sec.)

$$x\,\text{mL} = \frac{4\,\text{mL}}{\underset{4}{\cancel{60}\,\cancel{\text{sec}}}} \times \frac{\overset{1}{\cancel{15}\,\cancel{\text{sec}}}}{1}$$

**Alternate format:** To use 4 mL/min; however, you would need to add 1 min/60 sec to the equation and the setup would be as follows:

$$x\,\text{mL} = \frac{4\,\text{mL}}{1\,\cancel{\text{min}}} \times \frac{1\,\cancel{\text{min}}}{\underset{4}{\cancel{60}\,\cancel{\text{sec}}}} \times \frac{\overset{1}{\cancel{15}\,\cancel{\text{sec}}}}{1}$$

**Example 2:**  Order: Ativan 3 mg IV push stat

Available: Ativan 4 mg per mL

*The literature states: not to exceed 2 mg/min.*

a. How many mL of Ativan will you prepare? (Express answer in hundredths.)

b. How many min would it take to administer the medication as ordered?
   • a. First calculate the dosage to be administered using ratio and proportion, dimensional analysis, or formula method.

**Ratio and Proportion (Linear Format)**

$$4\,\text{mg} : 1\,\text{mL} = 3\,\text{mg} : x\,\text{mL}$$

$$4x = 3$$

$$\frac{4x}{4} = \frac{3}{4} = 0.75\,\text{mL}$$

$$x = 0.75\,\text{mL}$$

**Formula Method**

$$\frac{3 \text{ mg}}{4 \text{ mg}} \times 1 \text{ mL} = x \text{ mL}$$

**Dimensional Analysis**

$$x \text{ mL} = \frac{1 \text{ mL}}{4 \text{ mg}} \times \frac{3 \text{ mg}}{1}$$

**Ratio and Proportion (Fraction Format)**

$$\frac{4 \text{ mg}}{1 \text{ mL}} = \frac{3 \text{ mg}}{x \text{ mL}}$$

b.  Determine the time needed to administer the medication as ordered.

**Ratio and Proportion (Linear Format)**

$$2 \text{ mg} : 1 \text{ min} = 3 \text{ mg} : x \text{ min}$$

$$2x = 3$$

$$\frac{2x}{2} = \frac{3}{2} = 1.5 \ (1½)$$

$$x = 1½ \text{ min}$$

**Ratio and Proportion (Fraction Format)**

$$\frac{2 \text{ mg}}{1 \text{ min}} = \frac{3 \text{ mg}}{x \text{ min}}$$

1½ min would deliver the medication.

**Dimensional Analysis**

$$x \text{ min} = \frac{1 \text{ min}}{2 \text{ mg}} \times \frac{3 \text{ mg}}{1}$$

**Note:** Use the steps outlined in Example 1.

> ⚙ **POINTS TO REMEMBER**
>
> **IV Push Medications**
> - Always verify the compatibility of the medication and the IV solution when administering medications by IV push.
> - Never administer a medication by IV push at a rate faster than recommended. Always read package inserts and reputable medication resources for minimum time for IV administration and dilution.
> - Use ratio and proportion or dimensional analysis to determine the IV push time as recommended by a reputable reference.

## ▦ PRACTICE **PROBLEMS**

Calculate the IV push rate as indicated for problems 46-47.

46. Order: Valium 20 mg IV push stat at 5 mg/min for a client with seizures.

   Available: Valium 5 mg per mL

    a. How many milliliters will be
       needed to administer the dosage?    _____

    b. Determine the time it would take
       to infuse the dosage.    _____

    c. How many milligrams would you
       administer every 15 seconds?    _____

47. Order: Dilantin 150 mg IV push stat.

    Available: Dilantin 250 mg per 5 mL. Literature states IV infusion not to exceed
    50 mg/min.

    a. How much should you prepare
       to administer?    _____

    b. How much time is needed to
       administer the required dosage?    _____

**Answers on p. 543**

## 🗨 CLINICAL **REASONING**

**Scenario:** An elderly client has an order for 1,000 mL $D_5W$ at 100 mL/hr. The nurse assigned to the client attached IV tubing to the IV with a drop factor of 10 gtt/mL without checking the package of IV tubing. As a habit from a previous institution where she worked, the IV flow rate was calculated based on the drop factor of 20 gtt/mL. At the beginning of the next shift, the nurse making rounds noticed that the client was having difficulty breathing and seemed restless. When the nurse checked the IV rate, she discovered the rate was 33 macrogtt/min instead of 17 macrogtt/min.
a. What factors contributed to the error? _____
b. How did the IV rate contribute to the problem and why? _____
c. What should have been the action of the nurse who attached the IV tubing in relation
   to IV administration? _____

**Answers on p. 543**

## ⊙ CHAPTER **REVIEW**
Calculate the IV flow rate in gtt/min for the following IV administrations, unless another
unit of measure is stated.

1. 2,500 mL $D_5NS$ to infuse in 24 hr.
   Drop factor: 10 gtt/mL    _____

2. 500 mL $D_5W$ to infuse in 4 hr.
   Drop factor: 15 gtt/mL    _____

3. 300 mL NS to infuse in 6 hr.
   Drop factor: 60 gtt/mL    _____

4. 500 mL $D_5$ ½ NS over 12 hr.
   Drop factor: 20 gtt/mL    _____

5. A unit of whole blood (500 mL) to infuse in 4 hr. Drop factor: 10 gtt/mL

    _____

6. Infuse 2 L RL in 24 hr.
   Drop factor: 15 gtt/mL

    _____

7. 1,000 mL $D_5$ 0.45% NS in 6 hr.
   Drop factor: 20 gtt/mL

    _____

8. 250 mL $D_5W$ in 8 hr.
   Drop factor: 60 gtt/mL

    _____

9. 2 L $D_5RL$ at 150 mL/hr.
   Drop factor: 15 gtt/mL

    _____

10. 1,500 mL $D_5W$ in 24 hr.
    Drop factor: 15 gtt/mL

    _____

11. 250 mL $D_5W$ in 10 hr.
    Drop factor: 60 gtt/mL

    _____

12. Infuse 300 mL of $D_5W$ at 75 mL/hr.
    Drop factor: 60 gtt/mL

    _____

13. Infuse an IV medication with a volume of 50 mL in 45 minutes.
    Drop factor: 60 gtt/mL

    _____

14. Infuse 90 mL/hr of NS.
    Drop factor: 15 gtt/mL

    _____

15. Infuse an IV medication in 100 mL $D_5W$ in 30 minutes.
    Drop factor: 20 gtt/mL

    _____

16. Infuse 250 mL 0.45% NS in 5 hr.
    Drop factor: 20 gtt/mL

    _____

17. Infuse Kefzol 0.5 g in 50 mL $D_5W$ in 30 minutes. Drop factor: 60 gtt/mL

    _____

18. Infuse Plasmanate 500 mL over 3 hr.
    Drop factor: 10 gtt/mL

    _____

19. The prescriber orders the following IVs for 24 hr. Drop factor: 10 gtt/mL
    - 1,000 mL $D_5W$ c̄ 1 ampule multivitamin (MVI)
    - 500 mL $D_5W$
    - 250 mL $D_5W$

    _____

20. If 500 mL of $D_5W$ is to infuse in 8 hr, how many milliliters are to be administered per hour?

    _____

21. Infuse 500 mL Intralipids IV in 6 hr.
    Drop factor: 10 gtt/mL

    _____

22. An IV of 500 mL D$_5$W with 200 mg of minocycline is to infuse in 6 hr. Drop factor: 15 gtt/mL

_____

23. An IV of D$_5$W 500 mL was ordered to infuse over 10 hr at a rate of 13 gtt/min (13 macrogtt/min). Drop factor: 15 gtt/mL After 3 hr, you notice that 300 mL of IV solution is left. Recalculate the rate in gtt/min for the remaining solution

_____ gtt/min

Determine the percentage of change in IV rate, and state your course of action.

_____ %

24. An IV of D$_5$W 1,000 mL was ordered to infuse over 8 hr at a rate of 42 gtt/min (42 macrogtt/min). Drop factor: 20 gtt/mL After 4 hr, you notice that only 400 mL has infused. Recalculate the rate in gtt/min for the remaining solution.

_____ gtt/min

Determine the percentage of change, and state your course of action.

_____ %

25. An IV of 1,000 mL D$_5$ 1/2 NS has been ordered to infuse at 125 mL/hr. Drop factor: 15 gtt/mL The IV was hung at 7 AM. At 11 AM, you check the IV, and there is 400 mL left. Recalculate the rate in gtt/min for the remaining solution.

_____ gtt/min

Determine the percentage of change, and state your course of action.

_____ %

26. 900 mL of RL is infusing at a rate of 80 gtt/min (80 macrodrops/min). Drop factor: 15 gtt/mL How long will it take for the IV to infuse? (Express time in hours and minutes.)

_____

27. 1,000 mL of D$_5$W is infusing at 20 gtt/min (20 macrogtt/min). Drop factor: 10 gtt/mL How long will it take for the IV to infuse? (Express time in hours and minutes.)

_____

28. 450 mL of NS is infusing at 25 gtt/min (25 macrogtt/min). Drop factor: 20 gtt/mL How many hours will it take for the IV to infuse?

_____

29. An IV is regulated at 25 gtt/min
    (25 macrogtt/min).
    Drop factor: 15 gtt/mL
    How many milliliters of fluid will the
    client receive in 8 hr?                                   _____

30. An IV is regulated at 30 gtt/min
    (30 macrogtt/min).
    Drop factor: 15 gtt/mL
    How many milliliters of fluid will the
    client receive in 5 hr?                                   _____

31. 10 mEq of potassium chloride is placed
    in 500 mL of $D_5W$ to be administered
    at the rate of 2 mEq/hr. At what rate in
    mL/hr should the IV infuse?                               _____

32. Order: Humulin regular 7 units/hr.
    The IV solution contains 50 units of
    Humulin regular insulin in 250 mL
    of 0.9% NS. At what rate in mL/hr
    should the IV infuse?                                     _____

33. Order: Humulin regular U-100 11 units/hr.
    The IV solution contains 100 units of
    Humulin regular insulin in 100 mL
    of 0.9% NS. At what rate in mL/hr
    should the IV infuse?                                     _____

34. Infuse gentamicin 65 mg in 150 mL
    0.9% NS IVPB over 1 hr.
    Drop factor: 10 gtt/mL
    At what rate in gtt/min should the
    IV infuse?                                                _____

35. Infuse ampicillin 1 g that has been diluted
    in 40 mL 0.9% NS to infuse in 40 minutes.
    Drop factor: 60 gtt/mL
    At what rate in gtt/min should the
    IV infuse?                                                _____

36. 50 mL of 0.9% NS with 1 g ampicillin
    is infusing at 50 microgtt/min (50 gtt/min).
    Drop factor: 60 gtt/mL
    Determine the infusion time.                             _____

37. 500 mL RL is to infuse at a rate of
    80 mL/hr. If the IV was started at 7 PM,
    what time will the IV be completed?                       _____
    State time in military and traditional
    time.                                                     _____

38. A volume of 150 mL of NS is to
    infuse at 25 mL/hr.
    a. Calculate the infusion time.    _____
    b. The IV was started at 3:10 AM.
       What time will the IV be completed?
       State time in traditional and military
       time.    _____

39. The doctor orders 2.5 L of $D_5W$ to
    infuse at 150 mL/hr. Determine the
    infusion time.    _____

40. Order: Lasix 120 mg IV stat.
    Available: 10 mg per mL. The literature
    states IV not to exceed 40 mg/min.
    a. How many milliliters will you
       prepare?    _____
    b. Calculate the time required to
       administer the medication as ordered.    _____

41. 500 mL $D_5W$ with 30,000 units of
    heparin to infuse at 1,500 units per
    hour.
    Determine rate in mL/hr.    _____

42. Order: Humulin regular 20 units
    per hr. The IV solution contains
    100 units of Humulin Regular in
    500 mL of 0.9% NS.
    At what rate in mL/hr should the
    IV infuse?    _____

43. Order: Infuse Cefazolin 1 g in 100 mL
    0.9% NS over 40 min by infusion pump.    _____

44. Order: Infuse Vancomycin 1 g in 200 mL
    $D_5W$ over 90 min by infusion pump.    _____

45. An IV of 1,000 mL of $D_5W$ is started 1045
    to infuse over 8½ hr. What is the completion
    time of the IV? (State time in military and
    traditional time.)    _____

46. 1,000 mL 0.9% NS was started at 2100 to infuse
    at 80 mL/hr. Determine the infusion and
    completion time. (State in military and
    traditional time.)    _____

**Answers on pp. 543-547**

Ⓔvolve

# ⭐ ANSWERS

## Chapter 21

### Answers to Practice Problems

1. $x\text{ mL/hr} = \dfrac{1,800\text{ mL}}{24\text{ hr}}; x = 75\text{ mL/hr}$

2. $x\text{ mL/hr} = \dfrac{2,000\text{ mL}}{24\text{ hr}} = 83.3; x = 83\text{ mL/hr}$

3. $x\text{ mL/hr} = \dfrac{500\text{ mL}}{12\text{ hr}} = 41.6; x = 42\text{ mL/hr}$

4. $x\text{ mL/hr} = \dfrac{1,500\text{ mL}}{24\text{ hr}} = 62.5; x = 63\text{ mL/hr}$

5. $x\text{ mL/hr} = \dfrac{750\text{ mL}}{16\text{ hr}} = 46.8; x = 47\text{ mL/hr}$

6. macrodrop

7. microdrop

8. macrodrop

> ✏️ **NOTE**
> Some problems related to calculating gtt/min can be calculated using the formula method, dimensional analysis, or the formula method, with hours converted to minutes where indicated.

9. $x\text{ gtt/min} = \dfrac{75\text{ mL} \times 10\text{ gtt/mL}}{60\text{ min}} =$

$$\frac{75 \times 10}{60} = \frac{75 \times 1}{6} = \frac{75}{6}$$

$x = \dfrac{75}{6} = 12.5$

$x = 13\text{ gtt/min; 13 macrogtt/min}$

10. $x\text{ gtt/min} = \dfrac{30\text{ mL} \times 60\text{ gtt/mL}}{60\text{ min}} =$

$$\frac{30 \times 60}{60} = \frac{30 \times 1}{1} = \frac{30}{1}$$

$x = \dfrac{30}{1}; x = 30$

$x = 30\text{ gtt/min; 30 microgtt/min}$

11. Step 1: Calculate mL/ hr.

$x\text{ mL/hr} = \dfrac{1,000\text{ mL}}{6\text{ hr}} = 166.6$

$x = 167$

Step 2: Calculate gtt/min.

$x\text{ gtt/min} = \dfrac{167\text{ mL} \times 15\text{ gtt/mL}}{60\text{ min}} =$

$$\frac{167 \times 15}{60} = \frac{167 \times 1}{4} = \frac{167}{4}$$

$x = \dfrac{167}{4} = 41.7$

$x = 42\text{ gtt/min; 42 macrogtt/min}$

12. $x\text{ gtt/min} = \dfrac{60\text{ mL} \times 60\text{ gtt/mL}}{45\text{ min}} =$

$$\frac{60 \times 60}{45} = \frac{60 \times 4}{3} = \frac{240}{3}$$

$x = \dfrac{240}{3}; x = 80$

$x = 80\text{ gtt/min; 80 microgtt/min}$

13. Step 1: Calculate mL/ hr.

$x\text{ mL/hr} = \dfrac{1,000\text{ mL}}{16\text{ hr}} = 62.5; x = 63\text{ mL/hr}$

Step 2: Calculate gtt/min.

$x\text{ gtt/min} = \dfrac{63\text{ mL} \times 15\text{ gtt/mL}}{60\text{ min}} =$

$$\frac{63 \times 15}{60} = \frac{63 \times 1}{4} = \frac{63}{4}$$

$x = \dfrac{63}{4} = 15.7 = 16$

$x = 16\text{ gtt/min; 16 macrogtt/min}$

14. Step 1: Calculate mL/ hr.

$x\text{ mL/hr} = \dfrac{3,000\text{ mL}}{24\text{ hr}}; x = 125\text{ mL/hr}$

Step 2: Calculate gtt/min.

$x\text{ gtt/min} = \dfrac{125\text{ mL} \times 10\text{ gtt/mL}}{60\text{ min}} =$

$$\frac{125 \times 10}{60} = \frac{125 \times 1}{6} = \frac{125}{6}$$

$x = \dfrac{125}{6} = 20.8 = 21$

$x = 21\text{ gtt/min; 21 macrogtt/min}$

15. Step 1: Calculate mL/ hr.

$x\text{ mL/hr} = \dfrac{2,000\text{ mL}}{12\text{ hr}} = 166.6 = 167$

$x = 167\text{ mL/ hr}$

Step 2: Calculate gtt/min.

$$x \text{ gtt/min} = \frac{167 \text{ mL} \times 15 \text{ gtt/mL}}{60 \text{ min}} =$$

$$\frac{167 \times 15}{60} = \frac{167 \times 1}{4} = \frac{167}{4}$$

$$x = \frac{167}{4} = 41.7 = 42$$

$x = 42$ gtt/min; 42 macrogtt/min

16. Step 1: Determine the drop factor constant.

$$60 \div 10 = 6$$

Step 2: Calculate gtt/min.

$$x \text{ gtt/min} = \frac{200 \text{ mL/hr}}{6} = 33.3 = 33$$

$x = 33$ gtt/min; 33 macrogtt/min

17. Step 1: Determine the drop factor constant.

$$60 \div 10 = 6$$

Step 2: Calculate gtt/min.

$$x \text{ gtt/min} = \frac{140 \text{ mL/hr}}{3} = 46.6 = 47$$

$x = 47$ gtt/min; 47 macrogtt/min

18. Step 1: Determine mL/hr.

$$x \text{ mL/hr} = \frac{1,000 \text{ mL}}{10 \text{ hr}}; x = 100 \text{ mL/hr}$$

Step 2: Determine the drop factor constant.

$$60 \div 10 = 6$$

Step 3: Calculate gtt/min.

$$x \text{ gtt/min} = \frac{100 \text{ mL/hr}}{6} = 16.6 = 17$$

$x = 17$ gtt/min; 17 macrogtt/min

19. Remember that small volumes are multiplied and expressed in mL/hr.

Step 1: Determine mL/hr.

40 mL/20 min = $40 \times 3$ ($3 \times 20$ min)

$= 120$ mL/hr

Step 2: Determine the drop factor constant.

$$60 \div 10 = 6$$

Step 3: Calculate gtt/min.

$$x \text{ gtt/min} = \frac{120 \text{ mL/hr}}{6} = 20$$

$x = 20$ gtt/min; 20 macrogtt/min

20. Step 1: Determine mL/hr.

$$x \text{ mL/hr} = \frac{2,500 \text{ mL}}{16 \text{ hr}} = 156.2 = 156$$

Step 2: Calculate gtt/min.

$$x \text{ gtt/min} = \frac{156 \text{ mL} \times 10 \text{ gtt/mL}}{60 \text{ min}} =$$

$$\frac{156 \times 10}{60} = \frac{156 \times 1}{6} = \frac{156}{6}$$

$$x = \frac{156}{6} = 26$$

$x = 26$ gtt/min; 26 macrogtt/min

21. $$x \text{ gtt/min} = \frac{100 \text{ mL} \times 60 \text{ gtt/mL}}{60 \text{ min}} =$$

$$\frac{100 \times 60}{60} = \frac{100 \times 1}{1} = \frac{100}{1}$$

$$x = \frac{100}{1} = 100$$

$x = 100$ gtt/min; 100 microgtt/min

22. $$x \text{ gtt/min} = \frac{250 \text{ mL} \times 10 \text{ gtt/mL}}{60 \text{ min}} =$$

$$\frac{250 \times 10}{60} = \frac{250 \times 1}{6} = \frac{250}{6}$$

$$x = \frac{250}{6} = 41.6 = 42$$

$x = 42$ gtt/min; 42 macrogtt/min

23. a. 1 g : 10 mL = 1 g : $x$ mL

*or*

$$\frac{1 \text{ g}}{1 \text{ g}} \times 10 \text{ mL} = x \text{ mL}$$

$x = 10$ mL

Answer: 10 mL. The dosage ordered is contained in a volume of 10 mL. 10 mL of medication is added to the 50 mL of IV solution to give a total of 60 mL.

b. $$x \text{ gtt/min} = \frac{60 \text{ mL} \times 10 \text{ gtt/mL}}{45 \text{ min}} =$$

$$\frac{60 \times 10}{45} = \frac{60 \times 2}{9} = \frac{120}{9}$$

$$x = \frac{120}{9} = 13.3 = 13$$

$x = 13$ gtt/min; 13 macrogtt/min

24. a. 150 mg : 1 mL = 900 mg : $x$ mL

*or*

$$\frac{900 \text{ mg}}{150 \text{ mg}} \times 1 \text{ mL} = x \text{ mL}$$

$x = 6$ mL

Answer: 6 mL. The dosage ordered is more than the available strength; therefore more than 1 mL is needed to administer the dosage ordered.

Alternate solution:

$$300 \text{ mg} : 2 \text{ mL} = 900 \text{ mg} : x \text{ mL}$$

*or*

$$\frac{900 \text{ mg}}{300 \text{ mg}} \times 2 \text{ mL} = x \text{ mL}$$

This setup would net the same answer.

b. $x \text{ gtt/min} = \dfrac{75 \text{ mL} \times 10 \text{ gtt/mL}}{30 \text{ min}} =$

$$\frac{75 \times 10}{30} = \frac{75 \times 1}{3} = \frac{75}{3}$$

$$x = \frac{75}{3} = 25$$

$x = 25$ gtt/min; 25 macrogtt/min

25. a. $50 \text{ mg} : 1 \text{ mL} = 500 \text{ mg} : x \text{ mL}$

*or*

$$\frac{500 \text{ mg}}{50 \text{ mg}} \times 1 \text{ mL} = x \text{ mL}$$

$$x = 10 \text{ mL}$$

Answer: 10 mL. The dosage ordered is greater than the available strength; therefore you will need more than 1 mL to administer the ordered dosage. The volume of medication is added to the 100 mL of IV solution to get a total of 110 mL.

b. $x \text{ gtt/min} = \dfrac{110 \text{ mL} \times 15 \text{ gtt/mL}}{60 \text{ min}} =$

$$\frac{110 \times 15}{60} = \frac{110 \times 1}{4} = \frac{110}{4}$$

$$x = \frac{110}{4} = 27.5 = 28$$

$x = 28$ gtt/min; 28 macrogtt/min

26. a. $50 \text{ mg} : 10 \text{ mL} = 20 \text{ mg} : x \text{ mL}$

*or*

$$\frac{20 \text{ mg}}{50 \text{ mg}} \times 10 \text{ mL} = x \text{ mL}$$

Answer: 4 mL. The dosage ordered is less than the available strength; therefore you will need less than 10 mL to administer the ordered dosage.

b. Calculate mL/hr.

$$x \text{ mL/hr} = \frac{300 \text{ mL}}{6 \text{ hr}}; x = 50 \text{ mL/hr}$$

27. a. $16 \text{ mg} : 1 \text{ mL} = 300 \text{ mg} : x \text{ mL}$

*or*

$$\frac{300 \text{ mg}}{16 \text{ mg}} \times 1 \text{ mL} = x \text{ mL}$$

Answer: 18.8 mL (18.75 mL rounded to the nearest tenth). The dosage ordered is more than the available strength; therefore you will need more than 1 mL to administer the ordered dosage.

b. $x \text{ gtt/min} = \dfrac{318.8 \text{ mL} \times 10 \text{ gtt/mL}}{60 \text{ min}} =$

$$\frac{318.8 \times 10}{60} = \frac{318.8 \times 1}{6} = \frac{318.8}{6}$$

$$x = \frac{318.8}{6} = 53.1 = 53$$

$x = 53$ gtt/min; 53 macrogtt/min

Alternate solution:

$$160 \text{ mg} : 10 \text{ mL} = 300 \text{ mg} : x \text{ mL}$$

*or*

$$\frac{300 \text{ mg}}{160 \text{ mg}} \times 10 \text{ mL} = x \text{ mL}$$

28. a. $10 \text{ mg} : 1 \text{ mL} = 100 \text{ mg} : x \text{ mL}$

*or*

$$\frac{100 \text{ mg}}{10 \text{ mg}} \times 1 \text{ mL} = x \text{ mL}$$

$$x = 10 \text{ mL}$$

The dosage ordered is greater than the available strength; therefore you will need more than 1 mL to administer the ordered dose. 100 mL of IV fluid and medication volume gives a total of 110 mL.

b. $x \text{ gtt/min} = \dfrac{110 \text{ mL} \times 10 \text{ gtt/mL}}{60 \text{ min}} =$

$$\frac{110 \times 10}{60} = \frac{110 \times 1}{6} = \frac{110}{6}$$

$$x = \frac{110}{6} = 18.3 = 18$$

$x = 18$ gtt/min; 18 macrogtt/min

29. $15 \text{ mEq} : 1,000 \text{ mL} = 2 \text{ mEq} : x \text{ mL}$

$$\frac{15x}{15} = \frac{2,000}{15} = 133.3$$

$$x = 133 \text{ mL/hr}$$

*or*

$$\frac{15 \text{ mEq}}{1,000 \text{ mL}} = \frac{2 \text{ mEq}}{x \text{ mL}}$$

Answer: 133 mL/hr to deliver 2 mEq of potassium chloride per hour.

30. 50 units : 250 mL = 10 units : $x$ mL

$$\frac{50x}{50} = \frac{2,500}{50}$$

$$x = 50 \text{ mL/hr}$$

*or*

$$\frac{50 \text{ units}}{250 \text{ mL}} = \frac{10 \text{ units}}{x \text{ mL}}$$

Answer: 50 mL/hr must be administered for the client to receive 10 units/hr.

31. $60 \text{ microgtt/min} = \dfrac{150 \text{ mL} \times 60 \text{ gtt/mL}}{x \text{ min}}$

$$60 = \frac{150 \times 60}{x}$$

$$60 = \frac{9,000}{x}$$

$$\frac{60x}{60} = \frac{9,000}{60}$$

$$x = 150 \text{ minutes}$$

60 min = 1 hr; 150 min ÷ 60 = 2.5 hr

Answer: $2\frac{1}{2}$ hr

32. $35 \text{ macrogtt/min} = \dfrac{x \text{ mL} \times 15 \text{ gtt/mL}}{300 \text{ min}}$

$$35 = x \, (\times) \, \frac{\cancel{15}^{\,1}}{\cancel{300}_{\,20}}$$

$$35 = \frac{x}{20}$$

$$x = 35 \times 20 = 700$$

$$x = 700 \text{ mL}$$

33. $60 \text{ microgtt/min} = \dfrac{90 \text{ mL} \times 60 \text{ gtt/mL}}{x \text{ min}}$

$$60 = \frac{90 \times 60}{x}$$

$$60 = \frac{5,400}{x}$$

$$\frac{60x}{60} = \frac{5,400}{60}$$

$$x = 90 \text{ minutes}$$

60 min = 1 hr; 90 min ÷ 60 = 1.5 hr = $1\frac{1}{2}$ hr

34. Step 1: Determine mL/hr for the remaining solution.

$$x \text{ mL/hr} = \frac{250 \text{ mL}}{3 \text{ hr}}; x = 83.3 = 83 \text{ mL/hr}$$

Step 2: Calculate gtt/min.

$$x \text{ gtt/min} = \frac{83 \text{ mL} \times 15 \text{ gtt/mL}}{60 \text{ min}} =$$

$$\frac{83 \times 15}{60} = \frac{83 \times 1}{4} = \frac{83}{4} = 20.7 = 21$$

a. $x = 21$ gtt/min; 21 macrogtt/min

b. Determine the percentage of change.

$$\frac{21 - 16}{16} = \frac{5}{16} = 0.312 = 31\%$$

c. Percentage of change is greater than 25%. Assess client. Consult prescriber; order may need to be revised.

Determine the acceptable range for variation.

16 + (16 ÷ 4) = 16 + 4 = 20 gtt/min (macrogtt/min)

16 − (16 ÷ 4) = 16 − 4 = 12 gtt/min (macrogtt/min)

The safe range is 12–20 gtt/min (macrodrop/min). The recalculated rate is 21, although only out of range by 1 gtt. It is greater than 25%.

35. Step 1: Determine mL/hr for the remaining solution.

$$x \text{ mL/hr} = \frac{200 \text{ mL}}{1.5 \text{ hr}} = 133.3 = 133 \text{ mL/hr}$$

Step 2: Calculate gtt/min.

$$x \text{ gtt/min} = \frac{133 \text{ mL} \times 15 \text{ gtt/mL}}{60 \text{ min}} =$$

$$\frac{133 \times 15}{60} = \frac{133 \times 1}{4} = \frac{133}{4}$$

$$x = \frac{133}{4} = 33.2 = 33$$

a. $x = 33$ gtt/min; 33 macrogtt/min

b. Determine the percentage of change.

$$\frac{33 - 21}{21} = \frac{12}{21} = 0.571 = 57\%$$

c. Percentage of change is greater than 25%. Assess client. Consult prescriber; order may need to be revised.

Determine the acceptable range for variation.

21 + (21 ÷ 4) = 21 + 5.25 = 26.25 = 26 gtt/min (macrogtt/min)

21 − (21 ÷ 4) = 21 − 5.25 = 15.75 = 16 gtt/min (macrogtt/min)

The safe range is 16–20 gtt/min (macrogtt/min). The recalculated rate is 33 gtt/min (macrogtt). No, increasing the IV rate is greater than 25%.

36. Step 1: Determine mL/hr for the remaining solution.

$$x \text{ mL/hr} = \frac{750 \text{ mL}}{8 \text{ hr}} = 93.7 = 94$$

$$x = 94 \text{ mL/hr}$$

Step 2:  Calculate gtt/min.

$$x \text{ gtt/min} = \frac{94 \text{ mL} \times 20 \text{ gtt/mL}}{60 \text{ min}} =$$

$$\frac{94 \times 20}{60} = \frac{94 \times 1}{3} = \frac{94}{3}$$

$$x = \frac{94}{3} = 31.3 = 31$$

a.  $x = 31$ gtt/min; 31 macrogtt/min

b.  Determine the percentage of change.

$$\frac{31 - 28}{28} = \frac{3}{28} = 0.107 = 11\%$$

c.  The percentage of change is 11%. This is an acceptable increase. Assess if client can tolerate adjustment in rate. Check if allowed by institution policy.

Determine the acceptable range of variation.

$28 + (28 \div 4) = 28 + 7 = 35$ gtt/min (macrogtt/min)

$28 - (28 \div 4) = 28 - 7 = 21$ gtt/min (macrogtt/min)

The safe range is 21–35 gtt/min (macrogtt/min). The recalculated rate is 31. It is safe to increase the IV rate, which falls within the safe ±25% range.

37.  Step 1:  Determine mL/hr for remaining solution.

$$x \text{ mL/hr} = \frac{250 \text{ mL}}{3 \text{ hr}} = 83.3 = 83$$

$$x = 83 \text{ mL/hr}$$

Step 2:  Calculate gtt/min.

$$x \text{ gtt/min} = \frac{83 \text{ mL} \times 60 \text{ gtt/mL}}{60 \text{ min}} =$$

$$\frac{83 \times 60}{60} = \frac{83 \times 1}{1} = \frac{83}{1}$$

a.  $x = 83$ gtt/min; 83 microgtt/min

b.  Determine the percentage of change.

$$\frac{83 - 100}{100} = \frac{-17}{100} = -0.17 = -17\%$$

c.  The percentage of change is $-17\%$. This is an acceptable decrease. Assess client to see if able to tolerate adjustment in rate. Check if allowed by institution policy.

Determine the acceptable range for variation.

$100 + (100 \div 4) = 100 + 25 = 125$ gtt/min (microdrop)

$100 - (100 \div 4) = 100 - 25 = 75$ gtt/min (microdrop)

The safe range is 75–125 gtt/min (microdrop). The recalculated rate is 83 gtt/min (microdrop). It is safe to

decrease the rate to slow the rate to 83 gtt/min (microgtt), which is within the safe ±25% range.

38.  $\dfrac{500 \text{ mL}}{60 \text{ mL/hr}} = 8.33$ hr

0.33 hr $\times$ 60 min/hr $= 19.8 = 20$ min

a.  Answer: 8 hr + 20 min = infusion time

b.  Answer: 6:20 AM (10:00 PM + 8 hr + 20 min) *or* military time 0620 (2200 + 0820 = 3020 3020 − 2400 = 0620)

39.  $\dfrac{250 \text{ mL}}{80 \text{ mL/hr}} = 3.12$ hr

0.12 hr $\times$ 60 min/hr $= 7.2 = 7$ min

a.  Answer: 3 hr + 7 min = infusion time

b.  Answer: 5:07 AM (2:00 AM + 3 hr + 7 min) *or* military time 0507 (0200 + 0307 = 0507)

40.  $\dfrac{1,000 \text{ mL}}{60 \text{ mL/hr}} = 16.66$ hr

0.66 hr $\times$ 60 min/hr $= 39.6 = 40$ min

a.  Answer: 16 hr + 40 min = infusion time

b.  Answer: 10:40 PM (6:00 AM + 16 hr + 40 min) *or* military time 2240 (0600 + 1640 = 2240)

41.  $\dfrac{500 \text{ mL}}{75 \text{ mL/hr}} = 6.66$ hr

0.66 hr $\times$ 60 min/hr $= 39.6 = 40$ min

a.  Answer: 6 hr + 40 minutes = infusion time

b.  Answer: 8:40 PM (2:00 PM + 6 hr + 40 min) *or* military time 2040 (1400 + 0640 = 2040)

42.  Step 1:     15 gtt : 1 mL = 17 gtt : $x$ mL

$$\frac{15x}{15} = \frac{17}{15}$$

$$x = 17 \div 15 = 1.13 = 1.1 \text{ mL/min}$$

Step 2: 1.1 mL/min $\times$ 60 min/hr $= 66$ mL/hr

Step 3: $\dfrac{250 \text{ mL}}{66 \text{ mL/hr}} = 3.78$ hr

60 min/hr $\times$ 0.78 hr $= 46.8 = 47$ min

Answer: 3 hr + 47 min = infusion time

43.  Step 1: 10 gtt : 1 mL = 20 gtt : $x$ mL

$$\frac{10x}{10} = \frac{20}{10}$$

$$x = 2 \text{ mL/min}$$

Step 2: 2 mL/min $\times$ 60 min/hr $= 120$ mL/hr

Step 3: $\dfrac{1,000 \text{ mL}}{120 \text{ mL/hr}} = 8.33$ hr

60 min/hr $\times$ 0.33 hr $= 19.8 = 20$ min

Answer: 8 hr 20 min = infusion time

44. Step 1: 15 gtt : 1 mL = 10 gtt : $x$ mL

$$\frac{15x}{15} = \frac{10}{15} = 0.666 = 0.67$$

$$x = 0.67 \text{ mL/min}$$

Step 2: 0.67 mL/min × 60 min/hr =
40.2 mL/hr = 40 mL/hr

Step 3: $\dfrac{100 \text{ mL}}{40 \text{ mL/hr}} = 2.5 \text{ hr}$

Answer: 2 hr 30 min = infusion time

45. Step 1: 60 gtt : 1 mL = 35 gtt : $x$ mL

$$\frac{60x}{60} = \frac{35}{60}$$

$$x = 0.58 \text{ mL/min}$$

Step 2: 20 mL ÷ 0.58 mL/min = 34.4 = 34 min

Answer: 34 min = infusion time

46. a. 5 mg : 1 mL = 20 mg : $x$ mL

$$\frac{5x}{5} = \frac{20}{5}$$

$$x = 4 \text{ mL}$$

Answer: 4 mL. The dosage ordered is greater than the available strength; therefore more than 1 mL is needed to administer the dosage ordered.

*or*

$$\frac{20 \text{ mg}}{5 \text{ mg}} \times 1 \text{ mL} = x \text{ mL}$$

$$x \text{ mL} = \frac{1 \text{ mL}}{5 \text{ mg}} \times \frac{20 \text{ mg}}{1}$$

b. 5 mg : 1 min = 20 mg : $x$ min

$$\frac{5x}{5} = \frac{20}{5}$$

$$x = 4 \text{ min}$$

c. 5 mg : 60 sec = $x$ mg : 15 sec

$$\frac{60x}{60} = \frac{15}{60}$$

$$x = 1.25 \text{ mg per 15 sec}$$

47. a. 250 mg : 5 mL = 150 mg : $x$ mL

$$\frac{250x}{250} = \frac{750}{250}$$

$$x = 3 \text{ mL}$$

*or*

$$\frac{150 \text{ mg}}{250 \text{ mg}} \times 5 \text{ mL} = x \text{ mL}$$

Answer: 3 mL. The dosage ordered is less than the available strength; therefore you would need less than 5 mL to administer the dosage ordered.

b. 50 mg : 1 min = 150 mg : $x$ min

$$\frac{50x}{50} = \frac{150}{50}$$

$$x = 3 \text{ min}$$

## Answers to Clinical Reasoning Questions

a. The nurse was accustomed to using 20 gtt/mL and calculated the IV rate using 20 gtt/mL. The tubing used at the institution delivered 10 gtt/mL, and the nurse did not check the drop factor on the IV set package. Failure to check the drop factor of the IV tubing resulted in an incorrect IV rate.

b. Because of the excessive IV rate, the client developed signs of fluid overload and could have developed congestive heart failure.

c. The nurse should never assume what the drop factor for IV tubing is for macrodrop administration sets because they can vary. The nurse should have checked the IV tubing package for the drop factor, which is printed on the package.

## Answers to Chapter Review

> **NOTE**
> Many of the IV problems involving gtt/min could also be done by using the shortcut method or dimensional analysis.

> **NOTE**
> Some answers in the Chapter Review reflect the number of drops rounded to the nearest whole number and the rate in mL/hr.

1. a. Determine mL/hr.

   $$x \text{ mL/hr} = \frac{2,500 \text{ mL}}{24 \text{ hr}}; x = 104 \text{ mL/hr}$$

   b. Calculate gtt/min.

   $$x \text{ gtt/min} = \frac{104 \text{ mL} \times 10 \text{ gtt/mL}}{60 \text{ min}}$$

   $$x = 17 \text{ gtt/min}; 17 \text{ macrogtt/min}$$

2. a. Determine mL/hr.

   $$x \text{ mL/hr} = \frac{500 \text{ mL}}{4 \text{ hr}}; x = 125 \text{ mL/hr}$$

   b. Calculate gtt/min.

   $$x \text{ gtt/min} = \frac{125 \text{ mL} \times 15 \text{ gtt/mL}}{60 \text{ min}}$$

   $$x = 31 \text{ gtt/min}; 31 \text{ macrogtt/min}$$

3. a. Determine mL/hr.

$$x\,\text{mL/hr} = \frac{300\,\text{mL}}{6\,\text{hr}}; x = 50\,\text{mL/hr}$$

 b. Calculate gtt/min.

$$x\,\text{gtt/min} = \frac{50\,\text{mL} \times 60\,\text{gtt/mL}}{60\,\text{min}}$$

$x = 50$ gtt/min; 50 microgtt/min

4. a. Determine mL/hr.

$$x\,\text{mL/hr} = \frac{500\,\text{mL}}{12\,\text{hr}} = x = 42\,\text{mL/hr}$$

 b. Calculate gtt/min.

$$x\,\text{gtt/min} = \frac{42\,\text{mL} \times 20\,\text{gtt/mL}}{60\,\text{min}}$$

$x = 14$ gtt/min; 14 macrogtt/min

5. a. Determine mL/hr.

$$x\,\text{mL/hr} = \frac{500\,\text{mL}}{4\,\text{hr}}; x = 125\,\text{mL/hr}$$

 b. Calculate gtt/min.

$$x\,\text{gtt/min} = \frac{125\,\text{mL} \times 10\,\text{gtt/mL}}{60\,\text{min}}$$

$x = 21$ gtt/min; 21 macrogtt/min

6. 1 L = 1,000 mL

 2 L = 2,000 mL

 a. Determine mL/hr.

$$x\,\text{mL/hr} = \frac{2,000\,\text{mL}}{24\,\text{hr}}; x = 83\,\text{mL/hr}$$

 b. Calculate gtt/min.

$$x\,\text{gtt/min} = \frac{83\,\text{mL} \times 15\,\text{gtt/mL}}{60\,\text{min}}$$

$x = 21$ gtt/min; 21 macrogtt/min

7. a. Determine mL/hr.

$$x\,\text{mL/hr} = \frac{1,000\,\text{mL}}{6\,\text{hr}}; x = 167\,\text{mL/hr}$$

 b. Calculate gtt/min.

$$x\,\text{gtt/min} = \frac{167\,\text{mL} \times 20\,\text{gtt/mL}}{60\,\text{min}}$$

$x = 56$ gtt/min; 56 macrogtt/min

8. a. Determine mL/hr.

$$x\,\text{mL/hr} = \frac{250\,\text{mL}}{8\,\text{hr}}; x = 31\,\text{mL/hr}$$

 b. Calculate gtt/min.

$$x\,\text{gtt/min} = \frac{31\,\text{mL} \times 60\,\text{gtt/mL}}{60\,\text{min}}$$

$x = 31$ gtt/min; 31 microgtt/min

9. $x\,\text{gtt/min} = \dfrac{150\,\text{mL} \times 15\,\text{gtt/mL}}{60\,\text{min}}$

$x = 38$ gtt/min; 38 macrogtt/min

10. a. Determine mL/hr.

$$x\,\text{mL/hr} = \frac{1,500\,\text{mL}}{24\,\text{hr}}; x = 63\,\text{mL/hr}$$

 b. Calculate gtt/min.

$$x\,\text{gtt/min} = \frac{63\,\text{mL} \times 15\,\text{gtt/mL}}{60\,\text{min}}$$

$x = 16$ gtt/min; 16 macrogtt/min

11. a. Determine mL/hr.

$$x\,\text{mL/hr} = \frac{250\,\text{mL}}{10\,\text{hr}}; x = 25\,\text{mL/hr}$$

 b. Calculate gtt/min.

$$x\,\text{gtt/min} = \frac{25\,\text{mL} \times 60\,\text{gtt/mL}}{60\,\text{min}}$$

$x = 25$ gtt/min; 25 microgtt/min

12. $x\,\text{gtt/min} = \dfrac{75\,\text{mL} \times 60\,\text{gtt/mL}}{60\,\text{min}}$

$x = 75$ gtt/min; 75 microgtt/min

13. $x\,\text{gtt/min} = \dfrac{50\,\text{mL} \times 60\,\text{gtt/mL}}{45\,\text{min}}$

$x = 67$ gtt/min; 67 microgtt/min

14. $x\,\text{gtt/min} = \dfrac{90\,\text{mL} \times 15\,\text{gtt/mL}}{60\,\text{min}}$

$x = 23$ gtt/min; 23 macrogtt/min

15. $x\,\text{gtt/min} = \dfrac{100\,\text{mL} \times 20\,\text{gtt/mL}}{30\,\text{min}}$

$x = 67$ gtt/min; 67 macrogtt/min

16. a. Determine mL/ hr.

$$x\,\text{mL/hr} = \frac{250\,\text{mL}}{5\,\text{hr}}; x = 50\,\text{mL/hr}$$

 b. Calculate gtt/min.

$$x\,\text{gtt/min} = \frac{50\,\text{mL} \times 20\,\text{gtt/mL}}{60\,\text{min}}$$

$x = 17$ gtt/min; 17 macrogtt/min

17. $x\,\text{gtt/min} = \dfrac{50\,\text{mL} \times 60\,\text{gtt/mL}}{30\,\text{min}}$

$x = 100$ gtt/min; 100 microgtt/min

18. a. Determine mL/hr.

$$x\,\text{mL/hr} = \frac{500\,\text{mL}}{3\,\text{hr}}; x = 167\,\text{mL/hr}$$

 b. Calculate gtt/min.

$$x\,\text{gtt/min} = \frac{167\,\text{mL} \times 10\,\text{gtt/mL}}{60\,\text{min}}$$

$x = 28$ gtt/min; 28 macrogtt/min

19. a. Determine mL/hr.

$$x \, \text{mL/hr} = \frac{1{,}750 \, \text{mL}}{24 \, \text{hr}}; x = 73 \, \text{mL/hr}$$

  b. Calculate gtt/min.

$$x \, \text{gtt/min} = \frac{73 \, \text{mL} \times 10 \, \text{gtt/mL}}{60 \, \text{min}}$$

$$x = 12 \, \text{gtt/min; 12 macrogtt/min}$$

20. $x \, \text{mL/hr} = \dfrac{500 \, \text{mL}}{8 \, \text{hr}}; x = 63 \, \text{mL/hr}$

21. a. Determine mL/hr.

$$x \, \text{mL/hr} = \frac{500 \, \text{mL}}{6 \, \text{hr}}; x = 83 \, \text{mL/hr}$$

  b. Calculate gtt/min.

$$x \, \text{gtt/min} = \frac{83 \, \text{mL} \times 10 \, \text{gtt/mL}}{60 \, \text{min}}$$

$$x = 14 \, \text{gtt/min; 14 macrogtt/min}$$

22. a. Determine mL/hr.

$$x \, \text{mL/hr} = \frac{500 \, \text{mL}}{6 \, \text{hr}}; x = 83 \, \text{mL/hr}$$

  b. Calculate gtt/min.

$$x \, \text{gtt/min} = \frac{83 \, \text{mL} \times 15 \, \text{gtt/mL}}{60 \, \text{min}}$$

$$x = 21 \, \text{gtt/min; 21 macrogtt/min}$$

23. Time remaining = 7 hr

Volume remaining = 300 mL

  a. Determine mL/hr for remaining solution.

$$x \, \text{mL/hr} = \frac{300 \, \text{mL}}{7 \, \text{hr}}; x = 43 \, \text{mL/hr}$$

  b. Determine gtt/min (recalculated rate).

$$x \, \text{gtt/min} = \frac{43 \, \text{mL} \times 15 \, \text{gtt/mL}}{60 \, \text{min}}$$

$$x = 11 \, \text{gtt/min}$$

Answer: 11 macrogtt/min; 11 gtt/min

  c. Determine the percentage change.

$$\frac{11 - 13}{13} = \frac{-2}{13} = -0.153 = -15\%$$

The −15% is within the acceptable 25% variation. Assess if client can tolerate adjustment in rate.

Negative percentage of variation (−15%) indicates the adjusted rate will be decreased. Assess client, check institution policy, and continue to assess client during rate change.

Determine accepted range of variation.

$13 + (13 \div 4) = 13 + 3.25 = 16.25 = 16$ gtt/min (macrogtt/min)

$13 - (13 \div 4) = 13 - 3.25 = 9.75 = 10$ gtt/min (macrogtt/min)

The acceptable range is 10–16 gtt/min (macrogtt/min). The recalculated rate is 11 gtt/min (macrogtt/min). It is

safe to slow the IV rate to 11 gtt/min (macrogtt/min), which is in the safe range. It is below 25%.

24. Time remaining = 4 hr

Volume remaining = 600 mL

  a. Determine mL/hr for remaining solution.

$$x \, \text{mL/hr} = \frac{600 \, \text{mL}}{4 \, \text{hr}}; x = 150 \, \text{mL/hr}$$

  b. Determine gtt/min (recalculated rate).

$$x \, \text{gtt/min} = \frac{150 \, \text{mL} \times 20 \, \text{gtt/mL}}{60 \, \text{min}}$$

$$x = 50 \, \text{gtt/min}$$

Answer: 50 gtt/min; 50 macrogtt/min

  c. Determine the percentage change.

$$\frac{50 - 42}{42} = \frac{8}{42} = 0.190 = 19\%$$

The percentage of change is 19%. This is an acceptable increase. Assess if client can tolerate the adjustment in rate (42 gtt/min to 50 gtt/min). Check if allowed by institution policy. Assess client during rate change.

Determine accepted range of variation.

$42 + (42 \div 4) = 42 + 10.5 = 52.5 = 53$ gtt/min (macrodrop)

$42 - (42 \div 4) = 42 - 10.5 = 31.5 = 32$ gtt/min (macrodrop)

The acceptable range is 32–53 gtt/min (macrodrop). The recalculated rate is 50 gtt/min (macrodrop). The IV increase to 50 gtt/min (macrogtt) is within the safe range of 25%.

25. Time remaining = 4 hr

Volume remaining = 400 mL

  a. Determine mL/hr for remaining solution.

$$x \, \text{mL/hr} = \frac{400 \, \text{mL}}{4 \, \text{hr}}; x = 100 \, \text{mL/hr}$$

After determining mL/hr, gtt/min is recalculated.

  b. Determine gtt/min (recalculated rate).

$$x \, \text{gtt/min} = \frac{100 \, \text{mL} \times 15 \, \text{gtt/mL}}{60 \, \text{min}}$$

$$x = 25 \, \text{gtt/min}$$

Answer: 25 gtt/min; 25 macrogtt/min

  c. Determine the percentage change. The IV was ahead. The original IV order was 125 mL/hr = 31 gtt/min (31 macrogtt/min). The IV would have to be decreased from 31 gtt/min (31 macrogtt/min) to 25 gtt/min (25 macrogtt/min).

$$\frac{25 - 31}{31} = \frac{-6}{31} = -0.193 = -19\%$$

The −19% is within acceptable 25% variation. Assess if client can tolerate the adjustment in rate. Negative percentage of variation (−19%) indicates the adjusted rate will be decreased. Check institution policy. Assess client during rate change.

Determine accepted range of variation.

$31 + (31 \div 4) = 31 + 7.75 = 38.75 = 39$ gtt/min (macrogtt/min)

$31 - (31 \div 4) = 31 - 7.75 = 23.25 = 23$ gtt/min (macrogtt/min)

The accepted range is 23–39 gtt/min (macrogtt). The recalculated rate is 25 gtt/min (macrogtt/min). It is safe to slow the rate to 25 gtt/min (macrogtt/min) which is within the safe range of 25%.

26. 80 macrogtt/min (80 gtt/min) =
$$\frac{900 \text{ mL} \times 15 \text{ gtt/mL}}{x \text{ min}}$$
$$80 = \frac{900 \times 15}{x}$$
$$\frac{80x}{80} = \frac{13,500}{80}$$
$$x = 168.75 \text{ minutes}$$

60 min = 1 hr; 168.75 ÷ 60 = 2.81 hr

Time: 2.81 hr. Since 0.81 represents a fraction of an additional hour, 0.81 ~~hr~~ × 60 min/~~hr~~ 48.6 = 49 min.

Answer: 2 hr and 49 min

27. 20 macrogtt/min (20 gtt/min) =
$$\frac{1,000 \text{ mL} \times 10 \text{ gtt/mL}}{x \text{ min}}$$
$$20 = \frac{1,000 \times 10}{x}$$
$$\frac{20x}{20} = \frac{10,000}{20}$$
$$x = 500 \text{ min}$$

60 min = 1 hr; 500 ÷ 60 = 8.33 hr

Time: 8.33 hr

$0.33$ ~~hr~~ × 60 min/~~hr~~ = 19.8 = 20 min

Answer: 8 hr and 20 min

28. 25 macrogtt/min (25 gtt/min) =
$$\frac{450 \text{ mL} \times 20 \text{ gtt/mL}}{x \text{ min}}$$
$$25 = \frac{450 \times 20}{x}$$
$$\frac{25x}{25} = \frac{9,000}{25}$$
$$x = 360 \text{ min}$$

60 min = 1 hr; 360 ÷ 60 = 6 hr

**NOTE**
For problems 29-30: Formula, time expressed in minutes (60 min = 1 hr).

29. 25 macrogtt/min (25 gtt/min) =
$$\frac{x \text{ mL} \times 15 \text{ gtt/mL}}{480 \text{ min}}$$
$$25 = \frac{x \times 15}{480}$$
$$25 = \frac{15x}{480}$$
$$\frac{15x}{15} = \frac{25 \times 480}{15}$$
$$\frac{15x}{15} = \frac{12,000}{15}$$
$$x = 800 \text{ mL}$$

30. 30 macrogtt/min (30 gtt/min) = $\dfrac{x \text{ mL} \times 15 \text{ gtt/mL}}{300 \text{ min}}$
$$30 = \frac{x \times 15}{300}$$
$$30 = \frac{15x}{300}$$
$$\frac{15x}{15} = \frac{30 \times 300}{15}$$
$$\frac{15x}{15} = \frac{9,000}{15}$$
$$x = 600 \text{ mL}$$

**NOTE**
For problems 31-33, a ratio and proportion could be set up in a format other than the one shown in the problems.

31. 10 mEq : 500 mL = 2 mEq : x mL
$$10x = 500 \times 2$$
$$\frac{10x}{10} = \frac{1,000}{10}$$
$$x = 100 \text{ mL/ hr would be needed to infuse}$$
2 mEq/hr of potassium chloride

32. 50 units : 250 mL = 7 units : x mL
$$\frac{50x}{50} = \frac{1,750}{50}; x = 35 \text{ mL/ hr would be needed to}$$
infuse 7 units/hr of Humulin Regular insulin

33. 100 units : 100 mL = 11 units : x mL
$$\frac{100x}{100} = \frac{1,100}{100}; x = 11 \text{ mL/ hr of fluid would be}$$
needed to infuse 11 units/hr of Humulin Regular insulin

34. $x \text{ gtt/min} = \dfrac{150 \text{ mL} \times 10 \text{ gtt/mL}}{60 \text{ min}}$

    $x = 25 \text{ gtt/min}; 25 \text{ macrogtt/min}$

35. $x \text{ gtt/min} = \dfrac{40 \text{ mL} \times 60 \text{ gtt/mL}}{40 \text{ min}}$

    $x = 60 \text{ gtt/min}; 60 \text{ microgtt/min}$

36. Step 1: $60 \text{ gtt} : 1 \text{ mL} = 50 \text{ gtt} : x \text{ mL}$

    $\dfrac{60x}{60} = \dfrac{50}{60}$

    $x = 50 \div 60; x = 0.83 \text{ mL/min}$

    Step 2: $0.83 \text{ mL/}\cancel{\text{min}} \times 60 \cancel{\text{min}}\text{/hr} =$
    $49.8 = 50 \text{ mL/hr}$

    Step 3: $\dfrac{50 \cancel{\text{mL}}}{50 \cancel{\text{mL}}\text{/hr}} = 1 \text{ hr}$

    Answer: 1 hr = infusion time

37. Step 1: $\dfrac{500 \cancel{\text{mL}}}{80 \cancel{\text{mL}}\text{/hr}} = 6.25 \text{ hr}$

    Step 2: $60 \text{ min/}\cancel{\text{hr}} \times 0.25 \cancel{\text{hr}} = 15 \text{ min}$

    6 hr and 15 min = infusion time

    Step 3: $7{:}00 \text{ PM} + 6 \text{ hr} + 15 \text{ min}$ *or* $1900 + 0615 =$
    $2515 - 2400 = 0115$

    Answer: 1:15 AM; military time: 0115

38. $\dfrac{150 \cancel{\text{mL}}}{25 \cancel{\text{mL}}\text{/hr}} = 6 \text{ hr}$

    a. 6 hr = infusion time

    b. (3:10 AM + 6 hr = 9:10 AM). IV will be completed at 9:10 AM; military time: 0910.

39. Conversion is required. Equivalent:

    1 L = 1,000 mL

    Therefore 2.5 L = 2,500 mL

    Step 1: $\dfrac{2{,}500 \cancel{\text{mL}}}{150 \cancel{\text{mL}}\text{/hr}} = 16.66 \text{ hr}$

    Step 2: $60 \text{ min/}\cancel{\text{hr}} \times 0.66 \cancel{\text{hr}} = 39.6 = 40 \text{ min}$

    16 hr and 40 min = infusion time

40. a. $10 \text{ mg} : 1 \text{ mL} = 120 \text{ mg} : x \text{ mL}$

    $\dfrac{10x}{10} = \dfrac{120}{10}; x = 12 \text{ mL}$

    *or*

    $\dfrac{120 \text{ mg}}{10 \text{ mg}} \times 1 \text{ mL} = x \text{ mL}$

    Answer: 12 mL. The dosage ordered is more than the available strength; therefore more than 1 mL would be required to administer the dosage ordered.

    b. $40 \text{ mg} : 1 \text{ min} = 120 \text{ mg} : x \text{ min}$

    $\dfrac{40x}{40} = \dfrac{120}{40}; x = 3 \text{ min}$

    Answer: 3 min

41. $30{,}000 \text{ units} : 500 \text{ mL} = 1{,}500 \text{ units} : x \text{ mL}$

    $\dfrac{30{,}000x}{30{,}000} = \dfrac{750{,}000}{30{,}000}$

    $x = \dfrac{750{,}000}{30{,}000} = 25$

    $x = 25 \text{ mL/hr}$ of fluid would be needed to infuse 1,500 units/hr of heparin

42. $100 \text{ units} : 500 \text{ mL} = 20 \text{ units} : x \text{ mL}$

    $\dfrac{100x}{100} = \dfrac{10{,}000}{100} = 100$

    $x = 100 \text{ mL/hr}$ of fluid would be needed to infuse 20 units/hr of Humulin Regular insulin

43. $100 \text{ mL} : 40 \text{ min} = x \text{ mL} : 60 \text{ min}$

    $\dfrac{40 \, x}{40} = \dfrac{6000}{40}$

    $x = 150 \text{ mL/hr}$

    *or*

    $x \text{ mL/hr} = \dfrac{100 \text{ mL}}{\underset{2}{\cancel{40 \text{ min}}}} = \dfrac{\overset{3}{\cancel{60 \text{ min}}}\text{/hr}}{1}$

    $x = \dfrac{300}{2}$

    $x = 150 \text{ mL/hr}$

44. $x \text{ mL hr} = \dfrac{200 \text{ mL}}{1.5 \text{ hr}} = 133.3 = 133$

    $x = 133 \text{ mL/hr}$

45. 1045 start time

    $\dfrac{+0830}{1875}$ infusion time

    $\dfrac{-0060}{1815}$ (subtract 60 min; minutes greater than 60 min)

    $\dfrac{+0100}{1915}$ (addition of the hour that was subtracted)
    1915 (7:15 PM)

    Answer: 1915; 7:15 PM

    Alternate solution:

    1045 start time

    $\dfrac{+0830}{1875}$ infusion time

    Convert 75 min to 1 hr and 15 min and add to 1800.

    $\dfrac{+0115}{1915}$ (7:15 PM)

46. Step 1: Determine infusion time

    $\dfrac{1{,}000 \cancel{\text{mL}}}{80 \cancel{\text{mL}}\text{/hr}} = 12.5 \ (12\frac{1}{2} \text{ hr})$

    Step 2: Determine completion time.

    2100 start time

    $\dfrac{+1230}{3330}$ (time period greater than 24 hr)

    $\dfrac{-2400}{0930}$ or 9:30 AM the next day

    Answer: Infusion time 12½ hr (12.5 hr); completion time 0930; 9:30 AM

# CHAPTER 22
# Heparin Calculations

## Objectives

*After reviewing this chapter, you should be able to:*

1. State the importance of calculating heparin dosages accurately
2. Identify errors that have occurred with heparin administration
3. Calculate subcutaneous dosages of heparin
4. Calculate heparin dosages being administered intravenously (mL per hr, units per hr)
5. Calculate safe heparin dosages based on weight

## Heparin Errors

Heparin is an anticoagulant medication used to prevent the formation of blood clots, and it is identified as a ***high-alert*** medication because it carries a significant risk of causing serious injury or death to a client if misused. Despite the identification of heparin as being a high-alert medication, errors that involve the use of heparin have been well documented in the literature. Some of the cited causes of errors include mix-ups with concentrations of heparin, inadequate client monitoring, and calculation errors.

The occurrence of errors with anticoagulant medications prompted attention from organizations such as the Institute for Safe Medication Practices (ISMP), The Joint Commission (TJC), the Food and Drug Administration (FDA), and the United States Pharmacopeia (USP). The focus of these organizations was to minimize the potential for medication errors associated with anticoagulant therapy and reduce client harm from their use. TJC developed a National Patient Safety Goal (NPSG) [03.05.01] to address a hospital's responsibilities for the administration of anticoagulant therapy to reduce the likelihood of client harm. The NPSG includes client monitoring (baseline and ongoing laboratory tests) and the use of programmable infusion pumps when heparin is administered IV and continuously. The current National Patient Safety Goals (effective January 2020) can be viewed on TJC's website at www.jointcommission.org. The updated USP label standards for heparin became effective in 2013. The labeling standards for Heparin Sodium Injection, USP, and Heparin Lock Flush Solution, USP, were updated to clearly state the total dosage strength on the label, followed by the dosage strength per milliliter enclosed in parentheses. Other label enhancements will be discussed further in this chapter with the discussion of sample heparin labels.

There have been safety protocols instituted in many health care institutions related to the administration of heparin; these include (1) independent double-checks of heparin dosages (another nurse independently double-checking calculations before administration) and (2) the use of a weight-based protocol that uses the client's weight in kilograms (kg) as the basis for determining heparin bolus doses and infusion rates, which will be discussed later in this chapter. Although in some health care settings nurses prepare and mix IV heparin, the trend is to use premixed preparations of heparin from the manufacturer or have the pharmacy mix the solution. Strategies to reduce errors and therefore reduce the risk of harm to clients incorporate the Quality and Safety Education for Nurses (QSEN) competency of safety.

Heparin requires close monitoring of the client's blood work because of the bleeding potential associated with anticoagulant medications. Some heparin protocols also use the activated partial thromboplastin time (aPTT or APTT) to monitor the client's clotting values while receiving heparin. Another laboratory test being used is the measurement of anti-factor Xa levels.

As nurses, it is important to remember that even though heparin is commonly used in clinical practice, client safety during administration is an essential priority and needs to include correct calculations, client monitoring, and adherence to safety protocols to prevent errors and harm to a client.

## Heparin Administration

Heparin can be administered subcutaneously or intravenously; it is **never** administered intramuscularly because of the danger of hematomas (collections of extravasated blood trapped in tissues of skin or in an organ). Heparin therapy frequently consists of a combination of prescribed intermittent IV boluses (large doses to achieve a rapid therapeutic effect), followed by continuous IV infusion. When administered as a continuous IV infusion, the heparin dosage rate may be ordered in units/hr or mL/hr or individualized by weight as units per kilogram per hour (units/kg/hr). To maintain a constant rate, accurate dosing, and safe administration, IV heparin is always administered by an electronic infusion device. Only a syringe measured in milliliters should be used to measure a heparin dose. When calculating dosages of heparin, it is ordered in units and the medication is in units; there is no conversion of units.

## Heparin Dosage Strengths

Heparin is available in single-dose and multi-dose vials as well as in commercially prepared IV solutions and prefilled syringes. Heparin is available in various concentrations such as 1,000, 2,000, 5,000, and 10,000 units per mL and higher. Heparin Lock Flush Solution, which is used for flushing (e.g., med-locks, specialized IV lines), is available in 10 and 100 units per mL. The higher concentrations of heparin are used for anticoagulant therapy. Commercially prepared IV solutions with heparin are also available from pharmaceutical companies in several strengths. The dosage of heparin is written in red on IV bags to attract attention to the fact that the IV solution contains heparin.

> **(!) SAFETY ALERT!**
> The average heparin flush dosage strength is 10 units per mL and never exceeds 100 units per mL. Heparin sodium for injection and heparin lock flush solution can **never** be used interchangeably.

## Other Anticoagulant Medications

Low-molecular-weight heparins (LMWHs) are heparin derivatives that are used in clinical practice. They are prescribed for prevention and treatment of deep-vein thrombosis (DVT) following abdominal surgery, hip or knee replacement, unstable angina, and acute coronary syndromes. Examples are Lovenox (enoxaparin) and Fragmin (dalteparin). (See the labels for these medications in Figure 22.1.) Notice that the Lovenox label indicates the dosage strength in mg per 0.4 mL, and the Fragmin label indicates the dosage strength in international units (IU) per 0.3 mL; therefore Lovenox would be ordered in mg and Fragmin in IU.

## Reading Heparin Labels

As previously stated, heparin comes in various concentrations. Nurses **must always** carefully read the heparin label to verify that they have the correct concentration, which is critical to the prevention of lethal dosage errors with heparin. Refer to the labels shown in Figure 22.2 for Heparin Sodium Injection, USP, showing various heparin concentrations. Notice the following:
- Bolder, larger font
- Strength per total volume expressed (i.e., Label A, 10,000 units per 10 mL; Label B, 50,000 units per 10 mL), followed by dosage strength per mL in parentheses for both (Label A, 1,000 units per mL; Label B, 5,000 units per mL), Label C is a 1-mL size vial and states 1,000 units per mL.

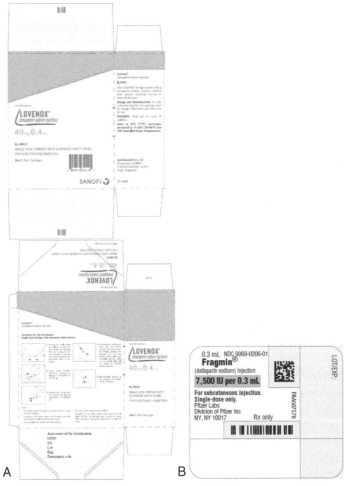

**Figure 22.1** (A) Lovenox label, 40 mg per 0.4 mL. (B) Fragmin label, 7,500 IU per 0.3 mL.

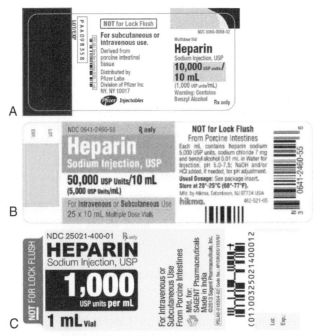

**Figure 22.2** (A) 10,000 units per 10 mL (1,000 units per mL). (B) 50,000 units per 10 mL (5,000 units per mL). (C) 1-mL vial, 1,000 units per mL.

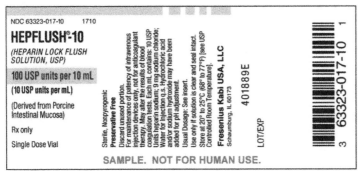

**Figure 22.3** Heparin Lock Flush Solution, 100 units per 10 mL (10 units per mL).

- The statement "Not for lock flush"

Figure 22.3 shows a label for Heparin Lock Flush Solution USP; notice the strength per total volume (100 units per 10 mL) and the dosage strength per mL (10 units per mL).

> **(!) SAFETY ALERT!**
>
> Heparin is available in different strengths; read labels carefully before administering to ensure the client's safety. Verify the dosage, vial, and amount to be given. Obtain an independent **double-check** from another nurse to ensure accuracy. Continuous monitoring of the client receiving heparin is essential because of the risk of hemorrhage or clots with an incorrect dose. To avoid misinterpretation of orders, whether written or done by computer entry or entered on the Medication Administration Record (MAR), the word *units* should not be abbreviated.

Now let's proceed with the calculation of heparin dosages.

## Calculation of Subcutaneous Dosages

Because of its inherent dangers and the need to ensure an accurate and exact dosage, when heparin is administered subcutaneously, a tuberculin syringe (1 mL) is used. Heparin is also available for use in prepackaged syringes. Institutional policies differ regarding the administration of heparin, and the nurse is responsible for knowing and following the policies. The methods of calculating presented in previous chapters are used to calculate subcutaneous (subcut) heparin, except the dosage is never rounded and is usually administered with a tuberculin syringe.

**Example:**  Order: Heparin 7,500 units subcut daily

Available: Heparin labeled 10,000 units per mL

What will you administer to the client?

**Setup:**
- No conversion is necessary. The order is in units and it is available in units.
- Think: What would be a logical dosage?
- Set up in ratio and proportion, the formula method, or dimensional analysis and solve.

**Ratio and Proportion (Linear Format)**

10,000 units : 1 mL = 7,500 units : $x$ mL

**Ratio and Proportion (Fraction Format)**

$$\frac{10{,}000 \text{ units}}{1 \text{ mL}} = \frac{7{,}500 \text{ units}}{x \text{ mL}}$$

$$\frac{10{,}000x}{10{,}000} = \frac{7{,}500}{10{,}000}$$

$$x = \frac{7{,}500}{10{,}000}$$

$$x = 0.75 \text{ mL}$$

**Formula Method**

$$\frac{7,500 \text{ units}}{10,000 \text{ units}} \times 1 \text{ mL} = x \text{ mL}$$
$$x = 0.75 \text{ mL}$$

**Dimensional Analysis**

$$x \text{ mL} = \frac{1 \text{ mL}}{10,000 \text{ units}} \times \frac{7,500 \text{ units}}{1}$$
$$x = \frac{7,500}{10,000}$$
$$x = 0.75 \text{ mL}$$

The dosage of 0.75 mL is reasonable because the dosage ordered is less than what is available. Therefore less than 1 mL will be needed to administer the ordered dosage. This dosage can be measured accurately with a tuberculin syringe (calibrated in tenths and hundredths of a milliliter). This dosage would not be rounded to the nearest tenth of a milliliter. Heparin is administered in exact dosages. A tuberculin syringe illustrating the dosage to be administered is shown in Figure 22.4.

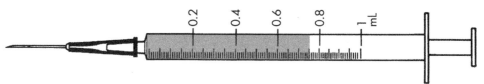

**Figure 22.4** Tuberculin syringe illustrating 0.75 mL drawn up.

## Calculation of IV Heparin Solutions

An infusion pump is **required** for the safe administration of IV heparin infusions. The nurse's primary responsibility is to administer the correct dosage and ensure that the dosage being administered is safe. When in doubt regarding a dosage ordered for a client or that the client is receiving, always check with the prescriber before administering it. Verify the dosage to be administered by obtaining an independent double-check (i.e., a second qualified person, such as another nurse, separately checking the calculation without knowing the result of their colleague). The ISMP does not recommend the use of an independent double-check for all high-alert medications. Independent double-checks should be based on careful assessment of processes and medications (e.g., IV heparin) that could pose the greatest risk of harm if an error occurs (June 2019; https://www.ismp.org/resources/independent-double-checks-worth-effort-if-used-judiciously-and-properly).

**The dosing guidelines for continuous heparin IV infusion for an adult are 20,000 to 40,000 units every 24 hours.** These guidelines are based on factors that include the client's condition, age, and test results, (i.e., aPTT).

Let's look at calculations with IV heparin

### Calculating Units per Hour

This can be done using ratio and proportion or dimensional analysis.

Example:  An IV solution of heparin is ordered for a client. $D_5W$ 1,000 mL containing 20,000 units of heparin is to infuse at 30 mL/hr. Calculate the dosage of heparin the client is to receive per hour.

Solution:
- If using ratio and proportion, the solution on hand (20,000 units in 1,000 mL) is the known ratio; for the rate of the infusion (in this problem, you want to determine the units that would be contained in 30 mL), $x$ units/30 mL would be the unknown ratio.

- For dimensional analysis, $x$ units/hr is what is being calculated. The **starting fraction** is 20,000 units per 1,000 mL, which is written with units in the numerator to match the units in the numerator being calculated. The rate, 30 mL/hr, is placed in the equation as the **second fraction** with 30 mL as the numerator, which matches the denominator of the starting fraction. Cancel the units to obtain the desired unit (units/hr). Reduce if possible and perform math operations.

### Ratio and Proportion (Linear Format)

20,000 units : 1,000 mL 5 $x$ units : 30 mL

*or*

### Ratio and Proportion (Fraction Format)

$$\frac{20,000\ units}{1,000\ mL} = \frac{x\ units}{30\ mL}$$

$$1,000\ x = 20,000 \times 30$$

$$\frac{1,000\ x}{1,000} = \frac{600,\cancel{000}}{1,\cancel{000}}$$

$$x = 600\ units/hr$$

### Dimensional Analysis

$$\frac{x\ units}{hr} = \frac{20,\cancel{000}\ units}{1,\cancel{000}\ \cancel{mL}} \times \frac{30\ \cancel{mL}}{1\ hr}$$

$$x = \frac{20 \times 30}{1}$$

$$x = \frac{600}{1}$$

$$x = 600\ units/hr$$

The client would receive **600 units/hr** from a solution containing 20,000 units in 1,000 mL of solution if the IV infusion is infusing at 30 mL/hr.

## Calculating mL/hr from Units/hr

Because heparin is ordered in units/hr and infused with an electronic infusion device, it is necessary to do calculations in mL/hr.

**Example 1:**  Order: Infuse heparin 850 units/hr from a solution containing 25,000 units in 500 mL $D_5W$.

## Solution:
- For ratio and proportion, the available solution (in this problem, 25,000 units/500 mL) is the known ratio, and the desired units/$x$ mL (in this problem 850 units/$x$ mL) is the unknown ratio.
- For dimensional analysis, mL/hr is being calculated. The **starting fraction** is 25,000 units per 500 mL, placing mL as the numerator to match the mL numerator of the units being calculated (500 mL/25,000 units). The **second fraction** is the 850 units/hr rate ordered, with units in the numerator, 850 units/1 hr. Cancel units; the desired unit mL/hr is left. Reduce if possible and perform math operations.

### Ratio and Proportion (Linear Format)

25,000 units : 500 mL 5 850 units : $x$ mL

**Ratio and Proportion (Fraction Format)**

$$\frac{25,000 \text{ units}}{500 \text{ mL}} = \frac{850 \text{ units}}{x \text{ mL}}$$

$$25,000\,x = 500 \times 85$$

$$\frac{25,000\,x}{25,000} = \frac{425,000}{25,000}$$

$$x = \frac{425}{25}$$

$$x = 17 \text{ mL/hr}$$

**Dimensional Analysis**

$$\frac{x \text{ mL}}{\text{hr}} = \frac{\overset{1}{\cancel{500}} \text{ mL}}{\underset{50}{\cancel{25,000}} \text{ units}} \times \frac{850 \cancel{\text{ units}}}{1 \text{ hr}}$$

$$x = \frac{850}{50}$$

$$x = \frac{85}{5}$$

$$x = 17 \text{ mL/hr}$$

To infuse 850 units/hr from a solution of 25,000 units of heparin in $D_5W$ 500 mL, the infusion pump would be set at 17 mL/hr.

**Example 2:** Order: Infuse 1,200 units of heparin per hour from a solution containing 20,000 units in 250 mL $D_5W$.

## Solution:
Refer to Example 1 for the steps for ratio and proportion and dimensional analysis.

**Ratio and Proportion (Linear Format)**

20,000 units : 250 mL 5 1,200 units : $x$ mL

**Ratio and Proportion (Fraction Format)**

$$\frac{20,000 \text{ units}}{250 \text{ mL}} = \frac{1,200 \text{ units}}{x \text{ mL}}$$

$$20,000\,x = 1,200 \times 250$$

$$\frac{20,000\,x}{20,000} = \frac{300,000}{20,000}$$

$$x = \frac{30}{2}$$

$$x = 15 \text{ mL/hr}$$

**Dimensional Analysis**

$$\frac{x\,\text{mL}}{\text{hr}} = \frac{\overset{1}{\cancel{250}\ \text{mL}}}{\underset{80}{\cancel{20{,}000}\ \text{units}}} \times \frac{1{,}200\ \cancel{\text{units}}}{1\ \text{hr}}$$

$$x = \frac{1{,}20\cancel{0}}{8\cancel{0}}$$

$$x = \frac{120}{8}$$

$$x = 15\ \text{mL/hr}$$

To infuse 1,200 units/hr of heparin from a solution containing 20,000 units in 250 mL D$_5$W, the infusion pump would be set at 15 mL/hr.

## Calculating Heparin Dosages Based on Weight

To prevent dosage and administration errors with heparin and increase client safety, many health care institutions have established **heparin protocols** to guide the administration of IV heparin dosages. The dosages of heparin are individualized based on the client's weight. The protocols are based on the client's weight in kilograms and their activated partial thromboplastin time APTT (sometimes written as aPTT). The APTT is a blood clotting value measured in seconds and is used as the criterion to titrate the heparin dosage, and adjustments are made accordingly. (See the sample protocol in Figure 22.5.) Heparin protocols consist of:

- The bolus or loading dose, which is the initial bolus based on the client's weight in kilograms
- The initial infusion rate based on the client's weight in kilograms
- Directions on what additional bolus and rate alterations must be made based on APTT results

Heparin protocols consist of **three** steps in the administration process in the following sequence:

1. **Bolus**
2. **Continuous infusion**
3. **Rebolus** and/or adjust infusion rate (increase, decrease, or discontinue)

It is imperative that nurses be familiar with the protocol at their individual institutions. The bolus and infusion rate can vary among institutions. According to Willihnganz, Gurevitz, and Clayton (2020), the bolus dosage is 70 to 100 units/kg, and the infusion rate is 15 to 25 units/kg/hr. These values can be different depending on the health care institution. For weight-based heparin calculations, the weight of the client is rounded to the nearest tenth of a kilogram or the exact number of kilograms. IV rates in mL/hr are rounded to the nearest whole number or nearest tenth depending on the infusion pump (some of which are capable of delivering IV fluids in tenths of a milliliter). Always check the equipment available at the institution before rounding IV flow rates to whole milliliters per hour (mL/hr). **Always be familiar with the values and protocol used for heparin administration at the institution to prevent errors that could be fatal and to ensure the safe administration of heparin to a client.** Also remember the importance of independent double-checks with IV heparin.

> **⚠ SAFETY ALERT!**
>
> For heparin to be therapeutically effective, the dosage **must** be accurate. A larger dosage than required can cause a client to hemorrhage, and an underdosage may not have the desired effect. Any questionable dosages should be verified with the prescriber **before** administration.

---

## Weight-Based Heparin Protocol

1. Bolus with heparin at 80 units/kg
2. Begin intravenous infusion of heparin at 18 units/kg/hr using 25,000 units heparin in 250 mL $D_5W$ or a concentration of 100 units per mL.
3. APTT 6 hours after rate change and then daily at 7am
4. Adjust intravenous heparin daily based on APTT results
   - APTT less than 35 sec, Bolus with 80 units/kg and increase rate by 4 units/kg/hr.
   - APTT 35-45 sec, Bolus with 40 units/kg and increase rate by 2 units/kg/hr.
   - APTT 46-70 sec, **No Change.**
   - APTT 71-90 sec, Decrease rate by 2 units/kg/hr.
   - APTT greater than 90 sec, **Stop** heparin infusion for 1 hour, and decrease rate by 3 units/kg/hr.

---

**Figure 22.5** Sample heparin weight-based protocol. *Note:* This protocol is for calculation purposes only.

In this text, for the purpose of calculating, round weight in kilograms to the nearest tenth. Milliliters per hour (mL/hr) are to be rounded to the whole number unless information is provided to do otherwise. Let's work through some examples of calculation of heparin dosages based on weight.

**Example 1:** A client weighs 160 lb.

Order: Administer a bolus of heparin sodium IV. The hospital protocol is 80 units/kg. Calculate the number of units to administer the bolus dosage.

**Solution:**

**Step 1:** Convert the client's weight to kilograms.

Conversion factor: 1 kg 5 2.2 lb
160 lb ÷ 2.2 = 72.72 = 72.7 kg (rounded to nearest tenth)

**Step 2:** Calculate the heparin bolus dosage.

$$80 \text{ units/kg} \times 72.7 \text{ kg} = 5,816 \text{ units}$$

The client should receive 5,816 units as a bolus dosage.

**Example 2:** A client weighs 165 lb.

Order: Bolus with heparin sodium 80 units/kg, then initiate IV infusion at 18 units/kg/hr.

Available: Heparin 25,000 units in 1,000 mL 0.9% NS

- Calculate the bolus dosage.
- Calculate the infusion rate.
- Determine the rate in mL/hr to set the infusion device.

**Solution:**

**Step 1:**    Convert the client's weight to kg.

Conversion factor:    1 kg = 2.2 lb

165 lb ÷ 2.2 = 75 kg

**Step 2:**    Calculate the heparin bolus dosage.

$$80 \text{ units/kg} \times 75 \text{ kg} = 6{,}000 \text{ units}$$

The client should receive 6,000 units as a bolus dosage.

**Step 3:**    Calculate the infusion rate.

$$18 \text{ units/kg/hr} \times 75 \text{ kg} = 1{,}350 \text{ units/hr}$$

**Step 4:**    Determine the rate in mL/hr at which to set the infusion device.

$$1{,}000 \text{ mL} : 25{,}000 \text{ units} = x \text{ mL} : 1{,}350 \text{ units}$$

$$25{,}000 \, x = 1{,}350 \times 1{,}000$$

$$\frac{25{,}000 \, x}{25{,}000} = \frac{1{,}350{,}000}{25{,}000}$$

$$x = \frac{1{,}350}{25} = 54$$

$$x = 54 \text{ mL/hr}$$

*or*

Use formula: $\dfrac{D}{H} \times Q = x$

$$\frac{1{,}350 \text{ units/hr}}{25{,}000 \text{ units}} \times 1{,}000 \text{ mL} = x \text{ mL/hr}$$

$$x = 54 \text{ mL/hr}$$

The infusion pump would be set at 54 mL/hr to deliver 1,350 units/hr.

*Note:* The problem only illustrates some of the methods that can be used for solving the problem.

Now let's do a problem illustrating the steps of calculating the bolus, continuous infusion, or rebolus and/or adjusting the infusion rate for a client weighing 198 lb using the sample protocol in Figure 22.5.

**Solution:**

**Step 1:**    Convert the client's weight to kilograms.

Conversion factor: 1 kg = 2.2 lb

198 lb ÷ 2.2 = 90 kg

**Step 2:**    Calculate the heparin bolus dosage.

$$80 \text{ units/kg} \times 90 \text{ kg} = 7{,}200 \text{ units}$$

The client should receive 7,200 units IV heparin as a bolus.

- To determine the volume (mL) the client would receive, remember that the concentration of heparin was indicated as 100 units per mL. This can be determined using the formula method, dimensional analysis, or ratio and proportion.

$$100 \text{ units} : 1 \text{ mL} = 7{,}200 \text{ units} : x \text{ mL}$$

$$100 \, x = 7{,}200$$

$$\frac{100 \, x}{100} = \frac{7{,}200}{100}$$

$$x = 72 \text{ mL (administer 72 mL to administer the bolus of 7,200 units)}$$

**Step 3:**    Calculate the infusion rate (18 units/kg/hr)

$$18 \text{ units/kg/hr} \times 90 \text{ kg} = 1{,}620 \text{ units/hr}$$

- Determine the rate in mL/hr at which to set the infusion pump to deliver 1,620 units/hr. Use the concentration of 100 units per mL.

$$100 \text{ units} : 1 \text{ mL} = 1{,}620 \text{ units} : x \text{ mL}$$

$$100 \, x = 1{,}620$$

$$\frac{100 \, x}{100} = \frac{1{,}620}{100} = 16.2$$

$$x = 16 \text{ mL/hr}$$

The pump would be set at 16 mL/hr to deliver 1,620 units/hr.

The client's APTT after 6 hours is reported as 43 seconds. According to the protocol, rebolus with 40 units/kg and increase the rate by 2 units/kg/hr. Let's look at how the rebolus and rate increase would be calculated.

**Step 4:**    Calculate the dosage (units/hr) of the continuous infusion increase based on the protocol using the client's weight in kg.

- Calculate the dosage (units) of heparin rebolus.

$$40 \text{ units/kg} \times 90 \text{ kg} = 3{,}600 \text{ units}$$

Determine the volume (mL) to administer 3,600 units.

$$100 \text{ units} : 1 \text{ mL} = 3{,}600 \text{ units} : x \text{ mL}$$

$$100 \, x = 3{,}600$$

$$\frac{100 \, x}{100} = \frac{3{,}600}{100}$$

$$x = 36 \text{ mL}$$

$$x = 36 \text{ mL (administer 36 mL to administer the rebolus of 3,600 units)}$$

**Step 5:**    Now determine the infusion rate increase (2 units/kg/hr 3 kg).

$$2 \text{ units/kg/hr} \times 90 \text{ kg} = 180 \text{ units/hr}$$

The infusion rate should be increased by 180 units/hr.

• Calculate the adjustment in the hourly infusion rate (mL/hr).

$$100 \text{ units} : 1 \text{ mL} = 180 \text{ units} : x \text{ mL}$$

$$100\,x = 180$$

$$\frac{100\,x}{100} = \frac{18\cancel{0}}{10\cancel{0}}$$

$$x = 1.8 \text{ mL/hr}$$

$x = 1.8$ mL/hr (adjustment that would be needed in the rate)

• Determine the increase rate:

16 mL/hr (current rate)
+ 1.8 mL/hr (increase)
17.8 = 18 mL/hr

Increase the rate on the pump to 18 mL/hr to increase the infusion by 180 units/hr.

---

### POINTS TO REMEMBER

• Heparin is a potent anticoagulant; it is often administered intravenously but can be administered subcutaneously.
• Heparin is measured in USP units. When orders are written, the word *units* is spelled out to prevent misinterpretation.
• Heparin dosages must be accurately calculated to prevent inherent dangers associated with the medication. Discrepancies in dosage should be verified with the prescriber before administration.
• Independent double-checks should be done for IV heparin before administration.
• When subcut heparin is administered, a tuberculin syringe is used (calibrated in tenths and hundredths of a milliliter). Answers are expressed in hundredths.
• Read heparin labels carefully because heparin comes in several strengths.
• There are several IV calculations that can be done (mL/hr, units/hr).
• Heparin is commonly ordered in units/hr and infused with an electronic infusion device.
• Heparin sodium for injection and heparin lock solution cannot be used interchangeably.
• The method of calculating IV heparin dosages can also be used to calculate IV dosages for other medications. Ratio and proportion and dimensional analysis can be used as well.
• Heparin dosages are individualized according to the weight of the client in kilograms and adjusted based on the APTT.
• Protocols for IV heparin vary from institution to institution; always know and follow the institution's policy. Heparin protocol consists of three steps in the administration process: (1) bolus, (2) continuous infusion, (3) rebolus and/or adjust infusion rate (increase, decrease, or discontinue).
• Monitoring a client's APTT while they are receiving heparin is a **must.**
• New heparin labels indicate the dosage strength (amount) per the entire container (vial) and the dosage strength per mL in parentheses.

---

### 🖩 PRACTICE **PROBLEMS**

Calculate the units of measure indicated by the problem.

1. Order: Infuse 1,000 units/hr of heparin IV
   from a solution of 1,000 mL 0.45% NS
   with 25,000 units of heparin. Calculate
   the rate in mL/hr.                                        _____

2. Order: Infuse $D_5$ 0.9% NS 1,000 mL
   with 25,000 units of heparin IV at 35 mL/hr.
   Calculate the dosage in units/hr. _____

3. Order: Infuse 750 mL $D_5$W with
   30,000 units of heparin IV at 25 mL/hr.
   Calculate the dosage in units/hr. _____

4. Order: Infuse $D_5$W 1,000 mL with
   25,000 units of heparin IV at 100 mL/hr.
   Determine the dosage in units/hr. _____

5. A client weighs 176 lb. Heparin infusion 20,000 units in 1,000 mL 0.9% sodium chloride.
   Order: Bolus with heparin sodium at 80 units/kg, then initiate drip at 18 units/kg/hr.
   (Round weight to the nearest tenth as indicated.) Calculate the following:

   a. _____ bolus dosage

   b. _____ infusion rate (initial)

   c. _____ mL/hr

Use the following weight-based heparin protocol for question 6. (Round weight to the nearest tenth as indicated; IV pump is calibrated in whole mL/hr.)

---

Bolus with heparin at 80 units/kg.
Begin intravenous infusion of heparin at 18 units/kg/hr using 25,000 units heparin in 500 mL $D_5$W for 50 units per mL.
Adjust intravenous heparin daily based on APTT results.
- APTT less than 35 seconds: Rebolus with 80 units/kg and increase rate by 4 units/kg/hr.
- APTT 35-45 seconds: Rebolus with 40 units/kg and increase rate by 2 units/kg/hr.
- APTT 46-70 seconds: **No change.**
- APTT 71-90 seconds: Decrease rate by 2 units/kg/hr.
- APTT greater than 90 sec. **Stop heparin** infusion for 1 hour and decrease rate by 3 units/kg/hr.

---

6. A client weighs 134.2 lb. Determine the bolus dose of heparin, the initial infusion rate, and then adjust the hourly infusion rate up or down based on the APTT results using the above weight-based heparin protocol. APTT is reported as 31 seconds.

**Answers on pp. 569-570**

---

## 🕹 CLINICAL **REASONING**

**Scenario:** A client has an order for heparin 3,500 units in 500 mL $D_5$W to infuse at a rate of 40 mL/hr. The nurse prepares the IV using the heparin labeled 100 units per mL and adds 35 mL of heparin to the IV.

a. What error occurred in the preparation of the IV solution and why? _____

_____

b. What preventive measures should the nurse have taken? _____

**Answers on p. 570**

## NGN Case Study

**Learning Outcomes:**
1. Calculate heparin dosages being administered intravenously (in mL/hr or units/hr).
2. Calculate safe heparin dosages based on weight.

**Case Scenario:** A client is admitted to the hospital with complaints of chest pain and shortness of breath. The client is diagnosed with a pulmonary embolism. The client weighs 192 lb. The physician writes an order for a heparin protocol (please see the heparin protocol below). Round the weight to the nearest tenth. The infusion pump can deliver medication to the tenths of an mL.

---

### Weight-Based Heparin Protocol

1. Bolus with heparin at 80 units/kg
2. Begin intravenous infusion of heparin at 18 units/kg/hr using 25,000 units heparin in 250 mL $D_5W$ or a concentration of 100 units per mL.
3. APTT 6 hours after rate change and then daily at 7am
4. Adjust intravenous heparin daily based on APTT results
   - APTT less than 35 sec, Bolus with 80 units/kg and increase rate by 4 units/kg/hr.
   - APTT 35-45 sec, Bolus with 40 units/kg and increase rate by 2 units/kg/hr.
   - APTT 46-70 sec, **No Change.**
   - APTT 71-90 sec, Decrease rate by 2 units/kg/hr.
   - APTT greater than 90 sec, **Stop** heparin infusion for 1 hour, and decrease rate by 3 units/kg/hr.

---

Use the scenario and heparin protocol to select the appropriate nursing actions from the list below.

| Potential Action | Appropriate Action |
|---|---|
| Calculate the client's weight as 87.3 kg. | |
| Calculate the client's weight as 422.4 kg. | |
| Calculate the client's weight as 192 kg. | |
| Give the client a bolus of 15,360 units. | |
| Give the client a bolus of 33,792 units. | |
| Give the client a bolus of 6,984 units. | |
| Begin the heparin drip at 7,603 units/hr. | |
| Begin the heparin drip at 1,571.4 units/hr. | |
| Begin the heparin drip at 3,456 units/hr. | |
| Program the electronic infusion device at 76 mL/hr. | |
| Program the electronic infusion device at 34.5 mL/hr. | |
| Program the electronic infusion device at 15.7 mL/hr. | |

**Reference:** Morris D: *Calculate with confidence,* ed 8, St Louis, Elsevier, copyright 2022.

*Case Study answers and rationales can be found on Evolve.*

---

### ⊙ CHAPTER **REVIEW**

For questions 1-7, calculate the dosage of heparin you will administer, use labels where provided, and shade the dosage on the syringe provided. For questions 8-30, calculate the units as indicated by the problem.

1. Order: Heparin 3,500 units subcut daily.

   Available:

   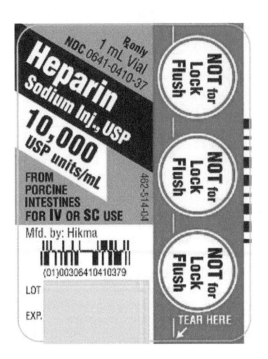

   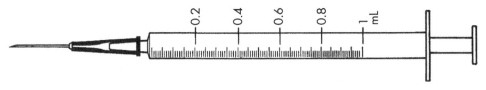

2. Order: Heparin 16,000 units subcut stat.

   Available:

   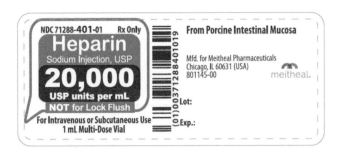

   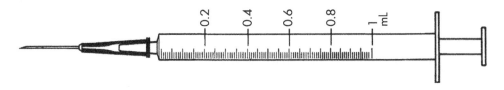

3. Order: Heparin 2,000 units subcut b.i.d.

   Available:

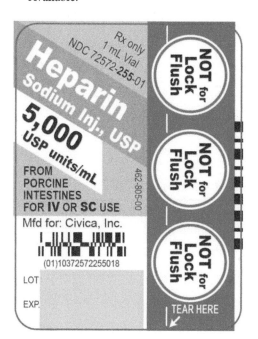

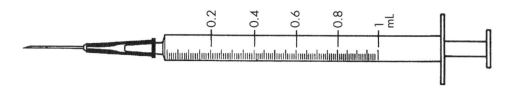

4. Order: Heparin flush 10 units every shift to flush a heparin lock.

   Available:

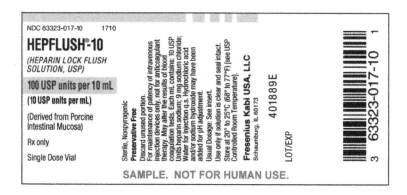

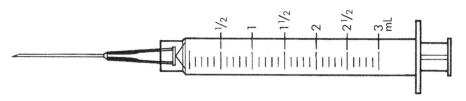

5. Order: Heparin 25,000 units IV in D$_5$W 500 mL.

   Available:

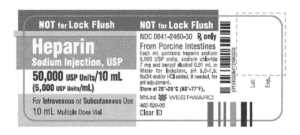

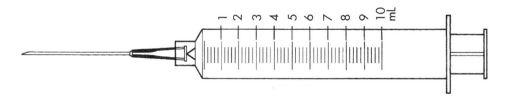

6. Order: Heparin 17,000 units subcut daily.

   Available:

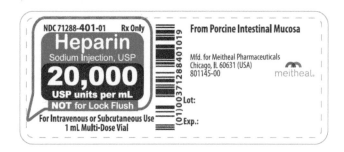

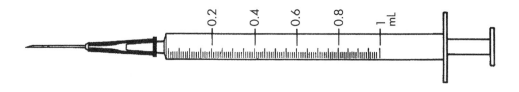

7. Order: Heparin 2,500 units subcut q12h.

   Available:

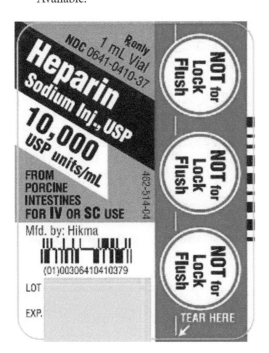

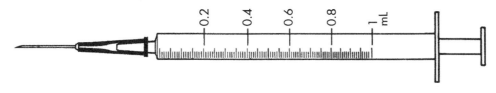

_____

8. Order: Heparin 2,000 units/hr IV. Available: 25,000 units of heparin in 1,000 mL of 0.9% NS.

   What rate in mL/hr will deliver
   2,000 units/hr?                    _____

9. Order: Heparin 1,500 units/hr IV. Available: 25,000 units of heparin in 500 mL $D_5W$.

   What rate in mL/hr will deliver
   1,500 units/hr?                    _____

10. Order: Heparin 1,800 units/hr IV. Available: 25,000 units heparin in 250 mL $D_5W$.

    What rate in mL per hr will deliver
    1,800 units/hr?                   _____

11. Order: 40,000 units heparin IV in 1 L 0.9% NaCl to infuse at 25 mL/hr.

    Calculate the hourly heparin dosage
    (units/hr).                       _____

12. Order: Heparin 40,000 units IV in 500 mL D₅W to infuse at 30 mL/hr.

   Calculate the hourly heparin dosage
   (units/hr).                                    _____

13. Order: 1 L of 0.9% NS with 40,000 units heparin IV over 24 hr. Calculate the following:

   a. mL/hr                                       _____

   b. units/hr                                    _____

14. Order: 1 L of D₅W with 15,000 units heparin IV over 10 hr. Calculate the following:

   a. mL/hr                                       _____

   b. units/hr                                    _____

15. Order: 500 mL of 0.9% NS with 10,000 units of heparin IV to infuse at 120 mL/hr.

   Calculate the hourly heparin dosage
   (units/hr).                                    _____

16. Order: Heparin 40,000 units IV in 1 L 0.9% NS to infuse at 1,000 units/hr.

   Calculate the rate in mL/hr.                   _____

17. Order: Heparin 25,000 units IV in 1 L 0.9% NS to infuse at 2,000 units/hr.

   Calculate the rate in mL/hr.                   _____

Calculate the hourly dosage of heparin (units/hr) for Questions 18-23.

18. Order: 50,000 units of heparin IV in 1,000 mL of D₅W to infuse at 60 mL/hr.

   _____

19. Order: 20,000 units of heparin IV in 500 mL D₅W to infuse at 20 mL/hr.

   _____

20. Order: 25,000 units of heparin IV in 1 L of D₅W to infuse at 56 mL/hr.

   _____

21. Order: 30,000 units of heparin IV in 500 mL
   of D₅W to infuse at 25 mL/hr.                  _____

22. Order: 40,000 units of heparin IV in 500 mL
   0.45% NS to infuse at 25 mL/hr.                _____

23. Order: 20,000 units of heparin IV in 1 L of
   D₅W to infuse at 80 mL/hr.                     _____

24. A central venous line requires flushing with heparin. Which of the two labels shown
   is appropriate for a heparin flush?

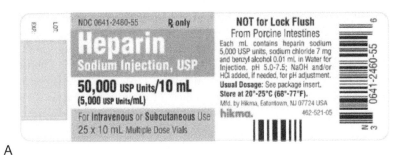

A

B

_____

For problems 25-27, round the weight to the nearest tenth as indicated. The pump delivers in whole mL/hr.

25. Order: Heparin drip at 18 units/kg/hr.

    Available: 25,000 units of heparin sodium in 1,000 mL of D$_5$W. The client weighs 80 kg. At what rate will you set the infusion pump?

    _____

26. A client weighs 210 lb. Heparin IV infusion: heparin sodium 25,000 units in 1,000 mL of 0.9% NS. Order is to give a bolus with heparin sodium 80 units/kg, then initiate drip at 14 units/kg/hr.

    Calculate the following:

    a. Heparin bolus dosage

    _____

    b. Infusion rate for the IV (initial)

    _____ units/hr

    c. At what rate will you set the infusion pump?

    _____

27. A client weighs 154 lb. Heparin IV infusion: heparin sodium 20,000 units in 1,000 mL D$_5$W. The hospital protocol is to give a bolus to the client with 80 units/kg and start drip at 14 units/kg/hr.

    Calculate the following:

    a. Heparin bolus dosage

    _____

    b. Infusion rate for the IV (initial)

    _____ units/hr

    c. Infusion rate in mL/hr

    _____

**Heparin Protocol for Questions 28-29**

> Bolus heparin at 80 units/kg.
>
> Begin intravenous infusion of heparin at 18 units/kg/hr using 25,000 units heparin in 250 mL $D_5W$ for 100 units per mL.
>
> Adjust intravenous heparin daily based on APTT results.
>
> - APTT less than 35 sec: Rebolus with 80 units/kg and increase rate by 4 units/kg/hr.
> - APTT 35-45 sec: Rebolus with 40 units/kg and increase rate by 2 units/kg/hr.
> - APTT 46-70 sec: **No change.**
> - APTT 71-90 sec: Decrease rate by 2 units/kg/hr.
> - APTT greater than 90 sec: **Stop heparin** infusion for 1 hour and decrease rate by 3 units/kg/hr.

28. A client weighs 100 kg. Determine the bolus dose of heparin, the initial infusion rate, and then adjust the hourly infusion rate up or down based on APTT results using the above weight-based heparin protocol. The APTT is reported as 71 seconds. The pump delivers in whole mL/hr.

29. A client weighs 162.8 lb. Determine the bolus dose of heparin, the initial infusion rate, and then adjust the hourly infusion rate up or down based on APTT results using the above weight-based protocol. The APTT is reported as 38 sec. The pump delivers in tenths of a mL.

30. **Directions for question 30:** Calculate the heparin dose in units/hr and the heparin infusion rate in mL/hr. (The pump is capable of delivering in tenths of a mL.)

    Order: Heparin 20 units/kg/hr. IV infusion for a patient/client who weighs 89 kg.
    Available: Heparin 25,000 units in 500 mL $D_5W$ (50 units per mL)
    a. Calculate dose in units/hr          _____
    b. Determine the rate in mL/hr          _____

**Answers on pp. 570-574**

For additional practice problems, refer to the Dosages Measured in Units section of the Elsevier's Interactive Drug Calculation Application, Version 1, on Evolve.

## ⭐ ANSWERS

### Chapter 22
### Answers to Practice Problems

1.  25,000 units : 1,000 mL = 1,000 units : $x$ mL

    *or*

    $$\frac{25,000 \text{ units}}{1,000 \text{ mL}} = \frac{1,000 \text{ units}}{x \text{ mL}}$$

    $$25,000x = 1,000 \times 1,000$$

    $$\frac{25,000x}{25,000} = \frac{1,000,000}{25,000}$$

    $$x = 40 \text{ mL/hr}$$

    Answer: 40 mL/hr

2.  25,000 units : 1,000 mL = $x$ units : 35 mL

    $$\frac{1,000x}{1,000} = \frac{875,000}{1,000}$$

    $$x = 875 \text{ units/hr}$$

    Answer: 875 units/hr.

3.  30,000 units : 750 mL = $x$ units : 25 mL

    $$\frac{750x}{750} = \frac{750,000}{750}$$

    $$x = 1,000 \text{ units/hr}$$

    Answer: 1,000 units/hr

4.  Calculate units/hr infusing.

    1,000 mL : 25,000 units = 100 mL : $x$ units

    $$\frac{1,000x}{1,000} = \frac{2,500,000}{1,000}$$

    $$x = \frac{2,500}{1}$$

    Answer: 2,500 units/hr

5.  Convert the weight to kilograms.

    Conversion factor: 2.2 lb = 1 kg

    176 lb ÷ 2.2 = 80 kg

    a.  Calculate the heparin bolus dosage.

    80 units/k̶g̶ × 80 k̶g̶ = 6,400 units

    Answer: 6,400 units

    b.  Calculate the infusion rate for the IV drip (initial).

    18 units/k̶g̶/hr × 80 k̶g̶ = 1,440 units/hr

    c.  Determine the rate in mL/hr at which to set the infusion rate.

    1,000 mL : 20,000 units = $x$ mL : 1,440 units

    $$\frac{20,000x}{20,000} = \frac{1,440,000}{20,000}$$

    $$x = \frac{144}{2}$$

    $$x = 72 \text{ mL/hr}$$

    Answer: 72 mL/hr

6.  **Step 1:** Convert the client's weight to kilograms.

    Conversion factor: 1 kg = 2.2 lb

    134.2 lb ÷ 2.2 = 61 kg

    **Step 2:** Calculate the heparin bolus dosage.

    80 units/k̶g̶ × 61 k̶g̶ = 4,880 units. The client should receive 4,880 units IV heparin as a bolus.

    Determine the volume (mL) the client would receive. The concentration of heparin is stated as 50 units per mL.

    50 units : 1 mL = 4,880 units : $x$ mL

    $$\frac{50x}{50} = \frac{4,880}{50}$$

    $$x = \frac{4,880}{50} = 97.6$$

    $$x = 98 \text{ mL (bolus is 98 mL)}$$

    **Step 3:** Calculate the infusion rate (18 units/kg/hr).

    18 units/k̶g̶/hr × 61 k̶g̶ = 1,098 units/hr. Determine the rate in mL/hr at which to set the infusion device (using the concentration of 50 units per mL).

    50 units : 1 mL = 1,098 units : $x$ mL

    $$\frac{50x}{50} = \frac{1,098}{50}$$

    $$x = \frac{1,098}{50} = 21.9$$

    $$x = 22 \text{ mL/hr}$$

    The client's APTT is 31 seconds. According to the protocol, rebolus with 80 units/kg and increase the rate by 4 units/kg/hr.

    **Step 4:** Calculate the dosage (units/hr) of the continuous infusion increase based on the protocol using the client's weight in kg.

    Calculate the dosage (units) of heparin rebolus.

    80 units/k̶g̶ × 61 k̶g̶ = 4,880 units

    Determine the volume (mL) to administer 4,880 units.

    50 units : 1 mL = 4,880 units : $x$ mL

    $$\frac{50x}{50} = \frac{4,880}{50}$$

    $$x = \frac{4,880}{50} = 97.6$$

    $$x = 98 \text{ mL bolus}$$

    Now determine the infusion rate increase (4 units/kg/hr × kg).

    4 units/k̶g̶/hr × 61 k̶g̶ = 244 units/hr

    The infusion rate should be increased by 244 units/hr.

    **Calculate the adjustment in the hourly infusion rate (mL/hr).**

50 units : 1 mL = 244 units : $x$ mL

$$\frac{50x}{50} = \frac{244}{50}$$

$$x = \frac{244}{50} = 4.8$$

$$x = 5 \text{ mL/hr}$$

**Increase rate:**

22 mL/hr (current rate)

+5 mL/hr (increase)

———————————

27 mL/hr (new infusion rate)

*Note:* This problem could also be done using the dimensional analysis or formula method.

## Answers to Clinical Reasoning Questions

a. The nurse used the incorrect concentration of heparin to prepare the IV solution. Heparin concentration of 100 units per mL is used for maintaining the patency of a line and for flushing.

b. The nurse should have read the label carefully because heparin comes in a variety of concentrations. The label indicates what the heparin flush is used for and that it is not for anticoagulant therapy. In addition, heparin is a high-alert medication and should have been double-checked with another nurse before administering. Heparin IV flushes are available in 10 units per mL and 100 units per mL. Heparin for IV flush is never used interchangeably with heparin sodium for injection.

## Answers to Chapter Review

For problems 4 and 5, an alternate solution might be to use the total amount (volume) in the vial and the number of mL to calculate the dose. Problems are shown using the dosage strength per mL.

1. 10,000 units : 1 mL = 3,500 units : $x$ mL

   *or*

   $$\frac{3,500 \text{ units}}{10,000 \text{ units}} \times 1 \text{ mL} = x \text{ mL}$$

   $x = 0.35$ mL. The dosage ordered is less than the available strength; therefore you will need less than 1 mL to administer the dosage.

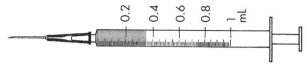

2. 20,000 units : 1 mL = 16,000 units : $x$ mL

   *or*

   $$\frac{16,000 \text{ units}}{20,000 \text{ units}} \times 1 \text{ mL} = x \text{ mL}$$

   Answer: 0.8 mL. The dosage ordered is less than the available strength; therefore you will need less than 1 mL to administer the dosage.

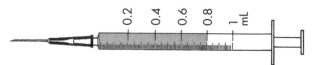

3. 5,000 units : 1 mL = 2,000 units : $x$ mL

   *or*

   $$\frac{2,000 \text{ units}}{5,000 \text{ units}} \times 1 \text{ mL} = x \text{ mL}$$

Answer: 0.4 mL. The dosage ordered is less than the available strength; therefore you will need less than 1 mL to administer the dosage.

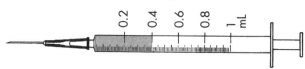

4. 10 units : 1 mL = 10 units : $x$ mL

   *or*

   $$\frac{10 \text{ units}}{10 \text{ units}} \times 1 \text{ mL} = x \text{ mL}$$

   1 mL contains 10 units, so you will need 1 mL to flush the heparin lock.

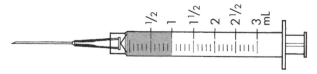

5. 5,000 units : 1 mL = 25,000 units : $x$ mL

   *or*

   $$\frac{25,000 \text{ units}}{5,000 \text{ units}} \times 1 \text{ mL} = x \text{ mL}$$

   Answer: 5 mL. The dosage ordered is more than the available strength; therefore you will need more than 1 mL to administer the dosage.

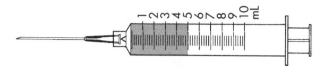

6. 20,000 units : 1 mL = 17,000 units : $x$ mL

*or*

$$\frac{17,000 \text{ units}}{20,000 \text{ units}} \times 1 \text{ mL} = x \text{ mL}$$

Answer: 0.85 mL. The dosage ordered is less than the available strength; therefore you will need less than 1 mL to administer the dosage.

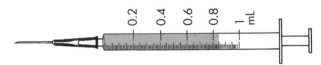

7. 10,000 units : 1 mL = 2,500 units : $x$ mL

*or*

$$\frac{2,500 \text{ units}}{10,000 \text{ units}} \times 1 \text{ mL} = x \text{ mL}$$

Answer: 0.25 mL. The dosage ordered is less than the available strength; therefore you will need less than 1 mL to administer the dosage.

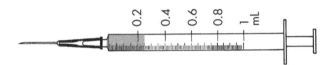

8. 25,000 units : 1,000 mL = 2,000 units : $x$ mL

$$\frac{25,000x}{25,000} = \frac{2,000,000}{25,000}$$

$x$ = 80 mL/hr. To administer 2,000 units of heparin per hour, 80 mL/hr must be given.

9. 25,000 units : 500 mL = 1,500 units : $x$ mL

$$\frac{25,000x}{25,000} = \frac{750,000}{25,000}$$

$x$ = 30 mL/hr. To administer 1,500 units of heparin per hour, 30 mL/hr must be given.

10. 25,000 units : 250 mL = 1,800 units : $x$ mL

$$\frac{25,000x}{25,000} = \frac{450,000}{25,000}$$

$x$ = 18 mL/hr. To administer 1,800 units of heparin per hour, 18 mL/hr must be given.

11. 1 L = 1,000 mL

40,000 units : 1,000 mL = $x$ units : 25 mL

$$\frac{1,000x}{1,000} = \frac{1,000,000}{1,000}$$

$$x = \frac{1,000,000}{1,000}$$

$$x = 1,000 \text{ units/hr}$$

12. 40,000 units : 500 mL = $x$ units : 30 mL

$$\frac{500x}{500} = \frac{1,200,000}{500}$$

$$x = 2,400 \text{ units/hr}$$

13. 1 L = 1,000 mL

a. Calculate mL/hr.

$$\frac{1,000 \text{ mL}}{24 \text{ hr}} = 41.6 = 42 \text{ mL/hr}$$

b. Calculate units/hr.

40,000 units : 1,000 mL = $x$ units : 42 mL

$$\frac{1,000x}{1,000} = \frac{1,680,000}{1,000}$$

$$x = \frac{1,680,000}{1,000}$$

$$x = 1,680 \text{ units/hr}$$

14. 1 L = 1,000 mL

a. Calculate mL/hr.

$$\frac{1,000 \text{ mL}}{10 \text{ hr}} = 100 \text{ mL/hr}$$

b. Calculate units/hr.

15,000 units : 1,000 mL = $x$ units : 100 mL

$$\frac{1,000x}{1,000} = \frac{1,500,000}{1,000}$$

$$x = \frac{1,500,000}{1,000}$$

$$x = 1,500 \text{ units/hr}$$

15. 10,000 units : 500 mL = $x$ units : 120 mL

$$\frac{500x}{500} = \frac{1,200,000}{500}$$

$$x = \frac{1,200,000}{500}$$

$$x = 2,400 \text{ units/hr}$$

16. 1 L = 1,000 mL

40,000 units : 1,000 mL = 1,000 units : $x$ mL

$$\frac{40,000x}{40,000} = \frac{1,000,000}{40,000}$$

$$x = \frac{1,000,000}{40,000}$$

$$x = 25 \text{ mL/hr}$$

17. 1 L = 1,000 mL

25,000 units : 1,000 mL = 2,000 units : $x$ mL

$$\frac{25,000x}{25,000} = \frac{2,000,000}{25,000}$$

$$x = \frac{2,000,000}{25,000}$$

$$x = 80 \text{ mL/hr}$$

18. 50,000 units : 1,000 mL = $x$ units : 60 mL

$$\frac{1,000x}{1,000} = \frac{3,000,000}{1,000}$$

$$x = \frac{3,000,000}{1,000}$$

$$x = 3,000 \text{ units/hr}$$

19. 20,000 units : 500 mL = $x$ units : 20 mL

$$\frac{500x}{500} = \frac{400,000}{500}$$

$$x = \frac{400,000}{500}$$

$$x = 800 \text{ units/hr}$$

20. 1 L = 1,000 mL

25,000 units : 1,000 mL = $x$ units : 56 mL

$$\frac{1,000x}{1,000} = \frac{1,400,000}{1,000}$$

$$x = \frac{1,400,000}{1,000}$$

$$x = 1,400 \text{ units/hr}$$

21. 30,000 units : 500 mL = $x$ units : 25 mL

$$\frac{500x}{500} = \frac{750,000}{500}$$

$$x = \frac{750,000}{500}$$

$$x = 1,500 \text{ units/hr}$$

22. 40,000 units : 500 mL = $x$ units : 25 mL

$$\frac{500x}{500} = \frac{1,000,000}{500}$$

$$x = \frac{1,000,000}{500}$$

$$x = 2,000 \text{ units/hr}$$

23. 1 L = 1,000 mL

20,000 units : 1,000 mL = $x$ units : 80 mL

$$\frac{1,000x}{1,000} = \frac{1,600,000}{1,000}$$

$$x = \frac{1,600,000}{1,000}$$

$$x = 1,600 \text{ units/hr}$$

24. Label "B" at 10 units per mL (100 units per 10 mL) is appropriate for flush. Heparin sodium for injection cannot be interchanged with heparin lock solution.

25. a. First determine units/kg the client should receive.

18 units/kg/hr × 80 kg = 1,400 units/hr

b. 1,000 mL : 25,000 units = $x$ mL : 1,440 units

$$\frac{25,000x}{25,000} = \frac{1,440,000}{25,000}$$

$$x = \frac{1,440}{25} = 57.6$$

$$x = 58 \text{ mL/hr}$$

Answer: 58 mL/hr

26. a. Convert the weight to kilograms.

Conversion factor: 2.2 lb = 1 kg

210 lb ÷ 2.2 = 95.45 kg = 95.5 kg

Calculate the heparin bolus dosage.

80 units/kg × 95.5 kg = 7,640 units

Answer: 7,640 units

b. Calculate the infusion rate for the heparin drip.

14 units/kg/hr × 95.5 kg = 1,337 units/hr

c. Calculate the infusion rate in mL/hr.

1,000 units : 25,000 units = $x$ mL : 1,337 units

$$\frac{25,000x}{25,000} = \frac{1,337,000}{25,000}$$

$$x = \frac{1,337}{25} = 53.4$$

$$x = 53 \text{ mL/hr}$$

Answer: 53 mL/hr

27. a. Convert the weight to kilograms.

Conversion factor: 2.2 lb = 1 kg

154 lb ÷ 2.2 = 70 kg

Calculate the heparin bolus dosage.

80 units/kg × 70 kg = 5,600 units

Answer: 5,600 units

b. Calculate the infusion rate for the heparin drip.

14 units/kg/hr × 70 kg = 980 units/hr

Answer: 980 units/hr

c. Calculate the infusion rate in mL/hr.

1,000 mL : 20,000 units = $x$ mL : 980 units

$$\frac{20,000x}{20,000} = \frac{980,000}{20,000}$$

$$x = \frac{98}{2}$$

$$x = 49 \text{ mL/hr}$$

28. **Step 1:** Calculate the heparin bolus dosage. (No weight conversion required; the weight is in kg.)

80 units/kg × 100 kg = 8,000 units. The client should receive 8,000 units IV heparin as a bolus.

Determine the volume (mL) the client would receive. The concentration is indicated as 100 units per mL.

100 units : 1 mL = 8,000 units : x mL

$$\frac{100x}{100} = \frac{8,000}{100}$$

$$x = \frac{8,000}{100}$$

$$x = 80 \text{ mL (bolus is 80 mL)}$$

**Step 2:** Calculate the infusion rate (18 units/kg/hr × kg).

18 units/kg/hr × 100 kg = 1,800 units/hr

Determine the rate in mL/hr at which to set the infusion device (using the concentration of 100 units per mL).

100 units : 1 mL = 1,800 units : x mL

$$\frac{100x}{100} = \frac{1,800}{100}$$

$$x = \frac{1,800}{100}$$

$$x = 18 \text{ mL/hr}$$

The client's APTT is reported as being 71 sec. (According to the protocol, decrease the rate by 2 units/kg/hr; there's no rebolus.)

**Step 3:** Determine the infusion decrease rate (2 units/kg/hr × kg).

2 units/kg/hr × 100 kg = 200 units/hr. The infusion rate should be decreased by 200 units/hr.

**Step 4:** Calculate the adjustment in the hourly infusion rate (mL/hr).

100 units : 1 mL = 200 units : x mL

$$\frac{100x}{100} = \frac{200}{100}$$

$$x = \frac{200}{100}$$

$$x = 2 \text{ mL/hr}$$

**Decrease rate:**

18 mL/hr (current rate)

−2 mL/hr (decrease)
_____

16 mL/hr (new infusion rate)

Decrease the rate on the pump to 16 mL/hr.

*Note:* This problem could also be done using dimensional analysis or formula method.

29. **Step 1:** Calculate the heparin bolus dosage.

Convert the weight to kg. Equivalent: 2.2 lb = 1 kg

162.8 lb ÷ 2.2 = 74 kg

80 units/kg × 74 kg = 5,920 units

The client should receive 5,920 units IV heparin as a bolus.

Determine the volume (mL) the client would receive. The concentration is indicated as 100 units per mL.

100 units : 1 mL = 5,920 units : x mL

$$\frac{100x}{100} = \frac{5,920}{100}$$

$$x = \frac{5,920}{100}$$

$$x = 59.2 \text{ mL (bolus is 59.2 mL)}$$

**Step 2:** Calculate the infusion rate (18 units/kg/hr × kg)

18 units/kg/hr × 74 kg = 1,332 units/hr

Determine the rate in mL/hr at which to set the infusion device (using the concentration of 100 units per mL).

100 units : 1 mL = 1,332 units : x mL

$$\frac{100x}{100} = \frac{1,332}{100}$$

$$x = \frac{1,332}{100}$$

$$x = 13.3 \text{ mL/hr (The pump delivers in tenths of a mL)}$$

The client's APTT is reported as being 38 sec (according to the protocol). Rebolus with 40 units/kg and increase rate by 2 units/kg/hr.

Rebolus: 40 units/kg × 74 kg = 2,960 units

100 units : 1 mL = 2,960 units : x mL

$$\frac{100x}{100} = \frac{2,960}{100}$$

$$x = 29.6 \text{ mL (bolus)}$$

**Step 3:** Determine the infusion increase rate.

2 units/kg/hr × kg

2 units/kg/hr × 74 kg = 148 units/hr

**Step 4:** Calculate the adjustment in the hourly infusion rate (mL/hr).

100 units : 1 mL = 148 units : x mL

$$\frac{100x}{100} = \frac{148}{100}$$

$$x = \frac{148}{100}$$

$$x = 1.48 = 1.5 \text{ mL/hr}$$

Increase rate:

13.3 mL/hr (current rate)

+1.5 mL/hr (increase)
_____

14.8 mL/hr (new infusion rate)

Increase the rate on the pump to 14.8 mL/hr.

*Note:* This problem could also be done using dimensional analysis or formula method.

30. No weight conversion required, the weight is in kg.

   a. Calculate the dose in units/hr

      20 units/kg/hr $\times$ 89 kg = 1,780 units/hr

      Answer: 1,780 units/hr

   b. Determine the rate in mL/hr to deliver 1,780 units/hr

      50 units : 1 mL = 1,780 units : $x$ mL

      $$\frac{50x}{50} = \frac{1,780}{50}$$

      $$x = \frac{1,780}{50}$$

      $x$ = 35.6 mL/hr (pump capable of delivering in tenths)

      Answer: 35.6 mL/hr. The pump would be set at 35.6 mL/hr to deliver 1,780 units/hr.

# CHAPTER 23
# Critical Care Calculations

## Objectives

*After reviewing this chapter, you should be able to:*

1. Calculate dosages in mcg/min, mcg/hr, and mg/min
2. Calculate dosages in mg/kg/hr, mg/kg/min, and mcg/kg/min

The content in this chapter may be required in nursing curriculums that have a critical care component or a specific component of advanced medical-surgical nursing that addresses this content. The content in this chapter can also be used as a reference for nurses working in specialty areas. This chapter provides basic information on medicated drips and titration. In the critical care setting, clients often receive medications to control vital functions that are potent and require close monitoring. These may include medications to maintain the client's blood pressure within normal range and antiarrhythmic medications to regulate the client's heart rate and/or rhythm. Other medications that may be given include sedatives and narcotics. Medications in the critical care setting may be given continuously IV at a constant rate, or the rate of the IV may be titrated (adjusted) to the client response. Examples of how medication dosages may be ordered include milliliters per hour (mL/hr), milligrams per hour (mg/hr), and micrograms per kilogram per minute (mcg/kg/min).

Although there have been instances in the past in which critical care medications were administered using volume-control tubing that has a microdrop calibration (60 gtt/mL), their use should only be in dire circumstances when an infusion pump is not available. Critical care medications should be administered using an electronic infusion pump. This text will focus on critical care medications administered using an infusion pump. As discussed in Chapter 20, pumps deliver in whole milliliters, and there are some pumps that deliver in tenths of a milliliter (usually used in the critical care setting). **Always** be familiar with the pump calibration at your institution. Because of the potency of the medications used, it is essential that nurses perform accurate calculation of dosages, correctly program the infusion pump, and perform continuous monitoring of the client for their response to the medications that are being administered. Despite the use of electronic infusion pumps, calculation errors, infusion pump malfunction, or errors in programming an infusion pump can occur. **Never assume;** to ensure client safety, always use an electronic infusion pump and verify calculations and programming of the pump with a second nurse before administering medications. Like insulin and heparin, many of the medications administered are high-alert medications. Errors in programming infusion pumps or administration of medications at a faster rate than specified or recommended can result in life-threatening effects.

> **! SAFETY ALERT!**
>
> Electronic infusion devices are routinely used to administer medications that are potent. Accurate calculations, correct programming of the pump, and client monitoring are crucial to prevent life-threatening effects, ensure the desired physiological response, and maintain client safety during administration of potent high-alert medications.

## Calculating Rate in mL/hr

The same methods shown in previous chapters involving medications in solution can be applied to critical care medications. Let's look at some examples.

**Example 1:** A solution of Morphine Sulfate 50 mg in 100 mL D₅W at 3.5 mg/hr. Calculate the rate in mL/hr using the solution strength available.

Solution:

### Ratio and Proportion (Linear Format)

$$50 \text{ mg} : 100 \text{ mL} = 3.5 \text{ mg} : x \text{ mL}$$

$$50x = 100 \times 3.5$$

$$\frac{50x}{50} = \frac{350}{50}$$

$$x = 7 \text{ mL/hr}$$

*or*

### Ratio and Proportion (Fraction Format)

$$\frac{50 \text{ mg}}{100 \text{ mL}} = \frac{3.5 \text{ mg}}{x \text{ mL}}$$

$$x = 7 \text{ mL/hr}$$

### Formula Method

$$\frac{3.5 \text{ mg/hr}}{50 \text{ mg}} \times 100 \text{ mL} = x \text{ mL/hr}$$

$$x = 7 \text{ mL/hr}$$

### Dimensional Analysis

As shown in previous chapters involving medications in solution, **isolate what is being calculated**. In this example, it is mL/hr. The **starting fraction** will be the information from the problem containing mL. (mL is placed in the numerator.) Set up **each fraction after** the starting fraction matching the previous denominator.

$$\frac{x \text{ mL}}{\text{hr}} = \frac{\overset{2}{\cancel{100} \text{ mL}}}{\underset{1}{\cancel{50 \text{ mg}}}} \times \frac{3.5 \text{ mg}}{1 \text{ hr}}$$

$$x = \frac{7}{1}$$

$$x = 7 \text{ mL/hr}$$

To infuse 3.5 mg/hr of Morphine Sulfate, set the infusion pump at 7 mL/hr.

**Example 2:** A solution of Isuprel (isoproterenol) 2 mg in 250 mL D₅W to infuse at a rate of 5 mcg/min. (The infusion pump is capable of delivering in tenths of an mL.)

Solution:

Step 1: Calculate the dose per hour.

$$60 \text{ min} = 1 \text{ hr}$$

$$5 \text{ mcg/min} \times 60 \text{ min/hr} = 300 \text{ mcg/hr}$$

Step 2: Convert 300 mcg to mg to match the available strength.
1,000 mcg = 1 mg; therefore 300 mcg = 0.3 mg

Step 3: Calculate the rate in mL/hr. (Use any of the methods shown in Example 1.)

### Ratio and Proportion (Linear Format *or* Fraction Format)

$$2 \text{ mg} : 250 \text{ mL} = 0.3 \text{ mg} : x \text{ mL}$$
$$2x = 250 \times 0.3$$
$$\frac{2x}{2} = \frac{75}{2} = 37.5$$

$$\frac{2 \text{ mg}}{250 \text{ mL}} = \frac{0.3 \text{ mg}}{x \text{ mL}}$$

$x = 37.5$ mL/hr (this is not rounded to the whole number; the pump delivers in tenths of an mL)

### Formula Method

$$\frac{0.3 \text{ mg/hr}}{2 \text{ mg}} \times 250 \text{ mL} = x \text{ mL}$$

### Dimensional Analysis

***Note:*** In this equation, you will need two additional conversion factors, 60 min = 1 hr and 1,000 mcg = 1 mg.

$$\frac{x \text{ mL}}{\text{hr}} = \frac{\overset{125}{\cancel{250} \text{ mL}}}{\underset{1}{\cancel{2} \text{ mg}}} \times \frac{1 \text{ mg}}{\underset{200}{\cancel{1,000} \text{ mcg}}} \times \frac{\overset{1}{\cancel{5} \text{ mcg}}}{1 \text{ min}} \times \frac{60 \text{ min}}{1 \text{ hr}}$$

$$x = \frac{125 \times 60}{200}$$

$$x = \frac{7,500}{200} = 37.5$$

$$x = 37.5 \text{ mL/hr}$$

To infuse 5 mcg/min of Isuprel, set the infusion pump at 37.5 mL/hr.

## Calculating Critical Care Dosages per Hour or per Minute

Example: Infuse dopamine 400 mg in 500 mL D$_5$W at 30 mL/hr. Calculate the dosage in mcg/min and mcg/hr.

Solution:

Step 1: Determine mg/hr.

$$400 \text{ mg} : 500 \text{ mL} = x \text{ mg} : 30 \text{ mL}$$
$$500x = 400 \times 30$$
$$\frac{500x}{500} = \frac{12,000}{500}$$
$$x = \frac{12,000}{500} = 24$$
$$x = 24 \text{ mg/hr}$$

Remember, ratio and proportion can be set up in linear or fraction format.

Step 2: The next step is to convert 24 mg to mcg because the question asks for mcg/min and mcg/hr. Change mg to mcg using the equivalent 1,000 mcg = 1 mg. Change mg to mcg by multiplying by 1,000 or moving the decimal point three places to the right.

$$24 \text{ mg/hr} = 24,000 \text{ mcg/hr}$$

Step 3: Now that you have the mcg/hr, change the mcg/hr to mcg/min using the equivalent 60 min = 1 hr.

Divide the number of mcg/hr by 60 to get the mcg/min.

$$24,000 \text{ mcg/hr} \div 60 \text{ min/hr} = 400 \text{ mcg/min}$$

**Note:** This is in mcg/min; however, these medications are usually delivered in mL/hr by pump, and you will need to take the calculation further. Later in the chapter you will see examples of changing mcg/min to mL/hr.

| Dimensional Analysis |
|---|

$$\frac{x \text{ mg}}{\text{hr}} = \frac{\overset{4}{\cancel{400}} \text{ mg}}{\underset{5}{\cancel{500} \text{ mL}}} \times \frac{30 \text{ mL}}{1 \text{ hr}}$$

$$x = \frac{120}{5}$$

$$x = 24 \text{ mg/hr}$$

To determine mg/min, 24 mg/hr ÷ 60 min/hr = 0.4 mg/min = 400 mcg/min

Dopamine infusing at 30 mL/hr = 24,000 mcg/hr; 400 mcg/min.

## Medications Ordered in Milligrams per Minute

Medications such as Lidocaine and Pronestyl are ordered in mg/min.

Example: A client is receiving Pronestyl 60 mL/hr. The solution available is Pronestyl 2 g in 500 mL $D_5W$. Calculate the mg/hr and the mg/min the client will receive.

Solution:

Step 1: A conversion is necessary; g must be converted to mg.
You are being asked for **(mg/min, mg/hr)**. Equivalent: 1 g = 1,000 mg.
Therefore 2 g = 2,000 mg. Multiply 2 by 1,000 or move decimal point three places to the right.

Step 2: Now determine the mg/hr by setting up a proportion. (Refer to problems earlier in the chapter illustrating the various methods that can be used.)

$$2,000 \text{ mg} : 500 \text{ mg} = x \text{ mg} : 60 \text{ mL}$$

$$500 x = 2,000 \times 60$$

$$\frac{500 x}{500} = \frac{120,000}{500}$$

$$x = \frac{1,200}{5}$$

$$x = 240 \text{ mg/hr}$$

Step 3:     Convert mg/hr to mg/min. Equivalent: 60 min = 1 hr.

$$240 \text{ mg/hr} \div 60 \text{ min/hr} = 4 \text{ mg/min}$$

### Dimensional Analysis

(**Note:** The starting fraction here is the conversion factor to match the desired numerator, and the solution strength is in g, with the conversion factor written so g is written in the numerator to match the denominator of the starting fraction.)

$$\frac{x \text{ mg}}{\text{hr}} = \frac{\overset{2}{\cancel{1,000}} \text{ mg}}{1 \cancel{g}} \times \frac{2 \cancel{g}}{\underset{1}{\cancel{500} \text{ mL}}} \times \frac{60 \cancel{\text{ mL}}}{1 \text{ hr}}$$

$$x = \frac{240}{1}$$

$$x = 240 \text{ mg/hr}$$

To determine mg/min, $240 \text{ mg/hr} \div 60 \text{ min/hr} = 4 \text{ mg/min}$.

Pronestyl infusing at 60 mL/hr is delivering 240 mg/hr; 4 mg/min.

## Calculating Dosages Based on mcg/kg/min

Medications are also ordered for clients based on dosage per kilogram per minute. These medications include Nipride, dopamine, and dobutamine. In these problems, the weight will be rounded to the nearest tenth as indicated for calculation.

Example:     Order: Dopamine 2 mcg/kg/min. The solution available is dopamine 400 mg in 250 mL $D_5W$. The client weighs 154 lb. (The pump is capable of delivering in tenths of an mL.)

Solution:

Step 1:     Convert the client's weight in pounds to kilograms.
            Equivalent: 2.2 lb = 1 kg
            To convert the weight, divide 154 lb by 2.2.
            154 lb ÷ 2.2 = 70 kg

Step 2:     Now that you have the client's weight in kg, determine the dosage per minute.

$$70 \cancel{\text{ kg}} \times 2 \text{ mcg/}\cancel{\text{kg}}\text{/min} = 140 \text{ mcg/min}$$

Converting mcg/min to mL/hr then would be easy using this example. (Equivalent: 1,000 mcg = 1 mg.)
a. Convert mcg/min to mcg/hr.

$$140 \text{ mcg/}\cancel{\text{min}} \times 60 \cancel{\text{ min}}\text{/hr} = 8,400 \text{ mcg/hr}$$

b. Convert mcg/hr to mg/hr.

$$8,400 \div 1,000 = 8.4 \text{ mg/hr}$$

c. Determine IV flow rate.

### Ratio and Proportion

$$400 \text{ mg} : 250 \text{ mL} = 8.4 \text{ mg} : x \text{ mL}$$

$$400x = 250 \times 8.4$$

$$\frac{400x}{400} = \frac{2,\cancel{100}}{\cancel{400}} = 5.25$$

$$x = 5.3 \text{ mL/hr}$$

**Dimensional Analysis**

$$\frac{x \text{ mL}}{\text{hr}} = \frac{\overset{5}{\cancel{250}} \text{ mL}}{\underset{8}{\cancel{400}} \text{ mg}} \times \frac{1 \cancel{\text{ mg}}}{1,000 \cancel{\text{ mcg}}} \times \frac{140 \cancel{\text{ mcg}}}{1 \cancel{\text{ min}}} \times \frac{60 \cancel{\text{ min}}}{1 \text{ hr}}$$

$$x = \frac{42,000}{8,000} = 5.25$$

$$x = 5.3 \text{ mL/hr}$$

The pump would be set at 5.3 mL/hr to administer the dose of dopamine at 2 mcg/kg/min.

## IV Flow Rates for Titrated Medications

Critically ill clients in the critical care area can receive potent medications by IV infusion using a process referred to as **titration**. **Titrated medications** are added to a specific volume of fluid and then adjusted accordingly to infuse at a rate at which the desired effect is attained. **The medications that are titrated include potent antiarrhythmic, vasopressor, and vasodilator medications; these must be monitored closely by the nurse.** IV medications that are titrated usually start at the lowest dosage and are increased and decreased as needed. Medications that are titrated are administered according to a protocol. Nurses **must** know the institution's protocol regarding administration of titrated medications. Because of the potency of medications used, minute changes in the infusion cause an effect on the client. Titrated medications are ordered within parameters to obtain a desirable outcome. The outcome desired depends on the medication. When a solution is titrated, **the lowest dosage of the medication is set first and increased or decreased as necessary. The higher dosage should not be exceeded without an order.** When a medication is to be titrated, the prescriber determines the titration for the individual client based on the desired outcome. The order for the titration of a medication includes the medication, the dosage in a specific volume of fluid, the dosage range (minimal dose and maximum dose), the starting dose for the medication (which is usually the minimal dose), and the desired outcome.

Dosage errors with titrated medications can result in dire consequences. Therefore, the nurse must have knowledge regarding the medication, the proper dosage adjustment, and the frequency of adjustments based on the client assessment and the prescribed parameters. Electronic infusion pumps are used with titrated medications.

There are also IV pumps available in the critical care setting, referred to as *smart pumps*. Smart pumps were discussed in Chapter 20. The sophistication of the smart pump depends on the software. Some smart pumps have incorporated calculating IV rates for specific medications. The nurse is able to select the medication from the IV pump "library" and enter the desired dose and concentration of the medication and the client's weight in kilograms; the pump then displays the IV rate in mL/hr.

Regardless of the type of infusion pump used, the nurse has the responsibility of having knowledge about the equipment to ensure safe medication administration of potent high-alert medications. The increase in sophistication of pumps do not relieve the nurse from his or her responsibility to think critically (i.e., Is the dosage reasonable? Is the rate correct to deliver the ordered dosage?). Pumps that have the ability to perform the needed calculations or a calculator should be used as a tool to check calculations and not as a tool for dosage calculation. Smart pumps should be used as a drive toward safe practice and used properly to ensure client safety. Remember that all pumps require human entry.

Because of the consequences associated with titrated medications, it is common practice at many institutions to have a double- or triple-check of medication dosages and the mathematical computations associated with them, even in instances where calculators may be used.

> **! SAFETY ALERT!**
> Know the equipment you are using and the institution's policy regarding the administration of titrated medications. **Never exceed** the prescribed upper dose limit. Notify the prescriber when the maximum limit is reached for a new order.

Let's look at some examples of titration of medications.

**Example 1:** Nipride has been ordered to titrate at 3 to 6 mcg/kg/min to maintain a client's systolic blood pressure below 140 mm Hg. The solution contains 50 mg Nipride in 250 mL D$_5$W. The client weighs 56 kg. Determine the rate to set the IV pump.

**Step 1:** Convert to **like units**.

Equivalent: 1,000 mcg = 1 mg
Therefore 50 mg = 50,000 mcg

**Step 2:** Calculate the concentration of solution in mcg/mL.

$$50,000 \text{ mcg} : 250 \text{ mL} = x \text{ mcg} : 1 \text{ mL}$$

$$\frac{250x}{250} = \frac{50,000}{250}$$

$$x = 200 \text{ mcg/mL}$$

The concentration of solution is 200 mcg/mL.

**Step 3:** Calculate the dosage range using the upper and lower dosages.

(Lower dosage) 3 mcg/kg/min × 56 kg = 168 mcg/min
(Upper dosage) 6 mcg/kg/min × 56 kg = 336 mcg/min

**Step 4:** Convert dosage range to mL/min.

(Lower dosage) 200 mcg : 1 mL = 168 mcg : $x$ mL

$$\frac{200x}{200} = \frac{168}{200}$$

$$x = 0.84 \text{ mL/min}$$

(Upper dosage) 200 mcg : 1 mL = 336 mcg : $x$ mL

$$\frac{200x}{200} = \frac{336}{200}$$

$$x = 1.68 \text{ mL/min}$$

**Step 5:** Convert mL/min to mL/hr.

(Lower dosage) 0.84 mL/min × 60 min/hr = 50.4 = 50 mL/hr
(Upper dosage) 1.68 mL/min × 60 min/hr = 100.8 = 101 mL/hr

A dosage range of 3 to 6 mcg/kg/min is equal to a flow rate of 50 to 101 mL/hr.
The client's condition has stabilized, and the flow rate is now maintained at 60 mL/hr. What dosage will be infusing per minute?

$$200 \text{ mcg} : 1 \text{ mL} = x \text{ mcg} : 60 \text{ mL}$$

$$x = 12,000 \text{ mcg/hr}$$

12,000 mcg/hr ÷ 60 min/hr = 200 mcg/min

## Solution to Example 1 Using Dimensional Analysis

**Step 1:** Calculate the dosage range first.

(Lower dosage) 3 mcg/kg/min × 56 kg = 168 mcg/min
(Upper dosage) 6 mcg/kg/min × 56 kg = 336 mcg/min

**Step 2:**     Calculate the IV rate in mL/hr for the lower dosage.

$$\frac{x\text{ mL}}{\text{hr}} = \frac{\overset{5}{\cancel{250}}\text{ mL}}{\underset{1}{\cancel{50}}\text{ mg}} \times \frac{1\text{ mg}}{1{,}000\text{ mcg}} \times \frac{168\text{ mcg}}{1\text{ min}} \times \frac{60\text{ min}}{1\text{ hr}}$$

$$x = 50.4 = 50\text{ mL/hr}$$

**Step 3:**     Calculate the IV rate in mL/hr for the upper dosage.

$$\frac{x\text{ mL}}{\text{hr}} = \frac{\overset{5}{\cancel{250}}\text{ mL}}{\underset{1}{\cancel{50}}\text{ mg}} \times \frac{1\text{ mg}}{1{,}000\text{ mcg}} \times \frac{336\text{ mcg}}{1\text{ min}} \times \frac{60\text{ min}}{1\text{ hr}}$$

$$x = 100.8 = 101\text{ mL/hr}$$

A dosage range of 3 to 6 mcg/kg/min is equal to a flow rate of 50 to 101 mL/hr.

The client's condition has stabilized, and the IV flow rate is now maintained at 60 mL/hr. What dosage will be infusing per minute?

$$\frac{x\text{ mcg}}{\text{min}} = \frac{\overset{4}{\cancel{1{,}000}}\text{ mcg}}{1\text{ mg}} \times \frac{50\text{ mg}}{\underset{1}{\cancel{250}}\text{ mL}} \times \frac{60\text{ mL}}{1\text{ hr}} \times \frac{1\text{ hr}}{60\text{ min}}$$

$$x = 200\text{ mcg/min}$$

## Developing a Titration Table

After calculating an initial IV rate for a medication being titrated, the client is monitored. If the desired response is not achieved, the dosage may have to be increased. This will require the nurse to find the corresponding IV rate in mL/hr for the new dosage. Any time the dosage is changed, recalculation of the corresponding IV rate is required. Rather than performing calculations each time a dosage is modified, the nurse can develop a titration table to provide the IV rate for any possible change in the medication dosage.

Let's look at the previous example (Example 1) and develop a titration table to increase the dosage by 1 mcg/min up to 6 mcg/min. Set up a ratio proportion to develop the titration table; use the minimum rate required to deliver 3 mcg/min to find the incremental flow rate that provides a dosage rate change of 1mcg/min.

The proportion is:

$$\frac{3\text{ mcg/min}}{50\text{ mL/hr}} = \frac{1\text{ mcg/min}}{x\text{ mL/hr}}$$

$$\frac{3x}{3} = \frac{50}{3} = 16.6$$

$$x = 17\text{ mL/hr}$$

So, for each change of 1 mcg/min, the incremental IV flow rate is 17 mL/hr.

| Titration Table | |
| --- | --- |
| **Dosage Rate (mcg/min)** | **Flow Rate (mL/hr)** |
| 3 mcg/min **(minimum)** | 50 mL/hr |
| 4 mcg/min | 67 mL/hr |
| 5 mcg/min | 84 mL/hr |
| 6 mcg/min **(maximum)** | 101 mL/hr |

Notice in this problem mL/hr was rounded to the nearest whole number. Remember, there are pumps capable of accepting one decimal place.

**Example 2:** Nitroglycerin has been ordered to titrate at 10 mcg/min to 60 mcg/min, and the rate should be increased by 10 mcg/min every 3-5 minutes for chest pain. The solution contains 50 mg nitroglycerin in 250 mL D$_5$W.

**Step 1:** Calculate the dose per hour using the upper and lower dosages.

$$10 \text{ mcg/\cancel{min}} \times 60 \text{ \cancel{min}/hr} = 600 \text{ mcg/hr}$$
$$60 \text{ mcg/\cancel{min}} \times 60 \text{ \cancel{min}/hr} = 3{,}600 \text{ mcg/hr}$$

**Step 2:** Convert mcg to mg to match the available strength.

$$1{,}000 \text{ mcg} = 1 \text{ mg}$$
$$600 \text{ mcg} = 0.6 \text{ mg}$$
$$3{,}600 \text{ mcg} = 3.6 \text{ mg}$$

**Step 3:** Calculate the rate in mL/hr.

$$50 \text{ mg} : 250 \text{ mL} = 0.6 \text{ mg} : x \text{ mL}$$
$$50x = 250 \times 0.6$$
$$\frac{50x}{50} = \frac{150}{50}$$

$$x = 3 \text{ mL/hr}$$

To infuse 10 mcg/min, set the IV rate at 3 mL/hr (minimum).

$$50 \text{ mg} : 250 \text{ mL} = 3.6 \text{ mg} : x \text{ mL}$$
$$50x = 250 \times 3.6$$
$$\frac{50x}{50} = \frac{900}{50}$$

$$x = 18 \text{ mL/hr}$$

To infuse 60 mcg/min, set the IV rate at 18 mL/hr (maximum). A dosage range of 10 to 60 mcg/min is equal to a flow rate of 3 to 18 mL/hr.

## Dimensional Analysis Setup for Example 2

Calculate the lower dosage.

$$\frac{x \text{ mL}}{\text{hr}} = \frac{\overset{5}{\cancel{250}} \text{ mL}}{\underset{1}{\cancel{50} \text{ \cancel{mg}}}} \times \frac{1 \text{ \cancel{mg}}}{1{,}000 \text{ \cancel{mcg}}} \times \frac{10 \text{ \cancel{mcg}}}{1 \text{ \cancel{min}}} \times \frac{60 \text{ \cancel{min}}}{1 \text{ hr}}$$

$$x = 3 \text{ mL/hr}$$

Calculate upper dosage.

$$\frac{x \text{ mL}}{\text{hr}} = \frac{\overset{5}{\cancel{250}} \text{ mL}}{\underset{1}{\cancel{50} \text{ \cancel{mg}}}} \times \frac{1 \text{ \cancel{mg}}}{1{,}000 \text{ \cancel{mcg}}} \times \frac{60 \text{ \cancel{mcg}}}{1 \text{ \cancel{min}}} \times \frac{60 \text{ \cancel{min}}}{1 \text{ hr}}$$

$$x = 18 \text{ mL/hr}$$

A dosage range of 10-60 mcg/min is equal to a flow rate of 3-18 mL/hr.

Develop a titration table using 10-mcg increments. Set up the proportion using the minimum to determine the dosage change of 10 mcg/min.

$$\frac{10 \text{ mcg/min}}{3 \text{ mL/hr}} = \frac{10 \text{ mcg/min}}{x \text{ mL/hr}}$$

$$\frac{10x}{10} = \frac{30}{10}$$

$$x = 3 \text{ mL/hr}$$

So, for each change of 10 mcg/min, the incremental IV flow rate is 3 mL/hr.

| Titration Table | |
|---|---|
| **Dosage Rate (mcg/min)** | **Flow Rate (mL/hr)** |
| 10 mcg/min (minimum) | 3 mL/hr |
| 20 mcg/min | 6 mL/hr |
| 30 mcg/min | 9 mL/hr |
| 40 mcg/min | 12 mL/hr |
| 50 mcg/min | 15 mL/hr |
| 60 mcg/min (maximum) | 18 mL/hr |

**Example 3:** Levophed (norepinephrine bitartrate) has been ordered to titrate at 3 mcg/min to 10 mcg/min, and the rate should be increased at 1 mcg/min to maintain blood pressure and keep systolic blood pressure greater than 100 mm Hg. The solution contains 2 mg Levophed in 250 mL D$_5$W. Develop a titration table at 1-mcg increments. The pump delivers in tenths.

**Step 1:** Calculate the dose per hour using the upper and lower dosages.

$$3 \text{ mcg/\cancel{min}} \times 60 \text{ \cancel{min}/hr} = 180 \text{ mcg/hr}$$
$$10 \text{ mcg/\cancel{min}} \times 60 \text{ \cancel{min}/hr} = 600 \text{ mcg/hr}$$

**Step 2:** Convert mcg to mg to match the available strength.

$$1,000 \text{ mcg} = 1 \text{ mg}$$
$$180 \text{ mcg} = 0.18 \text{ mg}$$
$$600 \text{ mcg} = 0.6 \text{ mg}$$

**Step 3:** Calculate the rate in mL/hr

$$2 \text{ mg} : 250 \text{ mL} = 0.18 \text{ mg} : x \text{ mL}$$
$$2x = 250 \times 0.18$$
$$\frac{2x}{2} = \frac{45}{2}$$
$$x = 22.5 \text{ mL/hr}$$

To infuse 3 mcg/min, set the IV rate at 22.5 mL/hr (minimum)

$$2 \text{ mg} : 250 \text{ mL} = 0.6 \text{ mg} : x \text{ mL}$$
$$2x = 250 \times 0.6$$
$$\frac{2x}{2} = \frac{150}{2}$$
$$x = 75 \text{ mL/hr}$$

To infuse 10 mcg/min, set the IV rate at 75 mL/hr. A dosage range of 3-10 mcg/min is equal to a flow rate of 22.5-75 mL/hr.

## Dimensional Analysis Setup for Example 3

Calculate the lower dosage.

$$\frac{x \text{ mL}}{\text{hr}} = \frac{\overset{125}{\cancel{250} \text{ mL}}}{\underset{1}{\cancel{2} \text{ mg}}} \times \frac{1 \cancel{\text{ mg}}}{1,000 \cancel{\text{ mcg}}} \times \frac{3 \cancel{\text{ mcg}}}{1 \cancel{\text{ min}}} \times \frac{60 \cancel{\text{ min}}}{1 \text{ hr}}$$

$$x = 22.5 \text{ mL/hr}$$

Calculate the upper dosage.

$$\frac{x \text{ mL}}{\text{hr}} = \frac{\overset{125}{\cancel{250} \text{ mL}}}{\underset{1}{\cancel{2} \text{ mg}}} \times \frac{1 \cancel{\text{ mg}}}{1,000 \cancel{\text{ mcg}}} \times \frac{10 \cancel{\text{ mcg}}}{1 \cancel{\text{ min}}} \times \frac{60 \cancel{\text{ min}}}{1 \text{ hr}}$$

$$x = 75 \text{ mL/hr}$$

A dosage range of 3-10 mcg/min is equal to a flow rate of 22.5-75 mL/hr.

Find the incremental flow rate for a dosage rate change of 1 mcg/min by setting up a ratio proportion.

The proportion is:

$$\frac{3 \text{ mcg/min}}{22.5 \text{ mL/hr}} = \frac{1 \text{ mcg/min}}{x \text{ mL/hr}}$$

$$\frac{3x}{3} = \frac{22.5}{3}$$

$$x = 7.5 \text{ mL/hr}$$

So, for each change of 1 mcg/min, the incremental IV flow rate is 7.5 mL/hr.

### Titration Table

| Dosage Rate (mcg/min) | Flow Rate (mL/hr) |
| --- | --- |
| 3 mcg/min **(minimum)** | 22.5 mL/hr |
| 4 mcg/min | 30 mL/hr |
| 5 mcg/min | 37.5 mL/hr |
| 6 mcg/min | 45 mL/hr |
| 7 mcg/min | 52.5 mL/hr |
| 8 mcg/min | 60 mL/hr |
| 9 mcg/min | 67.5 mL/hr |
| 10 mcg/min **(maximum)** | 75 mL/hr |

### POINTS TO REMEMBER

- Potent medications in the critical care setting should be administered by an electronic infusion device.
- Accurate calculation of dosages and client monitoring are essential when clients are receiving potent medications by IV infusion.
- Double-checking of calculations is essential to ensure correct dosage administration.
- Titration of medications requires careful adjustment of dosages to obtain a desirable client outcome.
- Know the institution's policy relating to titration of medications.
- **Do not** exceed the upper dose limit for titrated medications.
- **Always** be familiar with the calibration of the infusion pump being used to administer IV medications.
- The use of infusion pumps **does not** relieve the responsibility of the nurse to critically think.

## ⊞ PRACTICE **PROBLEMS**

Calculate the following as indicated. Unless stated otherwise, infusion pumps deliver in whole mL/hr.

1. A client weighing 50 kg is to receive a Dobutamine solution of 250 mg in 500 mL D5W ordered to titrate between 2.5 and 5 mcg/kg/min.

   a. Determine the flow rate setting for an infusion pump. _____

   b. If the IV flow rate is being maintained at 25 mL/hr after several titrations, what is the dosage infusing per minute? _____

2. Order: Epinephrine at 30 mL/hr. The solution available is 2 mg of epinephrine in 250 mL $D_5W$. Calculate the following:

   a. mg/hr _____

   b. mcg/hr _____

   c. mcg/min _____

3. Aminophylline 0.25 g is added to 500 mL $D_5W$ to infuse at 20 mL/hr. Calculate the following:

   mg/hr _____

4. Order: Pitocin at 25 mL/hr. The solution contains 20 units of Pitocin in 1,000 mL Ringer's Lactate.

   Calculate the number of units per hour the client is receiving. _____

5. Order: 3 mcg/kg/min of Nipride RTU.

   Available: 50 mg of Nipride RTU in 250 mL $D_5W$. Client's weight is 60 kg.

   Calculate the flow rate in mL/hr that will deliver this dosage. _____

6. A nitroglycerin drip is infusing at 3 mL/hr. The solution available is 50 mg of nitroglycerin in 250 mL $D_5W$. Calculate the following:

   a. mcg/hr _____

   b. mcg/min _____

7. Order: Procainamide to titrate at 2 mg/min to the maximum of 6 mg/min. The available solution is procainamide 2 g in 250 mL $D_5W$. Develop a titration table in 2-mg/min increments up to the maximum dose.

**Answers on pp. 593-594**

## 🔧 CLINICAL **REASONING**

**Scenario:** Isuprel is ordered for a client at the rate of 3 mcg/min with a solution containing Isuprel 1 mg in 250 mL D₅W. The nurse performed the following calculation to determine the rate by pump in mL/hr.

- Calculated the dosage per hour:

$$3 \text{ mcg/min} \times 60 \text{ min/hr} = 180 \text{ mcg/hr}$$

- Converted 180 mcg to milligrams to match the units in the solution strength:

$$180 \text{ mcg} = 0.018 \text{ mg}$$

- Calculated the rate in mL/hr:

$$1 \text{ mg} : 250 \text{ mL} = 0.018 \text{ mg} : x \text{ mL}$$
$$x = 250 \times 0.018$$
$$x = 4.5 = 5 \text{ mL/hr}$$

a. What error did the nurse make in her calculation to determine the rate in mL/hr?

_____

b. What could be the potential outcome of the error? _____

c. What should the rate be in mL/hr? _____

d. What preventive measures could have been taken by the nurse? _____

**Answers on p. 594**

## NGN Case Study

**Learning Objectives:**
1. Calculate dosages in mcg/min, mcg/hr, and mg/min.
2. Calculate dosages in mg/kg/hr, mg/kg/min, and mcg/kg/min, mcg/kg/hr.

**Case Scenario:** The client is in the intensive care unit for respiratory failure, is placed on a mechanical ventilator, and needs to be given sedation for comfort. Propofol is ordered for sedation at 15 mcg/kg/min. The client weighs 188 pounds. The solution available is Propofol 1,000 mg in 100 mL of D₅W. The electronic infusion device can be programed to tenths. Which actions are appropriate in planning care for this client? **Select all that apply.**

1. Calculate the client weight as 85.5 kg.
2. Calculate the patient weight as 413.6 kg.
3. Calculate the dose of propofol as 1282.5 mcg/min.
4. Calculate the dose of propofol as 6204 mcg/min.
5. Program the electronic infusion device for 7.7 mL/hr.
6. Program the electronic infusion device for 38.5 mL/hr.
7. Program the electronic infusion device for 16.9 mL/hr.

**Reference:** Morris: *Calculate with confidence*, ed 8, St Louis, Elsevier, copyright 2022.

*Case Study answers and rationales can be found on Evolve.*

## ⊙ CHAPTER **REVIEW**

Calculate the dosages as indicated. Use the labels where provided. Unless stated otherwise, pump is capable of delivering in a whole number of mL.

1. Client is receiving Isuprel at 30 mL/hr. The solution available is 2 mg of Isuprel in 250 mL D₅W. Calculate the following:

   a. mg/hr _____

   b. mcg/hr _____

   c. mcg/min _____

2. Infuse dopamine 800 mg in 500 mL D₅W at 30 mL/hr. Calculate the dosage in mcg/hr and mcg/min.

   Available:

   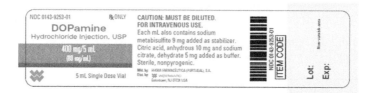

   a. mcg/hr _____

   b. mcg/min _____

   c. Calculate the number of milliliters
      you will add to the IV for this dosage. _____

3. Infuse Sodium Nitroprusside at 30 mL/hr. The solution available is 50 mg sodium nitroprusside in 250 mL 0.9% NS.

   Available:

   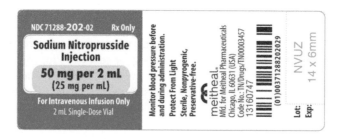

   Calculate the following:

   a. mcg/hr _____

   b. mcg/min _____

   c. Number of milliliters you will
      add to the IV for this dosage _____

4. Order: Lidocaine 2 g in 250 mL D₅W to infuse at 60 mL/hr. Calculate the following:

   a. mg/hr _____

   b. mg/min _____

5. Order: Aminophylline 0.25 g to be added to 250 mL of D₅W. The order is to infuse over 6 hr.

Available:

20 mL Single-dose
**Aminophylline**
**Injection, USP**
500 mg/20 mL (25 mg/mL)
Protect from light.
DO NOT USE IF CRYSTALS HAVE
SEPARATED FROM SOLUTION.

Rx only                    NDC 0409-5922-16
Each mL contains aminophylline (calculated as the
dihydrate) 25 mg (equivalent to 19.7 mg/mL of
anhydrous theophylline). May contain an excess of
ethylenediamine for pH adjustment. pH 8.8 (8.6 to
9.0). Sterile, nonpyrogenic. Use only if clear and
seal is intact and undamaged. Contains no
bacteriostat; use promptly; discard unused portion.
For intravenous use. Usual dosage: See insert.

Distributed by          RL-7074
Hospira, Inc., Lake Forest, IL 60045 USA   *Hospira*

   a. Calculate the dosage in mg/hr the
      client will receive.                    _____

   b. Calculate the number of milliliters you
      will add to the IV for this dosage.      _____

6. A client is receiving Pronestyl at 30 mL/hr. The solution available is 2 g Pronestyl in 250 mL D₅W. Calculate the following:

   a. mg/hr                                    _____

   b. mg/min                                   _____

7. Order: Pitocin (oxytocin) at 40 mL/hr. The solution available is 30 units of Pitocin in 1,000 mL of D₅W. Calculate the following:

   a. units/hr                                 _____

   b. units/min                                _____

8. A client is receiving bretylium at 45 mL/hr. The solution available is 2 g bretylium in 500 mL D₅W. Calculate the following:

   a. mg/hr                                    _____

   b. mg/min                                   _____

9. A client is receiving nitroglycerin 50 mg in 250 mL D₅W. The order is to infuse 500 mcg/min.

   What flow rate in mL/hr would be
   needed to deliver the ordered dosage?        _____

10. Dopamine has been ordered to maintain a client's blood pressure; 400 mg dopamine has been placed in 500 mL D₅W to infuse at 35 mL/hr.

    How many milligrams are being
    administered per hour?                       _____

11. A client is receiving Isuprel 2 mg in 250 mL D₅W. The order is to infuse at 20 mL/hr. Calculate the following:

a. mg/hr                          _____

b. mcg/hr                         _____

c. mcg/min                        _____

12. Order: 1 g of aminophylline in 1,000 mL D$_5$W to infuse over 10 hr.

Calculate the dosage in mg/hr the
client will receive.             _____

13. A client is receiving lidocaine 2 g in 250 mL D$_5$W. The solution is infusing at
22 mL/hr. Calculate the following:

a. mg/hr                          _____

b. mg/min                         _____

14. Order: Esmolol 2.5 g in 250 mL 0.9% NS at 30 mL/hr. Calculate the following:

a. mg/hr                          _____

b. mg/min                         _____

15. Order: Dobutamine 500 mg in 500 mL D$_5$W to infuse at 30 mL/hr.

Calculate the following:

a. mcg/hr                         _____

b. mcg/min                        _____

16. Order: Dopamine 400 mg in 500 mL 0.9% NS to infuse at 200 mcg/min.

Calculate the rate in mL/hr.      _____

17. Order: Magnesium sulfate 3 g/hr.

Available: 25 g of 50% magnesium sulfate in 300 mL D$_5$W.

What rate in mL/hr would be needed
to administer the required dose?  _____

18. Order: Nipride 50 mg in 250 mL D$_5$W to infuse at 2 mcg/kg/min. Client's weight is
120 lb.

Calculate the dosage per minute.  _____

19. Order: Dobutamine 250 mg in 500 mL of D$_5$W at 3 mcg/kg/min. The client weighs 80 kg.

What dosage in mcg/min should the
client receive?                   _____

20. Order: Infuse 1 g of aminophylline in 1,000 mL of D$_5$W at 0.7 mg/kg/hr. The client
weighs 110 lb.

a. Calculate the dosage in mg/hr. _____

    b. Calculate the dosage in mg/min. _____

    c. Reference states no more than
       20 mg/min. Is the order safe? _____

21. Norepinephrine (Levophed) 2 to 6 mcg/min has been ordered to maintain a
    client's systolic blood pressure at 100 mm Hg. The solution concentration is 2 mg
    in 500 mL $D_5W$.

    Determine the flow rate in mL/hr. _____

22. Esmolol is to titrate between 50 to 75 mcg/kg/min. The client weighs 60 kg. The solu-
    tion strength is 5,000 mg of esmolol in 500 mL $D_5W$.

    a. Determine the flow rate for an
       infusion pump. _____

    b. The titration rate is at 24 mL/hr.
       What is the dosage infusing per
       minute? _____

23. Order: Dobutamine 500 mg in 250 mL $D_5W$ to infuse at 10 mcg/kg/min. The client
    weighs 65 kg.

    Calculate the flow rate in mL/hr. _____

24. A client is receiving lidocaine 1 g in 500 mL $D_5W$ at a rate of 20 mL/hr. Calculate the
    following:

    a. mg/hr _____

    b. mg/min _____

25. Esmolol 1.5 g in 250 mL $D_5W$ has been ordered at a rate of 100 mcg/kg/min for a cli-
    ent weighing 102.4 kg. Determine the following:

    a. dosage in mcg/min _____

    b. rate in mL/hr _____

26. Order: Dopamine 400 mg in 500 mL $D_5W$ to infuse at 20 mL/hr. Determine the
    following:

    a. mg/min _____

    b. mcg/min _____

27. Order: Diltiazem HCl 125 mg in 100 mL $D_5W$ to infuse at 20 mg/hr.

    Available:

Determine the following:

a. How many milliliters will you
add to the IV?

_____

b. Determine the rate in mL/hr.
(Consider the medication in the
volume.)

_____

28. Order: 2 g Pronestyl in 500 mL D$_5$W to infuse at 2 mg/min.

Determine the rate in mL/hr.               _____

29. Dopamine is ordered at a rate of 3 mcg/kg/min for a client weighing 95.9 kg. The
solution strength is 400 mg dopamine in 250 mL D$_5$W. Determine the flow rate for an
IV pump. The pump is capable of delivering in tenths of an mL. _____

30. Infuse Dobutamine 250 mg in 500 mL D$_5$W at 5 mcg/kg/min. The client weighs
143 lb. Concentration of solution is 500 mcg per mL. How many mcg of dobutamine
will be infused per minute? _____ per hour? _____

31. A medication has been ordered at 2 to 4 mcg/min to maintain a client's systolic BP
greater than 100 mm Hg. The medication being titrated has 8 mg of medication in
250 mL D$_5$W. Determine the IV rate for 2 to 4 mcg range. Then assume that after
several changes in mL/hr have been made, the BP has stabilized at a rate of 5 mL/hr.
How many mcg/min is the client receiving at this rate? Determine the flow rate for
an IV pump capable of delivering in tenths of an mL.

a. _____ Flow rate for 2-4 mcg range

b. _____ mcg per/min at 5 mL /hr

32. Order: Nitroglycerin to titrate at 40 mcg/min for chest pain to a maximum of
100 mcg/min. The solution contains 40 mg of nitroglycerin in 250 mL D$_5$W. Develop
a titration table from minimum to maximum dose in 20-mcg/min increments.
The pump is capable of delivering in tenths.

33. Order: Levophed 4 mcg/min to maintain BP systolic greater than 100 mm Hg to
a maximum of 12 mcg/min. Available solution: Levophed 4 mg in 500 mL D$_5$W.
Develop a titration table in 2-mcg/min increments.

34. A solution of lorazepam 4 mg in 100 mL 0.9% NS to infuse at 1 mg/hr. Determine
the infusion rate.

35. A solution of Amiodarone 900 mg in 500 mL of D$_5$W to infuse at 0.5 mg/min.
Determine the infusion rate to deliver the ordered dosage. (The pump is capable of
delivering in tenths of an mL.)

**Answers on pp. 594-600**

evolve

For additional practice problems, refer to the Advanced Calculations section of the Critical Care Dosages section of the
Elsevier's Interactive Drug Calculation Application, Version 1, on Evolve.

### ⭐ ANSWERS

<u>**Chapter 23**</u>
**Answers to Practice Problems**

1. a. Step 1: Conversion: Equivalent: 1,000 mcg = 1 mg.
   Therefore 250 mg = 250,000 mcg.

   Step 2: 250,000 mcg : 500 mL = $x$ mcg : 1 mL

   $\dfrac{500x}{500} = \dfrac{250,000}{500}$; $x = 500$ mcg/mL

   Concentration of solution is 500 mcg/mL.

   Step 3: Calculate dosage range.

   Lower dosage:

   2.5 mcg/kg/min × 50 kg = 125 mcg/min

   Upper dosage:

   5 mcg/kg/min × 50 kg = 250 mcg/min

   Step 4: Convert dosage range to mL/min.

   Lower dosage:

   500 mcg : 1 mL = 125 mcg : $x$ mL

   $\dfrac{500x}{500} = \dfrac{125}{500}$

   $x = 0.25$ mL/min

   Upper dosage:

   500 mcg : 1 mL = 250 mcg : $x$ mL

   $\dfrac{500x}{500} = \dfrac{125}{500}$

   $x = 0.5$ mL/min

   Step 5: Convert mL/min to mL/hr.

   Lower dosage: 0.25 mL/min × 60 min/hr =
   15 mL/hr

   Upper dosage: 0.5 mL/min × 60 min/hr =
   30 mL/hr

   A dosage range of 2.5-5 mcg/kg/min is equal to a flow rate of 15-30 mL/hr.

   b. Determine dosage infusing per minute at 25 mL/hr:

   500 mcg : 1 mL = $x$ mcg : 25 mL

   $x = 12,500$ mcg/hr

   12,500 mcg ÷ 60 min = 208.3 mcg/min

2. a. 2 mg : 250 mL = $x$ mg : 30 mL

   $\dfrac{250x}{250} = \dfrac{60}{250}$

   $x = 0.24$ mg/hr

   b. Convert milligrams to micrograms
   (1,000 mcg = 1 mg).

   0.24 mg = 240 mcg/hr

   c. Convert mcg/hr to mcg/min.

   240 mcg/hr ÷ 60 min/hr = 4 mcg/min

3. a. Change grams to milligrams. (Note that you were asked to calculate mg/hr.)

   0.25 g = 250 mg (1 g = 1,000 mg)

   b. Calculate mg/hr.

   250 mg : 500 mL = $x$ mg : 20 mL

   $\dfrac{500x}{500} = \dfrac{5,000}{500}$

   $x = 10$ mg/hr

4. *Note:* Calculate units per hour only.

   20 units : 1,000 mL = $x$ units : 25 mL

   $\dfrac{1,000x}{1,000} = \dfrac{500}{1,000}$; $x = 0.5$ units/hr

   The client is receiving 0.5 units/hr.

5. Step 1: Determine the dosage per minute.

   60 kg × 3 mcg/kg/min = 180 mcg/min

   Step 2: Convert to dosage per hour.

   180 mcg/min × 60 min/hr = 10,800 mcg/hr

   Step 3: Convert to like units (1,000 mcg = 1 mg).

   10,800 mcg = 10.8 mg

   Calculate flow rate (mL/hr).

   50 mg : 250 mL = 10.8 mg : $x$ mL

   $50x = 250 × 10.8$

   $\dfrac{50x}{50} = \dfrac{2,700}{50}$

   $x = 54$ mL/hr

6. a. 50 mg : 250 mL = $x$ mg : 3 mL

   $\dfrac{250x}{250} = \dfrac{150}{250}$

   $x = 0.6$ mg/hr

   Convert to micrograms (1,000 mcg = 1 mg).

   0.6 mg/hr = 600 mcg/hr

   b. Convert mcg/hr to mcg/min.

   600 mcg/hr ÷ 60 min/hr = 10 mcg/min

7. Step 1: Calculate the dose per hour using the lower and upper dosages.

   2 mg/min × 60 min/hr = 120 mg/hr

   6 mg/min × 60 min/hr = 360 mg/hr

   Step 2: Convert mg to g to match the available strength.

   1,000 mg = 1 g

   120 mg = 0.12 g

   360 mg = 0.36 g

Step 3: Calculate the rate in mL/hr

$2 \text{ g} : 250 \text{ mL} = 0.12 \text{ g} : x \text{ mL}$

$2x = 250 \times 0.12$

$$\frac{2x}{2} = \frac{30}{2}$$

$x = 15 \text{ mL/hr}$

To infuse 2 mg/min, set the IV rate at 15 mL/hr (minimum).

$2 \text{ g} : 250 \text{ mL} = 0.36 \text{ g} : x \text{ mL}$

$2x = 250 \times 0.36$

$$\frac{2x}{2} = \frac{90}{2}$$

$x = 45 \text{ mL/hr}$

To infuse 6 mg/min, set the IV rate at 45 mL/hr (maximum).

A dosage range of 2-6 mg/min is equal to a flow rate of 15-45 mL/hr.

## Answers to Clinical Reasoning Questions

a. The nurse made the error in the second step (converting 180 mcg to mg to match the units in the solution strength). This led to the error in the mL/hr rate.

$180 \text{ mcg} = 0.18 \text{ mg} (1{,}000 \text{ mcg} = 1 \text{ mg})$

$180 \div 1{,}000 = 0.18 \text{ mg}$

b. The error would result in an incorrect IV rate in mL/hr; the answer obtained is used to determine the rate in mL/hr. Use of 0.018 mg would net an incorrect answer.

$1 \text{ mg} : 250 \text{ mL} = 0.018 \text{ mg} : x \text{ mL}$

$x = 250 \times 0.018$

$x = 4.5 = 5 \text{ mL/hr}$

## Answers to Chapter Review

1. a. Calculate the dosage per hr.

$2 \text{ mg} : 250 \text{ mL} = x \text{ mg} : 30 \text{ mL}$

$$\frac{250x}{250} = \frac{60}{250}$$

$$x = \frac{60}{250}$$

$x = 0.24 \text{ mg/hr}$

b. Convert milligrams to micrograms (1,000 mcg = 1 mg).

$1{,}000 \times 0.24 \text{ mg/hr} = 240 \text{ mcg/hr}$

c. Convert mcg/hr to mcg/min.

$240 \text{ mcg/hr} \div 60 \text{ min/hr} = 4 \text{ mcg/min}$

Set up proportion to determine the dosage of 2 mg/min.

$$\frac{2 \text{ mg/min}}{15 \text{ mL/hr}} = \frac{2 \text{ mg/min}}{x \text{ mL/hr}}$$

$$\frac{2x}{2} = \frac{30}{2}$$

$x = 15 \text{ mL/hr}$

So for a change of 2 mg/min, the incremental IV flow rate is 15 mL/hr.

| Titration Table | |
| --- | --- |
| **Dosage Rate (mcg/min)** | **Flow Rate (mL/hr)** |
| 2 mg/min **(minimum)** | 15 mL/hr |
| 4 mg/min | 30 mL/hr |
| 6 mg/min **(maximum)** | 45 mL/hr |

*Note:* This problem could also be done using dimensional analysis.

c. The rate in mL/hr should be 45 mL/hr and not 5 mL/hr.

$1 \text{ mg} : 250 \text{ mL} = 0.18 \text{ mg} : x \text{ mL}$

$x = 250 \times 0.18$

$x = 45 \text{ mL/hr}$

d. The nurse should have double-checked the math at each step. In addition, having another nurse check the calculation may have helped in recognizing the error in calculation.

2. Step 1: Determine dosage per hour.

$800 \text{ mg} : 500 \text{ mL} = x \text{ mg} : 30 \text{ mL}$

$$\frac{500x}{500} = \frac{24{,}000}{500}$$

$$x = \frac{24{,}000}{500}$$

$x = 48 \text{ mg/hr}$

a. Step 2: Convert milligrams to micrograms (1,000 mcg = 1 mg).

$48 \text{ mg/hr} \times 1{,}000 = 48{,}000 \text{ mcg/hr}$

b. Step 3: Convert mcg/hr to mcg/min.

$48{,}000 \text{ mcg/hr} \div 60 \text{ min/hr} = 800 \text{ mcg/min}$

c. 400 mg : 5 mL = 800 mg : $x$ mL

$$\frac{800 \text{ mg}}{400 \text{ mg}} \overset{or}{\times} 5 \text{ mL} = x \text{ mL}$$

Answer: 10 mL. The dosage ordered is greater than what is available. Therefore you will need more than 5 mL to administer the dosage.

Alternate solution:

80 mg : 1 mL = 800 mg : $x$ mL

$$\overset{or}{\frac{800 \text{ mg}}{80 \text{ mg}} \times 1 \text{ mL} = x \text{ mL}}$$

3. a. Determine dosage per hour.

50 mg : 250 mL = $x$ mg : 30 mL

$$\frac{250x}{250} = \frac{1,500}{250}$$

$$x = \frac{1,500}{250}$$

$$x = 6 \text{ mg/hr}$$

Convert milligrams to micrograms (1,000 mcg = 1 mg).

6 mg/hr × 1,000 = 6,000 mcg/hr

b. Convert mcg/hr to mcg/min.

6,000 mcg/h̶r̶ ÷ 60 min/h̶r̶ = 100 mcg/min

c. 50 mg : 2 mL = 50 mL : $x$ mL

$$\frac{50 \text{ mg}}{50 \text{ mg}} \times 2 \text{ mL} = x \text{ mL}$$

Answer: 2 mL. The dosage ordered is contained in a volume of 2 mL.

Alternate solution: 25 mg : 1 mL = 50 mg : $x$ mL

$$\overset{or}{\frac{50 \text{ mg}}{25 \text{ mg}} \times 1 \text{ mL} = x \text{ mL}}$$

4. a. Convert metric weight to the same as answer requested. Convert grams to milligrams.

1 g = 1,000 mg; therefore 2 g = 2,000 mg

2,000 mg : 250 mL = $x$ mg : 60 mL

$$\frac{250x}{250} = \frac{120,000}{250}$$

$$x = \frac{120,000}{250}$$

$$x = 480 \text{ mg/hr}$$

b. Convert mg/hr to mg/min.

480 mg/h̶r̶ ÷ 60 min/h̶r̶ = 8 mg/min

5. a. Step 1: Convert grams to milligrams (1,000 mg = 1 g).

0.25 g = 250 mg

Step 2: Calculate mg/hr.

250 mg : 6 hr = $x$ mg : 1 hr

$$\frac{6x}{6} = \frac{250}{6}$$

$$x = \frac{250}{6} = 41.66$$

$$x = 41.7 \text{ mg/hr}$$

b. 500 mg : 20 mL = 250 mg : $x$ mL

$$\overset{or}{\frac{250 \text{ mg}}{500 \text{ mg}} \times 20 \text{ mL} = x \text{ mL}}$$

Answer: 10 mL. The dosage ordered is less than the available strength; therefore you will need less than 20 mL to administer the dosage.

Alternate solution: 25 mg : 1 mL = 250 mg : $x$ mL

$$\overset{or}{\frac{250 \text{ mg}}{25 \text{ mg}} \times 1 \text{ mL} = x \text{ mL}}$$

6. a. Convert grams to milligrams (1,000 mg = 1 g).

2 g = 2,000 mg

Calculate mg/hr.

2,000 mg : 250 mL = $x$ mg : 30 mL

$$\frac{250x}{250} = \frac{60,000}{250}$$

$$x = \frac{60,000}{250}$$

$$x = 240 \text{ mg/hr}$$

b. Convert mg/hr to mg/min.

240 mg/h̶r̶ ÷ 60 min/h̶r̶ = 4 mg/min

7. a. Step 1: Calculate units/hr.

30 units : 1,000 mL = $x$ units : 40 mL

$$\frac{1,000 x}{1,000} = \frac{1,200}{1,000}$$

$$x = 1.2 \text{ units/hr}$$

b. Step 2: Calculate units/min.

1.2 units/h̶r̶ ÷ 60 min/h̶r̶ = 0.02 units/min

8. a. Change metric measures to same as question.

$$2 \text{ g} = 2,000 \text{ mg } (1 \text{ g} = 1,000 \text{ mg})$$

Calculate mg/hr.

$$2,000 \text{ mg} : 500 \text{ mL} = x \text{ mg} : 45 \text{ mL}$$

$$\frac{500x}{500} = \frac{90,000}{500}$$

$$x = \frac{90,000}{500}$$

$$x = 180 \text{ mg/hr}$$

b. Change mg/hr to mg/min.

$$180 \text{ mg/hr} \div 60 \text{ min/hr} = 3 \text{ mg/min}$$

9. Determine dosage per hour.

$$500 \text{ mcg/min} \times 60 \text{ min/hr} = 30,000 \text{ mcg/hr}$$

Convert micrograms to milligrams to match the available strength.

$$1,000 \text{ mcg} = 1 \text{ mg}$$

$$30,000 \text{ mcg/hr} = 30 \text{ mg/hr}$$

Calculate flow rate in mL/hr.

$$50 \text{ mg} : 250 \text{ mL} = 30 \text{ mg} : x \text{ mL}$$

$$\frac{50x}{50} = \frac{7,500}{50}$$

$$x = 150 \text{ mL/hr}$$

Set at 150 mL/hr to deliver 500 mcg/min.

10. $400 \text{ mg} : 500 \text{ mL} = x \text{ mg} : 35 \text{ mL}$

$$\frac{500x}{500} = \frac{14,000}{500}$$

$$x = 28 \text{ mg/hr}$$

11. a. Calculate mg/hr.

$$2 \text{ mg} : 250 \text{ mL} = x \text{ mg} : 20 \text{ mL}$$

$$\frac{250x}{250} = \frac{40}{250}$$

$$x = \frac{40}{250}$$

$$x = 0.16 \text{ mg/hr}$$

b. Convert milligrams to micrograms (1,000 mcg = 1 mg).

$$0.16 \text{ mg} \times 1,000 = 160 \text{ mcg/hr}$$

c. Convert mcg/hr to mcg/min (60 min = 1 hr).

$$160 \text{ mcg/hr} \div 60 \text{ min/hr} = 2.66 = 2.7 \text{ mcg/min}$$

12. Convert metric weight to same as question.

$$1,000 \text{ mg} = 1 \text{ g}$$

Calculate mg/hr.

$$1,000 \text{ mg} : 10 \text{ hr} = x \text{ mg} : 1 \text{ hr}$$

$$\frac{10x}{10} = \frac{1,000}{10}$$

$$x = 100 \text{ mg/hr}$$

13. a. Convert grams to milligrams.

$$2 \text{ g} = 2,000 \text{ mg } (1,000 \text{ mg} = 1 \text{ g})$$

$$2,000 \text{ mg} : 250 \text{ mL} = x \text{ mg} : 22 \text{ mL}$$

$$\frac{250x}{250} = \frac{44,000}{250}$$

$$x = \frac{44,000}{250}$$

$$x = 176 \text{ mg/hr}$$

b. Change mg/hr to mg/min.

$$176 \text{ mg/hr} \div 60 \text{ min/hr} = 2.93 = 2.9 \text{ mg/min}$$

14. Convert g to mg.

$$2.5 \text{ g} = 2,500 \text{ mg } (1 \text{ g} = 1,000 \text{ mg})$$

a. $2,500 \text{ mg} : 250 \text{ mL} = x \text{ mg} : 30 \text{ mL}$

$$\frac{250x}{250} = \frac{75,000}{250}$$

$$x = \frac{75,000}{250}$$

$$x = 300 \text{ mg/hr}$$

b. Convert mg/hr to mg/min.

$$300 \text{ mg/hr} \div 60 \text{ min/hr} = 5 \text{ mg/min}$$

15. a. Calculate mg/hr.

$$500 \text{ mg} : 500 \text{ mL} = x \text{ mg} : 30 \text{ mL}$$

$$\frac{500x}{500} = \frac{15,000}{500}$$

$$x = \frac{15,000}{500}$$

$$x = 30 \text{ mg/hr}$$

Convert milligrams to micrograms (1,000 mcg = 1 mg).

$$30 \text{ mg} = 30,000 \text{ mcg/hr}$$

b. Convert mcg/hr to mcg/min.

$$30,000 \text{ mcg/hr} \div 60 \text{ min/hr} = 500 \text{ mcg/min}$$

16. Determine dosage per hour.

$$200 \text{ mcg/min} \times 60 \text{ min/hr} = 12,000 \text{ mcg/hr}$$

Convert micrograms to milligrams (1,000 mcg = 1 mg).

$$12,000 \text{ mcg} \div 1,000 = 12 \text{ mg/hr}$$

Calculate the mL/hr.

$$400 \text{ mg} : 500 \text{ mL} = 12 \text{ mg} : x \text{ mL}$$

$$\frac{400x}{400} = \frac{6,000}{400}$$

$$x = 15 \text{ mL/hr}$$

17. $25 \text{ g} : 300 \text{ mL} = 3 \text{ g} : x \text{ mL}$

$$\frac{25x}{25} = \frac{900}{25}$$

$$x = \frac{900}{25}$$

$$x = 36 \text{ mL/hr; would administer 3 g}$$

18. Convert weight in pounds to kilograms (2.2 lb = 1 kg).

$$120 \text{ lb} \div 2.2 = 54.54 = 54.5 \text{ kg}$$

Calculate dosage per minute.

$$54.5 \text{ kg} \times 2 \text{ mcg/kg/min} = 109 \text{ mcg/min}$$

19. No conversion of weight is required.

$$80 \text{ kg} \times 3 \text{ mcg/kg/min} = 240 \text{ mcg/min}$$

20. a. Convert weight in pounds to kilograms (2.2 lb = 1 kg).

$$110 \text{ lb} \div 2.2 = 50 \text{ kg}$$

Calculate the dosage per hour.

$$50 \text{ kg} \times 0.7 \text{ mg/kg/hr} = 35 \text{ mg/hr}$$

b. Calculate the dosage per minute.

$$35 \text{ mg/hr} \div 60 \text{ min/hr} = 0.58 \text{ mg/min} = 0.6 \text{ mg/min}$$

c. The dosage is safe; it falls within the safe range.

21. Step 1: Convert to like units.

Equivalent: 1,000 mcg = 1 mg

Therefore 2 mg = 2,000 mcg

Step 2: Calculate the concentration of solution in mcg per mL.

$$2,000 \text{ mcg} : 500 \text{ mL} = x \text{ mcg} : 1 \text{ mL}$$

$$\frac{500x}{500} = \frac{2,000}{500}$$

$$x = 4 \text{ mcg per mL}$$

Lower dosage: $4 \text{ mcg} : 1 \text{ mL} = 2 \text{ mcg} : x \text{ mL}$

$$\frac{4x}{4} = \frac{2}{4}$$

$$x = 0.5 \text{ mL/min}$$

Upper dosage: $4 \text{ mcg} : 1 \text{ mL} = 6 \text{ mcg} : x \text{ mL}$

$$\frac{4x}{4} = \frac{6}{4}$$

$$x = 1.5 \text{ mL/min}$$

Step 3: Convert mL/min to mL/hr.

Lower dosage: $0.5 \text{ mL/min} \times 60 \text{ min/hr} = 30 \text{ mL/hr}$

Upper dosage: $1.5 \text{ mL/min} \times 60 \text{ min/hr} = 90 \text{ mL/hr}$

A dosage range of 2-6 mcg/min is equal to a flow rate of 30-90 mL/hr.

22. Step 1: Convert to like units of measurement.

Equivalent: 1,000 mcg = 1 mg

Therefore 5,000 mg = 5,000,000 mcg

Step 2: Calculate the concentration of solution in mcg per mL.

$$5,000,000 \text{ mcg} : 500 \text{ mL} = x \text{ mcg} : 1 \text{ mL}$$

$$\frac{500x}{500} = \frac{5,000,000}{500}$$

$$x = 10,000 \text{ mcg per mL}$$

The concentration of solution is 10,000 mcg per mL.

Step 3: Calculate the dosage range.

Lower dosage: $50 \text{ mcg/kg/min} \times 60 \text{ kg} = 3,000 \text{ mcg/min}$

Upper dosage: $75 \text{ mcg/kg/min} \times 60 \text{ kg} = 4,500 \text{ mcg/min}$

Step 4: Convert the dosage range to mL/min.

$$10,000 \text{ mcg} : 1 \text{ mL} = 1,000 \text{ mcg} : x \text{ mL}$$

Lower dosage: $10,000 \text{ mcg} : 1 \text{ mL} = 3,000 \text{ mcg} : x \text{ mL}$

$$\frac{10,000x}{10,000} = \frac{3,000}{10,000}$$

$$x = 0.3 \text{ mL/min}$$

Upper dosage: $10,000 \text{ mcg} : 1 \text{ mL} = 4,500 \text{ mcg} : x \text{ mL}$

$$\frac{10,000x}{10,000} = \frac{4,500}{10,000}$$

$$x = 0.45 \text{ mL/min}$$

Step 5: Convert mL/min to mL/hr.

Lower dosage: $0.3 \text{ mL/min} \times 60 \text{ min/hr} = 18 \text{ mL/hr}$

Upper dosage: $0.45 \text{ mL/min} \times 60 \text{ min/hr} = 27 \text{ mL/hr}$

a.  A dosage range of 50-75 mcg is equal to a flow rate of 18-27 mL/hr.

b.  Determine the dosage per minute infusing at 24 mL/hr.

$$10,000 \text{ mcg} : 1 \text{ mL} = x \text{ mcg} : 24 \text{ mL}$$

$$x = 10,000 \times 24 = 240,000 \text{ mcg/hr}$$

$$240,000 \text{ mcg/hr} \div 60 \text{ min/hr} = 4,000 \text{ mcg/min}$$

23.  Calculate the dosage per minute for the client.

$$65 \text{ kg} \times 10 \text{ mcg/kg/min} = 650 \text{ mcg/min}$$

Determine the dosage per hour.

$$650 \text{ mcg/min} \times 60 \text{ min/hr} = 39,000 \text{ mcg/hr}$$

Convert to like units.

$$1,000 \text{ mcg} = 1 \text{ mg}$$

$$39,000 \text{ mcg/hr} = 39 \text{ mg/hr}$$

Calculate mL/hr flow rate.

$$500 \text{ mg} : 250 \text{ mL} = 39 \text{ mg} : x \text{ mL}$$

$$\frac{500x}{500} = \frac{9,750}{500} = 19.5$$

$$x = 20 \text{ mL/hr}$$

Answer: To deliver a dosage of 10 mcg/kg/min, set the flow rate at 20 mL/hr (gtt/min).

24.  a.  Convert grams to milligrams.

$$1 \text{ g} = 1,000 \text{ mg}$$

Calculate mg/hr.

$$1,000 \text{ mg} : 500 \text{ mL} = x \text{ mg} : 20 \text{ mL}$$

$$\frac{500x}{500} = \frac{20,000}{500}$$

$$x = \frac{20,000}{500}$$

$$x = 40 \text{ mg/hr}$$

b.  Convert mg/hr to mg/min.

$$40 \text{ mg/hr} \div 60 \text{ min/hr} = 0.66 = 0.7 \text{ mg/min}$$

Answer: At the rate of 20 mL/hr, the client is receiving a dosage of 40 mg/hr or 0.7 mg/min.

25.  a.  10,240 mcg/min

b.  102 mL/hr

Calculate the dosage per minute.

$$100 \text{ mcg/kg/min} \times 102.4 \text{ kg} = 10,240 \text{ mcg/min}$$

Convert mcg/min to mg/min.

$$10,240 \text{ mcg} \div 1,000 = 10.24 = 10.2 \text{ mg/min}$$

Convert mg/min to mg/hr.

$$10.2 \text{ mg/min} \times 60 \text{ min/hr} = 612 \text{ mg/hr}$$

Calculate flow rate.

$$1 \text{ g} = 1,000 \text{ mg}; 1.5 \text{ g} = 1,500 \text{ mg}$$

$$1,500 \text{ mg} : 250 \text{ mL} = 612 \text{ mg} : x \text{ mL}$$

$$1,500 \, x = 250 \times 612$$

$$\frac{1,500x}{1,500} = \frac{153,000}{1,500}$$

$$x = 102 \text{ mL/hr}$$

26.  a.  0.27 mg/min

b.  270 mcg/min

Calculate the mg/hr infusing.

$$500 \text{ mL} : 400 \text{ mg} = 20 \text{ mL} : x \text{ mg}$$

$$500x = 400 \times 20$$

$$\frac{500x}{500} = \frac{8,000}{500}$$

$$x = 16 \text{ mg/hr}$$

Calculate the mg/min infusing.

$$16 \text{ mg/hr} \div 60 \text{ min/hr} = 0.266 = 0.27 \text{ mg/min}$$

Calculate the mcg/min.

$$1,000 \text{ mcg} = 1 \text{ mg}$$

$$0.27 \text{ mg/min} = 270 \text{ mcg/min}$$

27.  a.  5 mg : 1 mL = 125 mg : x mL

*or*

$$\frac{125 \text{ mg}}{5 \text{ mg}} \times 1 \text{ mL} = x \text{ mL}$$

Answer: 25 mL. The dosage ordered is more than the available strength. Therefore you will need more than 5 mL to administer the dosage.

Alternate solution:

$$25 \text{ mg} : 1 \text{ mL} = 125 \text{ mg} : x \text{ mL}$$

*or*

$$\frac{125 \text{ mg}}{25 \text{ mg}} \times 5 \text{ mL} = x \text{ mL}$$

b.  25 mL (med) + 100 mL IV solution = 125 mL (total fluid volume)

$$125 \text{ mg} : 125 \text{ mL} = 20 \text{ mg} : x \text{ mL}$$

$$125x = 125 \times 20$$

$$\frac{125x}{125} = \frac{2,500}{125}$$

$$x = 20 \text{ mL/hr}$$

28.  Calculate the dosage per hour.

$$2 \text{ mg/min} \times 60 \text{ min/hr} = 120 \text{ mg/hr}$$

Convert grams to milligrams.

$$1,000 \text{ mg} = 1 \text{ g}; 2 \text{ g} = 2,000 \text{ mg}$$

Calculate mL/hr.

$$2,000 \text{ mg} : 500 \text{ mL} = 120 \text{ mg} : x \text{ mL}$$

$$2,000\,x = 500 \times 120$$

$$\frac{2,000x}{2,000} = \frac{60,000}{2,000}$$

$$x = 30 \text{ mL/hr}$$

29. Calculate the dosage per minute.

$$3 \text{ mcg/kg/min} \times 95.9 \text{ kg} = 287.7 \text{ mcg/min}$$

Convert mcg/min to mcg/hr.

$$287.7 \text{ mcg/min} \times 60 \text{ min/hr} = 17,262 \text{ mcg/hr}$$

Convert mcg/hr to mg/hr (1,000 mcg = 1 mg).

$$17,262 \text{ mcg/hr} \div 1,000 = 17.26 = 17.3 \text{ mg/hr}$$

Calculate the IV flow rate.

$$400 \text{ mg} : 250 \text{ mL} = 17.3 \text{ mg} : x \text{ mL}$$

$$400x = 250 \times 17.3$$

$$\frac{400x}{400} = \frac{4,325}{400}$$

$$x = \frac{4,325}{400} = 10.81$$

$$x = 10.8 \text{ mL/hr}$$

To infuse 3 mcg/kg/min, set the rate at 10.8 mL/hr. The rate is not rounded to 11 mL/hr because the IV pump is capable of delivering in tenths of an mL.

30. Convert lb to kg (2.2 lb = 1 kg).

$$143 \text{ lb} \div 2.2 = 65 \text{ kg}$$

Find concentration per minute (mcg/min).

$$65 \text{ kg} \times 5 \text{ mcg/kg/min} = 325 \text{ mcg/min}$$

Find concentration per hour.

$$325 \text{ mcg/min} \times 60 \text{ min/hr} = 19,500 \text{ mcg/hr}$$

The concentration of dobutamine infused per minute is 325 mcg/min and 19,500 mcg/hr.

31. a. Convert mcg/min to mcg/hr.

$$2 \text{ mcg/min} \times 60 \text{ min/hr} = 120 \text{ mcg/hr}$$

Convert mcg/hr to mg/hr (1,000 mcg = 1 mg).

$$120 \text{ mcg/hr} \div 1,000 = 0.12 \text{ mg/hr}$$

Calculate the lower mL/hr flow rate.

$$8 \text{ mg} : 250 \text{ mL} = 0.12 \text{ mg} : x \text{ mL}$$

$$8\,x = 250 \times 0.12$$

$$\frac{8x}{8} = \frac{30}{8}$$

$$x = \frac{30}{8} = 3.75$$

$$x = 3.8 \text{ mL/hr}$$

The flow rate for the lower 2 mcg/min dosage is 3.8 mL/hr.

Calculate the upper 4 mcg/min flow rate.

Convert mcg/min to mcg/hr.

$$4 \text{ mcg/min} \times 60 \text{ min/hr} = 240 \text{ mcg/hr}$$

Convert mcg/hr to mg/hr (1,000 mcg = 1 mg).

$$240 \text{ mcg/hr} \div 1,000 = 0.24 \text{ mg/hr}$$

Calculate the upper mL/hr flow rate.

$$8 \text{ mg} : 250 \text{ mL} = 0.24 \text{ mg} : x \text{ mL}$$

$$8x = 250 \times 0.24$$

$$\frac{8x}{8} = \frac{60}{8}$$

$$x = \frac{60}{8}$$

$$x = 7.5 \text{ mL/h}$$

The flow rate for the upper 4 mcg/min = 7.5 mL/hr.

The flow rate range to titrate a dosage of 2-4 mcg/min is 3.8-7.5 mL/hr (mL/hr is not rounded; pump capable of delivering in tenths of an mL).

b. Calculate the dosage infusing at 5 mL/hr.

$$250 \text{ mL} : 8 \text{ mg} = 5 \text{ mL} : x \text{ mg}$$

$$\frac{250x}{250} = \frac{8 \times 5}{250}$$

$$x = \frac{40}{250}$$

$$x = 0.16 \text{ mg/hr}$$

Convert mg/hr to mcg/hr (1,000 mcg = 1 mg).

$$0.16 \text{ mg/hr} \times 1,000 = 160 \text{ mcg/hr}$$

Convert mcg/hr to mcg/min.

$$160 \text{ mcg/hr} \div 60 \text{ min/hr} = 2.66 = 2.7 \text{ mcg/min}$$

At the flow rate of 5 mL/hr, the client is now receiving 2.7 mcg/min.

32. Step 1: Calculate the dose per hour using the lower and upper dosages.

$$40 \text{ mcg/min} \times 60 \text{ min/hr} = 2,400 \text{ mcg/hr}$$
$$100 \text{ mcg/min} \times 60 \text{ min/hr} = 6,000 \text{ mcg/hr}$$

Step 2: Convert mcg to mg to match the available strength.

1,000 mcg = 1 mg
2,400 mcg = 2.4 mg
6,000 mcg = 6 mg

Step 3: Calculate the rate in mL/hr

$$40 \text{ mg} : 250 \text{ mL} = 2.4 \text{ mg} : x \text{ mL}$$

$$40x = 250 \times 2.4$$

$$\frac{40x}{40} = \frac{600}{40}$$

$$x = 15 \text{ mL/hr}$$

To infuse 40 mcg/min, set the IV rate at 15 mL/hr (minimum)

$$40 \text{ mg} : 250 \text{ mL} = 6 \text{ mg} : x \text{ mL}$$

$$40x = 250 \times 6 =$$

$$\frac{40x}{40} = \frac{1,500}{40}$$

$$x = 37.5 \text{ mL/hr}$$

To infuse 100 mcg/min, set the IV rate at 37.5 mL/hr (maximum).

A dosage of 40 to 100 mcg/min is equal to 15 to 37.5 mL/hr.

Set up proportion to determine the dosage change of 20 mcg/min.

$$\frac{40 \text{ mcg/min}}{15 \text{ mL/hr}} = \frac{20 \text{ mcg/min}}{x \text{ mL/hr}}$$

$$\frac{40x}{40} = \frac{300}{40}$$

$$x = 7.5 \text{ mL/hr}$$

So, for each change of 20 mcg/min, the incremental IV flow rate is 7.5 mL/hr.

| Titration Table | |
| --- | --- |
| **Dosage Rate (mcg/min)** | **Flow Rate (mL/hr)** |
| 40 mcg/min **(minimum)** | 15 mL/hr |
| 60 mcg/min | 22.5 mL/hr |
| 80 mcg/min | 30 mL/hr |
| 100 mcg/min **(maximum)** | 37.5 mL/hr |

33. Step 1: Calculate the dose per hour using the lower and upper dosages.

$$4 \text{ mcg/min} \times 60 \text{ min/hr} = 240 \text{ mcg/hr}$$

$$12 \text{ mcg/min} \times 60 \text{ min/hr} = 720 \text{ mcg/hr}$$

Step 2: Convert mcg/hr to available strength.

$$1,000 \text{ mcg} = 1 \text{ mg}$$

$$240 \text{ mcg} = 0.24 \text{ mg}$$

$$720 \text{ mcg} = 0.72 \text{ mg}$$

Step 3: Calculate the rate in mL/hr.

$$4 \text{ mg} : 500 \text{ mL} = 0.24 \text{ mg} : x \text{ mL}$$

$$4x = 500 \times 0.24$$

$$\frac{4x}{4} = \frac{120}{4}$$

$$x = 30 \text{ mL/hr}$$

To infuse 4 mcg/min, set the IV rate at 30 mL/hr (minimum).

$$4 \text{ mg} : 500 \text{ mL} = 0.72 \text{ mg} : x \text{ mL}$$

$$4x = 500 \times 0.72$$

$$\frac{4x}{4} = \frac{360}{4}$$

$$x = 90 \text{ mL/hr}$$

To infuse 12 mcg/min, set the IV rate at 90 mL/hr (maximum).

A dosage of 4-12 mcg/min is equal to 30-90 mL/hr.

Set up a proportion to determine the dosage change of 2 mcg/min.

$$\frac{4 \text{ mcg/min}}{30 \text{ mL/hr}} = \frac{2 \text{ mcg/min}}{x \text{ mL/hr}}$$

$$\frac{4x}{4} = \frac{60}{4}$$

$$x = 15 \text{ mL/hr}$$

For each change of 2 mcg/min, the incremental flow rate is 15 mL/hr.

| Titration Table | |
| --- | --- |
| **Dosage Rate (mcg/min)** | **Flow Rate (mL/hr)** |
| 4 mcg/min **(minimum)** | 30 mL/hr |
| 6 mcg/min | 45 mL/hr |
| 8 mcg/min | 60 mL/hr |
| 10 mcg/min | 75 mL/hr |
| 12 mcg/min **(maximum)** | 90 mL/hr |

34. $4 \text{ mg} : 100 \text{ mL} = 1 \text{ mg} : x \text{ mL}$

$$\frac{4x}{4} = \frac{100}{4}$$

$$x = 25 \text{ mL/hr}$$

35. Calculate the dosage per hr.

$$0.5 \text{ mg/min} \times 60 \text{ min/hr} = 30 \text{ mg/hr}$$

Calculate the mL/hr.

$$900 \text{ mg} : 500 \text{ mL} = 30 \text{ mg} : x \text{ mL}$$

$$900x = 500 \times 30$$

$$\frac{900x}{900} = \frac{1,500}{900} = 16.66$$

$$x = 16.7 \text{ mL/hr} \text{ (mL/hr is not rounded; pump capable of delivering in tenths of a mL)}$$

# CHAPTER 24
# Pediatric and Adult Dosage Calculations Based on Weight

## Objectives

*After reviewing this chapter, you should be able to:*

1. Convert body weight from pounds to kilograms
2. Convert body weight from kilograms to pounds
3. Calculate dosages based on milligram per kilogram
4. Determine whether a dosage is safe
5. Determine body surface area (BSA) using the West nomogram
6. Calculate BSA using formulas according to units of measure
7. Determine dosages using the BSA
8. Calculate the flow rates for pediatric IV therapy
9. Calculate the safe dosage ranges and determine if within normal range for medications administered IV in pediatrics
10. Calculate pediatric IV maintenance fluids

Nurses are accountable for ensuring that clients receive the "right dosage" of medication, as well as verifying that the dosage is appropriate and safe for a client before administration of medications. Information relating to the safe dosage for a medication is provided by the manufacturer. This information may be indicated on the medication label or package insert, or it may be found in a medication reference. Experts agree that medication administration and calculation of dosages for children provide uniques challenge for nurses and that children are a vulnerable population and have a higher potential for experiencing adverse effects and harm from medication errors than adults. Therefore accuracy in dosage calculation, determining if the dosage is in the safe dose range for the child, validating calculations, being knowledgeable about the medication being administered (e.g., about possible adverse reactions, indications for use) before administration of medications, and using appropriate measuring devices to administer medications safely to children becomes even more of a priority.

Causes of medication errors with pediatric clients that have been documented in literature include confusion between adult and pediatric formulation; calculation errors due to multiple calculations to individualize dosages on the basis of age, weight, mg/kg, or body surface area (BSA); and use of inaccurate measuring devices (e.g., household teaspoons) as opposed to devices such as oral dosing devices for small-volume doses. There are multiple factors that impact medication dosing for children and make them more susceptible to adverse effects of medication, including a higher percentage of water composing body weight; size; variable weight and body surface area (BSA); and physiological capabilities (e.g., immaturity of systems, differences in rate of medication absorption and excretion) that differ in comparison to adults.

To maximize drug effects and minimize adverse reactions before administering medications to children, the nurse must carefully calculate the dose and know whether the ordered dose is safe. Accuracy is always important when calculating medication dosages. For infants and children, exact and careful mathematics takes on even greater importance.

Nurses must adhere to pediatric protocols and guidelines and always use a reference to verify medication orders to ensure medications are correct and safe. In many health care institutions, the pharmacy supplies medications in unit doses to reduce the chance of error. This, however, does not alleviate the nurse's responsibility from verifying that the prescribed dose is accurate and safe.

> **! SAFETY ALERT!**
> There is a higher risk of death as a result of medication errors in children than in adults. The nurse is responsible for verifying that the dosage is correct and safe for administration.

The safe administration of medications to infants and children requires knowledge of the methods used in calculating dosages as well as application of the "six rights" of medication administration (right medication, right dosage, right time, right route, right client, right documentation) when working with pediatric clients and families. Nurses are also responsible for educating families regarding medication administration.

Dosages based on body weight are also referred to as weight-based dosing (based on the weight of the client). This is an important factor used to calculate medication dosages for children and adults, for oncology medications, and for specialized client populations such as older adults and critically ill clients. Dosing of medication is also done based on body surface area (BSA), measured in square meters ($m^2$) and based on height and weight of the client. Many oncology medications and medications used for children and the critically ill are based on the BSA.

Dosing based on body weight and BSA for adults and children will be discussed in this chapter.

## Older Adults (Geriatrics)

As already discussed (see Chapter 9), the increasing population of older adults (geriatrics) requires special consideration in medication administration. As with children, age-related physiological factors affect medication dosing; these include poor circulation, slower absorption, and decreased excretory function. Another factor is polypharmacy (the use of multiple medications by one person), which increases the chance of drugs interacting with one another and consequently affecting the action of a medication (i.e., minimizing or increasing the desired effect of a medication). Dosages of medications for a geriatric client are usually smaller. Nurses must check drug references and reliable internet sites for information related to the medications being administered. Package inserts for medications, which give recommended dosages for geriatric clients, should be checked.

As already stated, the nurse has the responsibility of determining whether a dose is safe for an individual client. This applies to both children and adults. The determination of a safe dose, which will be discussed later in this chapter, is done by comparing the ordered dosage of a medication to the recommended dosage provided by the drug manufacturer or from a reputable resource. If a dosage is higher than normal, it may be unsafe, and a dosage lower than normal may not produce the desired therapeutic effect. While it is not the responsibility of the nurse to order a medication dosage, **the nurse is legally responsible for notifying the prescriber regarding dosages that are incorrect or unsafe for administration.**

> **! SAFETY ALERT!**
> You are legally responsible for recognizing incorrect and unsafe dosages and for alerting the prescriber.

## Pediatric Medication Dosages

The nurse must be able to determine whether a prescribed pediatric dosage is within the recommended safe range. It is imperative that the nurse check reputable medication resources for specific dosage details. The recommended dose or dosage range can be found in the package insert, or on the medication label. Other references that may be checked for more in-depth and additional information on a medication are drug formularies at the institution, the Physician's Desk Reference (PDR), United States Pharmacopeia, medication guidebooks, and the manufacturer's website prescribing information. Various pocket-size pediatric medication handbooks are also available; one that is widely used is *The Harriett Lane Handbook* (Johns Hopkins Hospital, 2019).

> **! SAFETY ALERT!**
> To ensure safe practice, when in doubt, consult a reliable source. Always double-check dosages by comparing the prescribed dose with the recommended safe dose.

## Principles Relating to Basic Calculations

Before calculating medications for the child or infant, some guidelines are helpful.
- Calculation of pediatric dosages, as with adult dosages, involves the use of ratio and proportion, the formula method, or dimensional analysis to determine the amount of medication to administer.
- Pediatric dosages are much smaller than those for an adult. Micrograms are used a great deal. The tuberculin syringe (1-mL capacity) is used to administer very small dosages.
- Intramuscular (IM) dosages are usually not more than 1 mL for small children and older infants; however, this can vary with the size of the child. The recommended IM dosage for small infants is not more than 0.5 mL.
- The recommended subcutaneous (subcut) dosage for children is not more than 0.5 mL.
- Dosages that are less than 1 mL may be measured in tenths of a milliliter or with a tuberculin syringe in hundredths of a milliliter.
- Medications in pediatrics are not generally rounded off to the nearest tenth but may be administered with a tuberculin syringe (measured in hundredths) to ensure accuracy.
- All answers must be labeled.
- Know your institution's policy on the rounding of pediatric dosages.

## Calculation of Dosages Based on Body Weight

Most medications based on body weight are based on the client's weight in kilograms (kg). Therefore nurses must be competent in converting weights, including converting pounds, pounds and ounces, and grams to kilograms. Conversion of weights, as well as the methods used, were discussed in Chapter 8. The conversion factors related to weight are:
- 1 kg = 2.2 lb
- 1 lb = 16 oz
- 1 kg = 1,000 g

Because most medications are based on body weight in kilograms, it is essential to review again the conversion of weights to kilograms. Let's do some sample problems with weight conversions.

## Converting Pounds to Kilograms

> **RULE**
>
> To convert pounds to kilograms, use the conversion factor: 1 kg = 2.2 lb, divide by 2.2, and express the weight to the nearest tenth.

**Example 1:** Convert a child's weight of 30 lb to kilograms

**Solution:**

---

**Ratio and Proportion (Linear Format)**

$$2.2 \text{ lb} : 1 \text{ kg} = 30 \text{ lb} : x \text{ kg}$$

$$\frac{\cancel{2.2}\, x}{\cancel{2.2}} = \frac{30}{2.2}$$

$$x = \frac{30}{2.2} = 13.63$$

$x = 13.6$ kg (rounded to the nearest tenth)

Child's weight = 13.6 kg

---

**Ratio and Proportion (Fraction Format)**

$$\frac{2.2 \text{ lb}}{1 \text{ kg}} = \frac{30 \text{ lb}}{x \text{ kg}}$$

$$\frac{\cancel{2.2}\, x}{\cancel{2.2}} = \frac{30}{2.2}$$

$$x = \frac{30}{2.2} = 13.63$$

$$x = 13.6 \text{ kg}$$

---

**Dimensional Analysis**

$$x \text{ kg} = \frac{1 \text{ kg}}{2.2 \,\cancel{\text{lb}}} \times \frac{30 \,\cancel{\text{lb}}}{1}$$

$$x = \frac{30}{2.2} = 13.63$$

$$x = 13.6 \text{ kg}$$

**Example 2:** Convert an infant's weight of 14 lb and 6 oz to kilograms.

**Solution:**

**Ratio and Proportion (Linear Format)**

1. Convert oz to parts of a lb. Conversion factor 16 oz = 1 lb.

$$16 \text{ oz} : 1 \text{ lb} = 6 \text{ oz} : x \text{ lb}$$

$$\frac{\cancel{16}\,x}{\cancel{16}} = \frac{6}{16}$$

$$x = \frac{6}{16} = 0.37$$

$x = 0.4$ lb (rounded to the nearest tenth)

2. Add the computed lb to the total lb.

$$14 \text{ lb} + 0.4 \text{ lb} = 14.4 \text{ lb}$$
Infant's weight = 14.4 lb

3. Convert total lb to kg.

$$2.2 \text{ lb} : 1 \text{ kg} = 14.4 \text{ lb} : x \text{ kg}$$

$$\frac{\cancel{2.2}\,x}{\cancel{2.2}} = \frac{14.4}{2.2}$$

$$x = \frac{14.4}{2.2} = 6.54$$

$x = 6.5$ kg (rounded to the nearest tenth)
Infant's weight = 6.5 kg

**Dimensional Analysis**

$$x \text{ lb} = \frac{1 \text{ lb}}{16 \cancel{\text{ oz}}} \times \frac{6 \cancel{\text{ oz}}}{1}$$

$$x = \frac{6}{16} = 0.37$$

$x = 0.4$ lb (rounded to the nearest tenth)
Infant's weight = 14.4 lb

$$x \text{ kg} = \frac{1 \text{ kg}}{2.2 \cancel{\text{ lb}}} \times \frac{14.4 \cancel{\text{ lb}}}{1}$$

$$x = \frac{14.4}{2.2} = 6.54$$

$x = 6.5$ kg (rounded to the nearest tenth)
Infant's weight = 6.5 kg

**! SAFETY ALERT!**

Use caution when converting ounces to a fraction of a pound. Also, after converting the ounces to pounds, remember to add the answer to the remaining whole pounds to get the total pounds. Convert the total pounds to kg.

**Example 3:** Convert the weight of a 157-lb adult to kilograms.

Solution:

---

### Ratio and Proportion (Linear Format)

$$2.2 \text{ lb} : 1 \text{ kg} = 157 \text{ lb} : x \text{ kg}$$

$$\frac{\cancel{2.2} \, x}{\cancel{2.2}} = \frac{157}{2.2}$$

$$x = \frac{157}{2.2} = 71.36$$

$x = 71.4$ kg (rounded to the nearest tenth)

Adult's weight $= 71.4$ kg

---

### Dimensional Analysis

$$x \text{ kg} = \frac{1 \text{ kg}}{2.2 \cancel{\text{ lb}}} \times \frac{157 \cancel{\text{ lb}}}{1}$$

$$x = \frac{157}{2.2} = 71.36$$

$x = 71.4$ kg (rounded to the nearest tenth)

Adult's weight $= 71.4$ kg

---

## Converting Kilograms to Pounds

 **RULE**

To convert kilograms to pounds, use the conversion factor: 1 kg = 2.2 lb, multiply by 2.2, and express the weight to the nearest tenth.

**Example 1:** Convert a child's weight of 24.3 kg to pounds.

Solution:

---

### Ratio and Proportion (Linear Format)

$$2.2 \text{ lb} : 1 \text{ kg} = x \text{ lb} : 24.3 \text{ kg}$$

$$x = 24.3 \times 2.2 = 53.46$$

$x = 53.5$ lb (rounded to the nearest tenth)

Child's weight $= 53.5$ lb

---

### Dimensional Analysis

$$x \text{ lb} = \frac{2.2 \text{ lb}}{1 \cancel{\text{ kg}}} \times \frac{24.3 \cancel{\text{ kg}}}{1}$$

$$x = 2.2 \times 24.3 = 53.46$$

$x = 53.5$ lb (rounded to the nearest tenth)

Child's weight $= 53.5$ lb

**Example 2:** Convert an adult's weight of 70.2 kg to pounds.

Solution:

| Ratio and Proportion (Linear Format) |
| --- |

$$2.2 \text{ lb} : 1 \text{ kg} = x \text{ lb} : 70.2 \text{ kg}$$
$$x = 70.2 \times 2.2 = 154.44$$
$$x = 154.4 \text{ lb (rounded to the nearest tenth)}$$
Adult's weight $= 154.4$ lb

| Dimensional Analysis |
| --- |

$$x \text{ lb} = \frac{2.2 \text{ lb}}{1 \text{ kg}} \times \frac{70.2 \text{ kg}}{1}$$
$$x = 70.2 \times 2.2 = 154.44$$
$$x = 154.4 \text{ lb (rounded to the nearest tenth)}$$
Adult's weight $= 154.4$ lb

Infants 0 to 4 weeks old (neonates) and premature infants may also be given medications. The scale will convert the child's weight in grams, or the weight may be reported in grams, rather than kilograms. Therefore it may be necessary for the nurse to convert the weight in grams to kilograms.

## Converting Grams to Kilograms

**RULE**

To convert grams to kilograms, use the conversion factor 1 kg = 1,000 g, dividing the number of grams by 1,000 or moving the decimal point three places to the left. Round kilograms to the nearest tenth.

**Example 1:** Convert an infant's weight of 3,000 g to kilograms.

Solution:

| Ratio and Proportion (Linear Format) |
| --- |

$$1 \text{ kg} : 1,000 \text{ g} = x \text{ kg} : 3,000 \text{ g}$$
$$\frac{1,000\,x}{1,000} = \frac{3,000}{1,000}$$
$$x = \frac{3}{1} = 3$$
$$x = 3 \text{ kg}$$
Infant's weight $= 3$ kg
Decimal movement: $3000 = 3$ kg

**Dimensional Analysis**

$$x \, kg = \frac{1 \, kg}{1,000 \, g} \times \frac{3,000 \, g}{1}$$

$$x = \frac{3,000}{1,000}$$

$$x = \frac{3}{1} = 3$$

$$x = 3 \, kg$$

Infant's weight = 3 kg

**Example 2:** Convert an infant's weight of 1,350 g to kilograms.

Solution:

**Ratio and Proportion (Linear Format)**

$$1 \, kg : 1,000 \, g = x \, kg : 1,350 \, g$$

$$\frac{1,000 \, x}{1,000} = \frac{1,350}{1,000}$$

$$x = \frac{135}{100} = 1.35$$

$x = 1.4$ kg (rounded to the nearest tenth)

Infant's weight = 1.4 kg

Decimal movement: $1350 = 1.35 = 1.4$ kg

**Dimensional Analysis**

$$x \, kg = \frac{1 \, kg}{1,000 \, g} \times \frac{1,350 \, g}{1}$$

$$x = \frac{1,350}{1,000}$$

$$x = \frac{135}{100} = 1.35$$

$x = 1.4$ kg (rounded to the nearest tenth)

Infant's weight = 1.4 kg

*Note:* Remember that ratio and proportion can also be written in a fraction format and used to do conversions.

**Dimensional Analysis**

$$x \, lb = \frac{2.2 \, lb}{1 \, kg} \times \frac{10.2 \, kg}{1}$$

$$x = 2.2 \times 10.2 = 22.44$$

$$x = 22.4 \, lb$$

Child's weight = 22.4 lb

(rounded to the nearest tenth)

> **POINTS TO REMEMBER**
>
> - 2.2 lb = 1 kg, 1 kg = 1,000 g, 1 lb = 16 oz
> - To convert from pounds to kilograms, divide the number of pounds by 2.2. Carry the division to the hundredths place, and round the weight to the nearest tenth as indicated.
> - To convert from kilograms to pounds, multiply the number of kilograms by 2.2 and round the weight to the nearest tenth as indicated.
> - If the child's weight is in ounces and pounds, convert the ounces to the nearest tenth of a pound, and then add the answer to pounds to get the total pounds. Convert the total pounds to kilograms, and round to the nearest tenth as indicated.
> - To convert from grams to kilograms, divide by 1000 or move the decimal point three places to the left. Round kilograms to the nearest tenth as indicated.

# ▦ PRACTICE **PROBLEMS**

Convert the following weights in pounds to kilograms. Round to the nearest tenth as indicated.

1. 15 lb = _____ kg    6. 8 lb 4 oz = _____ kg

2. 68 lb = _____ kg    7. 5 lb 12 oz = _____ kg

3. 31 lb = _____ kg    8. 100¼ lb = _____ kg

4. 52 lb = _____ kg    9. 92¾ lb = _____ kg

5. 204.2 lb = _____ kg

Convert the following weights in kilograms to pounds. Round to the nearest tenth as indicated.

10. 21.3 kg = _____ lb    15. 71.4 kg = _____ lb

11. 17.7 kg = _____ lb    16. 73 kg = _____ lb

12. 22 kg = _____ lb    17. 98.3 kg = _____ lb

13. 15 kg = _____ lb

14. 34 kg = _____ lb

Convert the following weights in grams to kilograms. Round to the nearest tenth as indicated.

18. 1,450 g = _____ kg    20. 1,875 g = _____ kg

19. 2,900 g = _____ kg

**Answers on p. 646**

Before beginning to calculate dosages based on weight, let's review some terminology that will be used and that you will need to be familiar with.

---

**Recommended dosage** (also referred to as the *safe dosage*)—This information comes from a reputable medication reference, the medication label, or a package insert. The recommended dosage for children and adults is clearly indicated. The recommended dosage can be stated as weight based and usually in kilograms, such as mg/kg, mcg/kg, and so on. On occasion, the dosage may be expressed as mg/lb. The recommended dosage may also be stated in terms of the body surface area (BSA), which is measured in square meters (m$^2$). Recommended dosages may state, for example, mg/kg for a 24-hour period to be given in one or more divided dosages, or may specify other time intervals. A range is sometimes indicated for the recommended dosage and referred to as a safe dosage range (SDR). This is the minimum and maximum safe dosage for a medication as stated by an approved medication reference.

**Single dose**—A dose of medication administered one time or on an as-needed basis. It may be indicated as "per dose." For example, a medication in a medication reference guide may state 2 mg/kg/dose as the recommended dosage.

**Total daily dose**—The total amount of a medication that may be administered in a 24-hour period. Sometimes the total amount daily may be stated. "Daily" or "per day" is usually used to indicate a 24-hour period.

**Divided dosage**—Represents the dosage to be given at specific time intervals (e.g., "three divided dosages," "q6h," and so on). This is obtained by dividing the dosage for 24 hours by the frequency, or number of times, an individual will receive the medication.

**Dosage range**—The minimum to maximum dose for a medication (e.g., 10–20 mg/kg) to be therapeutic.

**Determining if the dosage is safe**—This is decided by comparing the ordered dosage with the recommended dosage.

---

Verification of safe doses recommended by body weight (for a child or adult) requires having the following information: weight of the client (usually in kg), the prescriber's order, and the weight-based information from a reputable reference. This information is used to determine whether a dose is safe or not following a systematic approach, such as the following:

- Convert the client's weight from lb to kg if necessary, and round kg to the nearest tenth.
- Calculate the safe dose by multiplying the weight of the client in kg by the recommended dosage from the reputable medication reference (rounded to the nearest tenth). This can be done also using ratio and proportion or dimensional analysis.
- Compare the recommended dosage for the individual client with the ordered dose.
- Determine if the dose is safe. If the dosage is safe, calculate the amount to give the ordered dosage. If the dosage is not safe (unsafe), notify the prescriber to verify the order before administering the medication.

Let's begin by looking at examples with children.

## Single-Dose Medications

This may be indicated in the reference as "per dose" or indicated with a slash (/) mark ("/dose").

Example 1:  The prescriber orders Narcan 1.2 mg IV stat for a child who weighs 12 kg.

According to *The Harriet Lane Handbook* (a reputable reference), the recommended dose for a child weighing less than 20 kg is 0.1 mg/kg/dose.

Step 1:  Convert weight to kg if necessary. No conversion of weight is required. The child's weight is in kg, and the recommended dosage is stated as 0.1 mg/kg.

Step 2:  Multiply the child's weight in kg by the recommended dose from the reference. 12 kg × 0.1 mg/kg/dose = 1.2 mg/dose. The safe dose of Narcan for the child weighing 12 kg is 1.2 mg/dose. The calculation of the safe dose could also be done by ratio and proportion or dimensional analysis. (Refer to the setup shown for this problem.)

Step 3:  Decide if the dose is safe by comparing the ordered and the recommended dosage. The dose ordered is 1.2 mg. **The dose is safe** because the dose that is ordered is the same as the safe dose recommended for the child.

Step 4:  Calculate the dosage to administer, using ratio and proportion, the formula method, or dimensional analysis.

### Ratio and Proportion (Linear Format)
The *known* ratio is the weight-based dose from the reference.

0.1 mg/dose : 1 kg = $x$ mg/dose : 12 kg

$x = 0.1 \times 12$

$x = 1.2$ mg/dose

The safe dose for a child weighing 12 kg is 1.2 mg/dose

### Ratio and Proportion (Fraction Format)

$$\frac{0.1 \text{ mg/dose}}{1 \text{ kg}} = \frac{x \text{ mg/dose}}{12 \text{ kg}}$$

$x = 0.1 \times 1.2$

$x = 1.2$ mg/dose

The safe dose for a child weighing 12 kg is 1.2 mg/dose.

### Dimensional Analysis
The recommended dose is the starting fraction (in this example, 0.1 mg/kg/dose).

$$\frac{x \text{ mg}}{\text{dose}} = \frac{0.1 \text{ mg}}{\text{kg/dose}} \times \frac{12 \text{ kg}}{1}$$

$x = 0.1 \times 12$

$x = 1.2$ mg/dose

The safe dose for a child weighing 12 kg is 1.2 mg/dose.

The safe dose of Narcan for a child weighing 12 kg is 1.2 mg/dose.
Now that we have determined the dose ordered for the child is safe, let's calculate the dosage to administer.

Order: Narcan (naloxone hydrochloride) 1.2 mg IV stat
Available:

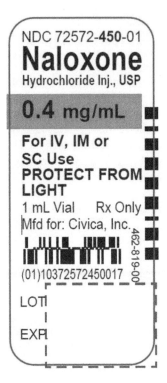

Solution:

| Ratio and Proportion (Linear Format) |
| --- |

$$0.4 \text{ mg} : 1 \text{ mL} = 1.2 \text{ mg} : x \text{ mL}$$

$$\frac{\cancel{0.4} \, x}{\cancel{0.4}} = \frac{1.2}{0.4}$$

$$x = \frac{1.2}{0.4} = 3$$

$$x = 3 \text{ mL}$$

| Ratio and Proportion (Fraction Format) |
| --- |

$$\frac{0.4 \text{ mg}}{1 \text{ mL}} = \frac{1.2 \text{ mg}}{x \text{ mL}}$$

$$x = \frac{1.2}{0.4} = 3$$

$$x = 3 \text{ mL}$$

| Formula Method |
| --- |

$$\frac{1.2 \text{ mg}}{0.4 \text{ mg}} \times 1 \text{ mL} = x \text{ mL}$$

$$x = \frac{1.2}{0.4} = 3$$

$$x = 3 \text{ mL}$$

**Dimensional Analysis**

$$x\,\text{mL} = \frac{1\;\text{mL}}{0.4\;\text{mg}} \times \frac{1.2\;\text{mg}}{1}$$

$$x = \frac{1.2}{0.4} = 3$$

$$x = 3\;\text{mL}$$

**Example 2:** The prescriber orders Ofirmev (acetaminophen) 700 mg IV q6h prn for pain for a child who weighs 94.6 lb. According to *The Harriet Lane Handbook*, for a child age 2-12 years or an adolescent/adult weighing less than 50 kg, the recommended dose is 15 mg/kg/dose q6h, or 12.5 mg/kg/dose q4h IV, up to a maximum of 75 mg/kg/24 hr.

Determine if the dosage ordered is safe. If the dosage is safe, calculate the number of milliliters to add to the IV.

Available:

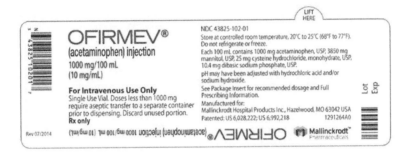

**Step 1:**    First, convert the child's weight from lb to kg using any of the methods already shown.

**Ratio and Proportion (Linear Format)**

$$2.2\;\text{lb} : 1\;\text{kg} = 94.6\;\text{lb} : x\;\text{kg}$$

$$\frac{\cancel{2.2}\,x}{\cancel{2.2}} = \frac{94.6}{2.2}$$

$$x = \frac{94.6}{2.2} = 43$$

$$x = 43\;\text{kg}$$

**Step 2:**    Calculate the recommended dosage. Note the recommended dosage from the reference you will be using is for q6h and for a weight less than 50 kg. Multiply the child's weight in kg by the recommended dose from the reference.

$$43\;\cancel{\text{kg}} \times 15\;\text{mg/}\cancel{\text{kg}}\text{/dose} = 645\;\text{mg/dose}$$

This can also be done using ratio and proportion or dimensional analysis. (Refer to Example 1.)

**Step 3:**    Compare the recommended safe dose for the child with the ordered dose and decide if the dose is safe. The recommended dose for the child weighing 43 kg is 645 mg/dose. The dose ordered is 700 mg q6h. The dosage is **not safe;** it is more than the recommended safe dosage for this child. The nurse would need to notify the prescriber to validate why the dose ordered is more than the recommended dosage; there may be factors that warrant a larger dose.

*Note:* **Because the dose ordered is not safe, we will not be calculating the number of mL to add to the IV.**

## Single-Dose Range Medications

Some single-dose medications can indicate a minimum and maximum range for a medication. The nurse will then need to calculate the minimum and maximum safe dosage.

**Example 3:** The prescriber orders Vistaril 15 mg IM q4h prn for nausea. The child weighs 38 lb. According to *The Harriet Lane Handbook,* the recommended dosage is 0.5 to 1 mg/kg/dose q4h prn. Determine if the dosage ordered is safe.

Solution:

**Step 1:**  First convert the child's weight in lb to kg and round to the nearest tenth of a kg.

---
**Ratio and Proportion (Linear Format)**

$$2.2 \text{ lb} : 1 \text{ kg} = 38 \text{ lb} : x \text{ kg}$$

$$\frac{\cancel{2.2}\, x}{\cancel{2.2}} = \frac{38}{2.2}$$

$$x = \frac{38}{2.2} = 17.27$$

$$x = 17.3 \text{ kg (rounded to the nearest tenth)}$$
---

*Note:* Refer to the conversion of weights at the beginning of the chapter if necessary for an alternate format for setting up a ratio and proportion and using dimensional analysis for converting weights.

**Step 2:**  Calculate the recommended dosage. Note the recommended dosage is stated as a range, 0.5 to 1 mg/kg/dose. Calculate the minimum and maximum safe dose range. Multiply the child's weight in kg by the mg/kg/dose.

**Minimum per dose:** 17.3 $\cancel{\text{kg}}$ × 0.5 mg/$\cancel{\text{kg}}$/dose = 8.65 = 8.7 mg/dose (rounded to the nearest tenth)

**Maximum per dose:** 17.3 $\cancel{\text{kg}}$ × 1 mg/$\cancel{\text{kg}}$/dose = 17.3 mg/dose

The safe dosage range of Vistaril for a child weighing 17.3 kg is 8.7 mg/dose-17.3 mg/dose.

The calculation of minimum and maximum dose can also be done using ratio and proportion or dimensional analysis.

---
**Ratio and Proportion (Linear Format)**

**Minimum per dose**

    0.5 mg/dose : 1 kg = $x$ mg/dose : 17.3 kg

    $x$ = 17.3 × 0.5 = 8.65 = 8.7

    $x$ = 8.7 mg/dose (rounded to the nearest tenth)

**Maximum per dose**

    1 mg/dose : 1 kg = $x$ mg/dose : 17.3 kg

    $x$ = 17.3 mg/dose

This could also be set up in a fraction format.
---

**Dimensional Analysis**

**Minimum per dose**

$$\frac{x\,mg}{dose} = \frac{0.5\,mg}{kg/dose} \times \frac{17.3\,kg}{1}$$

$$x = 17.3 \times 0.5 = 8.65 = 8.7$$

$$x = 8.7\,mg/dose\ \text{(rounded to the nearest tenth)}$$

**Maximum per dose**

$$\frac{x\,mg}{dose} = \frac{1\,mg}{kg/dose} \times \frac{17.3\,kg}{1}$$

$$x = 17.3\,mg/dose$$

**Step 3:** Decide if the dosage ordered is safe. The safe recommended dosage is 8.7 mg to 17.3 mg/dose. The dose is safe, because the ordered dose of 15 mg IM q4h falls within the range of 8.7 mg to 17.3 mg/dose.

**Step 4:** Calculate the dosage to administer the ordered dose.
Order: Vistaril 15 mg IM q4h prn for nausea

Available:

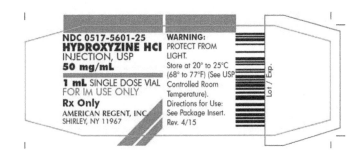

$$50\,mg : 1\,mL = 15\,mg : x\,mL$$

$$\frac{\cancel{50}\,x}{\cancel{50}} = \frac{15}{50}$$

$$x = \frac{15}{50} = 0.3$$

$$x = 0.3\,mL$$

*Note:* A ratio and proportion setup in fraction format, the formula method, or dimensional analysis could have been used to calculate the dose.

## Calculating Daily Doses

With some medications, the recommended dose is stated as a total daily dose, which can be indicated in the reference as "per day" with a slash mark, "/day," "/24 hr," or "daily," indicating that the total daily dose is divided into a number of individual doses throughout the day (e.g., "50 mg/kg/day in divided doses q8h," "four divided doses at q6h intervals"). When the total daily dosage indicates that the dose is divided at specific time intervals, in addition to calculating the total daily dosage, the total daily dose has to be divided to find the amount for a specific time interval (divided dose). The recommended divided dose is then compared to the ordered dose to determine whether the dose is safe.
Let's look at some examples.

**Example 4:** Order: Gentamicin 50 mg IVPB q8h for a child weighing 40 lb. According to *The Harriet Lane Handbook,* the recommended dosage for a child is 7.5 mg/kg/24 hr divided q8h. Determine if the dosage ordered is safe.

**Step 1:** Convert the child's weight from lb to kg using any of the methods for converting weights presented in this chapter and in earlier chapters on converting.

---

**Ratio and Proportion (Linear Format)**

2.2 lb : 1 kg = 40 lb : $x$ kg

$$\frac{\cancel{2.2}\,x}{\cancel{2.2}} = \frac{38}{2.2}$$

$$x = \frac{38}{2.2} = 17.27$$

$x = 18.2$ kg (rounded to the nearest tenth)

---

**Step 2:** Calculate the total daily dosage allowed for the child weighing 18.2 kg.
18.2 kg × 7.5 mg/kg/24 hr = 136.5 mg/24 hr

*Note:* 24 hr could be stated as daily or per day (/day).

This could also be calculated using ratio and proportion or dimensional analysis.

---

**Ratio and Proportion (Linear Format)**

7.5 mg/24 hr : 1 kg = $x$ mg/24 hr : 18.2 kg

$x = 18.2 × 7.5$

$x = 136.5$ mg/24 hr

*or*

---

**Ratio and Proportion (Fraction Format)**

$$\frac{7.5 \text{ mg/24 hr}}{1 \text{ kg}} = \frac{x \text{ mg/24 hr}}{18.2 \text{ kg}}$$

---

**Dimensional Analysis**

$$\frac{x \text{ mg}}{\text{dose}} = \frac{0.5 \text{ mg}}{\cancel{\text{kg}}/\text{dose}} \times \frac{17.3 \cancel{\text{kg}}}{1}$$

$x = 18.2 × 7.5$

$x = 136.5$ mg/day (24 hr)

*Note:* 24 hr was written as /day in the equation

The total daily dosage for this child is 136.5 mg/24 hr

**Step 3:** Now divide the total daily dosage by the number of times the medication will be administered to the client in 24 hours. In this example, the dose is to be given q8h, so the client would receive three (3) doses in a day (24 hr)
q8h = 24 ÷ 8 = 3
Total daily dosage: 136.5 mg ÷ 3 = 45.5 mg per dose

**Step 4:** Now compare the recommended dose for the child with the ordered dose and decide if the dose is safe. The ordered dose is 50 mg q8h, and the recommended dose is 45.5 mg/dose (or q8h). The dose is **not safe** because the ordered dose is more than the recommended safe dose. Remember to contact the prescriber to discuss the order. Factors such as the child's medical condition might warrant a larger dose.

*Note:* When dosages are compared for safety, it may be easier to calculate how many total milligrams or micrograms are ordered. This way usually involves multiplication rather than division. This will require one calculation, as opposed to two, and may decrease the chance of errors because fewer errors are usually made with multiplication than with division.

In this example, you could eliminate the division to find the amount per dose by using the total daily dosage.

Daily dosage according to this order, in this case:

50 mg q8h = 50 mg/dose × 3 doses/day = 150 mg/day (24 hr)

Decide if the ordered daily dose is safe. The ordered daily dosage is 150 mg, and the allowable safe daily dosage is 136.5 mg/24 hr. The dosage ordered is not safe, because 150 mg/day exceeds 136.5 mg/24 hr (per day).

**Example 5:** Order: Penicillin V Potassium 125 mg p.o. q6h for a child weighing 36 lb. According to *The Harriet Lane Handbook,* the recommended dose p.o for a child is 25-75 mg/kg/day divided q6-8hr. Determine if the dose ordered is safe. If the dose is safe, calculate the number of milliliters needed to administer the dose.

Available: Penicillin V Potassium oral solution 250 mg per 5 mL

**Step 1:** Convert the child's weight from lb to kg.

| Ratio and Proportion (Linear Format) |
| --- |

$$2.2 \text{ lb} : 1 \text{ kg} = 36 \text{ lb} : x \text{ kg}$$

$$\frac{\cancel{2.2}\, x}{\cancel{2.2}} = \frac{36}{2.2}$$

$$x = \frac{36}{2.2} = 16.36$$

$$x = 16.4 \text{ kg (rounded to the nearest tenth)}$$

**Step 2:** Calculate the recommended total daily dose for the child. (The recommended dosage range is 25-75 mg/kg/day.) Because the recommended dose is stated as a range, calculate the minimum and maximum dosage. (This can be done using ratio and proportion or dimensional analysis.)

**Minimum total daily dosage:** 16.4 $\cancel{\text{kg}}$ × 25 mg/$\cancel{\text{kg}}$/day = 410 mg/day

**Maximum total daily dosage:** 16.4 $\cancel{\text{kg}}$ × 75 mg/$\cancel{\text{kg}}$/day = 1,230 mg/day

The safe daily dosage range for a child weighing 16.4 kg is 410-1,230 mg/day.

**Step 3:** Now divide the minimum and maximum daily dosage by the number of times the medication will be administered in 24 hours. In this example, the medication is to be given q6h, so the child will receive four (4) doses in a day.

24 hr ÷ 6 = 4

**Minimum total daily dosage:** 410 mg ÷ 4 = 102.5 mg per dose (or q6h)

**Maximum total daily dosage:** 1,230 mg ÷ 4 = 307.5 mg per dose (of q6h)

The safe dose range for this child is 102.5-307.5 mg per dose (or q6h).

**Step 4:** Compare the recommended dose for the child with the ordered dose. The ordered dose is 125 mg q6h, and the recommended dose range is 102.5-307.5 mg/dose. The ordered **dose is safe** because it is within the range of the recommended safe dose.

**Alternate Solution:** Using the total daily dosage.

The dose ordered is 125 mg q6h (24 ÷ 6 = 4 doses per day).

125 mg/$\cancel{\text{dose}}$ × 4 $\cancel{\text{doses}}$/day = 500 mg/day. The ordered **dose is safe** because it falls within the range of 410-1,230 mg/day.

**Step 5:** The dose ordered is **safe**. Calculate the milliliters to administer the dose (using the formula method, ratio and proportion (linear or fraction format), or dimensional analysis).

**Ratio and Proportion (Linear Format)**

$$250 \text{ mg} : 5 \text{ mL} = 125 \text{ mg} : x \text{ mL}$$

$$250 \, x = 125 \times 5$$

$$\frac{250 \, x}{250} = \frac{625}{250}$$

$$x = \frac{625}{250} = 2.5$$

$$x = 2.5 \text{ mL}$$

To administer 125 mg of Penicillin V Potassium, the nurse will administer 2.5 mL.

**Example 6:** Amoxicillin 30 mg p.o. q12h for an infant weighing 2,600 g. According to *The Harriet Lane Handbook,* the recommended dosage is 20-30 mg/kg/day divided q12h. Determine if the dosage ordered is safe.

**Step 1:** Convert the weight in g to kg using any of the methods for weight conversion. g to kg is converting within the metric system (one metric unit to another metric unit); therefore movement of decimals can be used to convert the weight.
**Conversion factor:** 1 kg = 1,000 g; 2,600 = 2.6 kg

**Step 2:** Calculate the lowest and highest recommended total daily dosage for the infant.
The recommended dosage from the reference is a range.
**Minimum total daily dosage:** 2.6 kg × 20 mg/kg /day = 52 mg/day
**Maximum total daily dosage:** 2.6 kg × 30 mg/kg /day = 78 mg/day
The total daily dosage for an infant weighing 2.6 kg is 52-78 mg/day.

**Step 3:** Divide the minimum and maximum total daily dosage by the number of times the infant will receive doses in 24 hours. In this example, the dose is to be given q12h, so the infant will receive two (2) doses in a day.
24 hr ÷ 12 = 2
**Minimum total daily dose:** 52 mg ÷ 2 = 26 mg/dose (or q12h)
**Maximum total daily dose:** 78 mg ÷ 2 = 39 mg/dose (or q12h)
The safe dose range for the infant weighing 2.6 kg is 26-39 mg/dose.

**Step 4:** Compare the recommended dose for the infant with the ordered dose and determine if the dose is safe. The ordered dose is 30 mg q12h, and the recommended safe dose range is 26-39 mg/dose. The **dose is safe** because the ordered dose falls within the recommended safe range.

*Note:* The steps in this example could be calculated using ratio and proportion or dimensional analysis. Also, the total daily dosage could be used to determine whether the dose is safe. Refer to examples previously given for setup of problems using these methods.

> **⚠ SAFETY ALERT!**
> Remember that to avoid medication errors, it is imperative to calculate a safe dosage for a child and compare it to the dosage ordered. Verify dosages that are **lower or higher** than the recommended dosage with the prescriber **before** administering the medication. The nurse is legally liable for any medication administered.

## Adult Dosages Based on Body Weight

The information that has been provided regarding the calculation of dosages for children based on weight can also be applied to adults. The same methods (i.e., ratio and proportion, dimensional analysis) can be used. Let's look at some examples.

**Example 1:** Order: Gentamicin Sulfate 135 mg IV q8h for an adult client weighing 175 lb. According to *Clayton's Basic Pharmacology for Nurses* (2020), the recommended dosage is 3-5 mg/kg/day in two or three doses or 5-7 mg/kg once daily. Determine if the dosage ordered is safe.

**Step 1:** Convert the weight in lb to kg. Conversion factor: 2.2 lb = 1 kg.
175 lb ÷ 2.2 = 79.54 = 79.5 kg (rounded to the nearest tenth)

Step 2:   Calculate the recommended dosage (using 3-5 mg/kg/day; medication is ordered q8h; client would receive three doses in a day).
**Minimum total daily dosage:** 79.5 kg × 3 mg/kg/day = 238.5 mg/day
**Maximum total daily dosage:** 79.5 kg × 5 mg/kg/day = 397.5 mg/day

The recommended dosage per day for a client weighing 79.5 kg is 238.5-397.5 mg/day.

Step 3:   Determine the amount the client will receive per dose. Divide the total daily dosage by the number of times the medication will be administered. In this example, the medication is ordered q8h, so the client will receive three doses in a day.
**Minimum total daily dosage:** 238.5 mg ÷ 3 = 79.5 mg/dose
**Maximum total daily dosage:** 397.5 mg ÷ 3 = 132.5 mg/dose
The recommended dosage per dose is 79.5-132.5 mg/dose.

Step 4:   Compare the safe recommended dose to the ordered dose and determine if the dose is safe. The ordered **dose is not safe** because 135 mg q8h is outside of the dosage range (79.5-132.5 mg/dose). Remember that determining whether the dose is safe can also be done by using the total daily dosage. 135 mg q8h = 135 mg × 3 = 405 mg/day, which is outside the recommended dosage range of 238.5-397.5 mg/day. Therefore the ordered **dose is not safe**.

The nurse will need to contact the prescriber because the ordered dose is more than the recommended dose. Also, there may be a reason for the higher dose of medication (e.g., client condition).

Example 2:   Order: granisetron hydrochloride 0.75 mg IV 30 minutes before chemotherapy for an adult client weighing 165 lb. According to *Mosby's* 2020 *Nursing Drug Reference,* the recommended dosage is 10 mcg/kg over 5 min, 30 min before the start of cancer chemotherapy. Determine if the ordered dose is safe.

Step 1:   Convert the weight in lb to kg. Conversion factor: 2.2 lb = 1 kg.
165 lb ÷ 2.2 = 75 kg

Step 2:   Calculate the recommended dose.
75 kg × 10 mcg/kg = 750 mcg

The dose required for a client weighing 75 kg is 750 mcg.

Step 3:   Compare the safe recommended dose to the ordered dose and determine if the dose is safe. Conversion factor: 1,000 mcg = 1 mg.
0.75 mg = 750 mcg (0.75 × 1,000) (ordered dose converted to mcg to match the reference ([mcg/kg]).

The **dose is safe**. The ordered dose of 0.75 mg (750 mcg) is the same as the recommended safe dose.

---

### ⚙ POINTS TO REMEMBER

- Most weight-based medications are based on body weight in kg.
- To calculate dosages based on weight, the weight of the client is converted to the same unit of weight as the reference (e.g., lb to kg). The medication reference indicates the amount of medication per kg (e.g., 10 mg/kg).
- To calculate the dosage based on weight, there is a systematic approach:
  1. Convert the weight to kilograms if needed and round kilograms to the nearest tenth.
  2. Determine the total daily recommended dosage.
  3. To determine the dose that should be given each time (i.e., q6h), divide the total daily dosage by the number of times the medication will be administered in 24 hours.
  4. Compare the ordered dose with the safe recommended dose and determine if the dosage ordered is safe.
  5. Calculate the dosage to administer using ratio and proportion, the formula method, or dimensional analysis.
- Determining whether a dose is safe can also be determined by comparing the total daily dose.
- When the recommended dosage is stated in a range, calculate the minimum and maximum dosage for the medication.

- Ask the prescriber to verify any discrepancies in dosage that are less than the recommended dose and more than the recommended dose. Remember that factors such age, weight, and medical conditions can cause differences in the dosage of medications.
- Use appropriate resources to obtain the recommended dosage for a medication.
- Dosages less than the recommended dose may not be effective in achieving the therapeutic effect.
- For medications that are weight based, the calculations and steps are the same for adults and children.

## ▣ PRACTICE **PROBLEMS**

Round weights and dosages to the nearest tenth where indicated. Use labels where provided to answer the questions.

21. A child weighs 35 lb and has an order for Keflex (cephalexin) 150 mg p.o. q6h.

    Available:

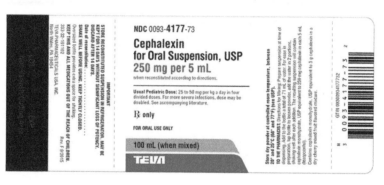

    a. What is the recommended dosage in mg/kg/day?            _____

    b. What is the child's weight in kilograms to nearest tenth?            _____

    c. What is the safe dosage range for this child?            _____

    d. Is the dosage ordered safe? (Prove mathematically.)            _____

    e. How many milliliters will you administer for each dosage?            _____

22. According to *The Harriet Lane Handbook*, the recommended dosage of clindamycin oral solution is 10-40 mg/kg/24 hr divided q6-8 hr. The child weighs 40 kg. (Base calculations on the medication being administered q6h.)

    a. What is the maximum dosage for this child in 24 hours?            _____

    b. What is the divided dosage range?            _____

23. The recommended initial dosage of mercaptopurine is 1.5-2.5 mg/kg/day p.o. The child weighs 44 lb.

    a. What is the child's weight in kilograms?    _____

    b. What is the initial safe daily dosage range for this child?    _____

24. A 44-lb child has an order for Erythromycin oral suspension 250 mg p.o. q6h. The usual dosage for children under 50 lb is 30 to 50 mg/kg/day in divided dosages q6h.

    a. What is the child's weight in kilograms?    _____

    b. What is the safe range of dosage for this child in 24 hours?    _____

    c. Is the dosage ordered safe? (Prove mathematically.)    _____

25. Refer to the Amphotericin B insert to calculate the dosage for an adult weighing 66.3 kg with good cardiorenal function.    _____

Partial Insert for Fungizone (Amphotericin B)

**DOSAGE AND ADMINISTRATION**
**CAUTION: Under no circumstances should a total daily dose of 1.5 mg/kg be exceeded. Amphotericin B overdoses can result in cardio-respiratory arrest (see OVERDOSAGE).**
FUNGIZONE Intravenous should be administered by *slow* Intravenous infusion. Intravenous infusion should be given over a period of approximately 2 to 6 hours (depending on the dose) observing the usual precautions for intravenous therapy (see PRECAUTIONS, General). The recommended concentration for intravenous infusion is 0.1 mg/mL (1 mg/10 mL).
Since patient tolerance varies greatly, the dosage of amphotericin B must be individualized and adjusted according to the patient's clinical status (e.g., site and severity of infection, etiologic agent, cardio-renal function, etc.).
A single intravenous **test dose** (1 mg in 20 mL of 5% dextrose solution) administered over 20-30 minutes may be preferred. The patient's temperature, pulse, respiration, and blood pressure should be recorded every 30 minutes for 2 to 4 hours.
In patients with **good cardio-renal function** and a **well tolerated test dose**, therapy is usually initiated with a daily dose of 0.25 mg/kg of body weight. However, in those patients having **severe and rapidly progressive fungal infection**, therapy may be initiated with a daily dose of 0.3 mg/kg of body weight. In patients with **impaired cardio-renal function** or a **severe reaction to the test dose**, therapy should be initiated with smaller daily doses (i.e., 5 to 10 mg).

26. A child with esophageal candidiasis weighs 12 lb, 6 oz. The recommended dose of IV fluconazole is 6 mg/kg on the first day, followed by 3 mg/kg once daily for 2 weeks.

    a. What is the child's weight in kilograms to the nearest tenth?    _____

    b. What is the first dosage for this child?    _____

    c. What is the subsequent dosage for this child?    _____

**Answers on p. 646**

## Calculating Dosages Using Body Surface Area

Body surface area (BSA) is used to calculate safe dosages for infants, children, and selected adult populations. Examples of types of medications that may require BSA-based dosing include chemotherapy medications and medications given to clients who have severe burns, receiving radiation treatment, and those with renal disease. BSA is the total surface area of the body expressed in square meters ($m^2$). BSA is calculated using the height and weight measurements. BSA can be determined using a special BSA slide ruler, BSA calculator, Nomogram chart, or a mathematical formula. BSA calculators can be found on the internet.

The two methods commonly used to calculate a BSA are the use of a nomogram and the use of a BSA formula. Both methods will be discussed in this text.

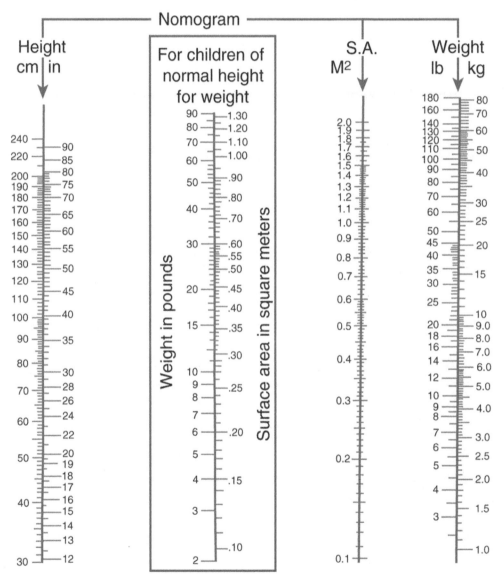

**Figure 24.1** West nomogram for estimation of body surface area. The surface area is indicated where a straight line that connects the height and weight levels intersects the surface area column or, if the patient is roughly of average size, from the weight alone *(enclosed area)*. (From Kliegman RM, St. Geme JW, Blum NJ, Shah SS, Tasker RC, Wilson KM: *Nelson textbook of pediatrics,* ed 21, Philadelphia, 2020, Saunders. Nomogram modified from the data of E. Boyd by C.D. West. See also Briars GL, Bailey BJ: Surface area estimation: pocket calculator v nomogram, *Arch Dis Child* 70:246–247, 1994.)

## Use of a Nomogram to Determine BSA

The nomogram provides an estimate of the BSA. The nomogram can be used to calculate the BSA for both children and adults for heights up to 240 cm (95 inches) and weights up to 180 lb. (There is an adult nomogram available for adults weighing more than 180 pounds.) The West nomogram is the best known BSA chart (Figure 24.1). The West nomogram has the height in inches and centimeters on the left and the weight in pounds and kilograms on the right. There is a box within the West nomogram that is used for children of normal height and weight. Normal height and weights are determined by growth and development charts. If the child is of a normal height and weight for his or her age, the BSA can be determined from weight alone. For example, a child weighing 70 lb and of normal height has a BSA of 1.10 m². To determine the BSA using the West nomogram, place a ruler extending from the height column on the left to the weight in the far right-hand column. The estimated BSA for the child is where the line intersects the surface area (SA) column. For example, by using the far right and left scales, you will find that a child who weighs 50 lb and is 36 in tall has a BSA of 0.8 m². If the ruler is slightly off the height or weight, the BSA will be incorrect. **Always** base the BSA on current height and weight measurements.

> **(!) SAFETY ALERT!**
>
> The increments and spaces on the BSA are **not consistent**. Be certain that you read the numbers and the calibration values between them carefully. To use the normal column on the West nomogram, check reliable resources such as a pediatric growth and development chart. **Do not** guess on the normal height and weight.

## ▣ PRACTICE **PROBLEMS**

Refer to the nomogram and determine the BSA (expressed in square meters) for the following children of normal height and weight.

27. For a child weighing 30 lb        _____

28. For a child weighing 42 lb        _____

29. For a child weighing 52 lb        _____

30. For a child weighing 44 lb        _____

31. For a child weighing 11 lb        _____

32. For a child weighing 20 lb        _____

Using the nomogram, calculate the following BSAs.

33. A child who is 90 cm long and weighs 50 lb        _____

34. A child who is 60 cm long and weighs 10 lb        _____

35. A baby who weighs 13 lb and is 19 inches long        _____

36. A child who weighs 30 lb and is 32 inches tall    _____

37. A child who weighs 13 kg and is 65 cm tall    _____

38. A child who is 19 inches long and weighs 5 lb    _____

**Answers on p. 647**

## Calculating BSA Using a Formula

The BSA can be calculated using a formula. To use the formula, you need the height and weight (adults and children) and a calculator that has the square root ($\sqrt{\phantom{x}}$) function. The formula used is based on the units in which the measurements are obtained. One formula uses metric measurements and the other household measurements. Notice that the difference in the formulas, in addition to the measurements used (metric versus household), is the difference in the denominators.

**Metric Formula**

$$\text{BSA (m}^2) = \sqrt{\frac{\text{Weight (kg)} \times \text{Height (cm)}}{3,600}}$$

**Household Formula**

$$\text{BSA (m}^2) = \sqrt{\frac{\text{Weight (lb)} \times \text{Height (in)}}{3,131}}$$

Let's look at examples using the metric formula.

---

**Example 1:**   Calculate the BSA for a child who weighs 23 kg and whose height is 128 cm. Express BSA to the nearest hundredth.
Problem setup:

$$\text{BSA (m}^2) = \sqrt{\frac{23\,(\text{kg}) \times 128\,(\text{cm})}{3,600}}$$

**Steps:**
1. Multiply the weight in kg by the height in cm.
2. Divide the product obtained in Step 1 by 3,600.

$$= \sqrt{\frac{2944}{3,600}} = \sqrt{0.817}$$

3. Enter the square root symbol ($\sqrt{\phantom{x}}$) into the calculator.

$$\sqrt{0.817} = 0.903$$

4. Round the final BSA in square meters to the nearest hundredth.
$$0.903 = 0.9\ \text{m}^2$$
$$\text{BSA} = 0.9\ \text{m}^2$$

---

**Example 2:**   Calculate the BSA for an adult who weighs 100 kg and whose height is 180 cm. Express BSA to the nearest hundredth. Follow the steps outlined in Example 1.

$$\text{BSA (m}^2) = \sqrt{\frac{100\,(\text{kg}) \times 180\,(\text{cm})}{3,600}} = \sqrt{5}$$

$$= \sqrt{5} = 2.236 = 2.24\ \text{m}^2$$

$$\text{BSA} = 2.24\ \text{m}^2$$

---

Now let's look at examples using household formula.

**Example 1:** Calculate the BSA for a child who weighs 25 lb and is 32 inches tall. Express the BSA to the nearest hundredth.
Problem setup:

$$\text{BSA (m}^2) = \sqrt{\frac{25\,(\text{lb}) \times 32\,(\text{in})}{3,131}}$$

**Steps:**
1. Multiply the weight in lb by the height in inches.
2. Divide the product obtained in step 1 by 3,131.

$$= \sqrt{\frac{800}{3,131}} = \sqrt{0.255}$$

3. Enter the square root symbol ($\sqrt{}$) into the calculator.

$$\sqrt{0.255} = 0.504$$

4. Round the final BSA in square meters to the nearest hundredth.
$$0.504 = 0.5 \text{ m}^2$$
$$\text{BSA} = 0.5 \text{ m}^2$$

**Example 2:** Calculate the BSA for an adult who weighs 143.7 lb and is 61.2 in tall. Express the BSA to the nearest hundredth. Follow the steps outlined in Example 1.

$$(\text{m}^2) = \sqrt{\frac{143.7\,(\text{lb}) \times 61.2\,(\text{in})}{3,131}} = \sqrt{2.808}$$

$$= \sqrt{2.808} = 1.675 = 1.68 \text{ m}^2$$

$$\text{BSA} = 1.68 \text{ m}^2$$

> ! **SAFETY ALERT!**
> Round the final answer **only** to the nearest hundredth to obtain a more accurate BSA for medication dosage. When using the calculator, don't forget the last step of pressing the square root function.

It is important to point out the slight variation in m$^2$ calculated by the metric and household methods because of rounding used to convert centimeters to inches: 1 inch = 2.54 cm, although it is rounded to 2.5 cm and used. Let's look at an example to illustrate this. Calculate the BSA of an adult whose weight is 95 kg (209 lb) and height is 180 cm (72 in).

**Metric BSA**

$$(\text{m}^2) = \sqrt{\frac{\text{Weight (kg)} \times \text{Height (cm)}}{3,600}} = \sqrt{\frac{95\,(\text{kg}) \times 180\,(\text{cm})}{3,600}} = \sqrt{4.75}$$

$$\sqrt{4.75} = 2.179 = 2.18 \text{ m}^2$$

**Household BSA**

$$(\text{m}^2) = \sqrt{\frac{\text{Weight (lb)} \times \text{Height (in)}}{3,131}} = \sqrt{\frac{209\,(\text{lb}) \times 72\,(\text{in})}{3,131}} = \sqrt{4.806}$$

$$\sqrt{4.806} = 2.192 = 2.19 \text{ m}^2$$

Notice that either metric or household measurement result in essentially the equivalent BSA.

**Technological Advances**

It is important to note that computer technology is being used more today and has made available applications that can be downloaded onto devices such as iPhones that can calculate the BSA after the data are input.

##  PRACTICE **PROBLEMS**

Determine the BSA for each of the following clients using a formula. Express the BSA to the nearest hundredth.

39. An adult whose weight is 95.5 kg and height is 180 cm

    _____

40. A child whose weight is 10 kg and height is 70 cm

    _____

41. A child whose weight is 4.8 lb and height is 21 inches

    _____

42. An adult whose weight is 170 lb and height is 67 inches

    _____

43. A child whose weight is 92 lb and height is 35 inches

    _____

44. A child whose weight is 24 kg and height is 92 cm

    _____

**Answers on p. 647**

---

⚙ **POINTS TO REMEMBER**

- The West nomogram provides an estimate of BSA using height and weight.
- There is a box within the West nomogram for children of normal height and weight based on growth and development charts; in this nomogram, the BSA can be determined from the weight alone.
- An error can be made in the BSA if the ruler is slightly off the height and weight.
- The formula method to calculate BSA is more accurate than use of the nomogram.
- The formulas used to calculate BSA are as follows:

$$\text{Metric BSA (m}^2) = \sqrt{\frac{\text{Weight (kg)} \times \text{Height (cm)}}{3,600}}$$

$$\text{Household BSA (m}^2) = \sqrt{\frac{\text{Weight (lb)} \times \text{Height (in)}}{3,131}}$$

**Determining BSA with a Formula Requires Use of a Calculator**

- Multiply height × weight (cm × kg, or lb × inches).
- Divide by 3,600 or 3,131, depending on the units of measure (divide by 3,600 if measures are in metric units [cm, kg] and by 3,131 if measures are in household units [inches, lb]).
- Enter the square root sign ($\sqrt{\ }$) to arrive at BSA in square meters.
- Round square meters to hundredths (two decimal places).
- There are applications available today that can be downloaded onto mobile devices that have computer programs that calculate the BSA.

## Dosage Calculation Based on BSA

As already mentioned, there are medications that provide the recommended dosages according to the BSA. The method used to determine the safe dosage based on weight are the same for calculating a dosage based on the BSA and determining whether the ordered dose is safe. To calculate the recommended dose based on the BSA, the nurse will need to do the following:

- Calculate the BSA or verify the client's BSA from a source such as the client's current medical record.
- Calculate the recommended dose using a reputable reference and a formula, ratio and proportion, or dimensional analysis.

  **Formula method**—The BSA of the client (adult or child) is multiplied by the recommended dosage from the reference to obtain the recommended dosage.

  **Ratio and proportion**—The known ratio is the BSA in square meters, obtained from an appropriate reference (e.g., medication insert, pediatric medication handbook).

  **Dimensional analysis**—The starting fraction is the BSA-based dosage from the reference.

- Compare the recommended dose to the ordered dose and decide whether the dosage is safe.

Let's look at some examples.

**Example 1:**   Order:  Vincristine 1.5 mg IV every Tuesday for a child who weighs 23 kg and is 126 cm tall.  According to *Mosby's 2020 Nursing Drug Reference,* the recommended dose for vincristine is 1-2 mg/m$^2$/wk. Determine if the dose is safe.

**Solution:**

**Step 1:**   Calculate the BSA using the metric formula.

$$\text{BSA (m}^2) = \sqrt{\frac{23\,(\text{kg}) \times 126\,(\text{cm})}{3,600}} = \sqrt{\frac{2,898}{3,600}} = \sqrt{0.805} = 0.897$$

BSA = 0.9 m$^2$

**Step 2:**   Calculate   the recommended dose. (**Note:** There is a range, so calculate the minimum and maximum dosage.) Multiply the child's BSA by the recommended dose from the medication reference.

**Formula Method:**

**Minimum dose:** 0.9 m$^2$ × 1 mg/m$^2$ = 0.9 mg

**Maximum dose:** 0.9 m$^2$ × 2 mg/m$^2$ = 1.8 mg

The safe dosage range for vincristine for this child is 0.9-1.8 mg /per week.

**Step 3:**   **The dosage is safe**, because the ordered dose of 1.5 mg falls within the recommended safe dose range of 0-9-1.8 mg per week.

Determining the recommended dose can also be done using ratio and proportion and dimensional analysis. The setup using those methods will be shown only for this example.

**Ratio and Proportion (Linear Format)**

Minimum dose:

$$1 \text{ mg}: 1 \text{ m}^2 = x \text{ mg} : 0.9 \text{ m}^2$$

Maximum dose:

$$2 \text{ mg} : 1 \text{ m}^2 = x \text{ mg} : 0.9 \text{ m}^2$$

**Ratio and Proportion (Fraction Format)**

Minimum dose: $\dfrac{1 \text{ mg}}{1 \text{ m}^2} = \dfrac{x \text{ mg}}{0.9 \text{ m}^2}$

Maximum dose: $\dfrac{2 \text{ mg}}{1 \text{ m}^2} = \dfrac{x \text{ mg}}{0.9 \text{ m}^2}$

**Dimensional Analysis**

Minimum dose:

$$x \text{ mg} = \frac{1 \text{ mg}}{1 \text{ m}^2} \times \frac{0.9 \text{ m}^2}{1}$$

Maximum dose:

$$x \text{ mg} = \frac{2 \text{ mg}}{1 \text{ m}^2} \times \frac{0.9 \text{ m}^2}{1}$$

**Example 2:** Carboplatin 500 mg IV has been ordered on Day 1 for a client with advanced ovarian cancer. The client weighs 125 lb and is 63 in tall, with a BSA of 1.59 m². According to *Mosby's 2020 Drug Reference* the recommended dosage is 300 mg/m². Determine if the dose ordered is safe.

**Step 1:** Although the BSA is given, it needs to be validated to make certain it is correct. Use the **household formula** to validate the BSA.

$$\text{BSA (m}^2) = \sqrt{\frac{125 \text{ (lb)} \times 63 \text{ (in)}}{3,131}} = \sqrt{\frac{7875}{3131}} = \sqrt{2.515} = 1.585$$

BSA = 1.59 m²

The BSA for the client is correct.

**Step 2:** Calculate the recommended dose using the client's BSA and the recommended dose from the reference.

1.59 m² × 300 mg/m² = 477 mg (single dose)

**Step 3:** Compare the recommended dose with the ordered dose. The recommended dose for this client is 477 mg (single dose), and the ordered dose is 500 mg (single dose). **The dose is not safe** for this client. Notify the prescriber to clarify the order before administering. The recommended dose could also be calculated using ratio and proportion or dimensional analysis. Refer to Example 1 for the setup using these methods.

> **POINTS TO REMEMBER**
>
> - Always check a dosage against BSA in square meter recommendations using appropriate resources (e.g., PDR, medication insert, drug reference book, pediatric medication handbook).
> - When you know the BSA, the dosage is determined by multiplying the BSA by the recommended dosage. (This is used when the recommended dosage is written by using the average dosage per square meter.) Ratio and proportion or dimensional analysis can also be used.
> - To determine whether a child's dosage is safe, a comparison must be made between what is ordered and the calculation of the dosage based on BSA.
> - If a dosage seems to be unsafe, consult the prescriber and verify the dosage before administering the dose.

## IV Therapy and Children
### Pediatric IV Administration

Administration of IV fluids to children is very specific because of their physiological development. Microdrop sets are used for infants and small children; electronic devices are used to control the rate of delivery. The rate of infusion for infants and children must be carefully monitored. The IV drop rate must be slow for small children to prevent complications such as cardiac failure because of fluid overload. Various IV devices decrease the size of the drop to "mini" or "micro" drop or 1/60 mL, thus delivering 60 minidrops or microdrops per milliliter. IV medications may be administered to a child over a period of time (several hours) or on an intermittent basis. For intermittent medication administration, several methods of delivery are used, including the following:

**Small-volume IV bags**—These may be used if the child has a primary IV line in place. A secondary tubing set is attached to a small-volume IV bag, and the piggyback method is used.

**Volume control sets**—Are used frequently to administer IV fluids hourly and intermittent IV medications to children. These are often referred to by their trade name which include: Buretrol, Volutrol, or Soluset. A volume control set consists of a calibrated chamber with a 150 mL capacity that connects to an IV solution. (Figure 24.2 shows a typical system that consists of a calibrated chamber.) When used to regulate IV fluid infusion, the nurse fills the chamber every 1 to 2 hours as needed with fluid directly from the IV solution. The chamber is calibrated in small increments. Small, prescribed amounts of fluid are added to the chamber, and the clamp above the chamber is fully closed. This protects the client from receiving more fluid than intended. This is especially important with children.

For the intermittent medication administration, the nurse injects the medication through the injection port at the top of the chamber, and adds an appropriate amount of IV fluid to dilute the medication, and it is infused over a specific period of time (see Figure 24.2). An IV flush (small amount of IV fluid) is administered immediately after the medication is infused.

An electronic controller or pump may also be used to administer intermittent IV medications. When used, the electronic device sounds an alarm when the Buretrol chamber is empty. Volume control devices may also be used in the adult setting for clients with fluid restrictions.

> ⚠ **SAFETY ALERT!**
>
> IV infusions should be monitored as frequently as every hour. A solution to flush the IV tubing is administered after the medication.

Regardless of the method used for medication administration in children, **a solution to flush the IV tubing is administered after the medication.** The purpose of the flush is to make sure the medication has cleared the tubing and the total dosage has been administered. Most institutions flush with normal saline solution as opposed to heparin. The amount of fluid used varies according to the length of the tubing from the medication source to the infusion site. **When IV medications are diluted for administration, the policy for including medication volume as part of the volume specified for dilution varies from institution to institution, as does the amount of flush. When flow rates (gtt/min, mL/hr) are calculated, it varies from institution to institution as to whether the flush is included. The nurse is responsible for checking the protocol at the institution to ensure that the correct procedure is followed.**

*Note:* In the sample calculations that follow, a 15-mL volume will be used as a flush unless otherwise specified, and the medication volume will be considered as part of the total dilution volume. The flush will not be considered in the total volume.

> ⚠ **SAFETY ALERT!**
>
> An excessively high concentration of an IV medication can cause vein irritation and potentially life-threatening effects. Dilution calculation is essential for the nurse.

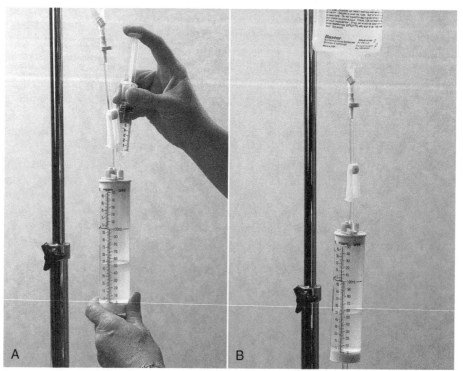

**Figure 24.2** Volume-controlled device (buretrol). (From Potter PA, Perry AG, Stockert P, Hall A: *Essentials for nursing practice,* ed 9, St Louis, 2019, Mosby.)

## Calculating IV Medications Using a Volume Control Set

A calibrated buretrol can be used to administer medications manually by using a roller clamp rather than a pump. In this case, it is necessary to use the formula presented in Chapter 21 or dimensional analysis and calculate gtt/min. Remember, buretrols are volume control devices and have a drop factor of 60 gtt/mL.

$$x \text{ gtt/min} = \frac{\text{Total volume (mL)} \times \text{drop factor (gtt/mL)}}{\text{Time in minutes}}$$

**Example:** An antibiotic dose of 100 mg in 2 mL is to be diluted in 20 mL of $D_5W$ to infuse over 30 minutes. A 15-mL flush follows. The administration set is a microdrop (buretrol). (The policy of the institution is to treat the medication volume as part of the total dilution volume.)

**Step 1:** Read the medication label, and determine what volume the 100-mg dosage is contained in. This is 2 mL.

**Step 2:** Allow 18 mL of $D_5W$ to run into the buretrol, and then add the 2 mL containing the 100 mg of medication. Roll the buretrol between your hands to allow medication to mix thoroughly. (2 mL + 18 mL = 20 mL for volume.)

**Step 3:** Determine the flow rate necessary to deliver the medication plus the flush in 30 minutes.

Total volume is 20 mL. Infusion time is 30 minutes.

$$x \text{ gtt/min} = \frac{20 \text{ mL (diluted medication)} \times 60 \text{ gtt/mL}}{30 \text{ min}}$$

$$x = \frac{20 \times \overset{2}{\cancel{60}}}{\underset{1}{\cancel{30}}} = 40 \text{ gtt/min}$$

Answer: $x = 40$ gtt/min; 40 microgtt/min

**Note:** If the flush is considered with the intermittent medication, note that the total volume will be diluted medication + flush, and then proceed with calculations (gtt/min, mL/hr).

### Dimensional Analysis

Refer to Chapter 21 if necessary to review setup.

$$\frac{x \text{ gtt}}{\text{min}} = \frac{\overset{20}{\cancel{60}} \text{ gtt}}{1 \text{ mL}} \times \frac{\overset{2}{\cancel{20}} \text{ mL}}{\underset{1}{\cancel{30}} \text{ min}}$$

$$x = \frac{40}{1}$$

$$x = 40 \text{ gt/min}; 40 \text{ microgtt/min}$$

**Step 4:** Adjust the IV flow rate to deliver 40 microgtt/min (40 gtt/min).

**Step 5:** Label the buretrol with the medication name, dosage, and medication infusing label.

**Step 6:** When administration of the medication is completed, add the 15-mL flush, and continue to infuse at 40 microgtt/min. Replace the label with a flush infusing label.

**Step 7:** When the flush is completed, restart the primary line and remove the flush infusing label. Document the medication according to institution policy on the medication administration record (MAR) or in the computer and the volume of fluid on the intake and output (I&O) sheet according to agency policy.

---

### TIPS FOR CLINICAL PRACTICE

To express the volume of gtt/min in mL/hr, remember that a microdrop administration set delivers 60 gtt/mL; therefore gtt/min = mL/hr. In this case, if the gtt/min = 40, then the mL/hr = 40.

---

As already mentioned, the buretrol can be used along with an electronic controller or pump. When used as previously stated, the electronic device will sound an alarm each time the buretrol empties. Let's examine the calculation necessary if the buretrol is used along with the pump or a controller. Calculations for which the buretrol is used with a pump or controller are done in mL/hr. Let's use the same example shown previously to illustrate the difference in calculation steps.

**Example 1:** An antibiotic dose of 100 mg in 2 mL is to be diluted in 20 mL of $D_5W$ to infuse over 30 minutes. A 15-mL flush follows. An infusion controller is used, and the tubing is a microdrop buretrol.

The same Steps 1 and 2 as shown in the previous example for buretrol only are followed.

**Step 1:** Calculate the flow rate for this microdrop.

Total volume is 20 mL; the flush is not considered in the volume.

**Step 2:** Total volume is 20 mL. Infusion time is 30 minutes. To calculate the IV rate in mL/hr, use ratio and proportion, dimensional analysis, or the formula method, as shown in Chapter 21. Refer to Chapter 21 if necessary to review the setup for the various methods. (Ratio and proportion and dimensional analysis are shown for Examples 1 and 2)

**Solution:**

---

### Ratio and Proportion (Linear Format)

$$20 \text{ mL} : 30 \text{ min} = x \text{ mL} : 60 \text{ min}$$

$$30x = 60 \times 20$$

$$\frac{\cancel{30}x}{\cancel{30}} = \frac{1,20\cancel{0}}{3\cancel{0}}$$

$$x = \frac{120}{3} = 40$$

$$x = 40 \text{ mL/hr}$$

**Answer:** Set the electronic infusion device to infuse at 40 mL/hr.

---

### Ratio and Proportion (Fraction Format)

$$\frac{20 \text{ mL}}{30 \text{ min}} = \frac{x \text{ mL}}{60 \text{ min}}$$

---

### Dimensional Analysis

$$\frac{x \text{ mL}}{\text{hr}} = \frac{20 \text{ mL}}{\cancel{30} \text{ min}_{1}} \times \frac{\cancel{60}^{2} \text{ min}}{1 \text{ hr}}$$

$$x = \frac{40}{1} = 40$$

$$x = 40 \text{ mL/hr}$$

**Example 2:** An antibiotic dose of 150 mg in 1 mL is to be diluted in 35 mL NS to infuse over 45 minutes. A 15-mL flush follows. A infusion pump will be used.

Total volume is 35 mL. Infusion time is 45 minutes. Calculate mL/hr rate.

**Solution:**

**Ratio and Proportion (Linear Format)**

$$35 \text{ mL} : 45 \text{ min} = x \text{ mL} : 60 \text{ min}$$

$$45x = 35 \times 60$$

$$\frac{\cancel{45}x}{\cancel{45}} = \frac{2,100}{45}$$

$$x = \frac{2,100}{45} = 46.6$$

$$x = 47 \text{ mL/hr}$$

**Answer:** Set the pump to infuse at 47 mL/hr

**Ratio and Proportion (Fraction Format)**

$$\frac{35 \text{ mL}}{45 \text{ min}} = \frac{x \text{ mL}}{60 \text{ min}}$$

**Dimensional Analysis**

$$\frac{x \text{ mL}}{\text{hr}} = \frac{35 \text{ mL}}{\overset{}{\underset{3}{\cancel{45} \text{ min}}}} \times \frac{\overset{4}{\cancel{60} \text{ min}}}{1 \text{ hr}}$$

$$x = \frac{140}{3} = 46.6$$

$$x = 47 \text{ mL/hr}$$

Set the pump to infuse at 47 mL/hr.

---

## 🖩 PRACTICE **PROBLEMS**

Determine the volume of solution that must be added to the buretrol in the following problems. Then determine the flow rate in gtt/min for each IV using a microdrop, and indicate mL/hr for a controller. (For all problems, use the medication volume as part of the total diluent volume.)

45. An IV medication dosage of 500 mg is ordered to be diluted to 30 mL and infuse over 50 minutes with a 15-mL flush to follow. The dosage of medication is contained in 3 mL. Determine the following:

a. Dilution volume    _____

b. Rate in gtt/min    _____

c. Rate in mL/hr    _____

46. The volume of a 20-mg dosage of medication is 2 mL. Dilute to 15 mL, and administer over 45 minutes with a 15-mL flush to follow. Determine the following:

a. Dilution volume  _____

b. Rate in gtt/min  _____

c. Rate in mL/hr  _____

**Answers on p. 647**

## Calculation of Daily Fluid Maintenance

Fluid overload or dehydration can pose a great threat to infants or young children. Nurses, therefore, must monitor not only the amount of medication but also the amount of fluid a child receives. The fluid a child receives over a 24-hour period is referred to as daily fluid maintenance needs (amount of fluid needed to maintain normal hydration). Daily fluid maintenance is also sometimes referred to as daily fluid requirements (DFR). The daily fluid maintenance includes both oral and parenteral fluids. The amount of maintenance fluid required depends on the weight of the child expressed in kilograms (kg). It does not include replacement for losses through vomiting, diarrhea, or fever. (See Table 24.1 for formula used to calculate the daily fluid maintenance.)

| TABLE 24.1 | Daily Fluid Maintenance Formula |
|---|---|

- 100 mL/kg/day for the first 10 kg of body weight
- 50 mL/kg/day for the next 10 kg of body weight
- 20 mL/kg/day for each kg above 20 kg of body weight

Let's look at examples calculating the daily fluid maintenance and the hourly rate. (The IV pump is programmable in whole numbers.)

---

**Example 1:** Child who weighs 7 kg

$$100 \text{ mL/kg/day} \times 7 \text{ kg} = 700 \text{ mL/day or per 24 hr}$$

$$x \text{ mL/hr} = \frac{700 \text{ mL}}{24 \text{ hr}} = 29.1$$

$$x = 29 \text{ mL/hr}$$

---

**Example 2:** Child weighs 14 kg

$$100 \text{ mL/kg/day} \times 10 \text{ kg} = 1,000 \text{ mL/day (for first 10 kg)}$$
$$50 \text{ mL/kg/day} \times 4 \text{ kg} = 200 \text{ mL/day (for remaining 4 kg)}$$

Total: 1,000 mL/day + 200 mL/day = 1,200 mL/day or per 24 hr

$$x \text{ mL/hr} = \frac{1,200 \text{ mL}}{24 \text{ hr}} = 50$$

$$x = 50 \text{ mL/hr}$$

---

---

**Example 3:**  A child weighs 35 lb

**Step 1:**      Convert 35 lb to kg. Conversion factor: 2.2 lb = 1 kg.

$$35 \text{ lb} \div 2.2 = 15.9 \text{ kg}$$

**Step 2:**      Apply formula to calculate the daily fluid maintenance.

$$100 \text{ mL/kg/day} \times 10 \text{ kg} = 1,000 \text{ mL/day (for first 10 kg)}$$
$$50 \text{ mL/kg/day} \times 5.9 \text{ kg} = 295 \text{ mL/day (for remaining 5.9 kg)}$$

Total: 1,000 mL/day + 295 mL/day = 1,295 mL/day or per 24 hr

$$x \text{ mL/hr} = \frac{1,295 \text{ mL}}{24 \text{ hr}} = 53.9$$
$$x = 54 \text{ mL/hr}$$

---

*Note:* In addition to the methods shown, ratio and proportion and dimensional analysis may be used to calculate the daily fluid maintenance.

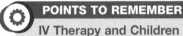 PRACTICE **PROBLEMS**

Determine the daily fluid maintenance and the hourly rate. (IV pump is programmable in whole numbers.)

47. Child weighs 13 kg

   a. Daily fluid maintenance _____ mL/day

   b. rate _____ mL/hr

48. Infant weighs 3,300 g

   a. Daily fluid maintenance _____ mL/day

   b. rate _____ mL/hr

**Answers on p. 647**

---

**⚙ POINTS TO REMEMBER**

**IV Therapy and Children**
- Pediatric IV medications are diluted for administration. It is important to know the institution's policy as to whether the medication volume is included as part of the total dilution volume.
- A flush is used after administration of IV medications in children. The volume of the flush will vary depending on the length of the IV tubing from the medication source.
- Check the institution's policy as to whether the volume of the flush is added to the diluted medication volume.
- Pediatric medication administration requires frequent assessment.
- Daily fluid maintenance is sometimes referred to as daily fluid requirements.
- The amount of maintenance fluid required is based on the child's weight in kg.
- Daily fluid maintenance formula:
  - 100 mL/kg/day for first 10 kg of body weight
  - 50 mL/kg/day for next 10 kg of body weight
  - 20 mL/kg/day for each kg above 20 kg of body weight

## Pediatric Oral and Parenteral Medications

Several methods have been presented to determine dosages for children in this chapter. It is important, however, to bear in mind that although the dosage may be determined according to weight, BSA, and other methods, the dosage to administer is calculated by using the same methods as for adults (ratio and proportion, the formula method, or dimensional analysis). It is important to remember the following differences with children's dosages.

### Remember:

- Dosages are smaller for children than for adults.
- Most oral medications for infants and small children come in liquid form to facilitate swallowing.
- The oral route is preferred; however, when necessary, medications are administered by the parenteral route.
- Not more than 1 mL is injected IM for small children and older infants; small infants should not receive more than 0.5 mL by IM injection.
- Parenteral dosages are frequently administered with a tuberculin syringe.

> **(!) SAFETY ALERT!**
> When in doubt, always double-check pediatric dosages with another nurse to decrease the chance of an error. Never assume! Think before administering.

## 🔲 CLINICAL **REASONING**

**Scenario:** According to *The Harriet Lane Handbook,* the recommended dosage for a child for ibuprofen as an antipyretic is 5-10 mg/kg/dose q6-8h p.o. The 7-month-old weighs $18\frac{1}{2}$ lb. The prescriber ordered 20 mg p.o. q6h for a temperature above 102° F. The infant's temperature is 102.8° F, and the nurse is preparing to administer the medication. The nurse believes the dosage is low but administers the medication based on the dosage being safe because it is below the safe dosage range. Several hours have passed, and the infant's temperature continues to increase.

a. What is the required single dosage for this infant?    _____

b. What should the nurse's actions have been and why?    _____

c. What preventive measures could have been taken by the nurse in this situation?    _____

**Answers on p. 647**

## NGN Case Study

**Learning Objectives:**
1. Convert body weight from pounds to kilograms.
2. Calculate dosages based on milligram per kilogram.
3. Determine whether a dosage is safe.

**Case Scenario:** The parents of an 18-month-old, bring their child into the emergency department because the child is fussy, not wanting to eat, and pulling at his left ear. An assessment is completed and the physician determines the child has an ear infection. The child weighs 20 pounds. The physician orders amoxicillin suspension 275 mg orally every 12 hours. Amoxicillin suspension is available as 250 mg per 5 mL. The recommended dose for amoxicillin is 20-40 mg/kg/day divided q12h po. Round weight to the nearest tenth.

Use an X to indicate which potential solutions are correct and incorrect based on the scenario provided.

| Potential Solution | Correct | Incorrect |
|---|---|---|
| The child weighs 9.1 kg. | | |
| The child weighs 44 kg. | | |
| The recommended dosage is 91 to 182 mg/dose q12h. | | |
| The recommended dosage is 440 to 880 mg/dose q12h. | | |
| The minimum total dosage is 182 mg/daily and the maximum total dosage is 364 mg/daily. | | |
| The minimum total dosage is 880 mg/daily and the maximum total dosage is 1760 mg/daily. | | |
| The dose is unsafe for the child. | | |
| The dose is safe for the child. | | |

**Reference:** Morris: *Calculate with confidence,* ed 8, St Louis, Elsevier, copyright 2022. (*Harriet Lane Handbook* for the dosage.)

*Case Study answers and rationales can be found on Evolve.*

## ⊙ CHAPTER **REVIEW**

Read the dosage information or label given for the following problems. Express body weight conversion to the nearest tenth where indicated and dosages to the nearest tenth.

1. Lasix 10 mg IV stat is ordered for a child weighing 22 lb. The recommended dose is 1–2 mg/kg/dose. Is the dosage ordered safe? (Prove mathematically.) _____

2. Furadantin oral suspension 25 mg p.o. q6h is ordered for a child weighing 37.4 lb. Recommended dosage is 5–7 mg/kg/24 hr divided q6h.

   Available: Furadantin oral suspension 25 mg per 5 mL.

   a. What is the child's weight in kilograms to the nearest tenth? _____

   b. What is the dosage range for this child? _____

   c. Is the dosage ordered safe? (Prove mathematically.) _____

   d. How many milliliters must be given per dosage to administer the ordered dosage? Calculate the dose if the order is safe. _____

3. Cefaclor 225 mg p.o. q8h is ordered for a child weighing 35 kg. _____

Available:

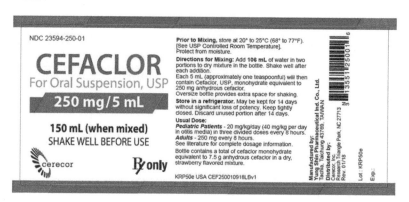

Is the dosage ordered safe?
(Prove mathematically.)

_____

4. Vibramycin 50 mg p.o. q12h is
   ordered for a child weighing 30 lb.
   The recommended dosage is
   2.2–4.4 mg/kg/day in two divided
   doses. Is the dose ordered safe?
   (Prove mathematically.)

   _____

5. Cleocin 150 mg p.o. q8h is
   ordered for a child weighing 36 lb. The
   recommended dosage is 10 to 40 mg/kg/day
   divided q6-8h.

   _____

   Available:

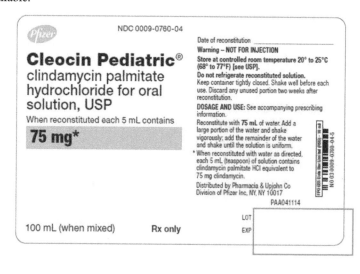

a. Is the dosage ordered safe?
   (Prove mathematically.)

   _____

b. How many milliliters would you need
   to administer one dosage? Calculate
   the dose if the order is safe.

6. Keflex (cephalexin) suspension 250 mg p.o. q6h is ordered for a child weighing 66 lb. The usual pediatric dosage is 25 to 50 mg/kg/day q6h.

   Available: Keflex suspension 250 mg per 5 mL.

   a. Is the dosage ordered safe? (Prove mathematically.) _____

   b. How many milliliters would you need to administer one dosage? Calculate the dose if the order is safe. _____

7. A 40-lb child who is 5 years old has an order for midazolam 1.5 mg IV stat. The recommended dose for a child 6 months-5 years is 0.05-0.1 mg/kg/dose. Is the dosage ordered safe? _____

Using the formula method for calculating BSA, determine the BSA in the following clients, and express answers to the nearest hundredth.

8. A 15-year-old who weighs 100 lb and is 55 inches tall _____

9. An adult who weighs 60.9 kg and is 130 cm tall _____

10. A child who weighs 55 lb and is 45 inches tall _____

11. An adult who weighs 65 kg and is 132 cm tall _____

12. An infant who weighs 6 kg and is 55 cm long _____

13. A child who weighs 42 lb and is 45 inches tall _____

14. An adult who weighs 74 kg and is 160 cm tall _____

15. An adult who weighs 150 lb and is 70 inches tall _____

Calculate the daily fluid maintenance and the hourly rate for questions 16-18: (Pump is programmed in whole milliliters unless otherwise indicated.)

16. Child weighing 25 kg

a. Daily fluid maintenance _____ mL/day

b. IV rate _____ mL/hr

17. Child weighing 77 lb

a. Daily fluid maintenance _____ mL/day

b. IV rate _____ mL/hr

18. Infant weighing 4,200 g

a. Daily fluid maintenance _____ mL/day

b. IV rate _____ mL/hr (pump capable of delivering in tenths).

For questions 19-20, round the answer in mg to the nearest tenth.

19. An adult weighs 72.7 kg and is 200 cm tall. The recommended dose for cisplatin is

50-70 mg per m$^2$ every 3-4 weeks for a client with advanced bladder cancer. Determine the BSA using the formula. Calculate the safe dosage range.

a. BSA_____

b. Dosage range _____ mg

20. A child weighs 21 lb and is 30 inches in height. The recommended dose for vincristine is 1-2 mg per m$^2$ once weekly. Determine the BSA using the formula. What is the dosage range for the child?

a. BSA _____

b. Dosage range _____ mg

Determine the flow rate in gtt/min for each IV using a microdrip, then indicate mL/hr for a controller. (Consider the medication volume as part of the total dilution volume, as shown in the chapter.)

21. A child is to receive 10 units of a medication. The dosage of 10 units is contained in 1 mL. Dilute to 30 mL and infuse in 20 minutes. A 15-mL flush is to follow. Medication is placed in a buretrol. Determine the rate in:

a. gtt/min_____

b. mL/hr _____

22. A child is to receive 80 mg of a medication. The dosage of 80 mg is contained in 2 mL. Dilute to 80 mL and infuse in 60 minutes. A 15-mL flush is to follow. Medication is placed in a buretrol. Determine the rate in:

a. gtt/min _____

b. mL/hr_____

23. A dosage of 250 mg in 5 mL has been ordered diluted to 40 mL and infused in 45 minutes. A 15-mL flush follows. Medication is placed in a buretrol. Determine the rate in:

a. gtt/min_____

b. mL/hr _____

24. Order: Digoxin 0.1 mg p.o. daily.

Available:

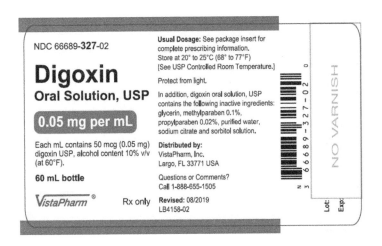

25. Order: Tegretol 0.25 g p.o. t.i.d.

Available:

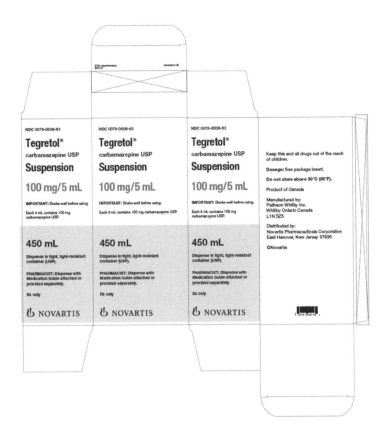

Calculate the dosages below. Use the labels where provided. Calculate to the nearest hundredth where necessary.

26. Order: Gentamicin 7.3 mg IM q12h.

    Available: 20 mg per 2 mL

NDC 63323-173-94   PRX17302
**GENTAMICIN**
*INJECTION, USP*
(PEDIATRIC)
equivalent to 10 mg/mL Gentamicin
**20 mg/2 mL**
**For IM or IV Use.**
**Must be diluted for IV use.**
**2 mL** Single Dose Vial
**Preservative Free   Rx only**

Manufactured by:
**Fresenius Kabi USA, LLC**
Lake Zurich, IL 60047

_____

27. Order: Nebcin (tobramycin sulfate) 60 mg IV q8h.

    Available:

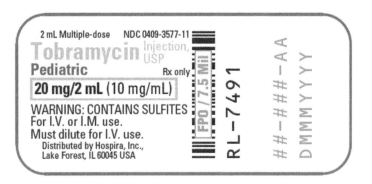

_____

Calculate the dosages to be given. Round answers to the nearest tenth as indicated (express answers in milliliters).

28. Order: Tylenol 0.4 g p.o. q4h p.r.n. for temp greater than 101° F.

    Available: Tylenol elixir labeled
    160 mg per 5 mL          _____

29. Order: Methotrexate 35 mg IV daily once a week (on Tuesdays).

    Available:

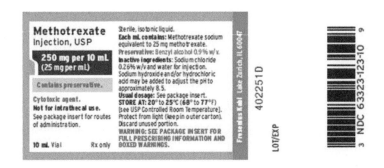

_____

30. Order: Amikacin 150 mg IV q8h.

    Available:

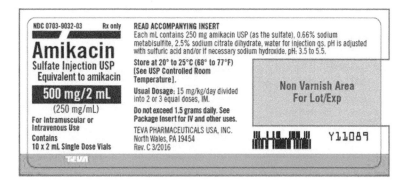

    _____

31. Order: Dilantin 62.5 mg p.o. b.i.d.

    Available: Dilantin oral suspension
    labeled 125 mg per 5 mL

    _____

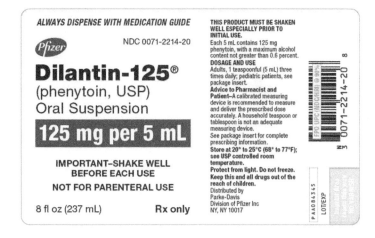

32. Order: Albuterol 3 mg p.o. b.i.d.

    Available:

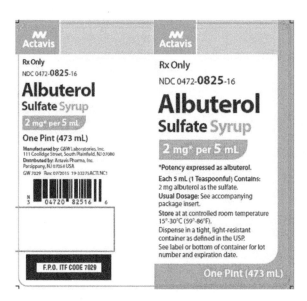

    _____

33. Order: Methylprednisolone 14 mg IV q6h.

    Available:

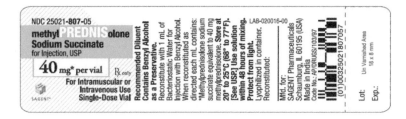

    _____

34. Order: Famotidine 20 mg p.o. b.i.d.

    Available:

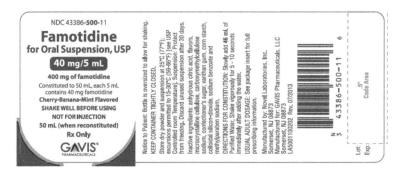

    _____

Round weights and dosages to the nearest tenth as indicated.

35. Order: Ceclor (cefaclor) 180 mg p.o. q12h. The infant weighs 10 lb.

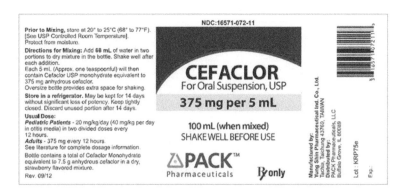

    a. Is the dosage ordered safe?
       (Prove mathematically.)                _____

    b. How many milliliters will you need
       to administer the dosage? Calculate
       the dose to administer if the dosage
       is safe.                                _____

36. Acetaminophen (Ofirmev) 525 mg IV q4h is ordered for a child weighing 92.4 lb. According to *The Harriet Lane Handbook,* the dosage for a child (age 2-12 years) or adolescent/adult weighing less than 50 kg is 15 mg/kg/dose q6h, or 12.5 mg/kg/dose q4h IV up to a maximum of 75 mg/kg/24 hr.

    a. What is the safe dosage for this child?  _____

    b. Is the dosage ordered safe?  _____

Round dosages and weights to the nearest tenth as indicated.

37. Order: Minoxidil for a child weighing 31 lb. The recommended dosage range is 0.1-0.2 mg/kg/24 hr.

    What is the safe dosage range for this child?  _____

38. A client weighs 140.8 lb. According to a reputable drug reference, the recommended initial dose of diltiazem is 0.25 mg/kg as a bolus.

    What is the initial dose for this client?  _____

39. A client weighs 147 lb and has an order for Amikacin 550 mg IV q12h. According to *Mosby's 2020 Nursing Drug Reference*, the recommended dosage for Amikacin is 15 mg/kg/day in two divided doses.

    Is the dose ordered for the client safe? (Provide a mathematical rationale.)  _____

40. A client with testicular cancer has a BSA of 1.7 m$^2$. According to *Mosby's 2020 Nursing Drug Reference*, the recommended dosage for Bleomycin IV 1-2 times a week is 10-20 units/m$^2$.

    Determine the recommended dosage for this client.  _____

**Answers on pp. 648-652**

For additional practice problems, refer to the Pediatric Dosages section of the Elsevier's Interactive Drug Calculation Application, Version 1, on Evolve.

## ⭐ ANSWERS

## Chapter 24
### Answers to Practice Problems

| | | | | | | |
|---|---|---|---|---|---|---|
| 1. 6.8 kg | 4. 23.6 kg | 7. 2.6 kg | 10. 46.9 lb | 13. 33 lb | 16. 160.6 lb | 19. 2.9 kg |
| 2. 30.9 kg | 5. 92.8 kg | 8. 45.6 kg | 11. 38.9 lb | 14. 74.8 lb | 17. 216.3 lb | 20. 1.9 kg |
| 3. 14.1 kg | 6. 3.8 kg | 9. 42.2 kg | 12. 48.4 lb | 15. 157.1 lb | 18. 1.5 kg | |

> **✎ NOTE**
> Any of the methods presented in Chapter 24 can be used to calculate dosages; not all are shown in the Answer Key.

21. a. 25 to 50 mg/kg/day

    b. Convert weight first (2.2 lb = 1 kg).
       35 ÷ 2.2 = 15.9 kg

    c. 25 mg : 1 kg = $x$ mg : 15.9 kg
       $x$ = 397.5 mg/day

       50 mg : 1 kg = $x$ mg : 15.9 kg
       $x$ = 795 mg/day

       *or*

       25 mg/kg/day × 15.9 kg = 397.5 mg/day

       50 mg/kg/day × 15.9 kg = 795 mg/day

       Dosage range is 397.5 to 795 mg/day.

    d. The dosage ordered falls within the range that is safe (150 mg × 4 = 600 mg). 600 mg/day falls within the 397.5 to 795 mg/day range.

    e. 250 mg : 5 mL = 150 mg : $x$ mL

       *or*

       $$\frac{150 \text{ mg}}{250 \text{ mg}} \times 5 \text{ mL} = x \text{ mL}$$

       $x$ = 3 mL

22. a. 10 mg : 1 kg = $x$ mg : 40 kg
       $x$ = 400 mg/day

       *or*
       10 mg/kg/day × 40 kg = 400 mg/day

       40 mg : 1 kg = $x$ mg : 40 kg
       $x$ = 1,600 mg/day

       *or*
       40 mg/kg/day × 40 kg = 1,600 mg/day

       Answer: 1,600 mg/day is the maximum dosage.

    b. q6h = 24 ÷ 4 = 4 doses per day
       400 mg ÷ 4 = 100 mg q6h
       1,600 mg ÷ 4 = 400 mg q6h

       Answer: 100-400 mg q6h is the divided dosage range (400 mg q6h is maximum divided dose).

23. Convert the child's weight to kilograms (2.2 lb = 1 kg).

    a. 44 lb ÷ 2.2 = 20 kg

    b. 1.5 mg/kg/day × 20 kg = 30 mg/day

    2.5 mg : 1 kg = $x$ mg : 20 kg
    $x$ = 50 mg/day

    *or*

    2.5 mg/kg/day × 20 kg = 50 mg/day

    30-50 mg/day (initial safe daily dosage range).

24. Convert weight (2.2 lb = 1 kg).

    a. 44 lb ÷ 2.2 = 20 kg

    b. 30 mg : 1 kg = $x$ mg : 20 kg
       $x$ = 600 mg/day

       *or*

       30 mg/kg/day × 20 kg = 600 mg/day

       50 mg : 1 kg = $x$ mg : 20 kg
       $x$ = 1,000 mg/day

       *or*

       50 mg/kg/day × 20 kg = 1,000 mg/day

       600-1,000 mg/day

    c. The dosage ordered is safe.
       250 mg × 4 = 1,000 mg. 1,000 mg falls within the safe range.

25. No weight conversion is required.

    0.25 mg : 1 kg = $x$ mg : 66.3 kg
    $x$ = 16.57 = 16.6 mg

    *or*

    0.25 mg/kg × 66.3 kg = 16.57 = 16.6 mg

    Answer: 16.6 mg is the dosage for the adult.

26. Convert weight (2.2. lb = 1 kg, 16 oz = 1 lb).

    6 oz ÷ 16 = 0.37 lb = 0.4 lb (to nearest tenth)

    Total weight in pounds = 12.4 lb

    a. 12.4 lb ÷ 2.2 = 5.63 = (5.6 kg to nearest tenth)

    b. 6 mg : 1 kg = $x$ mg : 5.6 kg
       $x$ = 33.6 mg

       *or*
       6 mg/kg × 5.6 kg = 33.6 mg

       Answer: 33.6 mg for the first dose.

    c. 3 mg : 1 kg = $x$ mg : 5.6 kg
       $x$ = 16.8 mg

       *or*
       3 mg/kg × 5.6 kg = 16.8 mg

       Answer: 16.8 mg daily for the subsequent dose.

27. $0.6 \text{ m}^2$

28. $0.78 \text{ m}^2$

29. $0.9 \text{ m}^2$

30. $0.8 \text{ m}^2$

31. $0.28 \text{ m}^2$

32. $0.44 \text{ m}^2$

33. $0.8 \text{ m}^2$

34. $0.28 \text{ m}^2$

35. $0.32 \text{ m}^2$

36. $0.58 \text{ m}^2$

37. $0.54 \text{ m}^2$

38. $0.18 \text{ m}^2$

39. $m^2 = \sqrt{\dfrac{95.5 \text{ (kg)} \times 180 \text{ (cm)}}{3{,}600}}$

$\sqrt{4.775} = 2.185 = 2.19 \text{ m}^2$

Answer: $2.19 \text{ m}^2$

40. $m^2 = \sqrt{\dfrac{10 \text{ (kg)} \times 70 \text{ (cm)}}{3{,}600}}$

$\sqrt{0.194} = 0.44 \text{ m}^2$

Answer: $0.44 \text{ m}^2$

41. $m^2 = \sqrt{\dfrac{4.8 \text{ (lb)} \times 21 \text{ (in)}}{3{,}131}}$

$\sqrt{0.032} = 0.178 = 0.18 \text{ m}^2$

Answer: $0.18 \text{ m}^2$

42. $m^2 = \sqrt{\dfrac{170 \text{ (lb)} \times 67 \text{ (in)}}{3{,}131}}$

$\sqrt{3.637} = 1.907 = 1.91 \text{ m}^2$

Answer: $1.91 \text{ m}^2$

43. $m^2 = \sqrt{\dfrac{92 \text{ (lb)} \times 35 \text{ (in)}}{3{,}131}}$

$\sqrt{1.028} = 1.014 = 1.01 \text{ m}^2$

Answer: $1.01 \text{ m}^2$

44. $m^2 = \sqrt{\dfrac{24 \text{ (kg)} \times 92 \text{ (cm)}}{3{,}600}}$

$\sqrt{0.613} = 0.783 = 0.78 \text{ m}^2$

Answer: $0.78 \text{ m}^2$

45. a. Dilution volume: 27 mL

b.

$x \text{ gtt/min} = \dfrac{30 \text{ mL (diluted medication)} \times 60 \text{ gtt/mL}}{50 \text{ min}}$

$x = \dfrac{30 \times 60}{50} = \dfrac{1800}{50} = 36 \text{ gtt/min}$

*or*

Use a ratio and proportion to determine mL/hr first. Remember that with a buretrol when a pump or controller is not used, mL/hr = gtt/min.

$30 \text{ mL} : 50 \text{ min} = x \text{ mL} : 60 \text{ min}$

*or*

$\dfrac{30 \text{ mL}}{50 \text{ min}} = \dfrac{x \text{ mL}}{60 \text{ min}}$

Answer: $x = 36 \text{ gtt/min}$; 36 microgtt/min

c. 36 mL/hr

46. a. Dilution volume: 13 mL

b.
$x \text{ gtt/min} = \dfrac{15 \text{ mL (diluted medication)} \times 60 \text{ gtt/mL}}{45 \text{ min}}$

$x = \dfrac{15 \times 60}{45} = \dfrac{900}{45} = 20 \text{ gtt/min}$

*or*

Use a ratio and proportion and determine mL/hr first.

$15 \text{ mL} : 45 \text{ min} = x \text{ mL} : 60 \text{ min}$

*or*

$\dfrac{15 \text{ mL}}{45 \text{ min}} = \dfrac{x \text{ mL}}{60 \text{ min}}$

Answer: $x = 20 \text{ gtt/min}$; 20 microgtt/min

c. 20 mL/hr

47. a. $100 \text{ mL/kg/day} \times 10 \text{ kg} = 1{,}000 \text{ mL/day}$
(for first 10 kg)

$50 \text{ mL/kg/day} \times 3 \text{ kg} = 150 \text{ mL/day}$
(for the remaining 3 kg)

Total: $1{,}000 \text{ mL/day} + 150 \text{ mL/day} = 1{,}150 \text{ mL/day}$

Answer: 1,150 mL/day or per 24 hr

b. $x \text{ mL/hr} = \dfrac{1{,}150 \text{ mL}}{24 \text{ hr}} = 47.9$

$x = 48 \text{ mL/hr}$

Answer: 48 mL/hr

48. Convert weight: Equivalent: 1 kg = 1,000 g

$3{,}300 \text{ g} \div 1{,}000 = 3.3 \text{ kg}$

a. $100 \text{ mL/kg/day} \times 3.3 \text{ kg} = 330 \text{ mL/day}$

Answer: 330 mL/day or per 24 hr

b. $x \text{ mL/hr} = \dfrac{330 \text{ mL}}{24 \text{ hr}} = 13.7$

$x = 14 \text{ mL/hr}$

Answer: 14 mL/hr

### Answers to Clinical Reasoning Questions

a. 42-84 mg/dose

b. Contact the prescriber; the dosage is too low. The dose is not safe because it is below the recommended therapeutic dose to be effective in decreasing the child's temperature.

c. The nurse should have notified the prescriber immediately so that the order could be revised. The child's temperature indicates an underdosage that is not safe. Do not assume it is safe because the dosage is lower than the recommended dosage.

## Answers to Chapter Review

1. Convert weight (2.2 lb = 1 kg).

   a. 22 lb ÷ 2.2 = 10 kg

   b. 1 mg/kg/dose × 10 kg = 10 mg/dose

   2 mg/kg/dose × 10 kg = 20 mg/dose

   The dosage ordered for this child is safe. 10 mg falls within the range of 10-20 mg per dose.

2. Convert child's weight in lb to kg.

   $$2.2 \text{ lb} = 1 \text{ kg}$$

   a. 37.4 lb ÷ 2.2 = 17 kg

   b. 5 mg/kg/24 hr × 17 kg = 85 mg/24 hr (day).

   7 mg/kg/24 hr × 17 kg = 119 mg/24 hr (day).

   Answer: The dosage range is 85-119 mg/day.

   $$q6h = 4 \text{ dosages}$$

   85 mg ÷ 4 = 21.25 mg = 21.3 mg per dose (q6h)

   119 mg ÷ 4 = 29.75 mg = 29.8 mg per dose (q6h)

   The divided dosage range is 21.3-29.8 mg per dose.

   The dosage ordered is 25 mg q6h.

   c. The dosage ordered is safe because 25 mg × 4 doses = 100 mg/day. It falls within the range of 85-119 mg/day. The dosage q6h also falls within the divided dosage range of 21.3-29.8 mg q6h.

   d. 25 mg : 5 mL = 25 mg : $x$ mL

   $$or$$

   $$\frac{25 \text{ mg}}{25 \text{ mg}} \times 5 \text{ mL} = x \text{ mL}$$

   $$x = 5 \text{ mL}$$

   Answer: Give 5 mL per dose. The dosage ordered is contained in 5 mL.

3. No conversion of weight is required. The child's weight is in kilograms, and the recommended dosage is expressed in kilograms (20 mg/kg/day).

   $$20 \text{ mg/kg/day} \times 35 \text{ kg} = 700 \text{ mg/day}$$

   $$q8h = 3 \text{ dosages}$$

   $$700 \text{ mg} \div 3 =$$

   $$233.33 = 233.3 \text{ mg per dosage}$$

   The dosage ordered is not safe. 225 mg × 3 = 675 mg/day. 675 mg/day is less than 700 mg/day and the dose being given q6h is less than 233.3 mg. Check with prescriber. Dose may be too low to be effective.

4. Convert the child's weight in pounds to kilograms. The recommended dosage is expressed in kilograms (2.2-4.4 mg/kg/day) (2.2 lb = 1 kg).

   $$30 \text{ lb} = 30 \div 2.2 = 13.6 \text{ kg}$$

   2.2 mg/kg/day × 13.6 kg = 29.9 mg/day

   4.4 mg/kg/day × 13.6 kg = 59.8 mg/day

   $$q12h = 2 \text{ dosages}$$

   29.9 mg ÷ 2 = 15 mg per dose.

   59.8 mg ÷ 2 = 29.9 mg per dose.

   50 mg × 2 = 100 mg/day. The dosage is not safe; notify the prescriber. 100 mg/day is greater than 29.9-59.8 mg/day. Also, the dose being administered q12h exceeds the recommended dosage.

5. Convert the child's weight in pounds to kilograms.

   a. The recommended dosage is stated in kilograms (10-40 mg/kg/day) (2.2 lb = 1 kg).

   $$36 \text{ lb} = 36 \div 2.2 = 16.4 \text{ kg}$$

   10 mg/kg/day × 16.4 kg = 164 mg/day

   40 mg/kg/day × 16.4 kg = 656 mg/day

   The medication is given q6-8h. The dosage in this problem is ordered q8h.

   $$24 \div 8 = 3 \text{ dosages}$$

   $$164 \text{ mg} \div 3 = 54.7 \text{ mg per dose}$$

   $$656 \text{ mg} \div 3 = 218.7 \text{ mg per dose}$$

   The dosage ordered is 150 mg q8h.

   $$150 \text{ mg} \times 3 = 450 \text{ mg/day.}$$

   The dosage is safe. 450 mg/day falls within the range of 164-656 mg/day. Also, the dose being administered q8h falls within the range of 54.7-218.7 mg per dose.

   b. 75 mg : 5 mL = 150 mg : $x$ mL

   $$or$$

   $$\frac{150 \text{ mg}}{75 \text{ mg}} \times 5 \text{ mL} = x \text{ mL}$$

   $$x = 10 \text{ mL}$$

   Answer: Give 10 mL per dose. The dosage ordered is more than the available dosage strength.

   Therefore you will need more than 5 mL to administer the dose.

6. a. Convert the child's weight in pounds to kilograms. The recommended dosage is expressed in kilograms (25-50 mg/kg) (2.2 lb = 1 kg).

   $$66 \text{ lb} = 66 \div 2.2 = 30 \text{ kg}$$

   25 mg/kg/day × 30 kg = 750 mg/day

   50 mg/kg/day × 30 kg = 1,500 mg/day

   The safe range is 750-1,500 mg/day.

   The medication is given in divided dosages.

   The dosage ordered is q6h.

   $$24 \div 6 = 4 \text{ dosages}$$

   750 mg ÷ 4 = 187.5 mg/per dosage

   1,500 mg ÷ 4 = 375 mg/per dosage

   The dosage range is 187.5-375 mg per dose q6h. 250 mg × 4 = 1,000 mg/day. This is a safe dosage because the total dosage falls within the safe range for 24 hr, and the divided dosage also falls within the safe range.

b. You would give 5 mL for one dosage.

$$250 \text{ mg} : 5 \text{ mL} = 250 \text{ mg} : x \text{ mL}$$

*or*

$$\frac{250 \text{ mg}}{250 \text{ mg}} \times 5 \text{ mL} = x \text{ mL}$$

$$x = 5 \text{ mL}$$

The dosage ordered is contained in 5 mL; therefore you will need to administer 5 mL.

7. Convert the child's weight in pounds to kilogram. The recommended dosage is expressed in kilograms (0.05-0.1 mg/kg/dose).

40 lb = 40 ÷ 2.2 = 18.2 kg

0.05 mg/kg/dose × 18.2 kg = 0.9 mg per dose

0.1 mg/kg/dose × 18.2 kg = 1.8 mg per dose

The dose range for this child is 0.9-1.8 mg per dose. The dose ordered is safe. 1.5 mg falls within the range of 0.9-1.8 mg per dose.

8. $m^2 = \sqrt{\dfrac{100 \text{ (lb)} \times 55 \text{ (in)}}{3,131}} = \sqrt{\dfrac{5,500}{3,131}} = \sqrt{1.756}$

$\sqrt{1.756} = 1.325$

Answer: 1.33 m$^2$

9. $m^2 = \sqrt{\dfrac{60.9 \text{ (kg)} \times 130 \text{ (cm)}}{3,600}} = \sqrt{\dfrac{7,917}{3,600}} = \sqrt{2.199}$

$\sqrt{2.199} = 1.482$

Answer: 1.48 m$^2$

10. $m^2 = \sqrt{\dfrac{55 \text{ (lb)} \times 45 \text{ (in)}}{3,131}} = \sqrt{\dfrac{2,475}{3,131}} = \sqrt{0.790}$

$\sqrt{0.790} = 0.888$

Answer: 0.89 m$^2$

11. $m^2 = \sqrt{\dfrac{65 \text{ (kg)} \times 132 \text{ (cm)}}{3,600}} = \sqrt{\dfrac{8,580}{3,600}} = \sqrt{2.383}$

$\sqrt{2.383} = 1.543$

Answer: 1.54 m$^2$

12. $m^2 = \sqrt{\dfrac{6 \text{ (kg)} \times 55 \text{ (cm)}}{3,600}} = \sqrt{\dfrac{330}{3,600}} = \sqrt{0.091}$

$\sqrt{0.091} = 0.301$

Answer: 0.3 m$^2$

13. $m^2 = \sqrt{\dfrac{42 \text{ (lb)} \times 45 \text{ (in)}}{3,131}} = \sqrt{\dfrac{1,890}{3,131}} = \sqrt{0.603}$

$\sqrt{0.603} = 0.776$

Answer: 0.78 m$^2$

14. $m^2 = \sqrt{\dfrac{150 \text{ (lb)} \times 70 \text{ (in)}}{3,131}} = \sqrt{\dfrac{10,500}{3,131}} = \sqrt{3.353}$

$\sqrt{3.353} = 1.831$

Answer: 1.81 m$^2$

15. $m^2 = \sqrt{\dfrac{150 \text{ (lb)} \times 70 \text{ (in)}}{3,131}} = \sqrt{\dfrac{10,500}{3,131}} = \sqrt{3.353}$

$\sqrt{3.353} = 1.831$

Answer: 1.83 m$^2$

16. a.

100 mL/kg/day × 10 kg = 1,000 mL/day (for the first 10 kg)

50 mL/kg/day × 10 kg = 500 mL/day (for the next 10 kg)

20 mL/kg/day × 5 kg = 100 mL/day (for remaining 5 kg)

Total: 1,000 mL/day + 500 mL/day + 100 mL/day = 1,600 mL/day

Answer: 1,600 mL/day or per 24 hr

b. $x \text{ mL/hr} = \dfrac{1,600 \text{ mL}}{24 \text{ hr}} = 66.6$

$x = 67 \text{ mL/hr}$

Answer: 67 mL/hr

17. Convert weight:

Equivalent: 2.2 lb = 1 kg

77 lb ÷ 2.2 = 35 kg

a.

100 mL/kg/day × 10 kg = 1,000 mL/day (for first 10 kg)

50 mL/kg/day × 10 kg = 500 mL/day (for next 10 kg)

20 mL/kg/day × 15 kg = 300 mL/day (for remaining 15 kg)

Total: 1,000 mL/day + 500 mL/day + 300 mL/day = 1,800 mL/day

Answer: 1,800 mL/day or per 24 hr

b. $x \text{ mL/hr} = \dfrac{1,800 \text{ mL}}{24 \text{ hr}}$

$x = 75 \text{ mL/hr}$

Answer: 75 mL/hr

18. Convert weight:

Equivalent: 1 kg = 1,000 g

4,200 g ÷ 1,000 = 4.2 kg

a. 100 mL/kg/day × 4.2 kg = 420 mL/day

Answer: 420 mL/day or per 24 hr

b. $x \text{ mL/hr} = \dfrac{420 \text{ mL}}{24 \text{ hr}} = 17.5$

$x = 17.5 \text{ mL/hr}$

Answer: 17.5 mL/hr (pump capable of delivering in tenths of an mL)

19. a.

$m^2 = \sqrt{\dfrac{72.7 \text{ (kg)} \times 200 \text{ (cm)}}{3,600}} = \sqrt{\dfrac{14,540}{3,600}} = \sqrt{4.038}$

$\sqrt{4.038} = 2.009$

Answer: 2.01 m$^2$

b. $2.01 \text{ m}^2 \times 50 \text{ mg/m}^2 = 100.5 \text{ mg}$

$2.01 \text{ m}^2 \times 70 \text{ mg/m}^2 = 140.7 \text{ mg}$

Answer: 100.5-140.7 mg q wk.

20. a. $m^2 = \sqrt{\dfrac{21 \text{ (lb)} \times 30 \text{ (in)}}{3,131}} = \sqrt{\dfrac{630}{3,131}} = \sqrt{0.201}$

$\sqrt{0.201} = 0.448$

Answer: $0.45 \text{ m}^2$

b. $0.45 \text{ m}^2 \times 1 \text{ mg/m}^2 = 0.5 \text{ mg}$

$0.45 \text{ m}^2 \times 2 \text{ mg/m}^2 = 0.9 \text{ mg}$

Answer: Dosage range is 0.5-0.9 mg.

21. $x \text{ gtt/min} = \dfrac{30 \text{ mL} \times 60 \text{ gtt/mL}}{20 \text{ min}}$

$x = \dfrac{1,800}{20}$

$x = 90 \text{ gtt/min}$

or

mL/hr determined with ratio and proportion

30 mL : 20 min = $x$ mL : 60 min

or

$\dfrac{30 \text{ mL}}{20 \text{ min}} = \dfrac{x \text{ mL}}{60 \text{ min}}$

a. 90 gtt/min; 90 microgtt/min

b. 90 mL/hr

22. $x \text{ gtt/min} = \dfrac{80 \text{ mL} \times 60 \text{ gtt/mL}}{60 \text{ min}}$

$x = \dfrac{4,800}{60}$

$x = 80 \text{ gtt/min}$

or

Determine mL/hr.

80 mL : 60 min = $x$ mL : 60 min

$\dfrac{80 \text{ mL}}{60 \text{ min}} = \dfrac{x \text{ mL}}{60 \text{ min}}$

a. 80 gtt/min; 80 microgtt/min

b. 80 mL/hr

23. $x \text{ gtt/min} = \dfrac{40 \text{ mL} \times 60 \text{ gtt/mL}}{45 \text{ min}}$

$x = \dfrac{2,400}{45}$

$x = 53 \text{ gtt/min}$

or

Determine mL/hr.

40 mL : 45 min = $x$ mL : 60 min

$\dfrac{40 \text{ mL}}{45 \text{ min}} = \dfrac{x \text{ mL}}{60 \text{ min}}$

a. 53 gtt/min; 53 microgtt/min

b. 53 mL/hr

24. 0.05 mg : 1 mL = 0.1 mg : $x$ mL

or

$\dfrac{0.1 \text{ mg}}{0.05 \text{ mg}} \times 1 \text{ mL} = x \text{ mL}$

Answer: 2 mL. The dosage ordered is more than the available strength; therefore you will need more than 1 mL to administer the dosage.

25. Conversion required. Equivalent: 1,000 mg = 1 g. Therefore 0.25 g = 250 mg.

100 mg : 5 mL = 250 mg : $x$ mL

or

$\dfrac{250 \text{ mg}}{100 \text{ mg}} \times 5 \text{ mL} = x \text{ mL}$

Answer: 12.5 mL. The dosage ordered is greater than the available strength; therefore you will need more than 5 mL to administer the dosage.

26. 20 mg : 2 mL = 7.3 mg : $x$ mL

or

$\dfrac{7.3 \text{ mg}}{20 \text{ mg}} \times 2 \text{ mL} = x \text{ mL}$

Answer: 0.73 mL. The dosage ordered is less than the available strength; therefore you will need less than 2 mL to administer the dosage.

27. 20 mg : 2 mL = 60 mg : $x$ mL

or

$\dfrac{60 \text{ mg}}{20 \text{ mg}} \times 2 \text{ mL} = x \text{ mL}$

Answer: 6 mL. The dosage ordered is more than the available strength; therefore you will need more than 2 mL to administer the dosage.

28. Conversion required. Equivalent: 1,000 mg = 1 g. Therefore 0.4 g = 400 mg.

160 mg : 5 mL = 400 mg : $x$ mL

or

$\dfrac{400 \text{ mg}}{160 \text{ mg}} \times 5 \text{ mL} = x \text{ mL}$

Answer: 12.5 mL. The dosage ordered is more than the available strength; therefore you will need more than 5 mL to administer the dosage.

29. 25 mg : 1 mL = 35 mg : $x$ mL

or

$\dfrac{35 \text{ mg}}{25 \text{ mg}} \times 1 \text{ mL} = x \text{ mL}$

Answer: 1.4 mL. The dosage ordered is more than the available strength; therefore you will need more than 1 mL to administer the dosage.

30. $250 \text{ mg} : 1 \text{ mL} = 150 \text{ mg} : x \text{ mL}$

    *or*

    $$\frac{150 \text{ mg}}{250 \text{ mg}} \times 1 \text{ mL} = x \text{ mL}$$

    Answer: 0.6 mL. The dosage ordered is less than the available strength; therefore you will need less than 1 mL to administer the dosage.

    Alternate solution: $500 \text{ mg} : 2 \text{ mL} = 150 \text{ mg} : x \text{ mL}$

    *or*

    $$\frac{150 \text{ mg}}{500 \text{ mg}} \times 2 \text{ mL} = x \text{ mL}$$

31. $125 \text{ mg} : 5 \text{ mL} = 62.5 \text{ mg} : x \text{ mL}$

    *or*

    $$\frac{62.5 \text{ mg}}{125 \text{ mg}} \times 5 \text{ mL} = x \text{ mL}$$

    Answer: 2.5 mL. The dosage ordered is less than the available strength; therefore you will need less than 5 mL to administer the dosage.

32. $2 \text{ mg} : 5 \text{ mL} = 3 \text{ mg} : x \text{ mL}$

    *or*

    $$\frac{3 \text{ mg}}{2 \text{ mg}} \times 5 \text{ mL} = x \text{ mL}$$

    Answer: 7.5 mL. The dosage ordered is more than the available strength; therefore you will need more than 5 mL to administer the dosage.

33. $40 \text{ mg} : 1 \text{ mL} = 14 \text{ mg} : x \text{ mL}$

    *or*

    $$\frac{14 \text{ mg}}{40 \text{ mg}} \times 1 \text{ mL} = x \text{ mL}$$

    Answer: 0.35 = 0.4 mL rounded to the nearest tenth. The dosage ordered is less than the available strength; therefore you will need less than 1 mL to administer the dosage.

34. $40 \text{ mg} : 5 \text{ mL} = 20 \text{ mg} : x \text{ mL}$

    *or*

    $$\frac{20 \text{ mg}}{40 \text{ mg}} \times 5 \text{ mL} = x \text{ mL}$$

    Answer: 2.5 mL. The dosage ordered is less than the available strength; therefore you will need less than 5 mL to administer the dosage.

35. a. Convert the child's weight in pounds to kilograms. The recommended dosage is expressed in kilograms (20 mg/kg/day) (2.2 lb = 1 kg).

    $10 \text{ lb} = 10 \div 2.2 = 4.5 \text{ kg}$

    $20 \text{ mg/kg/day} \times 4.5 \text{ kg} = 90 \text{ mg/day}$

The medication is given in two divided doses q12h. The dosage for the child is ordered q12h.

$24 \div 12 = 2$ doses.

$90 \text{ mg} \div 2 = 45 \text{ mg per dose}$

$180 \text{ mg} \times 2 = 360 \text{ mg/day}$

Notify the prescriber; the dosage is too high (not safe).

360 mg/day is greater than 90 mg/day. In addition, the dose the child is receiving q12h exceeds the dose recommended.

   b. The volume to be administered is not calculated because the dosage ordered is not safe.

36. a. Convert the child's weight in pounds to kilograms (2.2 lb = 1 kg). The recommended dosage is in kilograms, and the dosage is ordered q4h. The dosage is determined using 12.5 mg/kg/dose.

    $92.4 \text{ lb} = 92.4 \div 2.2 = 42 \text{ kg}$

    $12.5 \text{ mg/kg/dose} \times 42 \text{ kg} = 525 \text{ mg/dose}$

    The safe dosage for this child is 525 mg/dose.

   b. The dosage ordered for the child is safe. For this child's weight, 525 mg/dose is the recommended dosage, and 525 mg is the ordered dosage.

37. Convert the child's weight in pounds to kilograms. The recommended dosage is in kilograms 0.1-0.2 mg/kg/24 hr. Conversion factor: 2.2 lb = 1 kg.

    $31 \text{ lb} = 31 \div 2.2 = 14.1 \text{ kg}$

    $0.1 \text{ mg/kg/day} \times 14.1 \text{ kg} = 1.4 \text{ mg/day}$

    $0.2 \text{ mg/kg/day} \times 14.1 \text{ kg} = 2.8 \text{ mg/day}$

    The safe dosage range for this child is 1.4-2.8 mg/day.

38. a. Convert the client's weight to kg. Conversion factor: 2.2 lb = 1 kg.

    $140.8 \text{ lb} \div 2.2 = 64 \text{ kg}$

   b. Calculate the recommended initial dose for this client.

    $64 \text{ kg} \times 0.25 \text{ mg/kg} = 16 \text{ mg}$

    Answer: The initial dose for the client is 16 mg.

39. a. Convert the client's weight to kg. Conversion factor: 2.2 lb = 1 kg.

    $147 \text{ lb} \div 2.2 = 66.81 = 66.8 \text{ kg}$

   b. Calculate the recommended dose for the client.

    $66.8 \text{ kg} \times 15 \text{ mg/kg/day} = 1,002 \text{ mg/day}$

    The recommended daily dose for the client is 1,002 mg/day.

    Determine the divided dose (q12h = 2 × day; 24 hr ÷ 12 = 2).

    $1,002 \text{ mg} \div 2 = 501 \text{ mg}$

   c. Determine if the dose ordered for the client is safe.

The ordered dose is 550 mg q12h. 550 mg $\times$ 2 = 1,100 mg /day. The dose is not safe because the ordered dose (550 mg q12h) is more than the recommended dose. Also, the divided dose is more than what is recommended per dose. Contact the prescriber about the ordered dose and verify the order before administering.

40. Calculate the range of dosage from minimum to maximum.

1.7 $m^2$ $\times$ 10 units/$m^2$ = 17 units minimum dosage

1.7 $m^2$ $\times$ 20 units/$m^2$ = 34 units maximum dosage

The recommended dosage for this client is 17-34 units.

# Comprehensive Post-Test

Solve the following calculation problems. Remember to apply the principles learned in the text relating to dosages. Use labels where provided. Shade in the dosage on the syringe where provided.

1. Order: Amoxicillin and clavulanate potassium 300 mg p.o. q8h (ordered according to dose of amoxicillin).

   Available:

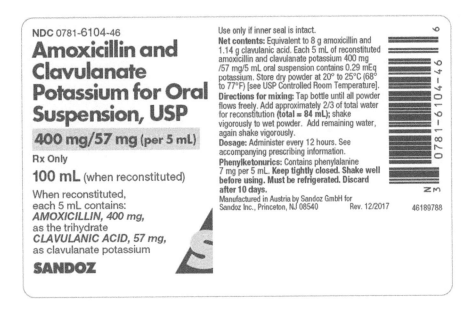

   NDC 0781-6104-46

   **Amoxicillin and Clavulanate Potassium for Oral Suspension, USP**

   400 mg/57 mg (per 5 mL)

   Rx Only

   **100 mL** (when reconstituted)

   When reconstituted,
   each 5 mL contains:
   *AMOXICILLIN, 400 mg,*
   as the trihydrate
   *CLAVULANIC ACID, 57 mg,*
   as clavulanate potassium

   **SANDOZ**

   Use only if inner seal is intact.
   **Net contents:** Equivalent to 8 g amoxicillin and 1.14 g clavulanic acid. Each 5 mL of reconstituted amoxicillin and clavulanate potassium 400 mg /57 mg/5 mL oral suspension contains 0.29 mEq potassium. Store dry powder at 20° to 25°C (68° to 77°F) [see USP Controlled Room Temperature].
   **Directions for mixing:** Tap bottle until all powder flows freely. Add approximately 2/3 of total water for reconstitution (**total = 84 mL**); shake vigorously to wet powder. Add remaining water, again shake vigorously.
   **Dosage:** Administer every 12 hours. See accompanying prescribing information.
   **Phenylketonurics:** Contains phenylalanine 7 mg per 5 mL. **Keep tightly closed. Shake well before using. Must be refrigerated. Discard after 10 days.**
   Manufactured in Austria by Sandoz GmbH for Sandoz Inc., Princeton, NJ 08540     Rev. 12/2017     46189788

   _____

2. Order: Latuda 60 mg p.o. daily.

   Available:

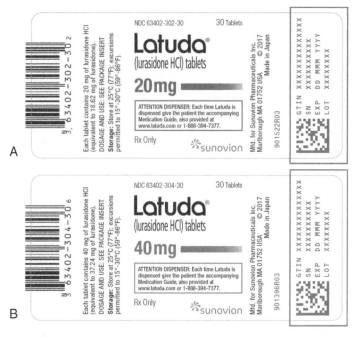

a. How many tablets of which dosage
   strength will you use to administer
   the ordered dosage?                    _____

b. Provide the rationale for your answer.    _____

3. Order: Bactrim DS 1 tab p.o. q12h for 14 days.

   Available:

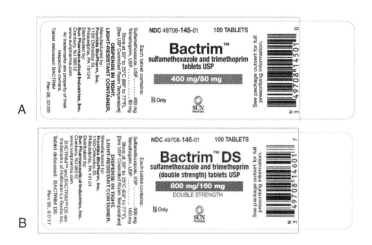

a. Indicate by letter which tablets the
   nurse would choose to administer to
   the client based on the order.          _____

b. Provide the rationale for your answer.    _____

4. Order: Heparin 6,500 units subcut daily. (Express your answer in hundredths.)

   Available:

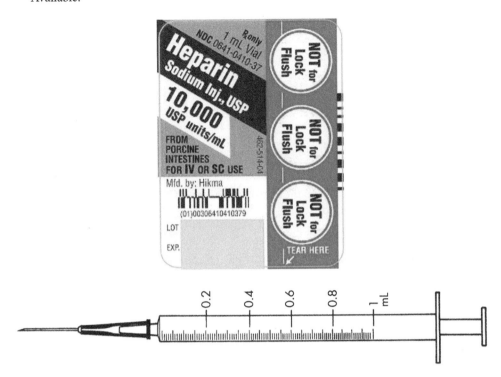

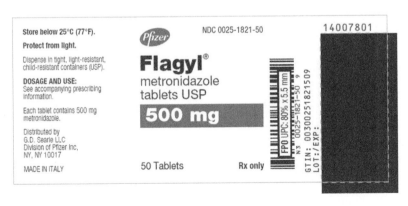

_____

5. Order: Flagyl 0.5 g p.o. b.i.d. for 7 days.

   Available:

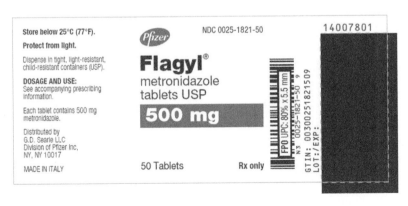

_____

6. Order: Amphotericin B 75 mg in 1,000 mL D$_5$W to infuse over 6 hr daily. The reconstituted solution contains 50 mg per 10 mL.

Available:

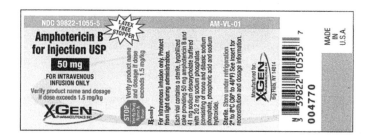

a. How many milliliters will the nurse add to the IV solution? _____

b. The IV is to infuse in 6 hr by infusion pump. Calculate the IV flow rate in mL/hr. _____

7. The recommended dose of Retrovir for adults with symptomatic HIV infection is 1 mg/kg infused over 1 hour q4h. Determine dosage for a client weighing 110 lb. _____

8. Order: Bosulif 0.5 g p.o. daily.

Available:

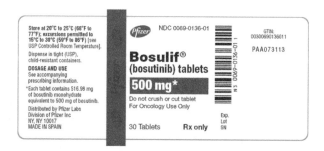

a. How many tablets will the nurse administer? _____

b. What are the directions for administration? _____

9.  Order: Tazicef 0.25 g IV q12h.

Available:

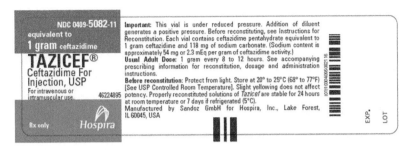

| Size | Amount of diluent to be added (mL) | Approximate available volume (mL) | Approximate ceftazidime concentration (mg/mL) |
|---|---|---|---|
| **Intramuscular** | | | |
| 1-gram vial | 3 | 3.6 | 280 |
| **Intravenous** | | | |
| 1-gram vial | 10 | 10.6 | 95 |
| 2-gram vial | 10 | 11.2 | 18 |

a.  Using the information provided, what concentration will the nurse prepare? _____

b.  How many milliliters will the nurse administer? _____

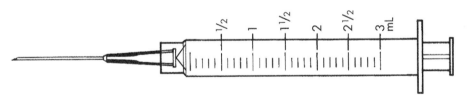

10. Order: Neurontin 900 mg p.o. b.i.d.

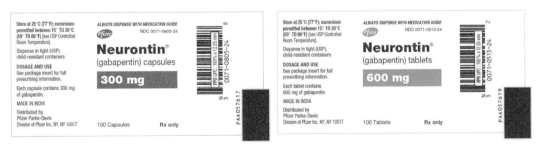

How many of which capsules would be best to administer to the client? _____

11. Order: Transfuse 1 unit packed red blood cells (250 mL) over 3 hr. The administration set delivers 10 gtt/mL. At what rate in gtt/min should the IV infuse?

_____

12. Order: Keytruda 200 mg in 100 mL 0.9% NS IV over 30 min by infusion pump.

Available:

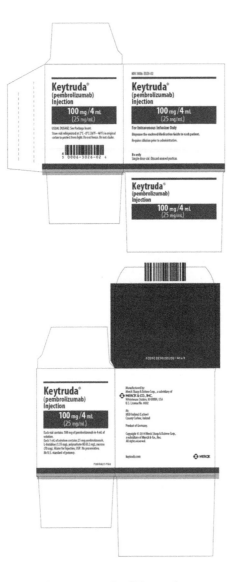

a. How many mL of Keytruda will you add to the IV bag?

_____

b. Determine the IV rate.

_____

13. Calculate the infusion time for an IV of 1,000 mL of $D_5NS$ infusing at 60 mL/hr. Express time in hours and minutes.

_____

14. The prescriber orders Septra Suspension
60 mg p.o. b.i.d. for a child weighing
12 kg. The pediatric medication reference
states that Septra Suspension contains
trimethoprim (TMP) 40 mg and
sulfamethoxazole (SMZ) 200 mg in
5 mL oral suspension, and the safe
dosage of the medication is based on
trimethoprim. According to *The Harriet
Lane Handbook,* the safe dosage is 8 to
12 mg/kg/day divided b.i.d. Is
the dosage ordered safe?           _____

15. A medicated IV of 100 mL is to infuse at a rate of 50 mL/hr.

   a. Determine the infusion time.        _____

   b. The IV was started at 10:00 AM.
      When will it be completed?
      (State time in military and
      traditional time.)                  _____

16. A client is to receive 10 mcg/min
nitroglycerin IV. The concentration
of solution is 50 mg of nitroglycerin in
250 mL $D_5W$. What should the flow rate
be (in mL/hr) to deliver 10 mcg/min?    _____

17. Order: Humulin Regular 6 units and Humulin NPH 16 units subcut at 7:30 AM.

   What is the total units the nurse will
   administer?                          _____

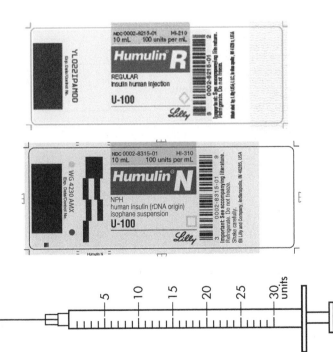

18. A dosage of 500 mg of a medication in a volume of 3 mL is to be diluted to 55 mL to
infuse over 50 minutes. A 20-mL flush is to follow.

    a. What is the dilution volume?    _____

    b. At what rate in gtt/min should the
       IV infuse? (Administration set is a
       microdrop.)    _____

    c. Indicate the rate in mL/hr.    _____

19. Calculate the body surface area (BSA),
    using the formula, for a child who weighs
    102 lb and is 51 inches tall. Calculate
    the BSA to the nearest hundredth.    _____

20. Acyclovir IV is to be administered to a child who has herpes simplex
    encephalitis. The child weighs 13.6 kg and is 60 cm tall. The recommended
    dosage is 500 mg/m$^2$. Use the formula to calculate the BSA.

    Available:

    a. What is the BSA? (Express your
       answer to the nearest hundredth.)    _____

    b. What will the dosage be?    _____

    c. Calculate the number
       of milliliters to administer.    _____

21. Prepare the following strength solution:
    2/5 strength Ensure Plus 250 mL.    _____

22. Calculate the amount of dextrose and NaCl in 2 L of $D_5$ $\frac{1}{4}$ NS.

    a. Dextrose    _____ g

    b. Sodium chloride    _____ g

23. 500 mL $D_5W$ was to infuse in 3 hours at 28 gtt/min (28 macrogtt/min). The drop fac-
    tor is 10 gtt/mL. After $1\frac{1}{2}$ hours, you notice 175 mL has infused.

    a. Recalculate the IV flow rate.    _____

    b. Determine the percentage of change.    _____

    c. State the course of action.    _____

24. Order: Infuse $D_5W$ 500 mL with 20,000 units heparin at 25 mL/hr. Determine the
    following:

    _____units/hr

25. Order: Morphine sulfate 80 mg in 250 mL of IV fluid to infuse at a rate of 20 mL/hr.

    Determine the dosage in mg/hr the client is receiving. _____

26. Order: Diltiazem HCl (cardizem) 25 mg IV over 2 minutes.

    Available:

    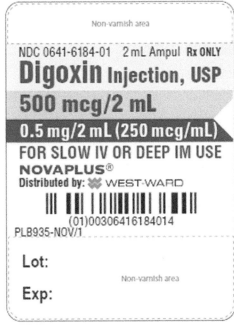

    a. How many milliliters will the nurse add to the IV? _____

    b. How many milliliters will the nurse infuse per minute? _____

27. Order: Cipro 0.5 g p.o. q12h.

    Available: Cipro tablets labeled 250 mg.

    How many tablets will be needed for 10 days of therapy? _____

28. Order: Lanoxin (digoxin) 0.375 mg p.o. stat.

    Available: Scored tablets labeled 125 mcg, 250 mcg, and 500 mcg.

    a. Which Lanoxin tablet(s) will the nurse use to prepare the dosage? _____

    b. How many tablets should the client receive? _____

29. Order: Digoxin 0.125 mg IV daily for 7 days.

    Available:

    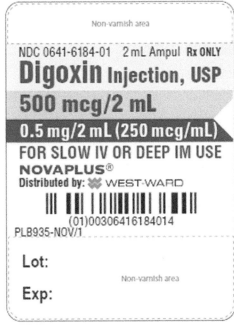

a. How many milliliters will the
   nurse administer?

_____

b. Shade the dosage in on the
   syringe provided.

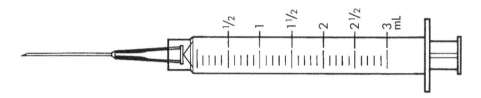

For problems 30-31, round weight to the nearest tenth as indicated.

30. The heparin protocol at an institution is: Bolus client with 80 units/kg of body weight and start drip at 14 units/kg/hr. Using the heparin protocol, determine the following for a client weighing 242 lb.

    a. Heparin bolus dosage

    _____

    b. Infusion rate for the heparin
       IV drip

    _____

31. Order: 20 units/kg/hr heparin IV. The client weighs 88 kg.

    How many units will the client
    receive per hour?

    _____

32. Order: Digoxin 0.375 mg IV push (infused slowly over 5 minutes).

    Available: Digoxin 0.25 mg per mL.

    a. How many milliliters should the
       nurse administer?

    _____

    b. At what rate in mL/min should the
       IV infuse?

    _____

33. Order: Morphine 8 mg IV q4h p.r.n. (infusion not to exceed 10 mg/4 min).

    Available: Morphine 10 mg per mL.

    a. How many milliliters will the
       nurse administer?

    _____

    b. How many minutes will it take
       for the IV to infuse?

    _____

34. Refer to the chart below and calculate the client's fluid intake in milliliters.

| ORAL INTAKE | IV INTAKE |
|---|---|
| 4 oz gelatin | 100 mL |
| 2 oz water | |
| 12 oz apple juice | |

What is the client's intake in mL? _____

Refer to the Heparin Weight-Based Protocol provided below to answer question 35.
1. Bolus heparin at 80 units/kg.
2. Begin intravenous infusion of heparin at 18 units/kg/hr using 25,000 units heparin in 250 mL D$_5$W for 1,000 units per mL.
3. Adjust intravenous heparin daily based on APTT results.
   - APTT less than 35 sec: Rebolus with 80 units/kg and increase rate by 4 units/kg/hr.
   - APTT 35-45 sec: Rebolus with 40 units/kg and increase rate by 2 units/kg/hr.
   - APTT 46-70 sec: **No change.**
   - APTT 71-90 sec: Decrease rate by 2 units/kg/hr.
   - APTT greater than 90 sec: **Stop heparin** infusion for 1 hour and decrease rate by 3 units/kg/hr.

35. Client weighs 187 lb. Determine the bolus dose of heparin and the initial intravenous rate of heparin. The APTT is reported as being 43 seconds. Determine the rebolus and adjust the intravenous rate based on the APTT results. (The pump is capable of delivering in tenths of a milliliter.)

36. A client is ordered to begin Levophed (norepinephrine bitartrate) at 4 mcg/min to maintain blood pressure and titrate to maintain systolic blood pressure greater than 100 mm Hg to a maximum of 12 mcg/min. Available solution is Levophed 8 mg in 1,000 mL D$_5$W. Develop a titration table from minimum to maximum dose in 2-mcg/min increments. (The IV pump is calibrated in whole mL.)

37. Versed (midazolam) 10 mcg/kg IV is ordered for sedation of a client. The client weighs 127.2 lb. How many mcg should the client receive? (Round weight to the nearest tenth.) _____

38. Order: Gemzar 900 mg IV weekly.

    Available:

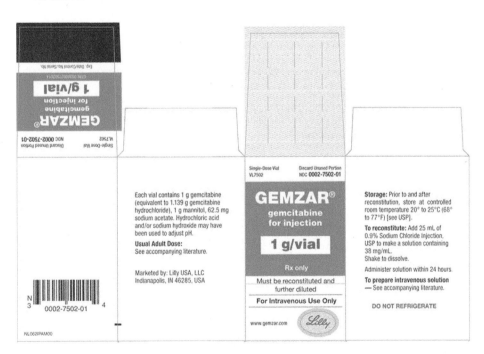

How many mL will the nurse add to the IV?    _____

39. Using a full-strength normal saline (0.9%) solution, prepare 180 mL of 1/3 strength normal saline solution, diluted with sterile water for wound care. Express answer in mL. _____

40. Refer to the following medication orders and correct them according to the ISMP published list of Error Prone Abbreviations and Symbols.

    a.  MS 4 mg sc q4h prn pain _____

    b.  Digoxin .375 mg p.o. qd _____

41. Order: Ultram 0.1 g po q6h prn for pain.

    Available:

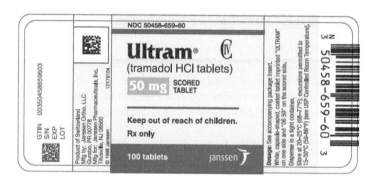

    How many tab(s) will the nurse administer? _____

42. Order: Vitamin K (phytonadione) 2.5 mg subcut stat.

    Available:

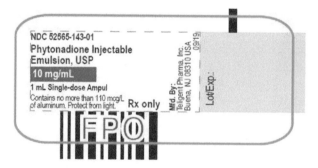

    a.  How many mL will the nurse administer? _____

    b.  Shade the dosage on the syringe provided.

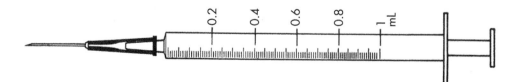

43. Order: Unasyn 1,550 mg IV q6h.

    Available: Refer to label and portion of the package insert.

    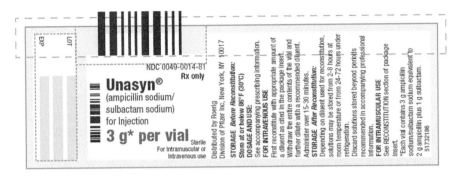

    | Unasyn Vial Size | Volume of Diluent to Be Added | Withdrawal Volume |
    |---|---|---|
    | 1.5 g | 3.2 mL | 4 mL |
    | 3 g | 6.4 mL | 8 mL |

    How many mL will the nurse administer? _____

44. Order: Demerol 40 mg IM and Vistaril 25 mg q4h prn for pain.

    Available: Demerol 50 mg per mL and Vistaril 50 mg per mL.

    a. What is the total dose in mL the nurse will administer? _____

    b. Shade the dosage on the syringe provided.

    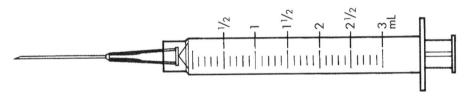

45. Order: Vincristine 4 mg IV q Thursday for a child who weighs 45 kg and is 155 cm. The recommended dose of Vincristine is 1-2 mg/m$^2$ in a single dose weekly. (Use the BSA Formula.) Round dosage to nearest tenth.

    Available:

    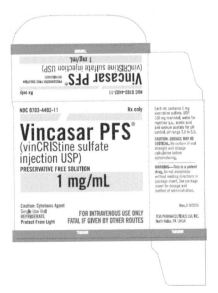

a. Is the dose ordered safe? (Prove mathematically.)

b. If the dosage ordered is safe, calculate the mL you would administer. _____

If not safe, explain why and describe what you should do. _____

_____

46. Calculate the I & O from 7 AM–3 PM.

A client has IV fluids $D_5$ $\frac{1}{2}$ NS with 20 mEq potassium chloride (KCl) infusing at 75 mL/hr at 7 AM. An order is received to increase the IV fluid to 100 mL/hr at 10 AM. The IV fluids are held for 1 hour while Ampicillin 1 g in 100 mL of 0.9% NS is infused from 12 PM to 1 PM. The client consumes the following:

**Breakfast:** $1\frac{1}{2}$ glasses of cranberry juice (glass = 6 oz)

$2\frac{1}{2}$ cups of tea (cup = 8 oz)

**Lunch:**   $\frac{3}{4}$ can of gingerale (can = 12 oz)

$\frac{1}{2}$ bowl of broth (bowl = 6 oz)

4 oz ice cream

The client voids four times during the shift: 375 mL, 250 mL, 400 mL, and 300 mL of urine.

Intake _____ mL

Output _____ mL

47. A continuous heparin infusion is to begin at 15 units/kg/hr for a client weighing 82 kg. Available: 25,000 units of heparin in 250 mL $D_5$W. Calculate the mL/hr (the pump is capable of delivering in tenths of an mL).

_____ mL/hr

For questions 48-50, calculate the daily fluid maintenance and hourly IV rate using the following formula:

| 100 mL/kg/day for the first 10 kg of body weight |
|---|
| 50 mL/kg/day for next 10 kg of body weight |
| 20 mL/kg/day for each kg of body weight above 20 kg |

48. Child weighs 32 kg

Infuse _____ mL of _____ mL/hr (pump delivers in tenths of an mL).

49. Infant weighs 2,500 g

Infuse _____ mL at _____ mL/hr (pump delivers in tenths of an mL)

50. Child weighs 78 lb (round weight to the nearest tenth)

    Infuse _____ mL at _____ mL/hr (pump delivers in
    whole mL)

For questions 51-52, determine BSA to the nearest hundredth and dosages to the nearest
tenth.

51. An adult client weighs 135 lb and is 62 in tall. The recommended dose for Gemzar IV
    for clients with ovarian cancer is 1,000 mg/m$^2$. Determine the BSA using the formula,
    and calculate the safe dose for the client.

    a. BSA                                _____

    b. Dosage in mg                       _____

52. An adult client weighs 92.7 kg and is 185 cm tall. The recommended dose for Bleo-
    mycin IV for the treatment of testicular carcinoma is 10-20 units/m$^2$ weekly or twice
    a week. The client is receiving 35 units IV weekly. Determine the BSA using the for-
    mula, and determine if the dose is safe.

    a. BSA                                _____

    b. Dosage range                       _____

    c. Is the dosage safe?
       (Provide a mathematical rationale.)   _____

**Answers on pp. 668-674**

## ⭐ ANSWERS

> **NOTE**
>
> Calculations may be performed using the formula method, ratio and proportion, or dimensional analysis.

1. 400 mg : 5 mL = 300 mg : $x$ mL

   *or*

   $$\frac{300 \text{ mg}}{400 \text{ mg}} \times 5 \text{ mL} = x \text{ mL}$$

   Answer: 3.8 mL

2. Answer: 2 tabs (1 40-mg tablet and 1 20-mg tablet). This would be the least number of tablets to administer the ordered dosage.

3. a. Tablets B: Bactrim DS.

   b. The prescriber's order indicates DS, which means double strength; therefore the client should be given the tabs that are labeled DS.

4. 10,000 units : 1 mL = 6,500 units : $x$ mL

   *or*

   $$\frac{6,500 \text{ units}}{10,000 \text{ units}} \times 1 \text{ mL} = x \text{ mL}$$

   Answer: 0.65 mL

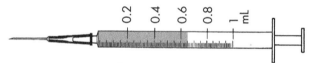

5. Conversion is required. Equivalent: 1,000 mg = 1 g

   Therefore 0.5 g = 500 mg

   500 mg : 1 tab = 500 mg : $x$ tab

   *or*

   $$\frac{500 \text{ mg}}{500 \text{ mg}} \times 1 \text{ tab} = x \text{ tab}$$

   Answer: 1 tab

6. a. 50 mg : 10 mL = 75 mg : $x$ mL

   *or*

   $$\frac{75 \text{ mg}}{50 \text{ mg}} \times 10 \text{ mL} = x \text{ mL}$$

   Answer: 15 mL

   b. Determine mL/hr.

   $$x \text{ mL/hr} = \frac{1,000 \text{ mL}}{6 \text{ hr}}; x = 166.6 = 167 \text{ mL/hr}$$

   Answer: 167 mL/hr

> **NOTE**
>
> Problem 6 could also be done by using a ratio and proportion, as illustrated in Chapter 21.

7. Convert weight in pounds to kilograms. Equivalent: 2.2 lb = 1 kg

   Therefore 110 lb ÷ 2.2 = 50 kg

   50 k̶g̶ × 1 mg/k̶g̶ = 50 mg

   Answer: 50 mg

8. a. Conversion is required. Equivalent: 1 g = 1,000 mg

   Therefore 0.5 g = 500 mg

   500 mg : 1 tab = 500 mg : $x$ tab

   *or*

   $$\frac{500 \text{ mg}}{500 \text{ mg}} \times 1 \text{ tab} = x \text{ tab}$$

   Answer: 1 tab

   b. Do not crush or cut tablet.

9. a. 95 mg per mL (Vial is 1 g.)

   b. Conversion is required. 1,000 mg = 1 g

   Therefore 0.25 g = 250 mg

   95 mg : 1 mL = 250 mg : $x$ mL

   *or*

   $$\frac{250 \text{ mg}}{95 \text{ mg}} \times 1 \text{ mL} = x \text{ mL}$$

   Answer: 2.63 mL = 2.6 mL

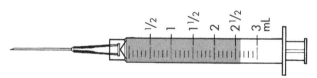

10. Answer: 2 caps: 1 300-mg cap and 1 600-mg cap). Administer the least amount of capsules to the client to administer the ordered dosage.

11. **Step 1:** Determine mL/hr.

    $$x \text{ mL/hr} = \frac{250 \text{ mL}}{3 \text{ hr}}; x = 83.3 = 83 \text{ mL/hr}$$

    **Step 2:** Calculate gtt/min.

    $$x \text{ gtt/min} = \frac{83 \text{ mL} \times 10 \text{ gtt/mL}}{60 \text{ min}}$$

    $$x = 13.8 = 14 \text{ gtt/min}$$

    Answer: 14 macrogtt/min; 14 gtt/min

    The shortcut method could also have been used to do the problem.

12. a. 25 mg : 1 mL = 200 mg : x mL

   *or*

   $$\frac{200 \text{ mg}}{25 \text{ mg}} \times 1 \text{ mL} = x \text{ mL}$$

   Answer: 8 mL

   Alternate solution:

   100 mg : 4 mL = 200 mg : x mL

   *or*

   $$\frac{200 \text{ mg}}{100 \text{ mg}} \times 4 \text{ mL} = x \text{ mL}$$

   b. 100 mL : 30 min = x mL : 60 min

   Answer: 200 mL/hr

   Alternate solution:

   $$x \text{ mL/hr} = \frac{100 \text{ mL}}{30 \text{ min}} \times 60 \text{ min/hr}$$

13. $$\frac{1,000 \text{ mL}}{60 \text{ mL/hr}} = 16.66$$

   60 min = 1 hr

   60 min/hr × 0.66 hr = 39.6 = 40 min

   Answer: 16 hr + 40 min

14. No weight conversion required. Weight is stated in kg.

   8 mg/kg/day × 12 kg = 96 mg/day

   12 mg/kg/day × 12 kg = 144 mg/day

   Divided dosage: 96 mg/day ÷ 2 = 48 mg b.i.d.

   144 mg/day ÷ 2 = 72 mg b.i.d.

   The safe dosage range is 96-144 mg/day.

   The divided dosage range is 48-72 mg b.i.d.

   Answer: The prescriber ordered 60 mg b.i.d. The dosage is safe (60 mg × 2 = 120 mg); it falls within the safe dosage range.

15. $$\frac{100 \text{ mL}}{50 \text{ mL/hr}} = 2 \text{ hr}$$

   a. 2 hr

   b. 12 noon or 12 PM (10:00 AM and 2 hours); military time: 1200

16. Determine the dosage per hour.

   10 mcg/min × 60 min = 600 mcg/hr

   Convert mcg to mg to match solution.

   1,000 mcg = 1 mg, therefore

   600 mcg = 0.6 mg

   Calculate mL/hr.

   50 mg : 250 mL = 0.6 mg : x mL

   *or*

   $$\frac{50 \text{ mg}}{250 \text{ mL}} = \frac{0.6 \text{ mg}}{x \text{ mL}}$$

   x = 3 mL/hr

Answer: To deliver 10 mcg/min, set the flow rate at 3 mL/hr (gtt/min).

17. 22 units (Humulin Regular 6 units + Humulin NPH 16 units)

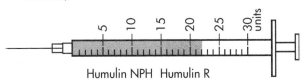

Humulin NPH   Humulin R

18. a. 52 mL

   b. $$x \text{ gtt/min} = \frac{55 \text{ mL} \times 60 \text{ gtt/mL}}{50 \text{ min}}$$

   x = 66 gtt/min

   Answer: 66 microgtt/min; 66 gtt/min. The shortcut method could also have been used to do this problem.

   c. 66 mL/hr (gtt/min with a microdrop = mL/hr)

19. $$\sqrt{\frac{102 \text{ (lb)} \times 51 \text{ (in)}}{3,131}} = \sqrt{1.66} = 1.288 = 1.29 \text{ m}^2$$

   Answer: 1.29 m²

20. a. $$\sqrt{\frac{13.6 \text{ (kg)} \times 60 \text{ (cm)}}{3,600}} = \sqrt{0.226} = 0.475$$

   $$= 0.48 \text{ m}^2$$

   Answer: 0.48 m²

   b. 0.48 m² × 500 mg/m² = 240 mg

   Answer: 240 mg

   c. 50 mg : 1 mL = 240 mg : x mL

   *or*

   $$\frac{240 \text{ mg}}{50 \text{ mg}} \times 1 \text{ mL} = x \text{ mL}$$

   Answer: 4.8 mL. The dosage ordered is greater than the available strength; therefore you will need more than 1 mL to administer the dosage.

   Alternate solution:

   1,000 mg : 20 mL = 240 mg : x mL

   *or*

   $$\frac{1,000 \text{ mg}}{20 \text{ mL}} = \frac{240 \text{ mg}}{x \text{ mL}}$$

   *or*

   $$\frac{240 \text{ mg}}{1,000 \text{ mg}} \times 20 \text{ mL} = x \text{ mL}$$

21. $$\frac{2}{5} \times 250 \text{ mL} = x \text{ mL}$$

   $$\frac{500}{5} = x$$

   x = 100 mL of Ensure Plus

   250 mL − 100 mL = 150 mL (water)

   Therefore you would add 150 mL of water to 100 mL of Ensure Plus to make 250 mL 2/5-strength Ensure Plus.

22. 1 L = 1,000 mL; therefore 2 L = 2,000 mL

   a. Dextrose: 5 g : 100 mL = x g : 2,000 mL

$$\frac{100x}{100} = \frac{10,000}{100}$$

*or*

$$\frac{5\ g}{100\ mL} = \frac{x\ g}{2,000\ mL}$$

   x = 100 g dextrose

   b. NaCl: 0.225 g : 100 mL = x g : 2,000 mL

$$\frac{100x}{100} = \frac{450}{100}$$

*or*

$$\frac{0.225\ g}{100\ mL} = \frac{x\ g}{2,000\ mL}$$

   x = 4.5 g NaCl

**NOTE**

Remember that ¼ NS (sodium chloride) is written as 0.225.

23. Time remaining: 3 hr − 1.5 hr = 1.5 hr (1½)

   Volume remaining: 500 mL − 175 mL = 325 mL

   a. **Step 1:** Calculate mL/hr.

      325 mL ÷ 1.5 hr = 216.6 = 217 mL/hr

**NOTE**

In problem 23, in addition to determining mL/hr, another method could be used to determine the drop factor constant and then gtt/min calculated using the drop factor constant.

24. Calculate the units/hr infusing.

   500 mL : 20,000 units = 25 mL : x units

$$\frac{500x}{500} = \frac{500,000}{500}$$

$$x = 1,000\ units/hr$$

   An IV of 500 mL containing 20,000 units of heparin infusing at 25 mL/hr is administering 1,000 units /hr.

25. 80 mg : 250 mL = x mg : 20 mL

$$\frac{250x}{250} = \frac{1,600}{250} = 6.4$$

   x = 6.4 mg/hr

26. a. 5 mg : 1 mL = 25 mg : x mL

$$\frac{25\ mg}{5\ mg} \times 1\ mL = x\ mL$$

   x = 5 mL

**Alternate solution:**

   25 mg : 5 mL = 25 mg : x mL

*or*

**Step 2:** Calculate the gtt/min.

$$x\ gtt/min = \frac{217\ mL \times 10\ gtt/mL}{60\ min}$$

$$x = \frac{217 \times 1}{6} = \frac{217}{6}$$

$$x = 36\ gtt/min;\ 36\ macrogtt/min$$

   The IV rate would have to be changed to 36 gtt/min (36 macrogtt/min).

   b. **Step 3:** Determine the percentage of change.

$$\frac{36 - 28}{28} = \frac{8}{28} = 0.285 = 29\%$$

   c. Course of action: Assess the client, and notify the prescriber. This increase is greater than 25%. The order may have to be revised.

Alternate calculation without percents:

Ordered rate ± (ordered rate ÷ 4) = acceptable IV readjustment rate

   28 (28 macrogtt/min) + (28 ÷ 4) = 28 + 7 = 35 gtt/min; 35 macrodrop per min

   28 (28 macrogtt/min) − (28 ÷ 4) = 28 − 7 = 21 gtt/min; 21 macrodrop per min

The safe range is 21 gtt/min (21 macrogtt/min) to 35 gtt/min (35 macrogtt/min). 36 macrogtt/min (36 gtt/min) is more than the acceptable range.

$$\frac{25\ mg}{25\ mg} \times 5\ mL = x\ mL$$

$$x = 5\ mL$$

This setup would yield the same answer of 5 mL.

   b. $\frac{5\ mL}{2\ min} = 2.5\ mL/min$

27. 1,000 mg = 1 g

   0.5 g = 500 mg

   Answer: 40 tabs (2 tabs per dose × 2 = 4 tabs; 4 tabs × 10 days = 40 tabs)

28. 1,000 mcg = 1 mg      0.375 mg = 375 mcg

   a. Give the client one 250-mcg tab and one 125-mcg tab.

      250-mcg tab

      + 125-mcg tab

      —————

      375 mcg

   b. 2 tabs (one 250-mcg tab and one 125-mcg tab) Give the least number of tablets without scoring.

29. a. No conversion necessary; use the dosage strength indicated on the label in mg (0.5 mg per 2 mL).

    0.5 mg : 2 mL = 0.125 mg : $x$ mL

    *or*

    $\dfrac{0.125 \text{ mg}}{0.5 \text{ mg}} \times 2 \text{ mL} = x \text{ mL}$

    $x = 0.5 \text{ mL}$

    b.

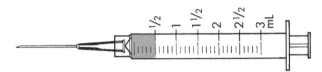

30. Convert weight: 2.2 lb = 1 kg

    242 lb ÷ 2.2 = 110 kg

    a. 80 units/kg × 110 kg = 8,800 units (bolus)

    b. 14 units/kg/hr × 110 kg = 1,540 units/hr

31. 20 units/kg/hr × 88 kg = 1,760 units/hr

32. a.    0.25 mg : 1 mL = 0.375 mg : $x$ mL

    *or*

    $\dfrac{0.375 \text{ mg}}{0.25 \text{ mg}} \times 1 \text{ mL} = x \text{ mL}$

    Answer: 1.5 mL

    b. 1.5 mL : 5 min = $x$ mL : 1 min

    5$x$ = 1.5

    $x$ = 0.3 mL/min

33. a. 10 mg : 1 mL = 8 mg : $x$ mL

    *or*

    $\dfrac{8 \text{ mg}}{10 \text{ mg}} \times 1 \text{ mL} = x \text{ mL}$

    Answer: 0.8 mL

    b. 10 mg : 4 min = 8 mg : $x$ min

    $\dfrac{10x}{10} = \dfrac{32}{10}$

    $x$ = 3.2 min

 **NOTE**

Any of the problems could also be done using dimensional analysis or the formula method.

34. Conversion is required. Equivalent: 30 mL = 1 oz

    Total oz = 18 oz

    18 oz × 30 = 540 mL

    540 mL (p.o.) + 100 mL (IV) = 640 mL

    Answer: 640 mL

35. **Step 1:** Convert the client's weight to kilograms.

    Equivalent: 1 kg = 2.2 lb

    187 lb ÷ 2.2 = 85 kg

    **Step 2:** Calculate the heparin bolus dosage.

    80 units/kg × 85 kg = 6,800 units. The client should receive 6,800 units IV heparin as a bolus.

    Determine the volume (mL) the client would receive. The concentration of heparin is 1,000 units per mL.

    1,000 units : 1 mL = 6,800 units : $x$ mL

    $\dfrac{1,000x}{1,000} = \dfrac{6,800}{1,000}$

    $x = \dfrac{6,800}{1,000}$

    $x$ = 6.8 mL (bolus is 6.8 mL)

    **Step 3:** Calculate the infusion rate (18 units/kg/hr).

    18 units/kg/hr × 85 kg = 1,530 units/hr. Determine the rate in mL/hr at which to set the infusion device using the concentration of 1,000 units per mL.

    1,000 units : 1 mL = 1,530 units : $x$ mL

    $\dfrac{1,000x}{1,000} = \dfrac{1,530}{1,000}$

    $x = \dfrac{1,530}{1,000}$

    $x$ = 1.53 = 1.5 mL/hr (not rounded to a whole number because the pump is capable of delivering in tenths of an mL)

    The client's APTT is 43 sec. According to the protocol, rebolus with 40 units/kg, and increase the rate by 2 units/kg/hr.

    **Step 4:** Calculate the dosage of heparin rebolus and the continuous infusion increase based on the APTT according to the protocol.

    Calculate the dosage (units) of heparin rebolus.

    40 units/kg × 85 kg = 3,400 units

    Determine the volume (mL) to administer 3,400 units.

    1,000 units : 1 mL = 3,400 units : $x$ mL

    $\dfrac{1,000x}{1,000} = \dfrac{3,400}{1,000}$

    $x = \dfrac{3,400}{1,000}$

    $x$ = 3.4 mL (bolus)

    Now determine the infusion rate increase (2 units/kg/hr × kg).

    2 units/kg/hr × 85 kg = 170 units/hr

The infusion rate should be increased by 170 units/hr.

Calculate the adjustment in hourly infusion rate (mL/hr).

$$1,000 \text{ units} : 1 \text{ mL} = 170 \text{ units} : x \text{ mL}$$

$$\frac{1,000x}{1,000} = \frac{170}{1,000}$$

$$x = \frac{170}{1,000}$$

$$x = 0.17 = 0.2 \text{ mL/hr}$$

The rate should be increased by 0.2 mL/hr.

**Increase rate:**

$$1.5 \text{ mL/hr (current rate)}$$

$$+ 0.2 \text{ mL/hr (increase)}$$

$$1.7 \text{ mL/hr (new infusion rate; not rounded to a whole number because pump is capable of delivering in tenths of an mL)}$$

36. **Step 1:** Calculate the dosage per hour using the upper and lower dosages.

$$4 \text{ mcg/min} \times 60 \text{ min/hr} = 240 \text{ mcg/hr}$$

$$12 \text{ mcg/min} \times 60 \text{ min/hr} = 720 \text{ mcg/hr}$$

**Step 2:** Convert mcg/hr to match the available strength.

Equivalent: 1,000 mcg = 1 mg

240 mcg = 0.24 mg

720 mcg = 0.72 mg

**Step 3:** Calculate rate in mL/hr for upper and lower dosage.

$$8 \text{ mg} : 1,000 \text{ mL} = 0.24 \text{ mg} : x \text{ mL}$$

$$\frac{8x}{8} = \frac{1,000 \times 0.24}{8}$$

$$\frac{8x}{8} = \frac{240}{8}$$

$$x = \frac{240}{8}$$

$$x = 30 \text{ mL/hr}$$

To infuse 4 mcg/min, set the infusion pump at 30 mL/hr.

$$8 \text{ mg} : 1,000 \text{ mL} = 0.72 \text{ mg} : x \text{ mL}$$

$$\frac{8x}{8} = \frac{1,000 \times 0.72}{8}$$

$$\frac{8x}{8} = \frac{720}{8}$$

$$x = \frac{720}{8}$$

$$x = 90 \text{ mL/hr}$$

To infuse 12 mcg/min, set the infusion pump at 90 mL/hr.

Dosage range of 4-12 mcg/min is equal to an IV flow rate of 30-90 mL/hr.

**Step 4:** Set up a proportion to determine the incremental flow rate for a dosage rate change of 2 mcg/min.

$$\frac{4 \text{ mcg/min}}{30 \text{ mL/hr}} = \frac{2 \text{ mcg/min}}{x \text{ mL/hr}}$$

$$\frac{4x}{4} = \frac{60}{4}$$

$$x = \frac{60}{4}$$

$$x = 15 \text{ mL/hr}$$

For each dosage change of 2 mcg/min, the incremental flow rate is 15 mL/hr.

Set up a titration table.

| Titration Table | |
| --- | --- |
| **Dosage Rate (mcg/min)** | **Flow Rate (mL/hr)** |
| 4 mcg/min **(minimum)** | 30 mL/hr |
| 6 mcg/min | 45 mL/hr |
| 8 mcg/min | 60 mL/hr |
| 10 mcg/min | 75 mL/hr |
| 12 mcg/min **(maximum)** | 90 mL/hr |

37. 1. Convert weight: Equivalent: 2.2 lb = 1 kg

$$127.2 \text{ lb} \div 2.2 = 57.8 \text{ kg}$$

2. $10 \text{ mcg/kg} \times 57.8 \text{ kg} = 578 \text{ mcg}$

Answer: 578 mcg

38. $38 \text{ mg} : 1 \text{ mL} = 900 \text{ mg} : x \text{ mL}$

*or*

$$\frac{900 \text{ mg}}{38 \text{ mg}} \times 1 \text{ mL} = x \text{ mL}$$

$$x = 23.68 = 23.7 \text{ mL}$$

Answer: 23.7 mL

39. No conversion required.

$$\frac{1}{3} \times 180 \text{ mL} = x \text{ mL}$$

$$x = \frac{180}{3}$$

$$x = 60 \text{ mL}$$

Answer: You need 60 mL of solute (normal saline) to prepare the desired solution (180 mL of 1/3 strength). The total to make is 180 mL. The amount of solvent needed, therefore, is:
180 mL − 60 mL = 120 mL (solvent/sterile water). To make 180 mL of 1/3 strength normal saline, mix 60 mL of full-strength normal saline and 120 mL of sterile water.

40. a. Morphine Sulfate 4 mg subcut q4h prn pain

b. Digoxin 0.375 mg p.o. daily (every day)

41. A conversion is required. Equivalent: 1,000 mg = 1 g

    0.1 g = 100 mg

    50 mg : 1 tab = 100 mg : x tab

    *or*

    $\dfrac{100 \text{ mg}}{50 \text{ mg}} \times 1 \text{ tab} = x \text{ tab}$

    Answer: 2 tabs

42. 10 mg : 1 mL = 2.5 mg : x mL

    *or*

    $\dfrac{2.5 \text{ mg}}{10 \text{ mg}} \times 1 \text{ mL} = x \text{ mL}$

    a. Answer: 0.25 mL. The available dosage strength is more than the ordered dosage. Therefore the nurse would need less than 1 mL to administer the ordered dosage.

    b.

    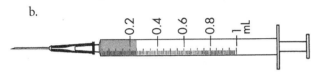

43. Conversion is required. Equivalent: 1 g = 1,000 mg

    1,550 mg = 1.55 g

    3 g : 8 mL = 1.55 g : x mL

    *or*

    $\dfrac{1.55 \text{ g}}{3 \text{ g}} \times 8 \text{ mL} = x \text{ mL}$

    $x = \dfrac{12.4}{3} = 4.13 = 4.1 \text{ mL}$

    Answer: 4.1 mL; 4.13 rounded to the nearest tenth. The available dosage strength is more than the ordered dosage. Therefore the nurse will need less than 8 mL to administer the ordered dosage.

44. **Step 1:** Calculate each medication:

    Demerol: 50 mg : 1 mL = 40 mg : x mL

    *or*

    $\dfrac{40 \text{ mg}}{50 \text{ mg}} \times 1 \text{ mL} = x \text{ mL}$

    Answer: 0.8 mL (Demerol)

    Vistaril: 50 mg : 1 mL = 25 mg : x mL

    *or*

    $\dfrac{25 \text{ mg}}{50 \text{ mg}} \times 1 \text{ mL} = x \text{ mL}$

    Answer: 0.5 mL (Vistaril)

    Answer: 0.8 mL of Demerol is needed and 0.5 mL of Vistaril. The available strengths for both medications is more than the dosage ordered. Therefore the nurse would need less than 1 mL to administer each medication.

**Step 2:** Add the two medications together to obtain the total volume you will administer.

a. Demerol 0.8 mL + Vistaril 0.5 mL = 1.3 mL. The total dose in mL the nurse will administer is 1.3 mL.

b.

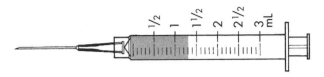

45. Determine the BSA.

    $$\text{m}^2 = \sqrt{\dfrac{45 \text{ (kg)} \times 155 \text{ (cm)}}{3,600}} = \sqrt{\dfrac{6,975}{3,600}} = \sqrt{1.937}$$

    $$\sqrt{1.937} = 1.391 = 1.39 \text{ m}^2$$

    $$1.39 \text{ m}^2 \times \dfrac{1 \text{ mg}}{\text{m}^2} = 1.39 = 1.4 \text{ mg}$$

    $$1.39 \text{ m}^2 \times \dfrac{2 \text{ mg}}{\text{m}^2} = 2.78 = 2.8 \text{ mg}$$

    a. Dosage not safe. 4 mg falls outside the range of 1.4 to 2.8 mg per (weekly) dose.

    b. Because the dosage is not safe, the milliliters to administer is not calculated, and the prescriber would be notified.

46. **Step 1:** Determine IV intake

    75 mL/hr (7a-10a) = 75 mL/hr × 3 hr = 225 mL

    100 mL/hr (10a–12p and 1p–3p) =

    　100 mL/hr × 4 hr = 400 mL

    Ampicillin 100 mL (12p–1p) =

    　100 mL × 1 hr = 100 mL

    Total IV intake = 725 mL

    **Step 2:** Determine p.o. intake

    　Cranberry juice 6 oz × 1½ = 9 oz

    　Tea 8 oz × 2½ = 20 oz

    　Gingerale 12 oz × ¾ = 9 oz

    　Broth 6 oz × ½ = 3 oz

    　Ice cream 4 oz

    　Total oz = 45 oz

    Convert oz to mL: Equivalent 1 oz = 30 mL

    　　45 oz × 30 = 1,350 mL

    **Step 3:** IV intake 725 mL + p.o. intake 1,350 mL = 2,075 mL

    Answer: Total intake = 2,075 mL

    **Step 4:** Total output: 375 mL + 250 mL + 400 mL + 300 mL = 1,325 mL

    Answer: Total output: 1,325 mL

47. **Step 1:**

    No weight conversion required; weight is in kilograms.

    Determine the number of units/hr based on client's weight in kilograms.

    15 units/kg/hr × 82 kg requires 1,230 units/hr of heparin.

    **Step 2:**

    Calculate the IV rate in mL/hr that delivers the client's hourly dose of heparin.

    25,000 units : 250 mL = 1,230 units : $x$ mL

    $$\frac{25,000x}{25,000} = \frac{307,500}{25,000}$$

    $$x = \frac{307,500}{25,000}$$

    $$x = 12.3 \text{ mL/hr}$$

    Answer: 12.3 mL/hr will deliver the client's hourly dose of 1,230 units. The rate is stated in tenths; the pump is capable of delivering in tenths of a milliliter.

48. No weight conversion required; child's weight is in kilograms.

    Child's weight = 32 kg

    **Step 1:** Determine the mL/day using the formula.

    100 mL/kg/day × 10 kg = 1,000 mL/day for first 10 kg

    50 mL/kg/day × 10 kg = 500 mL/day for next 10 kg

    20 mL/kg/day × 12 kg = <u>240 mL/day</u> for remaining 12 kg

    Total = 1,740 mL/day or per 24 hr

    Answer: 1,740 mL/day or per 24 hr

    **Step 2:** Determine ml/hr.

    $$x \text{ mL/hr} = \frac{1,740 \text{ mL}}{24 \text{ hr}} = 72.5 \text{ mL/hr}$$

    Answer: 72.5 mL/hr will deliver 1,740 mL/24 hr or per day. Pump capable of delivering in tenths of a milliliter.

49. **Step 1:** Weight conversion required. Convert weight to kilograms. Equivalent: 1 kg = 1,000 g

    2,500 g ÷ 1,000 = 2.5 kg

    **Step 2:** Select and apply appropriate formula.

    100 mL/kg/day × 2.5 kg = 250 mL/day or per 24 hr

    Answer: 250 mL/day or per 24 hr

**Step 3:** Determine mL/hr.

$$x \text{ mL/hr} = \frac{250 \text{ mL}}{24 \text{ hr}} = 10.41 = 10.4 \text{ mL/hr}$$

Answer: 10.4 mL/hr; 10.41 rounded to the nearest tenth of a milliliter. The pump is capable of delivering in tenths of a milliliter.

50. Weight conversion is required. Convert weight to kilograms. Equivalent: 2.2 lb = 1 kg

    78 lb ÷ 2.2 = 35.45 = 35.5 kg

    **Step 1:** Determine the mL/day using the formula.

    100 mL/kg/day × 10 kg = 1,000 mL/day for first 10 kg

    50 mL/kg/day × 10 kg = 500 mL/day for next 10 kg

    20 mL/kg/day × 15.5 kg = <u>310 mL/day</u> for remaining 15.5 kg

    Total = 1,810 mL/day or per 24 hr

    **Step 2:** Determine mL/hr

    $$x \text{ mL/hr} = \frac{1,810 \text{ mL}}{24 \text{ hr}} = 75.4 \text{ mL/hr} = 75 \text{ mL/hr}$$

    The pump is capable of delivering in whole mL; therefore mL/hr is rounded to a whole number.

51. a. BSA (m²) = $\sqrt{\dfrac{135 \text{ (lb)} \times 62 \text{ (in)}}{3,131}} = \sqrt{2.673}$

    = 1.634 = 1.63 m²

    Answer: 1.63 m²

    b. 1.63 m² × 1,000 mg/m² = 1,630 mg

    Answer: 1,630 mg

52. a. BSA (m²) = $\sqrt{\dfrac{92.7 \text{ (kg)} \times 185 \text{ (cm)}}{3,600}} = \sqrt{4.763}$

    = 2.182 = 2.18 m²

    Answer: BSA = 2.18 m²

    b. 2.18 m² × 10 units/m² = 21.8 units
       2.18 m² × 20 units/m² = 43.6 units

    Answer: The dosage range for this client is 21.8-43.6 units/wk.

    c. The dosage is safe; 35 units falls within the recommended dosage range of 21.8-43.6 units/wk.

# References

Administration on Aging: *2018 Profile of older Americans.* Retrieved from https://acl.gov/sites/default/files/Aging%20and%20Disability%20in%20America/2018OlderAmericansProfile.pdf.

*American Geriatrics Society 2019 updated AGS Beers Criteria for potentially inappropriate medication use in older adults.* Retrieved from https://www.whca.org/files/2020/09/Sept_18_BEERS-handout_Hecht.pdf.

American Hospital Association: *The Patient Care Partnership,* 2003. Retrieved from https://www.aha.org/system/files/2018-01/aha-patient-care-partnership.pdf.

DailyMed. Retrieved from https://dailymed.nlm.nih.gov.

ECRI Institute: *Culture of safety: An overview,* June 14, 2019. Retrieved from https://www.ecri.org/components/HRC/Pages/RiskQual21.aspx?tab=1.

*FDA and ISMP lists of look-alike drug names with recommended tall man letters.* Retrieved from https://www.ismp.org/sites/default/files/attachments/2017-11/tallmanletters.pdf.

*Guidelines for the safe use of automated dispensing cabinets,* February 7, 2019. Retrieved from https://www.ismp.org/resources/guidelines-safe-use-automated-dispensing-cabinets.

*Heparin dosage,* December 3, 2019. Retrieved from https://www.drugs.com/dosage/heparin.html.

*Humulin R U-500 (concentrated regular insulin).* Retrieved from https://www.ismp.org/sites/default/files/attachmens/2018-11/u-500-insulinfinal.pdf.

*Independent double checks: Worth the effort if used judiciously and properly,* June 6, 2019. Retrieved from https://www.ismp.org/resources/independent-double-checks-worth-effort-if-used-judiciously-and-properly.

*Infusion pump risk reduction strategies for clinicians,* February 2018. Retrieved from https://www.fda.gov/medical-devices/infusion-pumps/infusion-pump-risk-reduction-strategies-clinicians.

Institute for Safe Medication Practices: *ISMP guidelines for optimizing safe implementation and use of smart infusion pumps,* February 10, 2020. Retrieved from https://www.ismp.org/guidelines/safe-implementation-and-use-smart-pumps.

Institute for Safe Medication Practices: *ISMP guidelines for optimizing safe subcutaneous insulin use in adults,* June 2017. Retrieved from https://www.ismp.org/sites/default/files/attachments/2018-09/ISMP138D-Insulin%20Guideline-091318.pdf.

Institute for Safe Medication Practices: *ISMP guidelines for safe electronic communication of medication information,* January 16, 2019. Retrieved from https://www.ismp.org/node/1322.

Institute for Safe Medication Practices: *ISMP list of confused drug names.* Retrieved from https://www.ismp.org/recommendations/confused-drug-names-list.

Institute for Safe Medication Practices: *ISMP list of error-prone abbreviations, symbols, and dose designations.* Retrieved from https://www.ismp.org/recommendations/error-prone-abbreviations-list.

Institute for Safe Medication Practices: *ISMP list of high-alert medications in acute care settings.* Retrieved from https://www.ismp.org/sites/default/files/attachments/2018-10/highAlert2018new-Oct2018-v1.pdf.

Institute for Safe Medication Practices: *ISMP list of high-alert medications in community/ambulatory healthcare.* Retrieved from https://www.ismp.org/sites/default/files/attachments/2017-11/highAlert-community.pdf.

Institute for Safe Medication Practices: *Oral dosage forms that should not be crushed.* Retrieved from https://www.ismp.org/recommendations/do-not-crush.

Institute of Medicine, Committee on Identifying and Preventing Medication Errors, Board on Health Care Services: *Identifying and preventing medication errors* (Aspden P, Wolcott J, Bootman JL, Cronenwett LR, editors), Washington, DC, 2006, The National Academies Press.

Institute of Medicine, Committee on Quality of Health Care in America: *To err is human: Building a safer health system* (Kohn LT, Corrigan JM, Donaldson MS, editors), Washington, DC, 1999, National Academies Press. Summary retrieved from https://www.nap.edu/resource/9728/To-Err-is-Human-1999--report-brief.pdf.

John Hopkins Hospital: *The Harriet Lane handbook* (Hughes HK, Kahl LK, editors), ed 21, St Louis, 2018, Elsevier.

The Joint Commission: *Facts about Speak Up initiatives.* Retrieved from https://www.jointcommission.org/-/media/deprecated-unorganized/imported-assets/tjc/system-folders/topics-library/speak-up-initiatives-3-8-111pdf.pdf?db=web&hash=35207FD8591B82EFA5CD27D08D00A346&hash=35207FD8591B82EFA5CD27D08D00A346.

The Joint Commission: *Hospital: 2021 National Patient Safety Goals.* Retrieved from https://www.jointcommission.org/standards/national-patient-safety-goals/hospital-national-patient-safety-goals/.

The Joint Commission: *National Patient Safety Goals effective January 2020.* Retrieved from https://www.jointcommission.org/-/media/tjc/documents/standards/national-patient-safety-goals/2020/npsg_chapter_hap_jan2020.pdf?db=web&hash=6CC50D956B7AC5CF6BD22BDB7577B5A0.

The Joint Commission: *Official "do not use list."* Retrieved from https://www.jointcommission.org/-/media/tjc/documents/fact-sheets/do-not-use-list-8-3-20.pdf.

The Joint Commission: *Speak Up preventing medication errors.* Retrieved from https://www.jointcommission.org/resources/for-consumers/speak-up-campaigns/preventing-medicine-errors/.

*A pocket guide to the 2019 AGS Beers Criteria.* Retrieved from http://files.hgsitebuilder.com/hostgator257222/file/ags_2019_beers_pocket_printable_rh.pdf.

Potter PA, Perry AG, Stockert PA, Hall A: *Fundamentals of nursing,* ed 9, St Louis, 2017, Elsevier.

*Recommendations for the safe management of patients with an external subcutaneous insulin pump during hospitalization.* Retrieved from https://www.ismp.org/sites/default/files/attachments/2018-05/Insulin%20Pump%20Recommendations%2010-20-2016_0.pdf.

*A review of insulin errors,* October 29, 2019. Retrieved from http://www.diabetesincontrol.com/a-review-of-insulin-errors.

Skidmore-Roth L: *Mosby's 2020 nursing drug reference,* ed 33, St Louis, 2020, Elsevier.

*2018-2019 Targeted medication safety best practices for hospitals.* Retrieved from https://www.ismp.org/sites/default/files/attachments/2019-01/TMSBP-for-Hospitalsv2.pdf.

*2020-2021 Targeted medication safety best practices for hospitals.* Retrieved from https://www.ismp.org/sites/default/files/attachments/2020-02/2020-2021%20TMSBP-%20FINAL_1.pdf.

*U-500 insulin errors.* Retrieved from https://consumermedsafety.org/tools-and-resources/insulin-safety-center/u-500-insulin-errors.

US Food and Drug Administration: *Bar code label requirement for human drug products and biological products,* February 26, 2004. Retrieved from https://www.federalregister.gov/documents/2004/02/26/04-4249/bar-code-label-requirement-for-human-drug-products-and-biological-products.

Willihnganz M, Gurevitz SL, Clayton BD: *Clayton's basic pharmacology for nurses,* ed 18, St Louis, 2020, Elsevier.

# Appendix Table of Contents

Appendixes B, D, E, and F © Institute for Safe Medication Practices (ISMP), 2016. All rights reserved. Retrieved from http://www.ismp.org/Tools/errorproneabbreviations.pdf. Visit www.ismp.org for more medication safety information, or to report medication errors or near misses to the ISMP Medication Errors Reporting Program (MERP).

Appendix C © Joint Commission Resources: *"Do Not Use" abbreviation fact sheet.* Oakbrook Terrace, IL: Joint Commission on Accreditation of Healthcare Organizations, 2019. Retrieved from https://www.jointcommission.org/resources/news-and-multimedia/ fact-sheets/#first=10. Accessed May 4, 2020. Reprinted with permission.

As noted in Chapter 6, the **apothecary system** is an antiquated system of measurement. The system is sometimes referred to as the fraction system because parts of a unit are expressed by using fractions, with the exception of the fraction one-half, which is expressed as *ss* or $\overline{ss}$. The notations in this system are unusual and confusing, and errors have been identified from its use. The system also uses roman numerals and has inaccuracies that contribute to its use being unsafe. Recommendations from major national agencies focusing on client (patient) safety, including the Institute for Safe Medication Practices (ISMP), The Joint Commission (TJC), and the US Food and Drug Administration (FDA), included not using this system for safe practice, not using it in medication administration, and elimination of its use in favor of the metric system.

Some of the medication dosing cups used to administer liquid medications still have the apothecary measure drams (approximately the size of a teaspoon) indicated on them. The apothecary measures and symbols have been included on the ISMP's list of Error-Prone Abbreviations, Symbols, and Dose Designations. A brief discussion of apothecary units and their equivalents appears here so that they can be differentiated from acceptable units of measure. **Remember to use metric equivalents.**

**Apothecary Units:**
- The grain is the basic unit for weight.
- Volume measures include minim (approximately the size of a drop), dram (approximately the size of a teaspoon), and ounce (which is the same as the household ounce).
- Many of the household measures originated from the apothecary (e.g., ounce, which is still in use).

**Apothecary Units Abbreviation/Symbols**

| Unit | Abbreviation | Symbol |
| --- | --- | --- |
| grain | gr | N/A |
| ounce | oz | ℥ |
| dram | dr | ʒ |
| minim | m | N/A |

*ss, $\overline{ss}$—Apothecary symbol for $\frac{1}{2}$

Below is a partial listing of some of the common Apothecary–Metric Approximate Equivalents:

| Volume | Weight |
| --- | --- |
| 1 oz = 30 mL | 15 gr = 1 g (1,000 mg) |
| 15-16 m = 1 mL | 1 gr = 60-65 mg |
| 1 dr = 4-5 mL | gr $\frac{1}{2}$ or $\overline{ss}$ = 30 mg |
| | gr $\frac{1}{4}$ = 15 mg |
| 1 m = 1 gtt | gr $\frac{1}{6}$ = 10 mg |
| | gr $\frac{1}{100}$ = 0.6 mg |
| | gr $\frac{1}{150}$ = 0.4 mg |

**Apothecary/Metric Approximate Equivalent Clock**

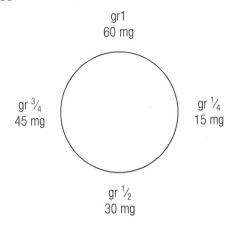

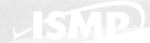

# FDA and ISMP Lists of
# Look-Alike Drug Names with Recommended Tall Man Letters

Since 2008, ISMP has maintained a list of drug name pairs and trios with recommended, **bolded** tall man (uppercase) letters to help draw attention to the dissimilarities in look-alike drug names. The list includes mostly generic-generic drug name pairs, although a few brand-brand or brand-generic name pairs are included. The US Food and Drug Administration (FDA) list of drug names with recommended tall man letters was initiated in 2001 with the agency's Name Differentiation Project (www.ismp.org/sc?id=520).

While numerous studies between 2000 and 2016 have demonstrated the ability of tall man letters alone or in conjunction with other text enhancements to improve the accuracy of drug name perception and reduce errors due to drug name similarity,[1-9] some studies have suggested that the strategy is ineffective.[10-12] The evidence is mixed due in large part to methodological differences and significant study limitations. Nevertheless, while gaps still exist in our full understanding of the role of tall man lettering in the clinical setting, there is sufficient evidence to suggest that this simple and straightforward technique is worth implementing as one among numerous strategies to mitigate the risk of errors due to similar drug names. To await irrefutable, scientific proof of effectiveness minimizes and undervalues the study findings and anecdotal evidence available today[13] that support this important risk-reduction strategy. As such, the use of tall man letters has been endorsed by ISMP, The Joint Commission (recommended but not required), the US Food and Drug Administration (as part of its Name Differentiation Project), as well as other national and international organizations, including the World Health Organization and the International Medication Safety Network (IMSN).[14]

**Table 1** provides an alphabetized list of FDA-approved established drug names with recommended tall man letters.

**Table 2** provides an alphabetized list of additional drug names with recommendations from ISMP regarding the use and placement of tall man letters. This is not an official list approved by FDA. It is intended for voluntary use by healthcare practitioners, drug information vendors, and medication technology vendors. Any product label changes by manufacturers require FDA approval.

To promote standardization regarding which letters to present in uppercase, ISMP follows a tested methodology whenever possible called the CD3 rule.[15] The methodology suggests working from the left of the drug name first by capitalizing all the characters to the right once 2 or more dissimilar letters are encountered, and then, working from the right, returning 2 or more letters common to both words to lowercase letters. When the rule cannot be applied because there are no common letters on the right side of the name, the methodology suggests capitalizing the central part of the word only. When application of this rule fails to lead to the best tall man lettering option (e.g., makes names appear too similar, makes names hard to read based on pronunciation), an alternative option is considered.

ISMP suggests that the **bolded**, tall man lettering scheme provided by FDA and ISMP for the drug name pairs listed in **Tables 1** and **2** be followed to promote consistency. continued on next page >

| Table 1. FDA-Approved List of Generic Drug Names with Tall Man Letters | |
|---|---|
| **Drug Name With Tall Man Letters** | **Confused With** |
| aceta**ZOLAMIDE** | aceto**HEXAMIDE** |
| aceto**HEXAMIDE** | aceta**ZOLAMIDE** |
| bu**PROP**ion | bus**PIR**one |
| bus**PIR**one | bu**PROP**ion |
| chlorpro**MAZINE** | chlorpro**PAMIDE** |
| chlorpro**PAMIDE** | chlorpro**MAZINE** |
| clomi**PHENE** | clomi**PRAMINE** |
| clomi**PRAMINE** | clomi**PHENE** |
| cyclo**SERINE** | cyclo**SPORINE** |
| cyclo**SPORINE** | cyclo**SERINE** |
| **DAUNO**rubicin | **DOXO**rubicin |
| dimenhy**DRINATE** | diphenhydr**AMINE** |
| diphenhydr**AMINE** | dimenhy**DRINATE** |
| **DOBUT**amine | **DOP**amine |
| **DOP**amine | **DOBUT**amine |
| **DOXO**rubicin | **DAUNO**rubicin |

continued on next page >

www.ismp.org

Institute for Safe Medication Practices

## FDA and ISMP Lists of Look-Alike Drug Names with Recommended Tall Man Letters

### Table 1. FDA–Approved List of Generic Drug Names with Tall Man Letters (continued)

| Drug Name With Tall Man Letters | Confused With |
| --- | --- |
| glipiZIDE | glyBURIDE |
| glyBURIDE | glipiZIDE |
| hydrALAZINE | hydrOXYzine – HYDROmorphone |
| HYDROmorphone | hydrOXYzine – hydrALAZINE |
| hydrOXYzine | hydrALAZINE – HYDROmorphone |
| medroxyPROGESTERone | methylPREDNISolone - methylTESTOSTERone |
| methylPREDNISolone | medroxyPROGESTERone - methylTESTOSTERone |
| methylTESTOSTERone | medroxyPROGESTERone - methylPREDNISolone |
| mitoXANTRONE | Not specified |
| niCARdipine | NIFEdipine |
| NIFEdipine | niCARdipine |
| prednisoLONE | predniSONE |
| predniSONE | prednisoLONE |
| risperiDONE | rOPINIRole |
| rOPINIRole | risperiDONE |
| sulfADIAZINE | sulfiSOXAZOLE |
| sulfiSOXAZOLE | sulfADIAZINE |
| TOLAZamide | TOLBUTamide |
| TOLBUTamide | TOLAZamide |
| vinBLAStine | vinCRIStine |
| vinCRIStine | vinBLAStine |

### Table 2. ISMP List of Additional Drug Names with Tall Man Letters***

| Drug Name With Tall Man Letters | Confused With |
| --- | --- |
| ALPRAZolam | LORazepam – clonazePAM |
| aMILoride | amLODIPine |
| amLODIPine | aMILoride |
| ARIPiprazole | RABEprazole |
| AVINza* | INVanz* |
| azaCITIDine | azaTHIOprine |
| azaTHIOprine | azaCITIDine |
| carBAMazepine | OXcarbazepine |
| CARBOplatin | CISplatin |
| ceFAZolin | cefoTEtan – cefOXitin – cefTAZidime – cefTRIAXone |
| cefoTEtan | ceFAZolin – cefOXitin – cefTAZidime – cefTRIAXone |
| cefOXitin | ceFAZolin – cefoTEtan – cefTAZidime – cefTRIAXone |
| cefTAZidime | ceFAZolin – cefoTEtan – cefOXitin – cefTRIAXone |
| cefTRIAXone | ceFAZolin - cefoTEtan – cefOXitin – cefTAZidime |
| CeleBREX* | CeleXA* |
| CeleXA* | CeleBREX* |
| chlordiazePOXIDE | chlorproMAZINE** |

\*  *Brand names always start with an uppercase letter. Some brand names incorporate tall man letters in initial characters and may not be readily recognized as brand names. An asterisk follows all brand names on the ISMP list.*

\*\*  *These drug names are also on the FDA list.*

\*\*\*  *The ISMP list is not an official list approved by FDA. It is intended for voluntary use by healthcare practitioners and drug information and technology vendors. Any manufacturers' product label changes require FDA approval.*

continued on next page >

www.ismp.org

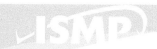

## FDA and ISMP Lists of Look-Alike Drug Names with Recommended Tall Man Letters

| Table 2. ISMP List of Additional Drug Names with Tall Man Letters*** (continued) | |
|---|---|
| **Drug Name With Tall Man Letters** | **Confused With** |
| chlorpro**MAZINE**** | chlordiaze**POXIDE** |
| **CIS**platin | **CARBO**platin |
| clo**BAZ**am | clonaze**PAM** |
| clonaze**PAM** | clo**NID**ine – clo**ZAP**ine – clo**BAZ**am – **LOR**azepam |
| clo**NID**ine | clonaze**PAM** – clo**ZAP**ine – Klono**PIN*** |
| clo**ZAP**ine | clonaze**PAM** – clo**NID**ine |
| **DACTIN**omycin | **DAPTO**mycin |
| **DAPTO**mycin | **DACTIN**omycin |
| DEPO-Medrol* | SOLU-Medrol* |
| diaze**PAM** | dil**TIAZ**em |
| dil**TIAZ**em | diaze**PAM** |
| **DOCE**taxel | **PACL**itaxel |
| **DOXO**rubicin** | **IDA**rubicin |
| **DUL**oxetine | **FLU**oxetine – **PAR**oxetine |
| e**PHED**rine | **EPINEPH**rine |
| **EPINEPH**rine | e**PHED**rine |
| epi**RUB**icin | eri**BUL**in |
| eri**BUL**in | epi**RUB**icin |
| fenta**NYL** | **SUF**entanil |
| flavox**ATE** | fluvoxa**MINE** |
| **FLU**oxetine | **DUL**oxetine – **PAR**oxetine |
| flu**PHENAZ**ine | fluvoxa**MINE** |
| fluvoxa**MINE** | flu**PHENAZ**ine - flavox**ATE** |
| guai**FEN**esin | guan**FACINE** |
| guan**FACINE** | guai**FEN**esin |
| Huma**LOG*** | Humu**LIN*** |
| Humu**LIN*** | Huma**LOG*** |
| hydr**ALAZINE**** | hydro**CHLORO**thiazide – hydr**OXY**zine** |
| hydro**CHLORO**thiazide | hydr**OXY**zine** – hydr**ALAZINE**** |
| **HYDRO**codone | oxy**CODONE** |
| **HYDRO**morphone** | morphine – oxy**MOR**phone |
| **HYDROXY**progesterone | medroxy**PROGESTER**one** |
| hydr**OXY**zine** | hydr**ALAZINE**** – hydro**CHLORO**thiazide |
| **IDA**rubicin | **DOXO**rubicin** – idaru**CIZU**mab |
| idaru**CIZU**mab | **IDA**rubicin |
| in**FLIX**imab | ri**TUX**imab |
| **INV**anz* | **AVIN**za* |
| **ISO**tretinoin | tretinoin |
| Klono**PIN*** | clo**NID**ine |
| La**MIC**tal* | Lam**ISIL*** |
| Lam**ISIL*** | La**MIC**tal* |

\*   Brand names always start with an uppercase letter. Some brand names incorporate tall man letters in initial characters and may
    not be readily recognized as brand names. An asterisk follows all brand names on the ISMP list.
\*\*  These drug names are also on the FDA list.
\*\*\* The ISMP list is not an official list approved by FDA. It is intended for voluntary use by healthcare practitioners and drug
    information and technology vendors. Any manufacturers' product label changes require FDA approval.

continued on next page >

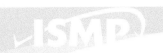

Institute for Safe Medication Practices

## FDA and ISMP Lists of Look-Alike Drug Names with Recommended Tall Man Letters

| Table 2. ISMP List of Additional Drug Names with Tall Man Letters*** (continued) | |
|---|---|
| **Drug Name With Tall Man Letters** | **Confused With** |
| lamiVUDine | lamoTRIgine |
| lamoTRIgine | lamiVUDine |
| levETIRAcetam | levOCARNitine – levoFLOXacin |
| levOCARNitine | levETIRAcetam |
| levoFLOXacin | levETIRAcetam |
| LEVOleucovorin | leucovorin |
| LORazepam | ALPRAZolam – clonazePAM |
| medroxyPROGESTERone** | HYDROXYprogesterone |
| metFORMIN | metroNIDAZOLE |
| methazolAMIDE | methIMAzole – metOLazone |
| methIMAzole | metOLazone – methazolAMIDE |
| metOLazone | methIMAzole – methazolAMIDE |
| metroNIDAZOLE | metFORMIN |
| metyraPONE | metyroSINE |
| metyroSINE | metyraPONE |
| miFEPRIStone | miSOPROStol |
| miSOPROStol | miFEPRIStone |
| mitoMYcin | mitoXANTRONE** |
| mitoXANTRONE** | mitoMYcin |
| NexAVAR* | NexIUM* |
| NexIUM* | NexAVAR* |
| niCARdipine** | niMODipine – NIFEdipine** |
| NIFEdipine** | niMODipine – niCARdipine** |
| niMODipine | NIFEdipine** – niCARdipine** |
| NovoLIN* | NovoLOG* |
| NovoLOG* | NovoLIN* |
| OLANZapine | QUEtiapine |
| OXcarbazepine | carBAMazepine |
| oxyCODONE | HYDROcodone – OxyCONTIN*– oxyMORphone |
| OxyCONTIN* | oxyCODONE – oxyMORphone |
| oxyMORphone | HYDROmorphone** – oxyCODONE – OxyCONTIN* |
| PACLitaxel | DOCEtaxel |
| PARoxetine | FLUoxetine – DULoxetine |
| PAZOPanib | PONATinib |
| PEMEtrexed | PRALAtrexate |
| penicillAMINE | penicillin |
| PENTobarbital | PHENobarbital |
| PHENobarbital | PENTobarbital |
| PONATinib | PAZOPanib |
| PRALAtrexate | PEMEtrexed |
| PriLOSEC* | PROzac* |

\* Brand names always start with an uppercase letter. Some brand names incorporate tall man letters in initial characters and may not be readily recognized as brand names. An asterisk follows all brand names on the ISMP list.
\*\* These drug names are also on the FDA list.
\*\*\* The ISMP list is not an official list approved by FDA. It is intended for voluntary use by healthcare practitioners and drug information and technology vendors. Any manufacturers' product label changes require FDA approval.

continued on next page >

www.ismp.org

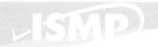

Institute for Safe Medication Practices

## FDA and ISMP Lists of Look-Alike Drug Names with Recommended Tall Man Letters

| Table 2. ISMP List of Additional Drug Names with Tall Man Letters*** (continued) | |
| --- | --- |
| Drug Name With Tall Man Letters | Confused With |
| PROzac* | PriLOSEC* |
| QUEtiapine | OLANZapine |
| quiNIDine | quiNINE |
| quiNINE | quiNIDine |
| RABEprazole | ARIPiprazole |
| raNITIdine | riMANTAdine |
| rifAMPin | rifAXIMin |
| rifAXIMin | rifAMPin |
| riMANTAdine | raNITIdine |
| RisperDAL* | rOPINIRole** |
| risperiDONE** | rOPINIRole** |
| riTUXimab | inFLIXimab |
| romiDEPsin | romiPLOStim |
| romiPLOStim | romiDEPsin |
| rOPINIRole** | RisperDAL* – risperiDONE** |
| SandIMMUNE* | SandoSTATIN* |
| SandoSTATIN* | SandIMMUNE* |
| sAXagliptin | SITagliptin |
| SEROquel* | SINEquan* |
| SINEquan* | SEROquel* |
| SITagliptin | sAXagliptin – SUMAtriptan |
| Solu-CORTEF* | SOLU-Medrol* |
| SOLU-Medrol* | Solu-CORTEF* – DEPO-Medrol* |
| SORAfenib | SUNItinib |
| SUFentanil | fentaNYL |
| sulfADIAZINE** | sulfaSALAzine |
| sulfaSALAzine | sulfADIAZINE** |
| SUMAtriptan | SITagliptin – ZOLMitriptan |
| SUNItinib | SORAfenib |
| TEGretol* | TRENtal* |
| tiaGABine | tiZANidine |
| tiZANidine | tiaGABine |
| traMADol | traZODone |
| traZODone | traMADol |
| TRENtal* | TEGretol* |
| valACYclovir | valGANciclovir |
| valGANciclovir | valACYclovir |
| ZOLMitriptan | SUMAtriptan |
| ZyPREXA* | ZyrTEC* |
| ZyrTEC* | ZyPREXA* |

\*    Brand names always start with an uppercase letter. Some brand names incorporate tall man letters in initial characters and may
      not be readily recognized as brand names. An asterisk follows all brand names on the ISMP list.
\*\*   These drug names are also on the FDA list.
\*\*\* The ISMP list is not an official list approved by FDA. It is intended for voluntary use by healthcare practitioners and drug
      information and technology vendors. Any manufacturers' product label changes require FDA approval.

www.ismp.org

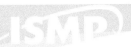

## FDA and ISMP Lists of Look-Alike Drug Names with Recommended Tall Man Letters

### References

1) DeHenau C, Becker MW, Bello NM, Liu S, Bix L. Tallman lettering as a strategy for differentiation in look-alike, sound-alike drug names: the role of familiarity in differentiating drug doppelgangers. *Appl Ergon.* 2016;52:77-84.

2) Filik R, Purdy K, Gale A, Gerrett D. Drug name confusion: evaluating the effectiveness of capital ("tall man") letters using eye movement data. *Soc Sci Med.* 2004;59(12):2597-601.

3) Filik R, Purdy K, Gale A, Gerrett D. Labeling of medicines and patient safety: evaluating methods of reducing drug name confusion. *Hum Factors.* 2006;48(1):39-47.

4) Grasha A. Cognitive systems perspective on human performance in the pharmacy: implications for accuracy, effectiveness, and job satisfaction (Report No. 062100). Alexandria (VA): NACDS. 2000.

5) Darker IT, Gerret D, Filik R, Purdy KJ, Gale AG. The influence of 'tall man' lettering on errors of visual perception in the recognition of written drug names. *Ergonomics.* 2011;54(1):21–33.

6) Or CK, Chan AH. Effects of text enhancements on the differentiation performance of orthographically similar drug names. *Work.* 2014;48(4):521–8.

7) Or CK, Wang H. A comparison of the effects of different typographical methods on the recognizability of printed drug names. *Drug Saf.* 2014;37(5):351–9.

8) Filik R, Price J, Darker I, Gerrett D, Purdy K, Gale A. The influence of tall man lettering on drug name confusion: a laboratory-based investigation in the UK using younger and older adults and healthcare practitioners. *Drug Saf.* 2010;33(8):677–87.

9) Gabriele S. The role of typography in differentiating look-alike/sound-alike drug names. *Healthc Q.* 2006; 9(Spec No):88-95.

10) Schell KL. Using enhanced text to facilitate recognition of drug names: evidence from two experimental studies. *Appl Ergon.* 2009;40(1):82–90.

11) Irwin A, Mearns K, Watson M, Urquhart J. The effect of proximity, tall man lettering, and time pressure on accurate visual perception of drug names. *Hum Factors.* 2013;55(2):253–66.

12) Zhong W, Feinstein JA, Patel NS, Dai D, Feudtner C. Tall man lettering and potential prescription errors: a time series analysis of 42 children's hospitals in the USA over 9 years. *BMJ Qual Saf.* Published Online First: November 3, 2015.

13) Leape LL, Berwick MB, Bates DW. What practices will most improve safety? Evidence-based medicine meets patient safety. *JAMA.* 2002;288(4):501-7.

14) Position statement on improving the safety of international non-proprietary names of medicines (INNs). Horsham (PA): International Medication Safety Network; November 2011.

15) Gerrett D, Gale AG, Darker IT, Filik R, Purdy KJ. Tall man lettering. Final report of the use of tall man lettering to minimise selection errors of medicine names in computer prescribing and dispensing systems. Loughborough University Enterprises Ltd; 2009.

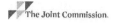 The Joint Commission.

# Official "Do Not Use" List

### The Joint Commission

# FACT SHEET

- This list is part of the Information Management standards
- Does not apply to preprogrammed health information technology systems (i.e. electronic medical records or CPOE systems), but remains under consideration for the future

Organizations contemplating introduction or upgrade of such systems should strive to eliminate the use of dangerous abbreviations, acronyms, symbols and dose designations from the software.

**For more information**

- Contact the Standards Interpretation Group at 630-792-5900.
- Complete the Standards Online Question Submission Form.

### Official "Do Not Use" List

| Do Not Use | Potential Problem | Use Instead |
|---|---|---|
| U, u (unit) | Mistaken for "0" (zero), the number "4" (four) or "cc" | Write "unit" |
| IU (International Unit) | Mistaken for IV (intravenous) or the number 10 (ten) | Write "International Unit" |
| Q.D., QD, q.d., qd (daily) | Mistaken for each other | Write "daily" |
| Q.O.D., QOD, q.o.d, qod (every other day) | Period after the Q mistaken for "I" and the "O" mistaken for "I | Write "every other day" |
| Trailing zero (X.0 mg)* Lack of leading zero (.X mg) | Decimal point is missed | Write X mg Write 0.X mg |
| MS | Can mean morphine sulfate or magnesium sulfate | Write "morphine sulfate" Write "magnesium sulfate" |
| MSO$_4$ and MgSO$_4$ | Confused for one another | |

¹ Applies to all orders and all medication-related documentation that is handwritten (including free-text computer entry) or on pre-printed forms.

**\*Exception:** A "trailing zero" may be used only where required to demonstrate the level of precision of the value being reported, such as for laboratory results, imaging studies that report size of lesions, or catheter/tube sizes. It may not be used in medication orders or other medication-related documentation.

### Development of the "Do Not Use" List

In 2001, The Joint Commission issued a *Sentinel Event Alert* on the subject of medical abbreviations. A year later, its Board of Commissioners approved a National Patient Safety Goal requiring accredited organizations to develop and implement a list of abbreviations not to use. In 2004, The Joint Commission created its "Do Not Use" List to meet that goal. In 2010, NPSG.02.02.01 was integrated into the Information Management standards as elements of performance 2 and 3 under IM.02.02.01.

6/19

# ISMP List of Error-Prone Abbreviations, Symbols, and Dose Designations

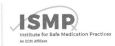

The abbreviations, symbols, and dose designations in the **Table** below were reported to ISMP through the ISMP National Medication Errors Reporting Program (ISMP MERP) and have been misinterpreted and involved in harmful or potentially harmful medication errors. These abbreviations, symbols, and dose designations should **NEVER** be used when communicating medical information verbally, electronically, and/or in handwritten applications. This includes internal communications; verbal, handwritten, or electronic prescriptions; hand-written and computer-generated medication labels; drug storage bin labels; medication administration records; and screens associated with pharmacy and prescriber computer order entry systems, automated dispensing cabinets, smart infusion pumps, and other medication-related technologies.

In the **Table**, error-prone abbreviations, symbols, and dose designations that are included on The Joint Commission's "**Do Not Use**" list (Information Management standard IM.02.02.01) are identified with a double asterisk (**\*\***) and must be included on an organization's "**Do Not Use**" list. Error-prone abbreviations, symbols, and dose designations that are relevant mostly in hand-written communications of medication information are highlighted with a dagger (†).

**Table.** Error-Prone Abbreviations, Symbols, and Dose Designations

| Error-Prone Abbreviations, Symbols, and Dose Designations | Intended Meaning | Misinterpretation | Best Practice |
|---|---|---|---|
| **Abbreviations for Doses/Measurement Units** | | | |
| cc | Cubic centimeters | Mistaken as u (units) | Use mL |
| IU\*\* | International unit(s) | Mistaken as IV (intravenous) or the number 10 | Use unit(s) (International units can be expressed as units alone) |
| l<br><br>ml | Liter<br><br>Milliliter | Lowercase letter l mistaken as the number 1 | Use L (UPPERCASE) for liter<br><br>Use mL (lowercase m, UPPERCASE L) for milliliter |
| MM or M<br><br>M or K | Million<br><br>Thousand | Mistaken as thousand<br><br>Mistaken as million<br><br>M has been used to abbreviate both million and thousand (M is the Roman numeral for thousand) | Use million<br><br>Use thousand |
| Ng or ng | Nanogram | Mistaken as mg<br><br>Mistaken as nasogastric | Use nanogram or nanog |
| U or u\*\* | Unit(s) | Mistaken as zero or the number 4, causing a 10-fold overdose or greater (e.g., 4U seen as 40 or 4u seen as 44)<br><br>Mistaken as cc, leading to administering volume instead of units (e.g., 4u seen as 4cc) | Use unit(s) |
| μg | Microgram | Mistaken as mg | Use mcg |
| **Abbreviations for Route of Administration** | | | |
| AD, AS, AU | Right ear, left ear, each ear | Mistaken as OD, OS, OU (right eye, left eye, each eye) | Use right ear, left ear, or each ear |
| IN | Intranasal | Mistaken as IM or IV | Use NAS (all UPPERCASE letters) or intranasal |

\*\* On The Joint Commission's "**Do Not Use**" list
† Relevant mostly in handwritten medication information

**List** — continued on page 2 ▶

List — continued from page 1

| Error-Prone Abbreviations, Symbols, and Dose Designations | Intended Meaning | Misinterpretation | Best Practice |
|---|---|---|---|
| IT | Intrathecal | Mistaken as intratracheal, intratumor, intratympanic, or inhalation therapy | Use intrathecal |
| OD, OS, OU | Right eye, left eye, each eye | Mistaken as AD, AS, AU (right ear, left ear, each ear) | Use right eye, left eye, or each eye |
| Per os | By mouth, orally | The os was mistaken as left eye (OS, oculus sinister) | Use PO, by mouth, or orally |
| SC, SQ, sq, or sub q | Subcutaneous(ly) | SC and sc mistaken as SL or sl (sublingual)<br><br>SQ mistaken as "5 every"<br>The q in sub q has been mistaken as "every" | Use SUBQ (all UPPERCASE letters, without spaces or periods between letters) or subcutaneous(ly) |
| **Abbreviations for Frequency/Instructions for Use** | | | |
| HS | Half-strength | Mistaken as bedtime | Use half-strength |
| hs | At bedtime, hours of sleep | Mistaken as half-strength | Use HS (all UPPERCASE letters) for bedtime |
| o.d. or OD | Once daily | Mistaken as right eye (OD, oculus dexter), leading to oral liquid medications administered in the eye | Use daily |
| Q.D., QD, q.d., or qd** | Every day | Mistaken as q.i.d., especially if the period after the q or the tail of a handwritten q is misunderstood as the letter i | Use daily |
| Qhs | Nightly at bedtime | Mistaken as qhr (every hour) | Use nightly or HS for bedtime |
| Qn | Nightly or at bedtime | Mistaken as qh (every hour) | Use nightly or HS for bedtime |
| Q.O.D., QOD, q.o.d., or qod** | Every other day | Mistaken as qd (daily) or qid (four times daily), especially if the "o" is poorly written | Use every other day |
| q1d | Daily | Mistaken as qid (four times daily) | Use daily |
| q6PM, etc. | Every evening at 6 PM | Mistaken as every 6 hours | Use daily at 6 PM or 6 PM daily |
| SSRI | Sliding scale regular insulin | Mistaken as selective-serotonin reuptake inhibitor | Use sliding scale (insulin) |
| SSI | Sliding scale insulin | Mistaken as Strong Solution of Iodine (Lugol's) | |
| TIW or tiw | 3 times a week | Mistaken as 3 times a day or twice in a week | Use 3 times weekly |
| BIW or biw | 2 times a week | Mistaken as 2 times a day | Use 2 times weekly |
| UD | As directed (ut dictum) | Mistaken as unit dose (e.g., an order for "dilTIAZem infusion UD" was mistakenly administered as a unit [bolus] dose) | Use as directed |

** On The Joint Commission's "**Do Not Use**" list
† Relevant mostly in handwritten medication information

List — continued on page 3 ▶

List — continued from page 2

| Error-Prone Abbreviations, Symbols, and Dose Designations | Intended Meaning | Misinterpretation | Best Practice |
|---|---|---|---|
| **Miscellaneous Abbreviations Associated with Medication Use** | | | |
| **BBA**<br><br>**BGB** | Baby boy A (twin)<br><br>Baby girl B (twin) | B in BBA mistaken as twin B rather than gender (boy)<br><br>B at end of BGB mistaken as gender (boy) not twin B | When assigning identifiers to newborns, use the mother's last name, the baby's gender (boy or girl), and a distinguishing identifier for all multiples (e.g., Smith girl A, Smith girl B) |
| **D/C** | Discharge or discontinue | Premature discontinuation of medications when D/C (intended to mean discharge) on a medication list was misinterpreted as discontinued | Use discharge and discontinue or stop |
| **IJ** | Injection | Mistaken as IV or intrajugular | Use injection |
| **OJ** | Orange juice | Mistaken as OD or OS (right or left eye); drugs meant to be diluted in orange juice may be given in the eye | Use orange juice |
| **Period following abbreviations (e.g., mg., mL.)†** | mg or mL | Unnecessary period mistaken as the number 1, especially if written poorly | Use mg, mL, etc., without a terminal period |
| **Drug Name Abbreviations** | | | |
| To prevent confusion, avoid abbreviating drug names entirely. Exceptions may be made for multi-ingredient drug formulations, including vitamins, when there are electronic drug name field space constraints; however, drug name abbreviations should NEVER be used for any medications on the *ISMP List of High-Alert Medications* (in Acute Care Settings [www.ismp.org/node/103], Community/Ambulatory Settings [www.ismp.org/node/129], and Long-Term Care Settings [www.ismp.org/node/130]). Examples of drug name abbreviations involved in serious medication errors include: | | | |
| **Antiretroviral medications (e.g., DOR, TAF, TDF)** | DOR: doravirine<br><br>TAF: tenofovir alafenamide<br><br>TDF: tenofovir disoproxil fumarate | DOR: Dovato (dolutegravir and lami**VUD**ine)<br><br>TAF: tenofovir disoproxil fumarate<br><br>TDF: tenofovir alafenamide | Use complete drug names |
| **APAP** | acetaminophen | Not recognized as acetaminophen | Use complete drug name |
| **ARA A** | vidarabine | Mistaken as cytarabine ("ARA C") | Use complete drug name |
| **AT II and AT III** | AT II: angiotensin II (Giapreza)<br><br>AT III: antithrombin III (Thrombate III) | AT II (angiotensin II) mistaken as AT III (antithrombin III)<br><br>AT III (antithrombin III) mistaken as AT II (angiotensin II) | Use complete drug names |
| **AZT** | zidovudine (Retrovir) | Mistaken as azithromycin, aza**THIO**prine, or aztreonam | Use complete drug name |
| **CPZ** | Compazine (prochlorperazine) | Mistaken as chlorpro**MAZINE** | Use complete drug name |
| **DTO** | diluted tincture of opium or deodorized tincture of opium (Paregoric) | Mistaken as tincture of opium | Use complete drug name |

** On The Joint Commission's **"Do Not Use"** list
† Relevant mostly in handwritten medication information

List — continued on page 4 ▶

4                                      Institute for Safe Medication Practices

**List** — continued from page 3

| Error-Prone Abbreviations, Symbols, and Dose Designations | Intended Meaning | Misinterpretation | Best Practice |
|---|---|---|---|
| HCT | hydrocortisone | Mistaken as hydro**CHLORO**-thiazide | Use complete drug name |
| HCTZ | hydro**CHLORO**thiazide | Mistaken as hydrocortisone (e.g., seen as HCT250 mg) | Use complete drug name |
| MgSO4** | magnesium sulfate | Mistaken as morphine sulfate | Use complete drug name |
| MS, MSO4** | morphine sulfate | Mistaken as magnesium sulfate | Use complete drug name |
| MTX | methotrexate | Mistaken as mito**XANTRONE** | Use complete drug name |
| Na at the beginning of a drug name (e.g., Na bicarbonate) | Sodium bicarbonate | Mistaken as no bicarbonate | Use complete drug name |
| NoAC | novel/new oral anticoagulant | Mistaken as no anticoagulant | Use complete drug name |
| OXY | oxytocin | Mistaken as oxy**CODONE**, Oxy**CONTIN** | Use complete drug name |
| PCA | procainamide | Mistaken as patient-controlled analgesia | Use complete drug name |
| PIT | Pitocin (oxytocin) | Mistaken as Pitressin, a discontinued brand of vasopressin still referred to as PIT | Use complete drug name |
| PNV | prenatal vitamins | Mistaken as penicillin VK | Use complete drug name |
| PTU | propylthiouracil | Mistaken as Purinethol (mercaptopurine) | Use complete drug name |
| T3 | Tylenol with codeine No. 3 | Mistaken as liothyronine, which is sometimes referred to as T3 | Use complete drug name |
| TAC or tac | triamcinolone or tacrolimus | Mistaken as tetracaine, Adrenalin, and cocaine; or as Taxotere, Adriamycin, and cyclophosphamide | Use complete drug names<br><br>Avoid drug regimen or protocol acronyms that may have a dual meaning or may be confused with other common acronyms, even if defined in an order set |
| TNK | TNKase | Mistaken as TPA | Use complete drug name |
| TPA or tPA | tissue plasminogen activator, Activase (alteplase) | Mistaken as TNK (TNKase, tenecteplase), TXA (tranexamic acid), or less often as another tissue plasminogen activator, Retavase (retaplase) | Use complete drug names |
| TXA | tranexamic acid | Mistaken as TPA (tissue plasminogen activator) | Use complete drug name |
| ZnSO4 | zinc sulfate | Mistaken as morphine sulfate | Use complete drug name |
| **Stemmed/Coined Drug Names** | | | |
| Nitro drip | nitroglycerin infusion | Mistaken as nitroprusside infusion | Use complete drug name |
| IV vanc | Intravenous vancomycin | Mistaken as Invanz | Use complete drug name |
| Levo | levofloxacin | Mistaken as Levophed (norepinephrine) | Use complete drug name |

** On The Joint Commission's "**Do Not Use**" list
† Relevant mostly in handwritten medication information

**List** — continued on page 5 ▶

List — continued from page 4

| Error-Prone Abbreviations, Symbols, and Dose Designations | Intended Meaning | Misinterpretation | Best Practice |
|---|---|---|---|
| **Neo** | Neo-Synephrine, a well known but discontinued brand of phenylephrine | Mistaken as neostigmine | Use complete drug name |
| **Coined names for compounded products (e.g., magic mouthwash, banana bag, GI cocktail, half and half, pink lady)** | Specific ingredients compounded together | Mistaken ingredients | Use complete drug/product names for all ingredients<br><br>Coined names for compounded products should only be used if the contents are standardized and readily available for reference to prescribers, pharmacists, and nurses |
| **Number embedded in drug name (not part of the official name) (e.g., 5-fluoro-uracil, 6-mercaptopurine)** | fluorouracil<br><br>mercaptopurine | Embedded number mistaken as the dose or number of tablets/capsules to be administered | Use complete drug names, without an embedded number if the number is not part of the official drug name |
| **Dose Designations and Other Information** | | | |
| **1/2 tablet** | Half tablet | 1 or 2 tablets | Use text (half tablet) or reduced font-size fractions (½ tablet) |
| **Doses expressed as Roman numerals (e.g., V)** | 5 | Mistaken as the designated letter (e.g., the letter V) or the wrong numeral (e.g., 10 instead of 5) | Use only Arabic numerals (e.g., 1, 2, 3) to express doses |
| **Lack of a leading zero before a decimal point (e.g., .5 mg)\*\*** | 0.5 mg | Mistaken as 5 mg if the decimal point is not seen | Use a leading zero before a decimal point when the dose is less than one measurement unit |
| **Trailing zero after a decimal point (e.g., 1.0 mg)\*\*** | 1 mg | Mistaken as 10 mg if the decimal point is not seen | Do not use trailing zeros for doses expressed in whole numbers |
| **Ratio expression of a strength of a single-entity injectable drug product (e.g., EPINEPHrine 1:1,000; 1:10,000; 1:100,000)** | 1:1,000: contains 1 mg/mL<br><br>1:10,000: contains 0.1 mg/mL<br><br>1:100,000: contains 0.01 mg/mL | Mistaken as the wrong strength | Express the strength in terms of quantity per total volume (e.g., **EPINEPH**rine 1 mg per 10 mL)<br><br>**Exception:** combination local anesthetics (e.g., lidocaine 1% and **EPINEPH**rine 1:100,000) |
| **Drug name and dose run together (problematic for drug names that end in the letter l [e.g., propranolol20 mg; TEGretol300 mg])** | propranolol 20 mg<br><br>**TEG**retol 300 mg | Mistaken as propranolol 120 mg<br><br>Mistaken as **TEG**retol 1300 mg | Place adequate space between the drug name, dose, and unit of measure |
| **Numerical dose and unit of measure run together (e.g., 10mg, 10Units)** | 10 mg<br><br>10 mL | The m in mg, or U in Units, has been mistaken as one or two zeros when flush against the dose (e.g., 10mg, 10Units), risking a 10- to 100-fold overdose | Place adequate space between the dose and unit of measure |

\*\* On The Joint Commission's "**Do Not Use**" list
† Relevant mostly in handwritten medication information

List — continued on page 6 ▶

**List** — continued from page 5

| Error-Prone Abbreviations, Symbols, and Dose Designations | Intended Meaning | Misinterpretation | Best Practice |
|---|---|---|---|
| Large doses without properly placed commas (e.g., 100000 units; 1000000 units) | 100,000 units<br><br>1,000,000 units | 100000 has been mistaken as 10,000 or 1,000,000<br><br>1000000 has been mistaken as 100,000 | Use commas for dosing units at or above 1,000 or use words such as 100 thousand or 1 million to improve readability<br><br>**Note:** Use commas to separate digits only in the US; commas are used in place of decimal points in some other countries |
| **Symbols** | | | |
| ʒ or<br><br>℩† | Dram<br><br>Minim | Symbol for dram mistaken as the number 3<br><br>Symbol for minim mistaken as mL | Use the metric system |
| **x1** | Administer once | Administer for 1 day | Use explicit words (e.g., for 1 dose) |
| **> and <** | More than and less than | Mistaken as opposite of intended<br><br>Mistakenly have used the incorrect symbol<br><br>< mistaken as the number 4 when handwritten (e.g., <10 misread as 40) | Use more than or less than |
| **↑ and ↓†** | Increase and decrease | Mistaken as opposite of intended<br><br>Mistakenly have used the incorrect symbol<br><br>↑ mistaken as the letter T, leading to misinterpretation as the start of a drug name, or mistaken as the numbers 4 or 7 | Use increase and decrease |
| **/ (slash mark)†** | Separates two doses or indicates per | Mistaken as the number 1 (e.g., 25 units/10 units misread as 25 units and 110 units) | Use per rather than a slash mark to separate doses |
| **@†** | At | Mistaken as the number 2 | Use at |
| **&†** | And | Mistaken as the number 2 | Use and |
| **+†** | Plus or and | Mistaken as the number 4 | Use plus, and, or in addition to |
| **°** | Hour | Mistaken as a zero (e.g., q2° seen as q20) | Use hr, h, or hour |
| **Φ or ∅†** | Zero, null sign | Mistaken as the numbers 4, 6, 8, and 9 | Use 0 or zero, or describe intent using whole words |
| **#** | Pound(s) | Mistaken as a number sign | Use the metric system (kg or g) rather than pounds<br><br>Use lb if referring to pounds |

**\*\*** On The Joint Commission's "**Do Not Use**" list
**†** Relevant mostly in handwritten medication information

**List** — continued on page 7 ▶

**List** — continued from page 6

| Error-Prone Abbreviations, Symbols, and Dose Designations | Intended Meaning | Misinterpretation | Best Practice |
|---|---|---|---|
| **Apothecary or Household Abbreviations** | | | |
| Explicit apothecary or household measurements may **ONLY** be safely used to express the directions for mixing dry ingredients to prepare topical products (e.g., dissolve 2 capfuls of granules per gallon of warm water to prepare a magnesium sulfate soaking aid). Otherwise, metric system measurements should be used. | | | |
| **gr** | Grain(s) | Mistaken as gram | Use the metric system (e.g., mcg, g) |
| **dr** | Dram(s) | Mistaken as doctor | Use the metric system (e.g., mL) |
| **min** | Minim(s) | Mistaken as minutes | Use the metric system (e.g., mL) |
| **oz** | Ounce(s) | Mistaken as zero or $0_2$ | Use the metric system (e.g., mL) |
| **tsp** | Teaspoon(s) | Mistaken as tablespoon(s) | Use the metric system (e.g., mL) |
| **tbsp or Tbsp** | Tablespoon(s) | Mistaken as teaspoon(s) | Use the metric system (e.g., mL) |

| Common Abbreviations with Contradictory Meanings | Contradictory Meanings | | Correction |
|---|---|---|---|
| For additional information and tables from Neil Davis (MedAbbrev.com) containing additional examples of abbreviations with contradictory or ambiguous meanings, please visit: www.ismp.org/ext/638. | | | |
| **B** | Breast, brain, or bladder | | Use breast, brain, or bladder |
| **C** | Cerebral, coronary, or carotid | | Use cerebral, coronary, or carotid |
| **D or d** | Day or dose (e.g., parameter-based dosing formulas using D or d [mg/kg/d] could be interpreted as either day or dose [mg/kg/day or mg/kg/dose]; or x3d could be interpreted as either 3 days or 3 doses) | | Use day or dose |
| **H** | Hand or hip | | Use hand or hip |
| **I** | Impaired or improvement | | Use impaired or improvement |
| **L** | Liver or lung | | Use liver or lung |
| **N** | No or normal | | Use no or normal |
| **P** | Pancreas, prostate, preeclampsia, or psychosis | | Use pancreas, prostate, preeclampsia, or psychosis |
| **S** | Special or standard | | Use special or standard |
| **SS or ss** | Single strength, sliding scale (insulin), signs and symptoms, or ½ (apothecary)  SS has also been mistaken as the number 55 | | Use single strength, sliding scale, signs and symptoms, or one-half or ½ |

**\*\*** On The Joint Commission's "**Do Not Use**" list
**†** Relevant mostly in handwritten medication information

While the abbreviations, symbols, and dose designations in the **Table** should **NEVER** be used, not allowing the use of **ANY** abbreviations is exceedingly unlikely. Therefore, the person who uses an organization-approved abbreviation must take responsibility for making sure that it is properly interpreted. If an uncommon or ambiguous abbreviation is used, and it should be defined by the writer or sender. Where uncertainty exists, clarification with the person who used the abbreviation is required.

# ISMP List of High-Alert Medications
## in Acute Care Settings

High-alert medications are drugs that bear a heightened risk of causing significant patient harm when they are used in error. Although mistakes may or may not be more common with these drugs, the consequences of an error are clearly more devastating to patients. We hope you will use this list to determine which medications require special safeguards to reduce the risk of errors. This may include strategies such as standardizing the ordering, storage, preparation, and administration of these products; improving access to information about these drugs; limiting access to high-alert medications; using auxiliary labels; employing clinical decision support and automated alerts; and using redundancies such as automated or independent double checks when necessary. (Note: manual independent double checks are not always the optimal error-reduction strategy and may not be practical for all of the medications on the list.)

### Classes/Categories of Medications

adrenergic agonists, IV (e.g., **EPINEPH**rine, phenylephrine, norepinephrine)

adrenergic antagonists, IV (e.g., propranolol, metoprolol, labetalol)

anesthetic agents, general, inhaled and IV (e.g., propofol, ketamine)

antiarrhythmics, IV (e.g., lidocaine, amiodarone)

antithrombotic agents, including:

- anticoagulants (e.g., warfarin, low molecular weight heparin, unfractionated heparin)
- direct oral anticoagulants and factor Xa inhibitors (e.g., dabigatran, rivaroxaban, apixaban, edoxaban, betrixaban, fondaparinux)
- direct thrombin inhibitors (e.g., argatroban, bivalirudin, dabigatran)
- glycoprotein IIb/IIIa inhibitors (e.g., eptifibatide)
- thrombolytics (e.g., alteplase, reteplase, tenecteplase)

cardioplegic solutions

chemotherapeutic agents, parenteral and oral

dextrose, hypertonic, 20% or greater

dialysis solutions, peritoneal and hemodialysis

epidural and intrathecal medications

inotropic medications, IV (e.g., digoxin, milrinone)

insulin, subcutaneous and IV

liposomal forms of drugs (e.g., liposomal amphotericin B) and conventional counterparts (e.g., amphotericin B desoxycholate)

moderate sedation agents, IV (e.g., dexmedetomidine, midazolam, **LOR**azepam)

moderate and minimal sedation agents, oral, for children (e.g., chloral hydrate, midazolam, ketamine [using the parenteral form])

opioids, including:

- IV
- oral (including liquid concentrates, immediate- and sustained-release formulations)
- transdermal

neuromuscular blocking agents (e.g., succinylcholine, rocuronium, vecuronium)

parenteral nutrition preparations

sodium chloride for injection, hypertonic, greater than 0.9% concentration

sterile water for injection, inhalation and irrigation (excluding pour bottles) in containers of 100 mL or more

sulfonylurea hypoglycemics, oral (e.g., chlorpro**PAMIDE**, glimepiride, gly**BURIDE**, glipi**ZIDE**, **TOLBUT**amide)

### Specific Medications

**EPINEPH**rine, IM, subcutaneous

epoprostenol (e.g., Flolan), IV

insulin U-500 (special emphasis*)

magnesium sulfate injection

methotrexate, oral, nononcologic use

nitroprusside sodium for injection

opium tincture

oxytocin, IV

potassium chloride for injection concentrate

potassium phosphates injection

promethazine injection

vasopressin, IV and intraosseous

*All forms of insulin, subcutaneous and IV, are considered a class of high-alert medications. Insulin U-500 has been singled out for special emphasis to bring attention to the need for distinct strategies to prevent the types of errors that occur with this concentrated form of insulin.

### Background

Based on error reports submitted to the ISMP National Medication Errors Reporting Program (ISMP MERP), reports of harmful errors in the literature, studies that identify the drugs most often involved in harmful errors, and input from practitioners and safety experts, ISMP created and periodically updates a list of potential high-alert medications. During June and July 2018, practitioners responded to an ISMP survey designed to identify which medications were most frequently considered high-alert medications. Further, to assure relevance and completeness, the clinical staff at ISMP and members of the ISMP advisory board were asked to review the potential list. This list of medications and medication categories reflects the collective thinking of all who provided input.

**Abbreviation definitions:** IV—intravenous   IM—intramuscular

# ISMP List of *High-Alert Medications* in Community/Ambulatory Healthcare

H igh-alert medications are drugs that bear a heightened risk of causing significant patient harm when they are used in error. Although mistakes may or may not be more common with these drugs, the consequences of an error are clearly more devastating to patients. We hope you will use this list to determine which medications require special safeguards to reduce the risk of errors and minimize harm.

This may include strategies like providing mandatory patient education; improving access to information about these drugs; using auxiliary labels and automated alerts; employing automated or independent double checks when necessary; and standardizing the prescribing, storage, dispensing, and administration of these products.

| Classes/Categories of Medications |
|---|
| antiretroviral agents (e.g., efavirenz, lamiVUDine, raltegravir, ritonavir, combination antiretroviral products) |
| chemotherapeutic agents, oral (excluding hormonal agents) (e.g., cyclophosphamide, mercaptopurine, temozolomide) |
| hypoglycemic agents, oral |
| immunosuppressant agents (e.g., azaTHIOprine, cycloSPORINE, tacrolimus) |
| insulin, all formulations |
| opioids, all formulations |
| pediatric liquid medications that require measurement |
| pregnancy category X drugs (e.g., bosentan, ISOtretinoin) |

| Specific Medications |
|---|
| carBAMazepine |
| chloral hydrate liquid, for sedation of children |
| heparin, including unfractionated and low molecular weight heparin |
| metFORMIN |
| methotrexate, non-oncologic use |
| midazolam liquid, for sedation of children |
| propylthiouracil |
| warfarin |

## Background

Based on error reports submitted to the ISMP Medication Errors Reporting Program (ISMP MERP), reports of harmful errors in the literature, and input from practitioners and safety experts, ISMP created a list of potential high-alert medications. During June-August 2006, 463 practitioners responded to an ISMP survey designed to identify which medications were most frequently considered high-alert drugs by individuals and organizations. In 2008, the preliminary list and survey data as well as data about preventable adverse drug events from the ISMP MERP, the Pennsylvania Patient Safety Reporting System, the FDA MedWatch database, databases from participating pharmacies, public litigation data, literature review, and a small focus group of ambulatory care pharmacists and medication safety experts were evaluated as part of a research study funded by an Agency for Healthcare Research and Quality (AHRQ) grant. This list of drugs and drug categories reflects the collective thinking of all who provided input. This list was created as part of the AHRQ funded project "Using risk models to identify and prioritize outpatient high-alert medications" (Grant # 1P20HS017107-01).

INSTITUTE FOR SAFE MEDICATION PRACTICES
www.ismp.org

# Index

# Drug Label Index